P9-BYC-872

Medical and Dental Space Planning
for the 1990s

Medical and Dental Space Planning
for the 1990s

Jain Malkin

VNR VAN NOSTRAND REINHOLD
New York

Copyright © 1990 by Van Nostrand Reinhold

I(T)P™ Van Nostrand Reinhold is a division of International Thomson Publishing, Inc.
The ITP logo is a trademark under license

Printed in the United States of America

For more information, contact:

Van Nostrand Reinhold
115 Fifth Avenue
New York, NY 10003

Chapman & Hall
2-6 Boundary Row
London
SE1 8HN
United Kingdom

Thomas Nelson Australia
102 Dodds Street
South Melbourne, 3205
Victoria, Australia

Nelson Canada
1120 Birchmount Road
Scarborough, Ontario
Canada M1K 5G4

Chapman & Hall GmbH
Pappelallee 3
69469 Weinheim
Germany

International Thomson Publishing Asia
221 Henderson Road #05-10
Henderson Building
Singapore 0315

International Thomson Publishing Japan
Hirakawacho Kyowa Building, 3F
2-2-1 Hirakawacho
Chiyoda-ku, 102 Tokyo
Japan

International Thomson Editores
Campos Eliseos 385, Piso 7
Col. Polanco
11560 Mexico D.F. Mexico

All rights reserved. No part of this work covered by the copyright hereon may be reproduced or used in any form or by any means—graphic, electronic, or mechanical, including photocopying, recording, taping, or information storage and retrieval systems—without the written permission of the publisher.

96 97 98 99 QEB KP 10 9 8 7 6 5 4 3

Library of Congress Cataloging-in-Publication Data
Malkin, Jain.
Medical and dental space planning for the 1990s.
Includes index.
1. Medical offices—Design and construction. 2. Dental offices—Design and construction. I. Title.
R728.M235 1989 725'.5 89-5625
ISBN 0-442-26485-2

To Stuart,
for his good cheer and encouragement
throughout the many months
of writing this book.

Contents

Preface **xi**

Introduction Changing Perspectives **xiii**

Chapter 1 Psychology: Implications for Health Care Design **1**

Chapter 2 General Parameters of Medical Space Planning **6**

Chapter 3 The Practice of Medicine: Primary Care **19**

General Practice, Internal Medicine, and Pediatrics

Chapter 4 Medicine: Specialized Suites **92**

Obstetrics & Gynecology, Women's Centers, Otolaryngology, Ophthalmology, Dermatology, Plastic Surgery, Allergy, Psychiatry, Neurology, Neurosurgery, General Surgery, Urology, Orthopedic Surgery

Chapter 5 Diagnostic Medicine **186**

Radiology, Clinical Laboratory

Chapter 6 Group Practice **249**

Chapter 7 Ambulatory Surgical Centers **265**

Chapter 8 Sports Medicine **294**

Chapter 9 Paramedical Suites **314**

Physical Therapy, Pharmacy

Chapter 10 The Practice of Dentistry **332**

General Dentistry, Orthodontics, Pediatric Dentistry, Oral Surgery, Endodondics, Periodontics

Chapter 11 The Impact of Color on the Medical Environment **408**

Chapter 12 Interior Finishes and Furniture **422**

Chapter 13 Lighting **433**

Chapter 14 Construction Methods and Building Systems **445**

Chapter 15 Researching Codes and Reference Materials **451**

Appendixes Handicapped Toilet • View Box Illuminators • Specimen Pass-Through • Interview Questionnaires (Medical and Dental) **457**

Index **469**

Color Plates

Figure 3-2. Waiting room.

Figure 3-3. Pediatric play area.

Figure 3-56. Waiting room, cardiac surgery suite.

Figure 3-77. Pediatric examination room.

Figure 3-79. Reception window, pediatric clinic.

Figure 4-3. Children's area.

Figure 4-12. Waiting room, OB-GYN suite.

Figure 4-13. Waiting room, women's clinic.

Figure 4-14. Corridor, women's clinic.

Figure 4-39. Waiting room, ophthalmology.

Figure 4-40. Reception window, ophthalmology suite.

Figure 4-49. Waiting room, dermatology.

Figure 4-54. Plastic surgery examination room for hands, also serves as a recovery room.

Figure 4-62. Waiting room, plastic surgery.

Figure 4-63. Corridor, plastic surgery suite.

Figure 4-64. Waiting room, plastic surgery.

Figure 4-74. Diplomas, imaginatively framed.

Figure 4-75. Consultation room, psychiatry.

Figure 4-76. Consultation room, psychiatry (opposite view).

Figure 4-106. Waiting room, orthopedic surgery.

Figure 6-14. Corridor, group practice clinic. Note indirect lighting details and signage.

Figure 6-15. Waiting room, family practice module, group practice clinic.

Figure 7-4. Patient prep corridor. Note use of sandblasted glass detail to add interest to corridor, and visually open up examination rooms, on other side of wall.

Figure 7-9. Operating room. Note vinyl inset wallgraphic.

Figures 7-22 & 7-23. Recovery area, with view into private recovery rooms. Note use of color, glass block, and oak detailing.

Figure 8-3. Pool and spa. Note interesting architectural features, lighting, and use of color.

Figure 8-8. Trompe l'oeil (*fool-the-eye*) mural expands, and adds dimension, to the room.

Figure 8-9. Sophisticated mural gives illusion of looking through panes of glass, at the bay.

Figure 8-10. Skillfully executed trompe l'oeil mural gives person exercising the illusion of riding along the boardwalk.

Figure 8-17. Snack bar/lounge, Western Montana Sports Medicine & Fitness Center.

Figure 10-39. Waiting room, general dentistry office.

Figure 10-40. Reception area with patient education room.

Figure 10-57. Orthodontic treatment bay.

Figure 10-62. Waiting room, children's dental clinic.

Figure 10-63. Pre-flight check-in, children's dental clinic.

Figure 10-64. Pedodontic bay.

Figure 10-67. Operatory bay, orthodontics.

Figure 10-68. Corridor, orthodontic office. Note architectural detailing of ceiling.

Figure 10-81. Waiting room, periodontics office.

Figure 10-82. Operatory, periodontics.

Figure 11-1. The old color wheel.

Figure 11-2. The new color wheel.

Figure 11-3. Simultaneous contrast.

Figure 11-4. Successive contrast/afterimage.

Figure 13-9. Corridor, dermatology suite, indirect lighting.

Preface

*I*n 1970 I decided to specialize in health care design. I spent many weeks at the library researching the literature on medical and dental space planning, color and its effect on patients, and the psychological aspects of illness — how do patients and visitors react to hospitals? Why do people fear a visit to the doctor or dentist? What role does lighting play in patient rooms?

Much to my surprise, very little had been written on these topics. I found nothing in architecture or design publications, but did come across an occasional article in obscure publications sometimes dating from the 1940s. There were a few articles in the *American Journal of Occupational Therapy* on the effect of the environment on the patient, and there were numerous articles on color preferences of various ethnic groups or cultural taboos with respect to color. A handful of articles on limited aspects of office space planning were scattered in medical or dental practice management magazines and Department of Health, Education, and Welfare publications. Here was a field with few resources and vast potential.

Most medical and dental offices in 1970 were either colorless and clinical or drab and dreary. There was no middle ground. Clinical offices had high levels of illumination, easy-to-clean shiny surfaces, and a lot of medical or dental instruments in view — *clean and clinical.* At the other end of the spectrum, were offices with brown shag carpeting, residential pendant lights, nubby, earth tone upholstery fabric that wouldn't show soil, and poorly styled wood furniture that appeared to have been rescued from a Salvation Army truck. Waxy plastic plants completed this dingy and unhygienic environment.

I concluded that I would have to do my own empirical research to gather enough data on which to base my design work. I spent the better part of a year visiting hospitals, interviewing staff and patients, and observing how patients were handled. I also visited many physicians and dentists and asked about their practices — what kinds of instruments they used; what size treatment room would be efficient; what kinds of changes would make their offices more efficient; and what critical adjacencies existed between rooms or treatment areas.

I documented my visits with photographs of confusing signage, waiting rooms furnished with Goodwill rejects, dismal lighting, corridors jammed with medical equipment, and examination rooms that resembled Dr. Jekyll's laboratory. At the end of my research, I had accumulated over 2000 photos and reams of notes which I analyzed and formulated my design philosophy. My dual major, Psychology and Environmental Design, gave me a certain theoretical background with which to interpret the data. This data base, combined with my 19 years of experience designing hundreds of medical and dental offices, has resulted in this book.

A person with no prior experience in health care design can study this book and become familiar not only with current philosophical issues, but also with medical procedures, equipment associated with each medical or dental specialty, room sizes, traffic flow, construction methods, codes, interior finishes, and more. I have attempted to synthesize my research and experience so that others will not have to follow such a laborious course of study in order to enter this rapidly expanding field.

Today, probably more than a thousand architects and designers across the country list health care as one of their specialities. In its infancy when I started out, the field has reached maturity. No longer concerned with discovering the basic rules and principles, specialists can devote themselves to refining what has been learned and to innovation.

The first edition of this book was published in 1982 and featured exclusively my own work. However, this new, revised edition, to give a broader perspective, includes examples of work by other practitioners who are credited under each photo. I thank each of these designers and photographers for sharing their work. The revised edition includes new chapters on the design of sports medicine facilities, ambulatory surgical centers, and the use of lasers; expanded chapters on diagnostic imaging and on dentistry; and it contains dozens of new space plans for all specialties. The text has been revised to include new developments in medical treatment and to familiarize readers with state-of-the-art medical and dental equipment.

I offer special thanks to my colleagues, architect David Schoenherr and Mark Reilly, for their assistance in producing all of the illustrations on CADD, and to my assistant, Mary Anne Jones, for her help in preparing the manuscript.

Introduction: Changing Perspectives

Dramatic changes have occurred in the delivery of health care since the first edition of this book. Some might even call it a revolution. The long-term effects of this upheaval are so pervasive that designers, to satisfy the needs of medical clients, must understand the economic climate in which today's physician practices.

The seminal event that kicked off a series of radical changes in the traditional fee structure began in 1984, with the federal government's prospective pricing program, whereby Medicare and Medicaid reimbursements were made on a fixed, flat-fee basis, rather than as a percentage of an individual physician's fee. Based upon a list of some 470 diagnosis-related groups (DRGs) of procedures, the physician/provider receives a flat fee, regardless of actual cost. Since Medicare and Medicaid compose approximately 40 percent of the national health care budget, hospitals and physicians were forced to take a hard look at ways to reduce costs.

Following the lead of the federal government, some states also initiated prospective pricing programs, and insurance companies followed suit, issuing guidelines and directives making physicians feel that third-party payers, rather than they, were managing their patients' care. As an example, an insurance company may stipulate that certain procedures will be paid for only if done on an outpatient basis.

Health insurance used to be simple. People chose their own doctors, and visited them whenever they wished. Insurance companies rarely asked questions, regardless of frequency or costs. Insurance companies received the medical bills and paid them, less the deductible, or a percentage of out-of-pocket costs.

Today, however, medical insurance is complicated and has become a battleground wherein health care providers, consumers, employers, and insurance companies are each trying to retain control of their respective interests. Spiraling health care costs have forced insurance companies and physician groups to develop alternative health care delivery systems. Chief among these are new types of group health insurance programs designed to reduce employers' health care expenditures while controlling insurance companies' costs.

These insurance plans include a number of safeguards to discourage unnecessary use. For example, specialists usually must be referred by a member's primary care physician, also known as a *gatekeeper.* Small patient co-payments at the time treatment is received are a part of many plans. On a local level, each plan's utilization review committee evaluates whether certain treatments, visits, and charges are medically necessary in order to control payments to physicians. They also set rates physicians can charge for office visits or certain procedures.

The most common *alternative delivery systems* are

health maintenance organizations (HMOs) and preferred provider organizations (PPOs). An HMO offers a range of health and medical benefits to subscribers for a prepaid fixed fee. Members must accept service from physicians and hospitals within the HMO's established network. Based on the principle of prevention, HMOs pay for screening examinations to keep people healthy. They contend that it is cheaper to keep people healthy than to treat them when sick. These plans generally offer many benefits to subscribers including routine physicals, immunizations, X-rays, complete surgical coverage, and discounts on prescription drugs, all for the fixed monthly fee. The only restriction is that one may not go outside the physician/hospital network for treatment, unless specifically referred there by the plan.

The two main types of HMOs are the *Independent Practice Association* (IPA) and the *group practice* model. The latter usually employs its own physicians or engages them on a contract basis. Care is delivered through a number of clinics owned and operated by the HMO. At the primary care level, subscribers generally accept care from any available physician; however, Kaiser, the nation's largest HMO, encourages members to request and select their own primary care physician.

HMOs may or may not be large enough to own their own hospitals. When they do not, they contract with hospitals and medical specialists to service their subscribers, with the understanding that treatment protocols and costs will be evaluated by the HMO. IPA-type HMOs are usually developed by groups of physicians to service employers. A big difference between these and group practice models is that IPAs allow physicians to remain in private practice and to treat subscribers from their own offices. Therefore, IPA physicians are not employees of the HMO, and they are reimbursed either through a flat fee or capitation system, or on a fee-for-service basis.

With *capitation,* the physician receives a set monthly fee for caring for each patient regardless of the amount of care required. If less care is provided, the physician can keep the difference, but if more care is required, the physician must absorb the loss. Obviously, volume is a requirement for this system's success.

The fee-for-service reimbursement is less of a gamble. Physicians are reimbursed for all services at negotiated discounted rates. These rates, however, may be up to 40 percent less than their customary fee.

On the other hand, a Preferred Provider Organization allows members to chose any physician, specialist, or hospital they wish, but they receive a discounted rate only if they select a provider within the specified network. Employers' costs with a PPO plan are generally higher, because there is no cap on payment for care. Physicians, while they must discount fees, in return receive a high volume of patients.

The 1980s will be known for a restructuring of the health care system. It was estimated that by 1990 there would be 750 HMOs in operation with a total of 40 million enrollees,[1] and that by 1997, 50 percent of the private-pay healthcare population will be members of an HMO.[2] However, many HMOs are losing money, and industry analysts predict there will be a major shakeout, accompanied by a number of fatalities. A major consolidation led by industry giants, such as Blue Cross, Blue Shield, Aetna, Prudential, and Cigna, will force poorly managed or undercapitalized plans out

[1]*Hospitals* Magazine, February 5, 1986. "HMOs: A shake-up (and shakeout) on the horizon?" edited by Maria Traska.

[2]"Managed care will dominate within a decade — experts," by Sanford C. Bernstein & Co. as reported in *Modern Healthcare,* July 29, 1988.

of the market. The nation's largest insurance carriers are now getting involved in *providing,* rather than just paying for, health care. These companies have already created their own HMOs or PPOs, or have arranged joint ventures with existing plans. In some cities hospitals are developing their own HMO and PPO plans by forming networks with loyal physicians.

Hospitals, experiencing the same kinds of economic and market-driven pressures that affect physicians, are setting up marketing exchanges with physicians to establish mutually beneficial, long-term relationships. Hospitals offer targeted physicians incentives for their loyalty and for referring patients to that hospital. Physicians gain access to sophisticated marketing and strategic planning studies commissioned by the hospital. They may also receive patients from a physician referral system set up by the hospital. In a hospital/physician network, physicians receive help in maintaining and enhancing their practices, and hospitals increase their admissions and bond physicians to their hospital.

Crystal ball gazers aside, it's difficult to predict what the health care delivery system will look like ten years from now. The incredible number of alternatives competing for validation will no doubt be reduced by normal economic forces. Nevertheless, industry analysts do agree that traditional indemnity plans wherein physicians are reimbursed their "usual and customary charges" will be replaced by plans that are more cost-effective for employers.

Physicians will become more aggressively involved in developing new delivery systems, including ownership or partnership. However, physicians will have to practice a different type of medicine, with the emphasis and incentive on keeping the patient healthy, and when the patient needs treatment, doing the right thing the first time.

Some predict that by 1995, the vast majority of Americans will be under some form of *managed care* or capitation plan. Regardless of individual differences, it is likely to be a marriage between physicians and competent, professional managers. Some wonder whether managed care will limit access to new diagnostic and therapeutic technologies. Will efforts to reduce costs limit access to sophisticated imaging equipment, lasers, and use of new interventional cardiovascular procedures and drugs? Will the development of new technologies be slowed by loss of incentives? New technologies increase costs, but improve the quality of care. Perhaps an individual health plan's future success may depend upon a statement of policy regarding utilization of these new technologies when deemed appropriate for a patient's care.

Some startling figures reveal just how pervasive managed care will be in the 1990s:*

- Traditional fee-for-service (indemnity coverage) will drop to about 5 percent of the nongovernmental market; it represented 72 percent of that market in 1985.
- Managed fee-for-service coverage will represent about 25 percent of the nongovernmental market. However, managed fee-for-service eventually will be rolled into HMO and PPA (preferred provider arrangement) hybrids.
- HMOs will represent 30 percent of that market, with IPA-model plans capturing 22 percent of the market. Group-model HMOs will repesent about 8 percent.
- PPAs will take up at least 40 percent of the nongovernmental market. In 1985, they accounted for only 4 percent.

**Hospitals Magazine,* in an article by Peter Boland, April 5, 1988.

However significant these economic changes have been, they are not the only forces reshaping the traditional doctor-patient relationship. Emphasis has shifted from the treatment of disease to keeping people healthy. The focus on wellness pervades our culture as an increasing number of people become interested in fitness, nutrition, and disease prevention.

The new consumer is wiser and more educated about health care, and shops for health care services. The traditional "doctor knows best" approach has been challenged by consumers who put the responsibility for their health in their own hands.

Health education centers, as adjuncts to hospitals and other health service agencies, have sprung up in storefronts and shopping malls, making wellness information accessible to the community. At the same time, these ventures promote hospitals' names and services.

Mobile vans carry health information and screening to residential and rural areas. Frequently parked at shopping centers, they do cholesterol screening, blood pressure checks, blood tests for diabetes, measurements of body fat, or take chest X-rays.

Future social, economic, and political considerations are certain to change the character of health delivery systems. Industry analysts find it difficult to predict what types of services the market will demand; therefore, health care designers are expected to build into each facility as much flexibility as possible, to accommodate change. What is known, however, is that two significant issues will drive health care delivery in new directions. These issues are AIDS and the elderly.

The treatment of AIDS patients has placed a tremendous financial burden on health care systems, the community, and insurance companies. Treatment and care of AIDS patients are bankrupting our hospitals and taxing community social service agencies. Scientists predict that the development of a vaccine to control the spread of AIDS may be eight years away. By that time, owing to the eight-year gestation period, those who have been exposed to the virus or those with symptoms will constitute an AIDS population requiring treatment for the next 20 to 30 years.

Precautions that must be taken by health care workers, including those who work in hospitals, medical offices, and dental offices, have increased the costs of treating all patients. Surgeons and operating room personnel are at high risk because of open wounds and the spattering of blood. Surgeons wear protective eyewear and double gloves. They often work more slowly during procedures to minimize any unexpected events that might increase contact with blood. Longer operating room time means greater expense for every procedure.

Dentists and chairside assistants are especially at risk to hepatitis B virus (HBV) and to HIV virus. Stringent infection control procedures in dental offices prevent cross-contamination to dentists, technicians, and patients. These extra measures to control asepsis require extra time between each and every patient. In fact, compliance with Center for Disease Control recommendations is no longer left to the discretion of individual practitioners, but is mandated by OSHA. Failure to comply is against the law and bears a heavy penalty.

All these factors indicate that designers of health care facilities must be very aware of asepsis control in all health care environments. The irony is that new medical and dental offices are going to look more clinical, as they looked many years ago, before practitioners realized that patients were comforted by carpeted examination rooms and textured wallcoverings. This could amount to a giant step backward, aesthetically, unless the designer is clever and innovative in utilizing smooth, easy-to-clean materials.

The "graying of America," the other significant issue driving health care today, assures that gerontology will become a major specialty. There will be an extraordinary number of skilled nursing facilities, personal care or assisted living units, and congregate care facilities constructed. Care and housing of the elderly has become an enormous industry, challenging architects, sociologists, gerontologists, and developers to satisfy the many and diverse needs of what may become the largest segment of the population.

There will be an increased need for highly specialized facilities such as cancer centers, chemical dependency treatment units, burn centers, mental health facilities, and rehabilitation units. The 1980s have seen a proliferation of rehabilitation units and mental health facilities, influenced by the fact that this type of treatment is not subject to fixed-fee DRG reimbursement.

It is likely that rehabilitation units located in or near general hospitals will focus their attention on making patients more independent and able to provide better home care for themselves. These patients include diabetics, arthritics, the orthopedically handicapped, amputees, cancer patients, stroke victims, and brain-injured individuals.

Home health care has become a major industry, owing to the aging population and the emphasis on cost containment. Bringing health care services to people in their homes is, at the same time, better for the patient and less expensive for the agency paying for that care.

The trend toward outpatient care will continue, with approval for many more procedures to be done on an outpatient basis. For example, cardiac catheterizations are now being performed in ambulatory surgical centers. MRI (Magnetic Resonance Imaging) technology makes it possible to examine and diagnose many diseases with noninvasive techniques, where heretofore invasive procedures were required. One example is arthroscopy of the knee.

All of this suggests that the medical space planner will need to become familiar with an increasing number of medical procedures and techniques, to accommodate them properly in new outpatient facilities.

Although the 1990s will bring enormous changes in health care delivery, health care will continue to be one of the fastest growing categories of nonresidential construction, offering architects and interior designers an unlimited number of challenging projects.

CHAPTER 1

Psychology: Implications for Health Care Design

OVERVIEW

A visit to the physician or dentist traumatizes many people. The basis for the fear, even more than lack of familiarity with procedures and a feeling of helplessness, may stem from the invasion of one's personal space.

Americans maintain larger territorial boundaries than most other cultures. For example, an American may maintain an imaginary barrier 24 inches in front of him or her as a safe conversational distance for strangers, while a person from the Middle East may reduce that safe boundary to 12 inches. Furthermore, studies show that Americans will tolerate a person at a closer distance to the side than in front of them.

Another curious fact is that Americans physically remove themselves from a situation when they want solitude or privacy. Middle Easterners, by contrast, simply stop talking and ignore the presence of others nearby, allowing themselves to be isolated even when physically surrounded by others. The Japanese employ similar tactics to gain privacy in a crowd.

Nowhere is a person's privacy violated more than in a medical or dental examination. One's territorial limits are invaded by strangers who poke, probe, and prod. And when the examination demands that the patient be naked, even the barrier of clothing ceases to protect. Is it any wonder that a visit to the dentist or physician can intimidate even the most stouthearted among us? How, then, can practitioners break through this barrier to examine and treat patients without arousing fear and anxiety?

First, the patient must perceive the positive aspects of the care he or she is receiving through an understanding of the procedures and how they will enhance his or her enjoyment of life. The relief of pain or the prevention of disease are joys in themselves. Second, the diagnostic and therapeutic milieu must *promote health* rather than aggravate illness and cause anxiety. The environment must be clean, cheerful, and nonthreatening, with contemporary furnishings, pleasing colors, and interesting textures. The staff must be neatly groomed, well trained, and interested in the patients' well-being.

PATIENT SATISFACTION

Patient satisfaction is the new buzzword. It's the difference between providing what a patient *needs,* and what a patient *wants.* It is important not only to satisfy clinical needs, but also to meet psychological expectations.

Principal components of patient satisfaction are a warm and caring staff, attractive nonclinical surroundings, and the ability for patients and visitors to easily find their way around the medical center without getting lost.

THE NEW CONSUMERISM

The new consumerism has radically changed patient/physician relationships. There was a time when people never dared to question a physician's diagnosis or recommendations for treatment. Physicians and other health professionals were placed on a pedestal, and even malpractice suits were infrequent. Sociologists attribute this loss of innocence to the Vietnam war, the Watergate scandal, the dumping of toxic waste, environmental pollution, and other issues that have caused many to question whether those in authority actually have our well-being in mind. Added to this are the efforts of people like Ralph Nader, who educated consumers to examine critically the safety of products and practices commonly in use. The result is a new group of consumers who focus on wellness, who put responsibility for health in their own hands, who play an active role in keeping themselves fit, and who shop for health care services with a critical eye.

Shopping for health care services is a new concept. Formerly, people visited the family doctor with whom they had grown up, or they selected a practitioner in the neighborhood. However, with the type of mobility that characterizes our society, people move frequently, and long-term relationships with health care providers are often not possible. This fact and the upsurge of interest in holistic medicine and the proliferation of public information regarding the prevention of disease combine to create a consumer-driven market.

This has spawned great competition among health care providers, who look for ways to differentiate themselves. Many medical and dental specialists are increasingly image-conscious, which prompts them to engage marketing consultants as well as design professionals to help them achieve their goals.

First Impressions Count

Once the patient walks into the office, the waiting room should establish immediate rapport and put the patient at ease. First impressions are very important. Out-of-date furniture, worn upholstery, tables with cigarette burns, and dirty spots on walls and woodwork give the patient a message that the doctor does not care about patient comfort, or that he or she is reluctant to replace things when they wear out. It further suggests that the doctor may be a person who is outdated on medical matters as well. *Lack of confidence in the doctor breeds anxiety in the patient.*

WAITING: A FRUSTRATING INCONVENIENCE

Waiting, unhappily, is one of the frustrations that often accompanies a visit to the doctor. Patients who are in pain or who are alarmed about an undiagnosed illness will accept waiting, realizing that doctors cannot always schedule appointments accurately. Well patients, however, such as those in a screening facility, have a different attitude and are not willing to accept discomfort or inconvenience without registering complaints.

Few wait with pleasure. In fact, waiting tends to concentrate one's attention on the details of the surroundings, making the presence or lack of good interior design more noticeable. Burned-out light bulbs, waxy plastic plants, and the crooked magazine rack become exaggerated irritants. In the words of the inimitable architecture critic Ada Louise Huxtable, "Doctors' offices are where Danish modern went to die."

Many people visit a physician or dentist during their work day. Excessive waiting leads to anxiety and hostility, with worries about time away from the office and being late for meetings. An emergency at the hospital or the delivery of a baby are situations that people will forgive. They understand medical emergencies. But physicians who make a continual practice of overbooking, disregarding their patients' time schedules are, perhaps without realizing it, not taking their patients seriously.

Seating Arrangements

Americans, in particular, do not like to be touched by strangers. Middle Eastern and Latin cultures, by contrast, encourage closeness and touching. In the Arab world, olfaction, as expressed by breathing in the face of a friend, is considered a necessary part of social grace. To deny a friend the smell of one's breath is a cause of shame. Middle Easterners and Latins will huddle together much more closely than will Americans in a crowd.

Thus seating arrangements in a waiting room designed for Americans should not force strangers to sit together — this only intensifies the stress of visiting the physician or dentist. Individual chairs should be provided and arranged so that strangers do not have to face one another with a distance of less than eight feet between them. Chairs should be placed against walls or in configurations that offer a degree of security, so that seated persons do not feel they are in jeopardy of being approached from behind. Careful planning in this regard will assure patient comfort.

Cultural Differences

If the medical office or clinic serves an ethnic population, it is important to research how that group uses space. Some cultural groups, for example, tend to bring many relatives when one family member has to visit the doctor. Perhaps this is due to a distrust of "modern medicine" or the need for emotional support provided by the presence of the family. People who do not speak English well or those from rural areas might easily become intimidated by modern technology. Books by Robert Summer and Edward T. Hall are excellent resources for the cultural use of space.

PERCEIVED STATUS DIFFERENCE

One of the main reasons patients feel intimidated may be due to the perceived status difference between the physician or technician and themselves. The patient sits in a powerless position while being acted upon by others. Feelings of helplessness are accelerated when physicians are protected by fortress-type desks and imposing executive chairs from which they appear to talk down to the patient, who is seated at a "safe" distance in a simple chair with no protective barrier. Physicians most likely do not intend to set up their consultation room to intimidate the patient, but the effect is there nonetheless.

Another example of patient intimidation occurs when a radiologist issues instructions via a loudspeaker from a remote control room to a semi-naked patient splayed on the X-ray table — a humiliating experience. Every effort should be made to treat the patient as an equal, to explain each step of a medical or dental procedure, to make the patient a partner in his or her treatment, and to allow the patient as much dignity as possible during what can best be described as humiliating medical examinations: gastrointestinal X-ray studies, proctologic examinations, and so forth. An individual's most private bodily functions are scrutinized by strangers, causing great psychological stress.

PRIVACY IS IMPORTANT

Examination rooms should have a dressing area where patients may disrobe, confident that the nurse or doctor will not barge in on them while naked. A dressing area also provides a place for patients to hang their undergarments out of view of strangers. It should have a mirror, a chair, and hooks to hang clothes. Similarly, radiology suites should have dressing rooms and a safe place to leave or lock up valuables. The floors should be carpeted so that patients do not have to walk barefoot on cold floors to the radiography rooms.

Subliminal Cues

There is no substitute for live green plants in a waiting room. Plastic plants suggest that live plants probably could not survive the environment, and the patient may fare no better. Healthy, lustrous greenery, on the other hand, promotes feelings of well-being.

A poorly illuminated waiting room not only makes it difficult to read, but subliminally suggests to patients that the doctor is trying to hide something — perhaps poor housekeeping, dust-encrusted baseboards, soiled carpet, finger-marked glass, or faded draperies. Burned-out light bulbs are the ultimate insult, indicating a consummate inattention to detail.

A closed, sliding glass window with a buzzer for service tells patients that they are not really welcome — that they are intruding on the staff's privacy. The receptionist should always be in view of patients and accessible to them.

Body Language Indicates Stress

The patient's body language can indicate when the patient is uncomfortable with the physician, dentist, or technician. Averted eyes — looking away from the doctor — is one sign. Body positioned away from the doctor is another. Stereotyped behavior (tapping toes, shaking a leg, or rocking) is another. At these signs, the doctor must reestablish contact with the patient and break the perceived-status-difference barrier. Taking the patient's hand and asking if he or she is okay is both friendly and reassuring. It also establishes the kind of rapport that discourages malpractice suits.

SEEING THE DOCTOR AS A PERSON

The consultation room (and sometimes the waiting room) may contain the doctor's personal memorabilia. Such items help the patient to see the doctor as a person with a family, hobbies, and interests outside of medicine. This reassures the patient that the doctor is a real person, not just a white coat with a stethoscope.

Style of Furnishings Should Not Be Trendy

There is considerable opportunity for the doctor to express his or her personality and style preferences in furniture. Indeed, for obstetricians, gynecologists, plastic surgeons, and pediatricians, the sky is the limit. But most physicians, surgeons in particular, must carefully select furniture that will convey a solid, conservative image. Patients need to feel that their surgeon is not impulsive — that he or she is a serious person not subject to frivolities and trendy decor.

Even if patients are not consciously aware of the message they are getting from the office interior design, they are subconsciously reading it. The body language of the office environment tells patients things that might subconsciously undermine their confidence in the physician or dentist. Confidence can be reinforced through attention to the patients' comfort.

Although patients sometimes abuse nice furnishings by putting their feet on the chairs or placing gum on the upholstery, that is the price that must be paid to make patients feel comfortable. The replacement factor should be built into the office overhead. The fact is, most patients do not abuse the pleasant surroundings provided for them, so why make the many suffer for the transgressions of the few? Needless to say, the psychological benefits of an office designed to serve the patients far outweigh any drawbacks.

CHAPTER 2

General Parameters of Medical Space Planning

BUILDING SHELL DESIGN

Efficient medical offices begin with an intelligently designed building shell. All too often medical office buildings (MOBs) are planned by designers or architects who are unfamiliar with the special requirements of medical tenants; thus, the structure of the building does not lend itself to an efficient layout of suites. Structural column locations, stair placement, elevators, electrical room, mechanical shafts, public restrooms (if provided), and window modules either impede of facilitate layout of individual suites.

Other factors that influence the design of an MOB are the shape and size of the site, the specific requirements of a particular tenant or client, a beautiful view, or the architect's desire to impose a unique design on the project. All of these factors have to be weighed and balanced along with applicable codes, zoning restrictions, and the client's budget. A building that is completely functional and efficient, but totally insensitive to aesthetics may not rent as quickly as the owners may wish. But an MOB designed primarily for aesthetic merit, with only secondary concern for internal planning efficiency, will also be difficult to rent.

Floor Area Efficiency

To begin with, an MOB should contain at least 11,000 to 12,000 square feet of rentable space per floor in order to accommodate suites of varying sizes and configurations as well as to increase the efficiency of stairs and elevators. The elevator, mechanical equipment room, electrical room, and public restrooms can be placed in the core with rental space wrapped around the perimeter (Figures 2-1 and 2-2) or the services may be located at the ends of a double-loaded public corridor (Figure 2-4). Figure 2-1 gives 80 percent rentable space and Figure 2-3 gives 89 percent rentable space, but it must be noted that Figure 2-1 includes restrooms. Medical buildings usually are designed to an 85 percent efficiency, but architectural features such as an atrium or a large lobby can reduce the efficiency to 80 percent.

The core factor is 12 percent in Figure 2-2, reflecting the gain in efficiency due to the large floor plate. The building shell in Figure 2-2 is designed to accommodate large users on the 60-foot-bay depth side. If the building is leased to smaller tenants, public corridors penetrating the 60-foot depth may have to be added, thereby reducing somewhat the potential rentable area.

Often, it is most efficient to place stairs and other intrusions into the rental space at the ends of the building as shown in Figures 2-3 and 2-4. Special attention must be paid to locating stairwells when one tenant intends to lease an entire floor or half a floor. In such case, the public exit stairwell may fall within an individual suite — a nonpublic space. One way to handle this is to provide a third stair in the center of the building so that, even if one tenant takes half a floor, two stairs remain accessible for tenants on the other half of the floor (Figure 2-4).

Figure 2-2 shows a layout with one stair set in, to allow a 52-foot-bay depth between it and the end of the building, so that a large suite can run across the end of the building either at the 52-foot depth, or a 32-foot depth utilizing a 20-foot "allowable" dead-end corridor, extending from the stairwell. One must remember, however, when locating a suite across the end of a building: If the occupancy load is high enough, two exits may be required, with a separation equal to one-half the distance of the diagonal of the suite. In a large suite, this would be achieved by extending another corridor perpendicular to the public corridor for the secondary exit.

In spite of these issues, especially with a floor plate as large as that shown in Figure 2-2, setting in the stair on one end provides great flexibility with respect to the size of suites that may be accommodated. It should be noted that the stairwells themselves must be located with a separation (generally measured to the center of each door) of one-half the diagonal of the floor.

Structural Support

The structural support system for the building should allow as much flexibility as possible for the layout of tenant spaces. For a multi-story building, a moment-resistant steel frame offers considerably more flexibility in space planning and window placement than does a building supported with "K" braces, for example. Of course, moment-resistant steel is a considerably more expensive option. Regardless of the type of system used, it is imperative that the structural engineer work very closely with the medical space planner, so that structural elements can be accommodated within the planning grid.

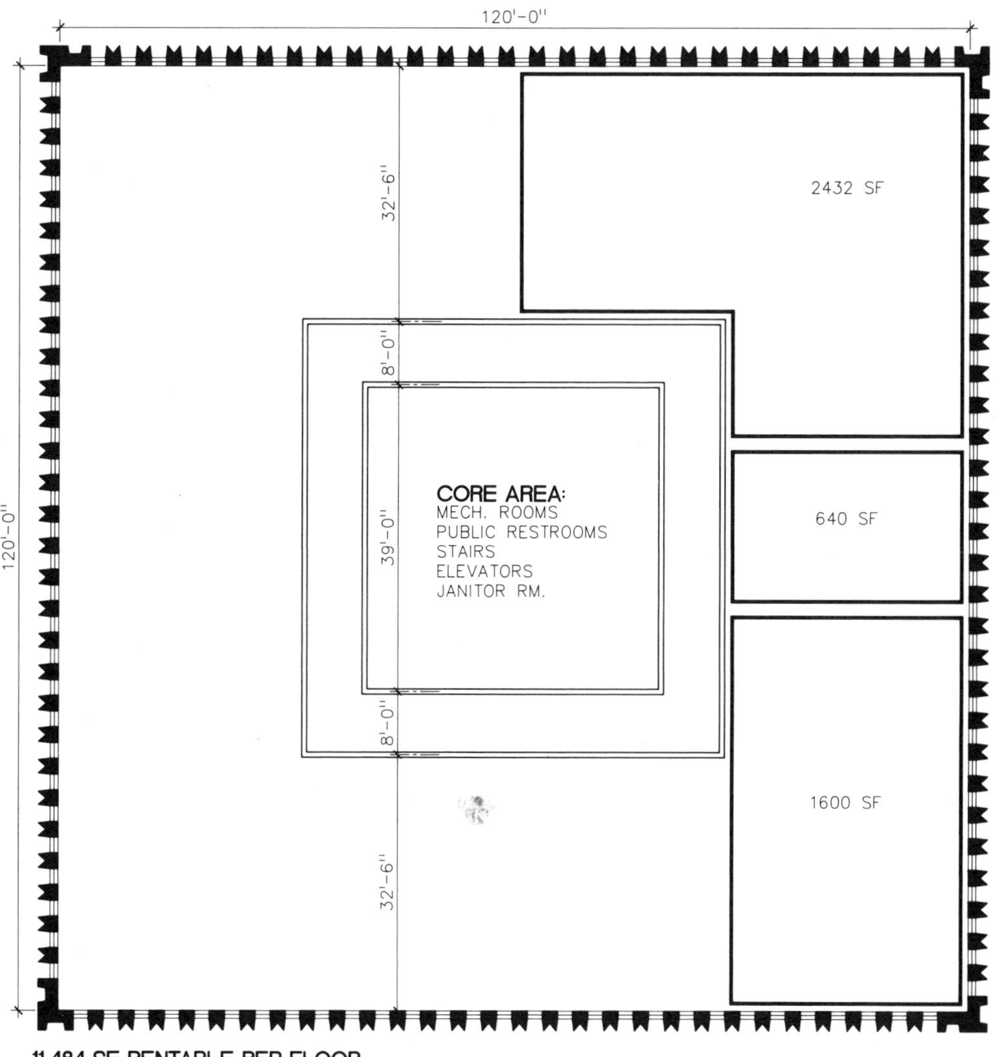

Figure 2-1. Floor plan, building shell.

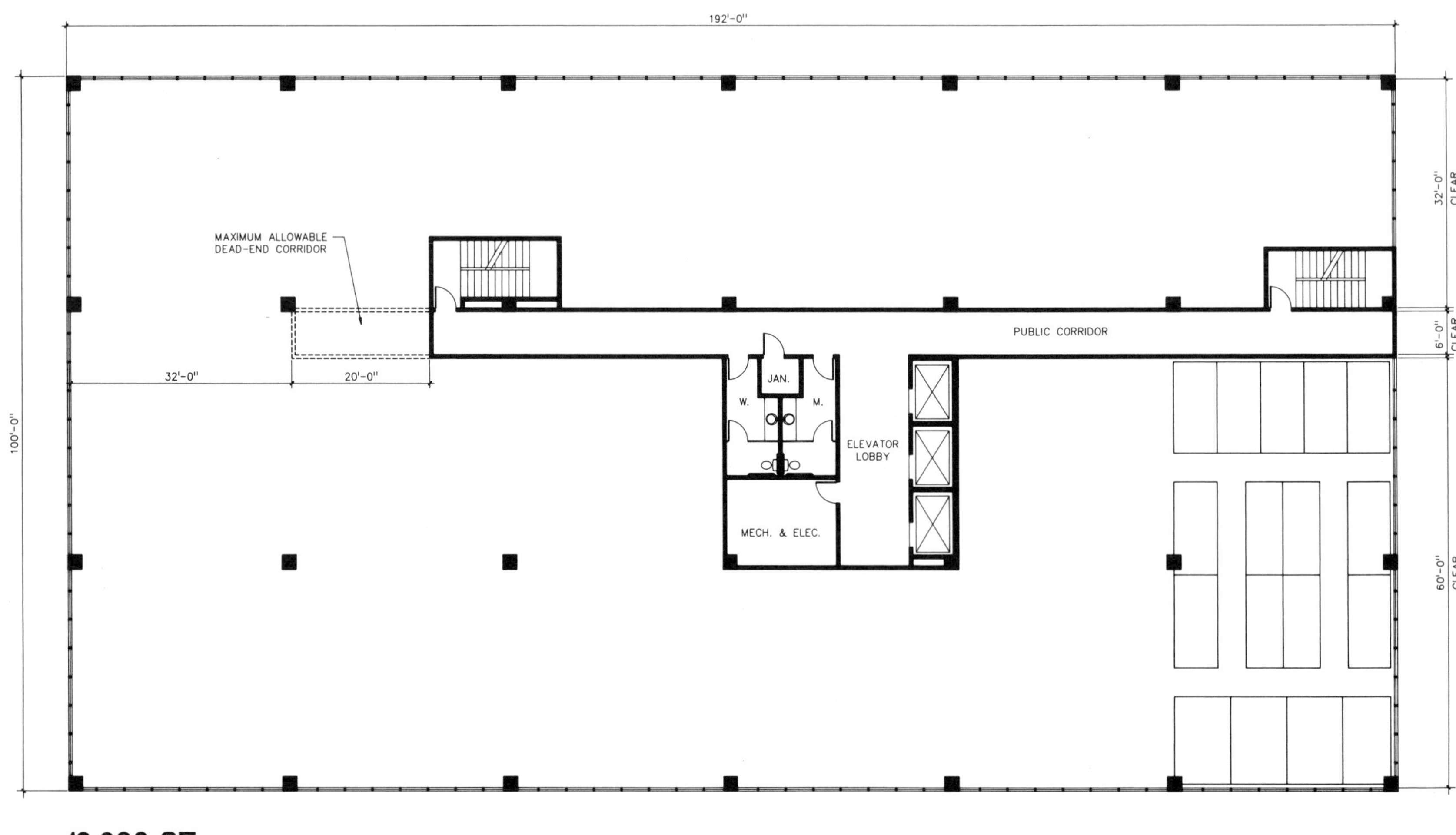

Figure 2-2. Floor plan, building shell.

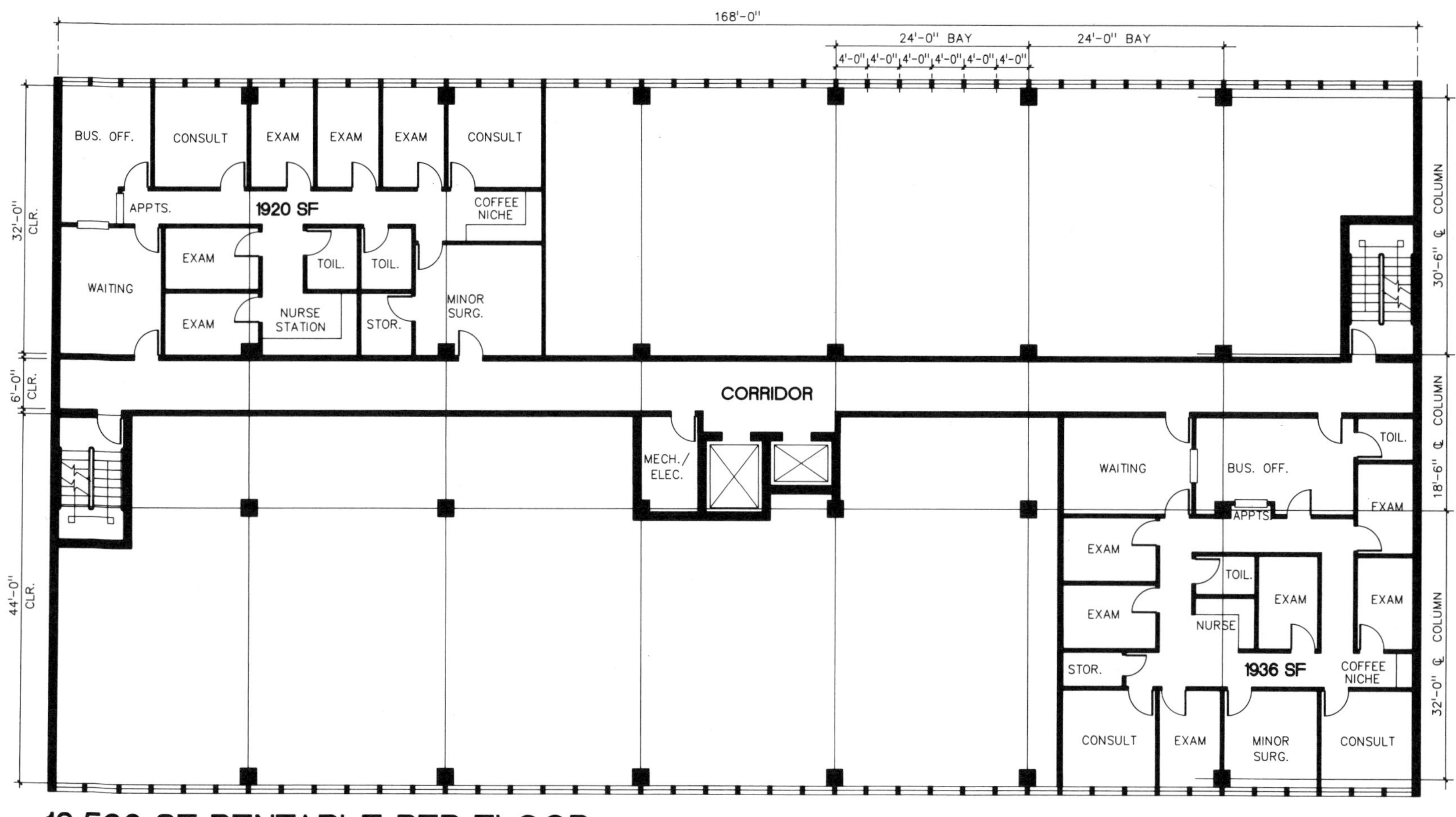

13,500 SF RENTABLE PER FLOOR

Figure 2-3. Floor plan, building shell.

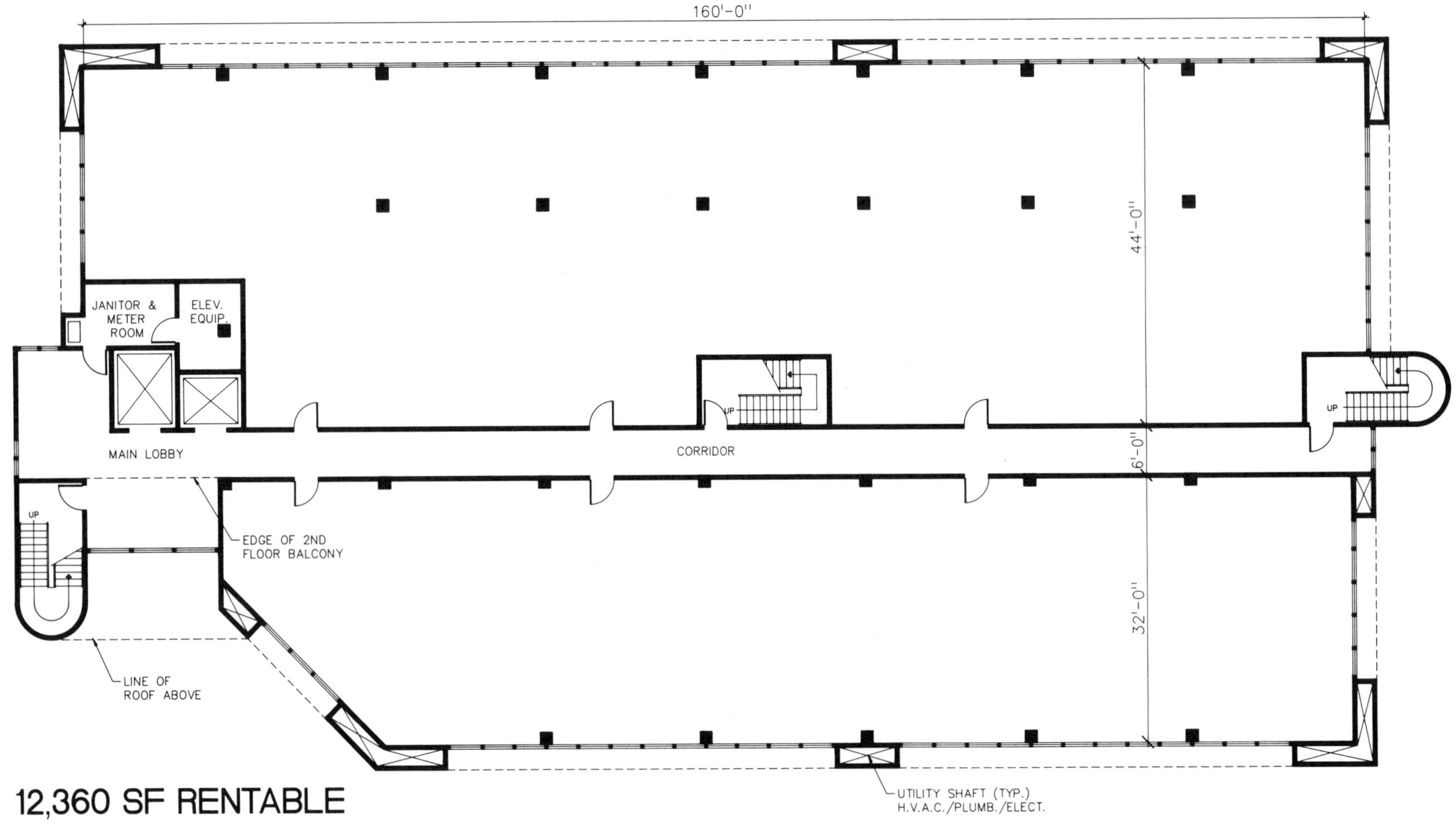

Figure 2-4. Floor plan, building shell.

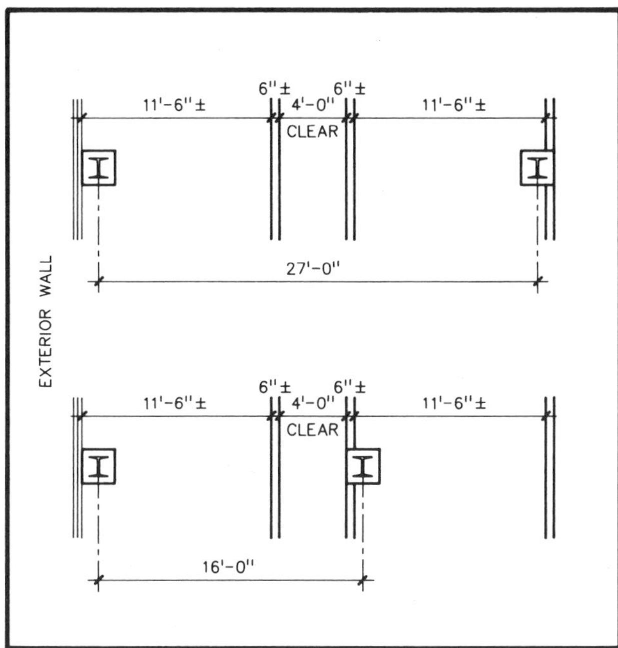

Figure 2-5. Location of columns.

Perimeter columns, ideally, would be flush with the inside face of the exterior wall (Figure 2-2), so that they do not protrude into the room or, at the least, be flush with the exterior face of the building so that protrusion into the room is minimized. On the interior, columns for a 32-foot-bay depth would fall as shown in Figure 2-3 on the inside face of the public corridor wall, spanning 30 feet 6 inches center to center, creating a column free space in between.

For a 44-foot-bay depth, the intermediate column should occur either 16 feet or 17 feet on-center, measured from the column on the exterior wall, and depending upon whether it is flush with the exterior face or extends totally from the inside of the exterior wall (Figures 2-4 and 2-5). Here, there will be a 12-foot-deep row of rooms across the exterior wall. There would then be a 4-foot-wide corridor, and the column should fall on the far side of the corridor, extending into the center row of rooms. Obviously, one would not want that intermediate column to fall within the corridor space.

Another option for locating the intermediate column in a 44-foot-bay depth is illustrated in Figure 2-3. It occurs in the wall of the business office or waiting room, making it 32 feet on center, measured from the column on the exterior wall.

It is difficult to give absolute dimensions for locating columns, because there are so many variables. The "box-in" size of the columns, whether one uses 4-foot-wide or 5-foot-wide interior corridors, and the fact that high-rise buildings have larger columns affect the spacing between them.

Locations of structural columns should not adversely affect the flexibility of the space if the building is engineered properly. Most rooms are small; thus, the density of partitions is high. Long spans are not necessary. A tradeoff inevitably arises here. Reducing the span between columns makes it possible to use lighter-weight beams, thereby reducing the cost of the building. However, more columns, closer together, reduce space planning flexibility. The occurrence of perimeter columns at intervals creating 20-foot-wide or 24-foot-wide bays, and interior columns spaced as shown in Figure 2-4, often works well. Where the spaces on both sides of the corridor are a 32-foot depth, all columns may be contained in the perimeter walls with none occurring within tenant spaces.

PLANNING MODULE

A considerable amount of standardization exists in the sizes of rooms in a medical suite. For the most part, suites can be laid out on either a 4-foot or 4-foot 6-inch planning grid. Having said that, however, one must acknowledge the odd-sized treatment rooms, toilets, and specialty rooms such as radiology.

The author prefers a 4-foot planning module. Based on this, there are four common bay depths that accommodate efficiently suites of certain sizes. To begin with, a *28-foot-bay depth* works well for small suites anywhere from 500 to 1500 square feet. It can even accommodate an 1800-square-foot suite as shown in Figure 2-6. These suites are extremely easy to plan because they involve two 12-foot-deep rows of rooms separated by a 4-foot-wide corridor.

A *32-foot-bay depth* is the most common and accommodates suites anywhere from 1200 to 3000 square feet. This is similar to the 28-foot-bay depth in that it is also a double-loaded corridor, except that the row of rooms closest to the public corridor is 16 feet deep. This is where the waiting room and business office would generally be located. A 3000-square-foot suite, at a 32-foot-bay depth, would be 92 feet long and would involve long walking distances. Therefore, a 3000-square-foot suite would be accommodated better in a 44-foot-bay depth where a center core, or island, may be used.

A *44-foot-bay depth* works well for suites between 1800 to 4000 square feet. Figures 2-3 and 2-6 illustrate how a central core may be used. With suites less than 1800 square feet, a 44-foot-bay depth does not allow enough windows. It creates a narrow, deep suite.

Suite Bay Depths

28 feet	• suites	500 to 1500 square feet
32 feet	• suites	1200 to 3000 square feet
44 feet	• suites	1800 to 4000 square feet
60 feet	• suites	4000 to 10,000 square feet

For purposes of illustration, an identical suite is created in a 28-foot-bay depth and a 44-foot-bay depth in Figure 2-6, and in a 32-foot-bay depth in Figure 2-3. Consultation rooms are 12 × 12 feet, and exam rooms are usually 8 × 12 feet in size. Minor surgery rooms are generally 12 × 12 feet. Thus a fairly predictable layout of rooms can be expected.

If suites are laid out with a storage room at the end of a corridor, as shown in the 798-square-foot suite in Figure 2-6 and in the suites in Figure 2-3, a tenant can expand into an adjoining suite by eliminating the storage room and continuing the corridor, with no other remodeling necessary in the existing suite.

Suites over 4000 square feet work well in a 60-foot-bay depth. Starting at the public corridor wall and moving toward the exterior wall, this allows for a 16-foot-deep row of rooms, a 4-foot-wide corridor, two 12-foot-deep rows of rooms back to back, another 4-foot corridor, and a 12-foot-deep row of rooms parallel to the exterior wall. One may have a number of transverse corridors running perpendicular to the two aforementioned ones, as illustrated in the block diagram in Figure 2-2. This bay depth works for suites anywhere from 4000 to 10,000 square feet. It is not impossible to design a suite less than 4000 square feet in a 60-foot-bay depth; however, unless it is a corner suite with windows on two sides as shown in Figure 2-2, it becomes a narrow, deep suite with few windows.

Suites over 10,000 square feet, depending upon the size of the building, may become a full-floor tenant. In this case, if they were a tenant in the building shown in Figure 2-3, the suite would have a bay depth of 83 feet. In the building shown in Figure 2-4, the tenant could take one-half of the floor and achieve a large square space. The third stair, centrally located, would provide the two required exits for the tenants on the other half of the floor.

One cannot state unequivocally, for example, that a 4000-square-foot suite would be more efficient in a 44-foot-bay depth than a 60-foot-bay depth. The type of medical specialty, penetrations of stairs and elevators,

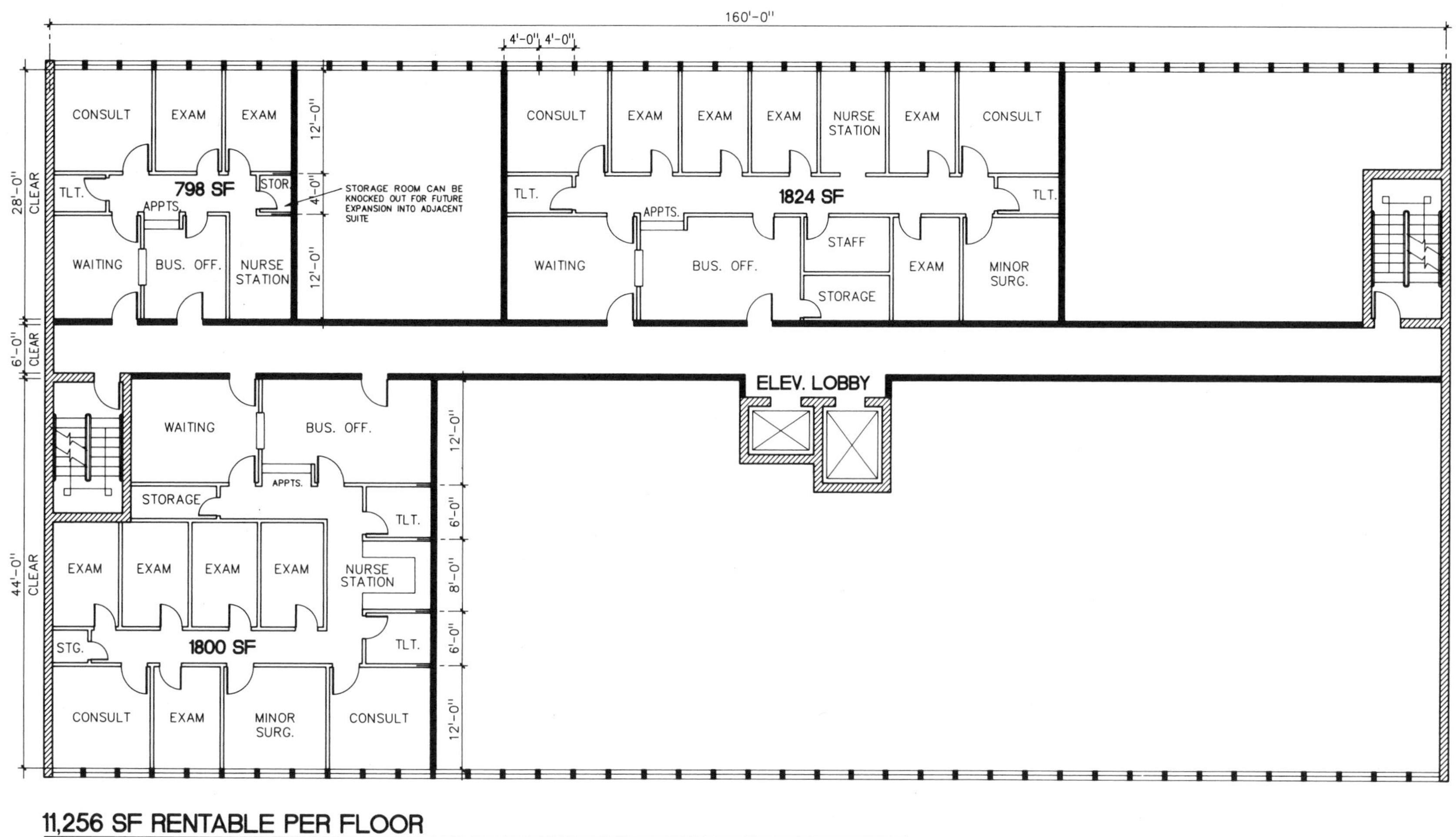

Figure 2-6. Floor plan, building shell.

and the spacing between columns may, in an individual building, make one bay depth preferable to another. If both are available in the building, it would be wise to provide alternate layouts to see which works best. The reader is referred to the radiology suite in Figure 5-2 for an example of a 6600-square-foot suite that runs in an "L" shape along the 44-foot-bay depth and continues across the end of the building.

If one designs a medical building so that suites on one side of the public corridor have a depth of 32 feet, and the other, a depth of 44 feet (Figures 2-3 and 2-4), one would have considerable flexibility to place tenants where the suites can be laid out most efficiently. If feasibility studies prepared prior to the design of the building shell show that there is a considerable need for large suites, then one side of the building might be designed at a 60-foot-bay depth. Sometimes a suite can be laid out equally well in two different bay depths, and the only difference may be that one requires more circulation area than another.

The average medical suite for a solo practitioner would be 1200 square feet. Few suites are smaller than that. The bulk of suites the designer will encounter fall in the range of 1200 to 2500 square feet. There may be large orthopedic or internal medicine suites ranging from 3500 to 8000 square feet. Since the terms of financing often specify that the building must be 50 percent preleased before construction begins, it is often possible to know who the large tenants with special needs will be, and the building can be shaped with those requirements in mind.

An MOB constructed purely on speculation with little preleasing would be difficult to plan without a profile or feasibility study of physicians in the area, their space needs were they to lease space, and their respective specialties.

Window Placement

Window placement is a significant issue in a medical office building. With so many small rooms, it is important that windows fall in the right place and that structural columns occur on the coordinates of the planning module so that they can be buried in the walls. Windows with mullions at 4 feet on-center function well when a 4-foot planning grid is utilized. This permits exam rooms to be 8 feet wide (7-foot 6-inch clear) and consultation rooms to be 12 feet wide (11-foot 6-inch clear) along the window wall. The 4-foot window module can be reduced to a 2-foot module to permit even greater flexibility, but this amounts to an increased construction cost. When windows are irregularly sized, or something other than the 4-foot module, partitions have to jog in order to meet a mullion.

It is important that windows start at 42 inches off the floor so that cabinets can be put under them, and patient privacy in an exam room is not violated. Even in a waiting room or lobby, windows should not start at the floor because it limits the area of seating. The glazing color should be gray, not bronze, because the latter tends to make skin look jaundiced.

Ceiling Heights

An 8-foot or 8-foot 6-inch ceiling height is suitable for individual suites with the exception of a few individual rooms such as radiology, outpatient surgery, or physical therapy, which require a 9- or 10-foot-high ceiling. A standard suspended acoustic ceiling works well, but ideally, for acoustical reasons, should be laid out individually in each room with interior partitions extending above the finished ceiling 6 to 9 inches.

AMENITIES

When a dentist or physician evaluates one building against another, various factors are considered in addition to lease terms and a possible equity position. Amenities such as a health club, a conference center, dedicated parking for physicians, and a coffee shop or deli may make one building more attractive than another. A building's image is important, but less so than for corporate users, who will generally seek out the most upscale building their budgets will allow.

Physicians try to tailor the image to their patient profile. Plastic surgeons and other specialists who perform largely elective procedures may be more interested in a high-profile building. However, a primary care physician with a broad spectrum of patients may choose a more modest building that will not make low-income patients feel uncomfortable. This physician would be more interested in other attributes of the building such as freeway access, convenient parking for patients, and proximity to the hospital.

BUILDING SHELL CONFIGURATIONS

The building shell configurations illustrated in this chapter are straightforward and highly functional. Other considerations sometimes prevail. The site may be best suited to a square building, a cruciform building, or perhaps one in a T-shape. If located on a prominent corner, the part of the building that faces the corner might be sculpted or articulated in such a way as to make it more dramatic.

Sometimes, in an attempt to make an architectural statement, the exterior of the building will have a stair-step configuration. This can greatly reduce the efficiency of the suites unless careful consideration is given to the length of each staggered section to make sure that a row of rooms will fit within it. Niches in the exterior wall can be even more of a problem, resulting in very irregular room shapes. Buildings that are oval or have a circular configuration are next to impossible to utilize for medical office buildings.

BUILDING STANDARDS

It is important to define building standards for tenant improvements in order to establish an acceptable level of quality for construction items. These building standards would normally be prepared by the medical space planner for review by the owner and tenant improvement contractor. The items included are construction details for each type of partition, sound attenuation, suite entry hardware, door closers, interior doors, casework style and details, plumbing fixtures, ceiling system, light fixtures, electrical hardware, interior finishes, design of reception window, and so forth.

These items are generally accepted by all tenants in the building. Some may wish to upgrade light fixtures, add wallcoverings, or upgrade the carpet, but the basic construction items will be consistent throughout the building. This assures the owner, who has to maintain the building, that replacement parts will be on hand, and, if a tenant moves out, the owner won't be left with a suite having French Provincial residential hardware, for example.

TENANT IMPROVEMENT ALLOWANCES

Owners or developers offer tenants a *tenant improvement allowance,* expressed as a per-square foot amount, to build their suites. These amounts vary from building to building and also reflect geographical differences in construction costs. At the lower end of the spectrum, tenants cannot build even a simple suite without adding $15 to $20 per foot, from their own pocket, to the allowance. At the upper end of the spectrum, tenants may be able to build a "plain vanilla" suite (one with minimum casework, building standard lighting, and painted walls) at the tenant improvement allowance, without adding money to it.

Generally speaking, tenants don't expect to be able to build a medical or dental suite within the tenant improvement allowance. Suites such as family practice, pediatrics, and dermatology, however, would be less expensive to build than an ophthalmology suite, for example, which has a great deal of electrical work.

At the upper end in terms of construction cost would be radiology suites, oral surgery, ambulatory surgical centers, and many dental suites. All of these contain a great deal of plumbing, electrical, and special construction details that make them extremely expensive to construct. For this reason, physicians and dentists are highly desirable tenants. They invest so much in tenant improvements that they move infrequently. Commercial office tenants often move every few years, whereas it is not unusual for a physician to occupy a space for 10 to 15 years.

An alternate method of dealing with tenant improvements is to present tenants with a *work letter* stipulating exactly how many of each item (i.e., lineal feet of casework, number of electrical outlets, number of doors, lineal feet of partitions) they will receive per 1000 square feet of rentable space. These quantities are tied to the per-square-foot allowance. In theory, if the tenant did not exceed those quantities of each item, per 1000 square feet, the suite would be built with no out-of-pocket expenses.

POLITICS

When designing tenant suites, one becomes aware of a fundamental issue: conflicting goals of various parties regarding tenant privileges and limitations. Of particular concern are ownership of the building (whether the tenants may participate in ownership), tenant improvement allowances offered by the owners, whether tenants may have their own radiology equipment, and whether tenants will be permitted to engage their own contractors.

In essence, owners generally want to give as little as possible but lease the building quickly and at high rents, and tenants want to move into custom suites, designed according to their every whim, without having to foot any out-of-pocket expenses. The tug-of-war usually continues until the tenant actually takes occupancy of the suite, and then, little by little, the issues seem to resolve themselves. However, the space planner is often caught in the middle.

If retained by the owner of the building to do space planning for the tenants, the designer's obligation is to protect the rights of the owner; when employed by an individual tenant, the designer is charged with negotiating with the building owner to secure the greatest number of goods for the tenant. When one is the space planner for the building and also engaged to provide custom interior design services for a tenant, one must wear two hats and represent both parties well.

LEASING CONSIDERATIONS

Leasing a medical building requires a great deal of strategy. It is helpful if the leasing agent is experienced in dealing with physicians. Targeting one or two key physician groups is the best way to kick off the leasing effort. Physicians are often reluctant to be the first to lease space in a new building. It takes a couple of leaders who are not afraid to risk being first in order to interest other physicians. The strategy involves determining who those key physicians are and going after them. Their interest in the project signals the seal of approval to others in the medical community.

Strategy also comes into play when determining optimum locations for various suites within the building. Some of this is a factor of the building shell itself, as suites of a certain size might be better accommodated in one location than another. Apart from that consideration, however, high-volume suites are best located, if not on the ground floor, then at least near the elevator, to limit foot traffic down the corridor.

Radiology, due to the weight of the equipment, would usually be found on the ground floor and, for ease of access, so would the clinical lab. Specialties such as general practice or internal medicine, which use radiology and lab services a great deal, would wisely be located adjacent to those suites. Low-volume specialties such as plastic surgery, neurology, or cardiac surgery might be located on upper floors, perhaps in a corner suite.

For corner suites, one would not locate a 1500-square-foot tenant in a choice corner. These suites should be saved to use as an inducement to woo a prime tenant. Remember, however, when a suite is located across the end of a building, if the suite is of sufficient size to require two exits, there will have to be a separation between them. This is sometimes difficult to achieve at the end of a building.

Another issue to think about when laying out suites on a floor and taking into account the tenant's preference for location is that it is important to not leave any "holes" or unleasable size spaces between suites. In order to avoid this, tenants cannot always be located exactly where they would wish to be. This is where the space planner's skill as a mediator comes into play.

The first tenants to express interest in a new medical building are often radiology, clinical lab, and pharmacy, but they are often the last actually to confirm a lease since they depend on the other tenants for their livelihood. If the building is only 50 percent leased upon completion and these tenants have to move in, they will suffer. Furthermore, they will want to know, in advance of signing a lease, who the major tenants are, so that they can project whether the composition of the building will net enough revenue for them. A fully equipped radiology suite represents an investment of several million dollars in equipment and construction costs. Such equipment is not easily relocated. Understandably, such tenants want very specific information on the other tenants in the building before committing to a lease.

HOSPITAL-BASED MOBs

Medical office buildings that are adjacent to and affiliated with hospitals have very special needs that will be touched on only briefly in this discussion. The major consideration lies in the interface with the hospital. Will the hospital actually be occupying space in the MOB? If so, and if inpatients have access to these facilities, the MOB may be subject to more stringent standards and codes, thereby greatly increasing construction costs.

If the MOB is to be physically connected to the hospital, great thought must be given to the configuration of each floor with regard to stairwells, elevators, and point of entry to the hospital, so that future expansion is not hampered, and circulation between the hospital and the MOB is efficient. One disadvantage to physicians in a hospital-affiliated MOB is that sometimes the hospital imposes limitations upon individual tenants whose services or practices are likely to compete with hospital departments. This is particularly true of diagnostic radiology, clinical lab, physical therapy, and pharmacy services.

Hospitals benefit by having on-campus MOBs to provide a core group of admitting physicians who are loyal to the hospital. This also increases utilization of the hospital's ancillary services.

CHAPTER 3

The Practice of Medicine: Primary Care

The field of medicine is continually expanding as new knowledge and concepts are put into practice. But at the base level of the health care delivery system, we begin with the primary fields of medicine: General Practice, Pediatrics, Family Practice, and Internal Medicine. Physicians in these areas are responsible for the total health care needs of their patients. They are termed "primary" medical specialties because they are normally the entry-level physician one would consult about a medical problem.

If the problem requires a specialist, the general practitioner or internist will then refer the patient to a specialist — perhaps to a urologist, a neurologist, orthopedist, or allergist. There are certain obvious exceptions to this primary care referral system. People frequently consult allergists, plastic surgeons, dermatologists, obstetricians and gynecologists, or orthopedists on their own if they feel certain they have a problem that falls into that specialist's domain.

While a primary physician may refer patients to a specialist to consult on a special problem, he or she will be in contact with the specialist and will retain overall responsibility for the patient's care. This provides for continuity of care — one physician who records a continuing health history for a patient and who oversees and coordinates total health care over a period of years. This is particularly important for patients with long-term disabilities such as diabetes, heart disease, or hypertension.

A general practitioner is a doctor who, having completed medical school and an internship, began his or her medical practice. A G.P. gains a broad general knowledge through experience that enables him or her to treat most medical disorders encountered by his or her patients. Doctors in family practice, a relatively new medical specialty, have had at least three years' training and service in all major areas of medicine such as surgery, obstetrics and gynecology, pediatrics, internal medicine, and psychiatry. For the purpose of space planning, the needs of general practice and family practice physicians are identical.

GENERAL PRACTICE

The individual rooms that compose this suite, with modifications, form the specialized suites to be discussed in future chapters. Together, these rooms constitute the basic medical suite.

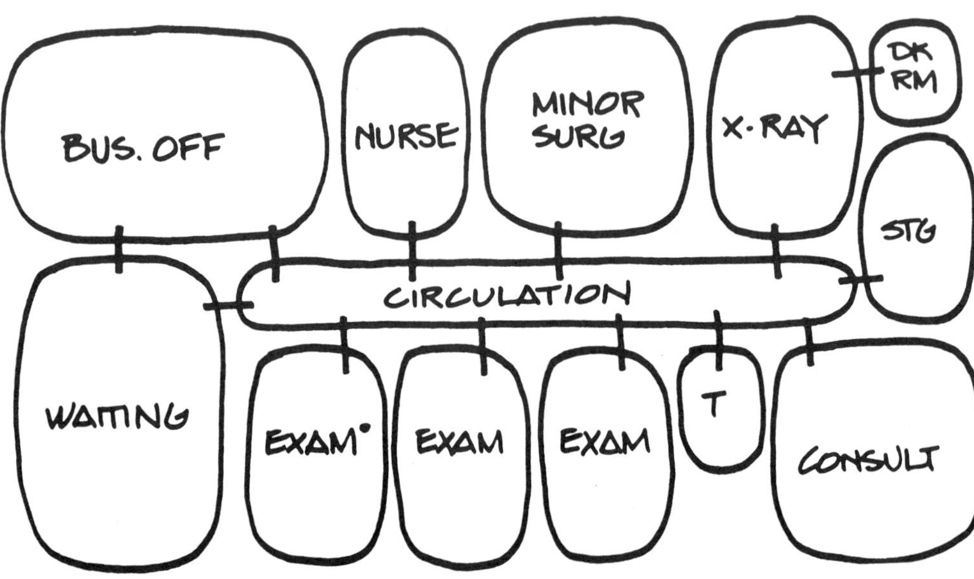

Figure 3-1. Schematic diagram of a general practice suite.

Therefore the philosophy behind the design of these individual rooms (waiting room, business office, exam room, consultation room, nurse station) will be discussed in depth in this chapter.

The Functions of a Medical Suite

1. Administrative
   A. Waiting and Reception
   B. Business (Appointments, Bookkeeping, Insurance, Clerical)
   C. Medical Records
2. Patient Care
   A. Examination
   B. Treatment/Minor Surgery
   C. Consultation
3. Support Services
   A. Nurse Station/Laboratory
   B. X-ray, Darkroom
   C. Storage
   D. Staff Lounge

The schematic diagram (Figure 3-1) shows the relationship of rooms. The patient enters the waiting room, checks in with the receptionist via a communicating window between the business office and waiting room, and takes a seat in the waiting room. Since most medical offices require advance appointments (as opposed to walk-ins), the nurse will have pulled the patient's medical record prior to the patient entering the office.

Later, a nurse or assistant calls the patient to the examination area. Usually the nurse or assistant will then weigh the patient, sometimes take a urine sample, record blood pressure, and take a short history. This is done either at the nurse station or in the exam room. The nurse may also record the patient's temperature.

In the exam room, the nurse or aide prepares the patient for the examination and arranges the instruments the physician will need. The doctor enters the room, washes hands, chats with the patient about symptoms, makes notes in the patient's chart, and proceeds to examine the patient, often with a nurse or assistant in attendance. After examination, the patient is asked to dress and meet the physician in the consultation room, where a diagnosis and recommended treatment are discussed. The patient leaves the office, passing an appointment desk or window where future appointments may be booked and where payment for services may be made or arranged.

Obvious deviations to the above may occur when, for example, a patient breaks a limb. In this case, a patient may be sent to an X-ray room first, and then proceed to a minor surgery room to have a cast applied without ever entering an exam room. In high-volume practices, it slows down the physician to have to return repeatedly to a consultation room with each patient, so the doctor usually diagnoses and prescribes right in the exam room. With this brief outline, we shall turn to a detailed analysis of each area.

Waiting Room

The waiting room is the patient's introduction to a physician or dentist. One forms a first impression of the practitioner by the image projected in the waiting room. This is where psychology plays a significant role. Outdated furniture with torn and faded upholstery may simply be the result of a doctor's busy schedule or his or her reluctance to focus on it as an important aspect of patient care.

But, whatever the actual reason, such a neglected waiting room conveys to a patient that this is a doctor who may be as outdated in his or her medical studies and technology as the waiting room shows. The neglect of the waiting room generalizes to other areas,

Table 3-1. Analysis of Program. General Practice

No. of Physicians:	1	2	3
Consultation	12 × 12 = 144	2 @ 12 × 12 = 288	3 @ 12 × 12 = 432
Exam Rooms	3 @ 8 × 12 = 288	6 @ 8 × 12 = 576	9 @ 8 × 12 = 864
Waiting Room	12 × 14 = 168	14 × 18 = 252	20 × 24 = 480
Business Office	12 × 14 = 168	14 × 16 = 224	18 × 30 = 540[a]
Nurse Station	8 × 10 = 80	10 × 12 = 120	12 × 12 = 144
Toilets	2 @ 5 × 6 = 60	2 @ 5 × 6 = 60	3 @ 5 × 6 = 90
Storage	4 × 6 = 24	6 × 8 = 48	8 × 10 = 80
Cast Room	Use Minor Surgery	Use Minor Surgery	12 × 12 = 144
EKG	Use Minor Surgery	Use Minor Surgery	8 × 12 = 96
Staff Lounge	—	8 × 12 = 96	10 × 12 = 120
Minor Surgery	12 × 12 = 144	12 × 12 = 144	12 × 12 = 144
X-ray Area[b]	—	12 × 20 = 240	12 × 20 = 240
Laboratory	—	8 × 10 = 80	16 × 16 = 256[c]
Subtotal	1076 ft^2	2128 ft^2	3630 ft^2
15% Circulation	161	319	545
Total	1237 ft^2	2447 ft^2	4175 ft^2

[a]Includes insurance clerk, bookkeeper, and office manager.

[b]Includes darkroom, control, film filing, and dressing area.

[c]Includes lab, waiting, and blood draw.

and patients tend to feel that this is a physician who might be neglectful in their care — one who manages to slide along with minimum standards. Designing the waiting room as a comfortable, cheerful space with appealing colors, soft lighting, and attractive furnishings is paramount (Color Plate 1, Figure 3-2). These items are discussed in greater detail in Chapter 12.

In addition to the psychological aspects of the waiting room design, it must above all be functional. Unless the office is located in a warm climate, the waiting room should include a secure space for hanging coats and stashing boots and umbrellas.

A patient must be able to enter the room and proceed directly to the receptionist's window without tripping over people or furniture. After checking in, the patient should be able to select a magazine from a conveniently located rack, and find a seat. When called, the seated patient should be able to move quickly into the examination area without disturbing other patients. Should the patient be handicapped, traffic aisles must be wide enough to accommodate a wheelchair, and there must be an open space in the room where the person in a wheelchair can comfortably remain, without clogging the traffic flow. The handicapped do not like to be made to feel they are a burden to the nonhandicapped population. They prefer to be independent, and they must be considered in the planning stages of a project so their needs and rights to access can be humanely and sympathetically handled.

The size of the waiting room can be determined after interviewing the physician and staff (see Appendix for client interview form). The composition of the doctor's patient population and his or her work habits will dictate parameters the designer must follow. Common sense dictates that a physician who sees people without advance appointments will need a much larger waiting room than one who follows an appointment schedule.

Low-volume practices such as surgical specialties or psychiatry require smaller waiting rooms than do high-volume specialties such as general practice, orthopedics, pediatrics, internal medicine, and OB-GYN. In addition, practices that accommodate a large number of emergencies need a larger waiting room. Accident cases will frequently be brought through the staff private entrance to avoid parading what might be a gory sight through the waiting room. The larger the patient volume, the larger the waiting room needs to be. A convenient formula for determining the number of seats follows.

$$2P \times D - E = S \qquad \frac{2P \times D}{2} = L$$

Where

P = Average number of patients per hour (per physician)

D = Number of doctors

E = Number of exam rooms

S = Seating

L = Late factor

The waiting room must accommodate at least one hour's patients. If each doctor sees an average of four patients per hour, and each G.P. has three examining rooms, and it is assumed that each patient is accompanied by one friend or relative, a solo practitioner would require five seats in the waiting room:

$$2(4) \times 1 - 3 = 5$$

Because this is a one-physician practice, it would be wise to assume that the doctor will run half an hour late, so the waiting room must accommodate one and one-half hour's patients. This expansion factor can be expressed as:

$$\frac{2P \times D}{2} = L \qquad \frac{2(4) \times 1}{2} = 4$$

Thus the waiting room should accommodate $S + L$, or nine persons, plus an area for children, if space permits. The late factor can generally be reduced as the number of physicians is increased. It is important to understand that these formulas are only a guide. The specifics of each practice and space limitations of the suite will often dictate waiting room capacity. The formula, and good common sense, may tell you that ideally 45 seats should be provided, but the physical limitations of the space and the physicians' intent to squeeze in as many exam rooms as possible may limit seating capacity to 25.

In medical space planning, as in life, rarely does the ideal prevail. The designer has to skillfully juggle the client's requests, the client's budget, building codes, structural limitations of the given space, and the principles of medical space planning. Tradeoffs and compromises are the reality from which suites are built.

Once the number of waiting room seats has been estimated, the size of the room can be determined, allowing 15 to 20 square feet per person. The author has found 18 square feet per person a workable guide for the average medical office. Nevertheless, the amount of space required for a comfortable waiting room will vary according to the room's configuration, the location of the entry foyer, and the reception window.

An area may be provided for children (Color Plate 1, Figure 3-3). A table and chairs or a toy box is welcomed by parents. Special furniture can be fabricated (see Pediatrics), which will keep children occupied, quiet, and out of danger of being stepped on. Keep in mind that a children's corner must be located away from door swings or other hazards on which children might injure themselves. The children's area must be in sight of the receptionist, who is charged with keeping order.

A large aquarium (Figure 3-4) is a nice addition to a waiting room. It is restful and enjoyed by adults and children alike.

Some physicians prefer maximum communication between front office staff and patients and favor a waiting room separated from the business office by only a low partition. Although this may comfort the patient

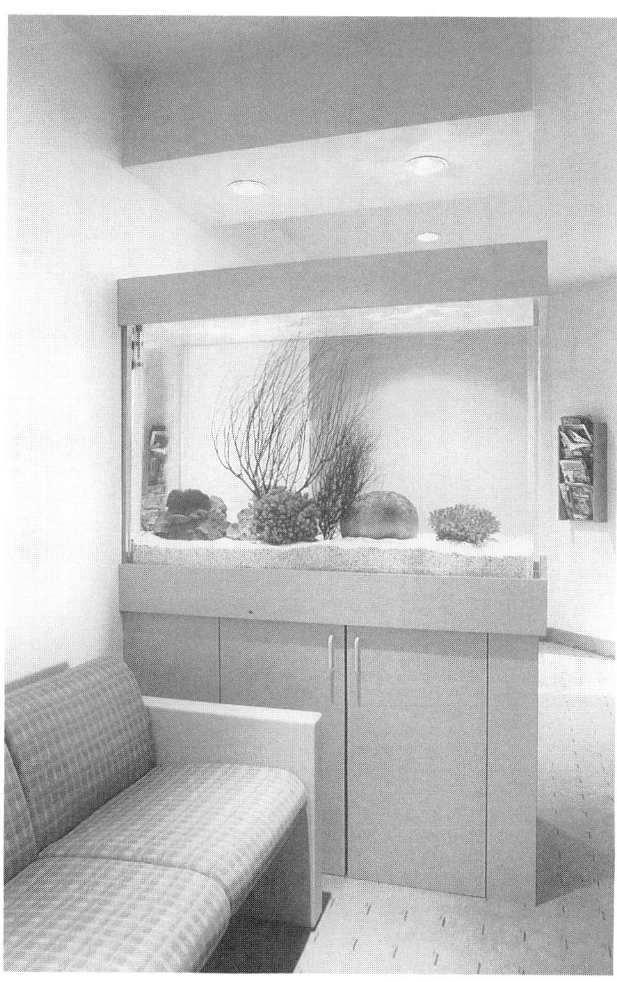

Figure 3-4. Aquarium adds interest to waiting room.
(Design: Jain Malkin Inc.; Photographer: John Christian.)

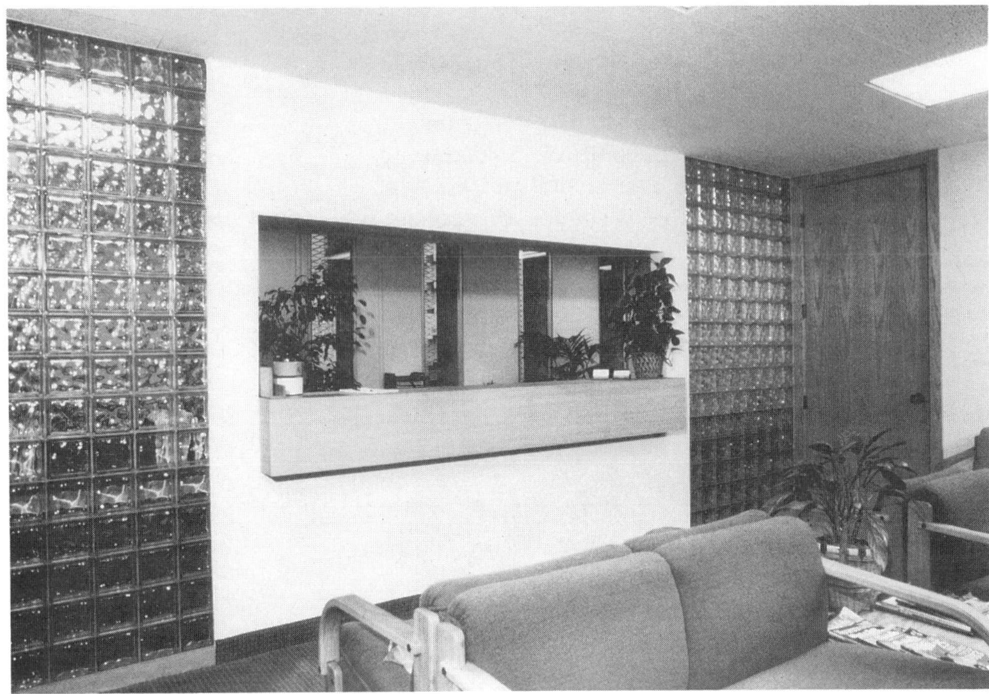

Figure 3-5a. Reception window, internal medicine suite. *(Design: Jain Malkin Inc.; Photographer: Jain Malkin.)*

psychologically, it often results in a loss of privacy for staff, who frequently have to discuss delicate matters with a patient. The patient might suffer embarrassment, knowing that the adjacent waiting patients may overhear the conversation.

For this reason, many offices use a 4- to 6-foot-wide window with a plastic laminate shelf, starting at 42 inches off the floor (Figures 3-5*a* and 3-5*b*). A sliding glass window may be added for additional staff privacy, but it does convey a negative image of closing out the patients. (If glass is used, it should always be clear, not obscure, so that patients have visual contact with staff.)

To deal effectively with these issues when designing the waiting room, do not place chairs too close to the reception window; position the receptionist's telephone to the side of the window opening to help mask conversations, and provide an area, in the front office, where staff and patients may discuss a sensitive topic without it being overheard.

There is disagreement as to the practicality of providing a toilet room in the waiting area. It saves staff the trouble of frequently directing patients into the bathroom of the examination area, but it has the disadvantage of patients emptying their bladders before the nurse can request a urine specimen. In pediatric offices, however, a toilet in the reception area is desirable to enable mothers to change a baby's diaper.

Reception

Since the receptionist maintains the appointment book, she must see the patient on arrival and just before leaving. She must also have a good view of the waiting room from her seat so that she can see who is waiting (Figure 3-6). The appointment book is usually quite large, particularly when open. Thus she needs approximately 6 lineal feet of countertop work surface located in front of the reception window with a recess for a typewriter, a place for the phone and to write messages, a place for the appointment book, and if possible, an L-shaped return facing the corridor appointment "good-bye" window so that while remaining seated, she can swivel around, greet an exiting patient, book an appointment, or accept payment for services (Figure 3-7).

In an office with two or three front office staff, the appointments/cashier station and reception window may be separated (Figures 3-7*a* and 3-8) to provide greater privacy for the exiting patient.

Front office personnel may also help in the back office, assisting the doctor in the examining room at times, weighing patients, or recording histories, but usually their duties will be confined to the business office.

It is desirable to design the business office in such a way that staff can easily cover one another's station. An efficient layout can sometimes mean that one fewer person is required, considerably reducing the overhead.

Patient Education

Patient education is an important part of health care, which most physicians try to accommodate in their suite design. It is generally located at the front of the suite, and may even be an alcove off the waiting room. For reasons of privacy, however, it is advisable to create a room, perhaps 8 × 10 feet, and build carrels or partitions between patients.

A 30-inch high countertop would have a small television monitor, and a VCR would be housed in an open compartment underneath (see Figure 4-105). Shallow cabinets provide storage space for videotapes. Tapes cover all sorts of topics: presurgical instructions, information about various diseases or injuries, ways to

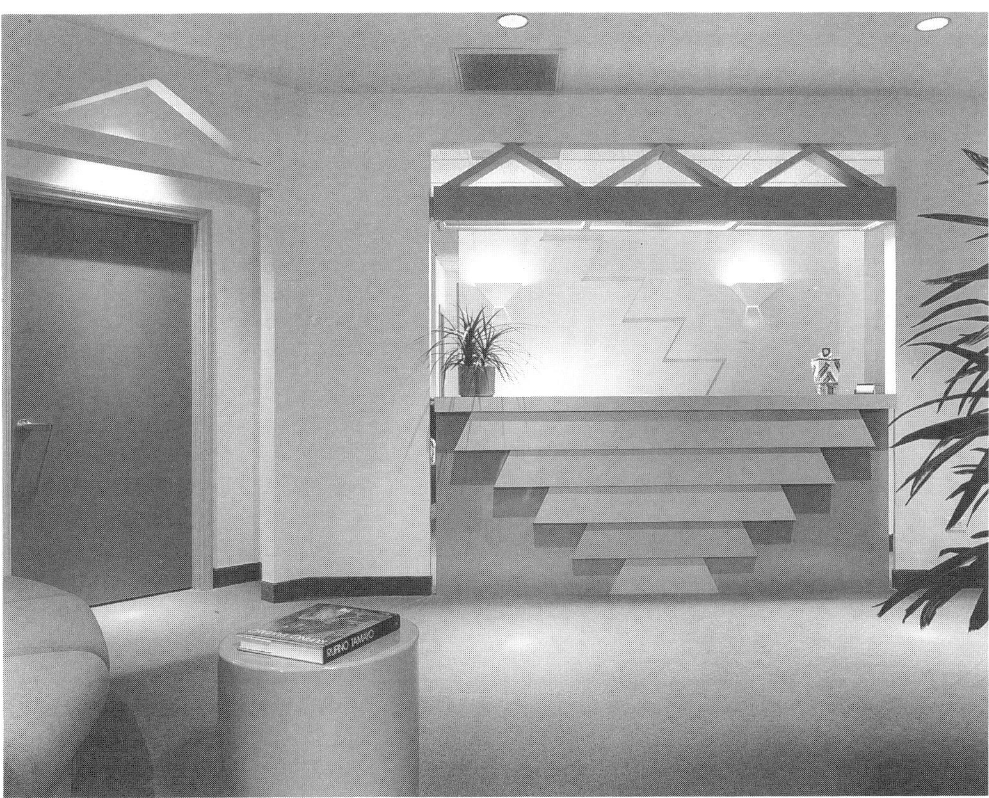

Figure 3-5b. Reception window, women's health center. (*Design: Jain Malkin Inc.; Photographer: Kim Brun.*)

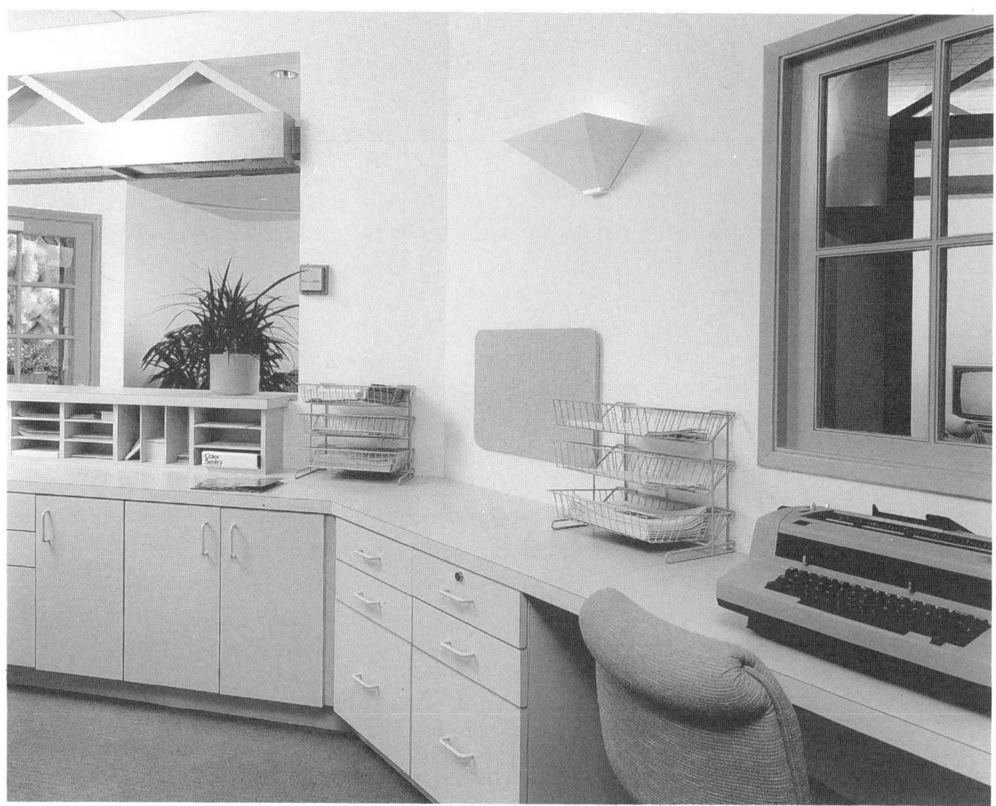

Figure 3-6. Business office, reception area. (*Design: Jain Malkin Inc.; Photographer: Kim Brun.*)

lower health risks, and they may even allow a patient to view his or her own surgery. The use of videotapes allows the doctor to communicate a great deal of information, in a professional manner, without having to explain each concept or procedure personally.

Business Office

Frequently referred to as the *front office* in medical jargon (versus the *back office* or examination area), this is the heart of the medical office. Appointments are scheduled here; patients are billed; medical records are stored here; patients are greeted from this room; and routine insurance and bookkeeping duties are performed here.

In a small practice, one or two people may perform all these tasks. In a large practice, three or more persons may occupy the business office. A convenient rule of thumb is one secretary for each two doctors in a low-volume practice and one secretary per physician in a high-volume practice. If a physician is seeing four to five patients per hour, the secretary may be spending more time with patients than the doctor does, since her work would involve arranging and rescheduling patient appointments on the telephone whenever the doctor is delayed or has to rearrange his or her daily schedule, filing medical charts, typing reports to referring physicians, billing patients, collecting money, filling out insurance forms, answering the phone, and ordering supplies.

A convenience in the business office is a gate door (just the lower portion) or a Dutch door (two halves that operate independently). In either case, the lower half of the door should have a 42-inch high shelf on it. This permits communication with patients as they are exiting the office and suffices for brief greetings or a routine discussion about a bill without the patient having to enter the bookkeeper's or the business office.

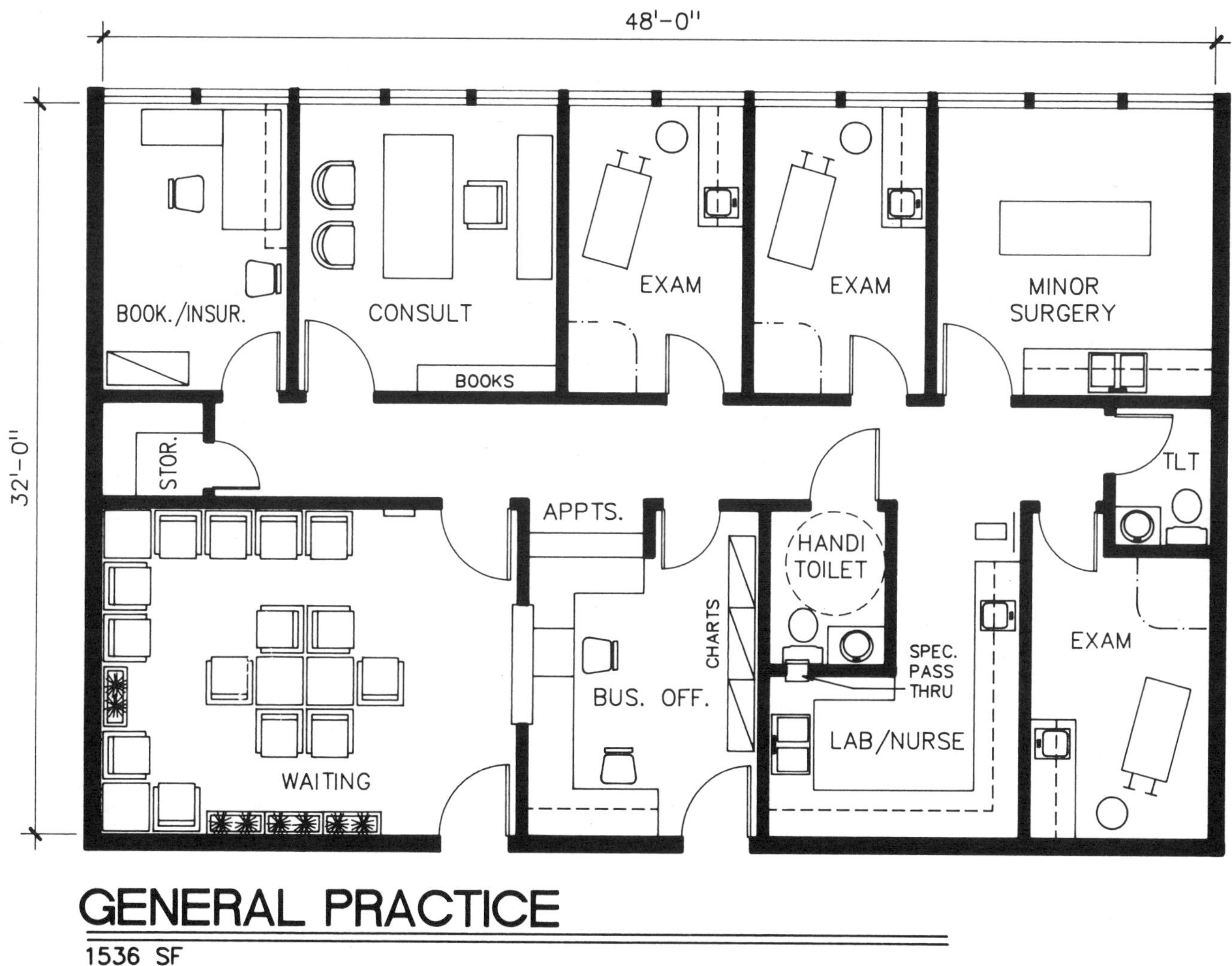

Figure 3-7. Suite plan for general practice, 1536 square feet.

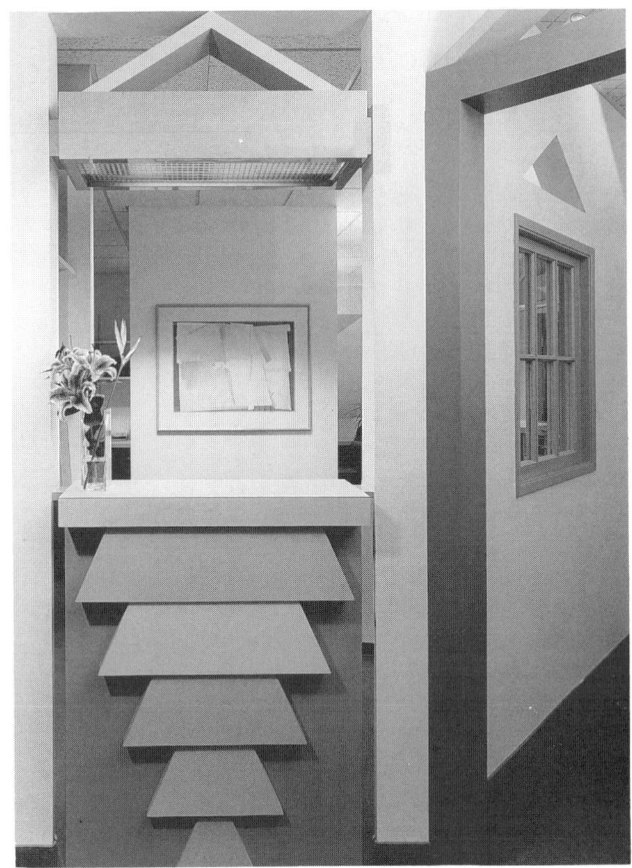

Figure 3-7a. Cashier/appointments window, women's clinic. (*Design: Jain Malkin Inc.; Photographer: Kim Brun.*)

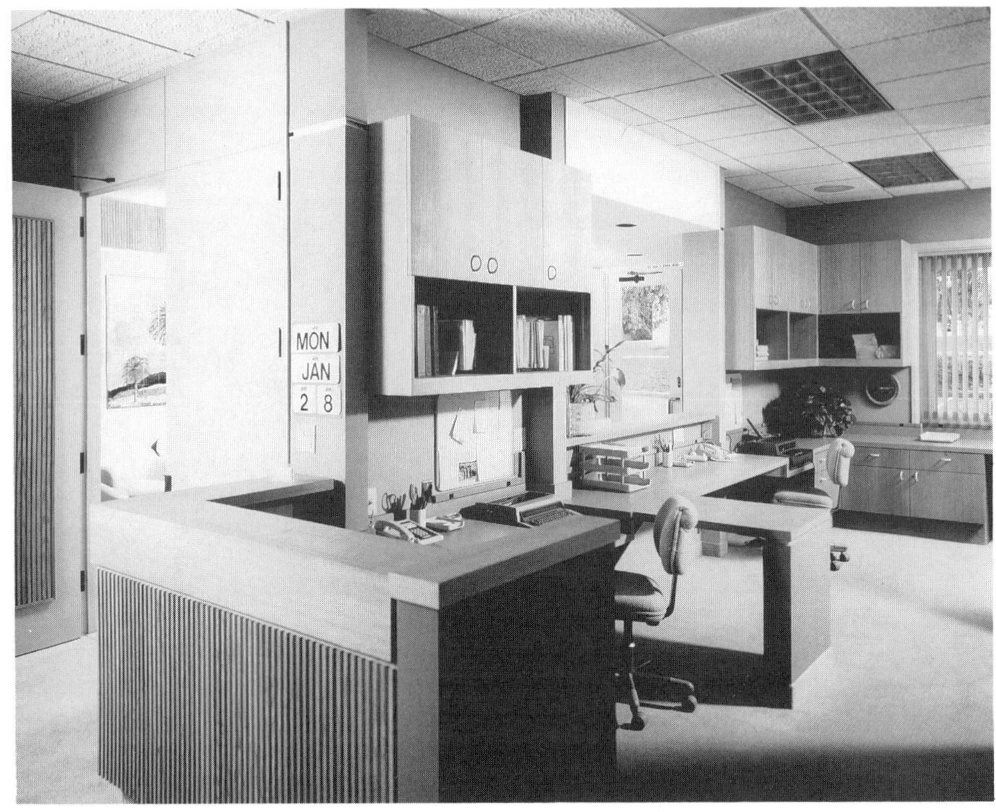

Figure 3-8. Business office, cashier/appointments desk. (*Photo courtesy: Jain Malkin Inc.; Photographer: Michael Denny.*)

The shelf on the gate door serves several purposes. It can be a convenient place to rest one's elbows when chatting; one can use it to write a check; or medical charts can be passed back and forth over it. Sometimes a box or container might be fastened to the shelf in which medical charts for patients who have already been seen might be placed for refiling.

Depending upon the width of the corridor (standard corridor width is 48 inches clear), the Dutch or gate door might be located in a recess or alcove so that a patient who stops to chat will not be blocking corridor traffic. However, for longer conversations and more privacy, the patient would enter through that door and proceed to the bookkeeper's office. A guest chair should be provided in the bookkeeper's office for this purpose.

Bookkeeping

Computer Systems. Today, many medical and dental offices are computerized. Some offices use computers only for word processing and for billing. Others use computers to link their offices with the hospital and with support services such as a laboratory or radiology group. This enables a doctor to pre-admit a patient to the hospital, book radiology procedures, or schedule surgery, and receive an immediate reply.

Practitioners with a totally computerized office will have sophisticated software that handles appointment scheduling, patient accounting, patient histories, patient and insurance billing, revenue projections, collection letters, referring physician reports, patient medication data reports, statements, and insurance claims tracking. With an integrated software system, patient data can be tabulated to produce a variety of reports that allow the practitioner to analyze the practice. These may include cross-referencing of diagnoses and procedures, and demographic analysis of marketing efforts (Figure 3-9).

Since computer systems vary considerably in size and number of components, the designer must study the specific system the client plans to use before determining the space to be allotted and the relationship of personnel and machines. Basically, computers are either micro, mini, or mainframe, in size. Personal computers are "micro," with the computer generally sitting on the countertop with the VDT (video display terminal) above (Figure 3-10). The keyboard is off to one side or may be on a narrow slide-out shelf under the countertop. This has the advantage of lowering the keyboard to a standard typing height.

Minicomputers are larger than micros and sit on the floor under or alongside of the desk (Figure 3-11). In this case, the VDT sits directly on the countertop or may be mounted on an adjustable arm. Mainframes come in a variety of sizes generally starting with the size of a large, floor-model copy machine (Figure 3-12). These are usually placed in a small dedicated room with individually controlled air conditioning. A raised floor for access to cables may be required. One mainframe can link or network many remote terminals.

Regardless of brand or system, there are always these items: a computer, a printer (Figure 3-13), and one or more video display terminals. Data is input to and accessed from the computer via the keyboard. There is also a need for storage of computer printouts, computer paper, floppy disks, and other magnetic media. The printer may sit on a countertop or on its own stand, and it may be connected to several computers.

It is important to be aware of the effects of glare from overhead lighting and from windows when laying out workstations using VDTs. Glare causes reflections on the screen that lead to eye strain and stress.

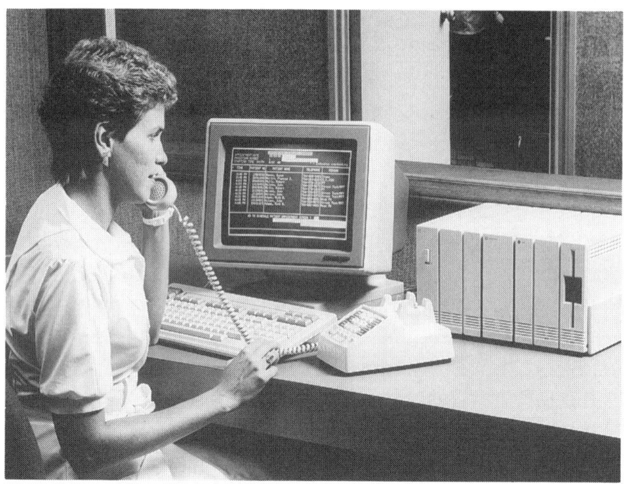

Figure 3-9. Total Practice Management Solution (TPMS) System. (*Courtesy UNISYS, Charlotte, NC.*)

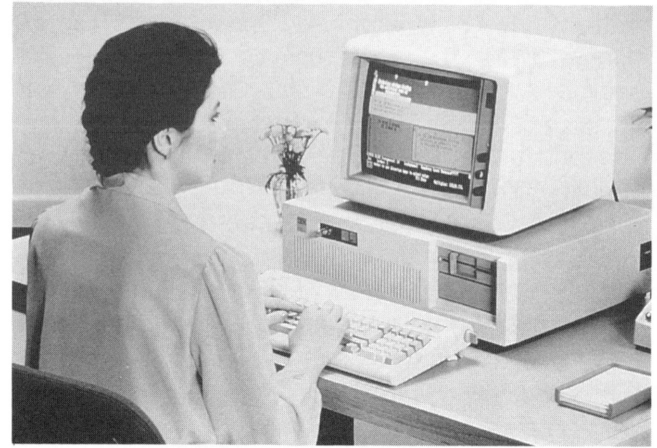

Figure 3-10. Desktop personal computer. (*Courtesy IBM Corp., White Plains, NY.*)

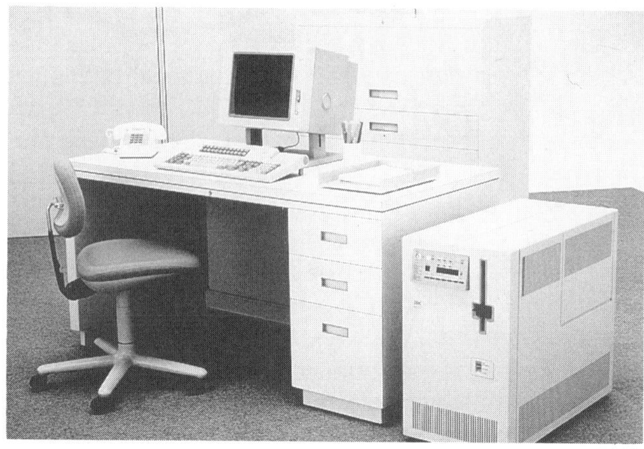

Figure 3-11. Workstation with computer alongside desk. (*Courtesy IBM Corp., White Plains, NY.*)

Traditional Methods. While computers are indispensable for data management, many offices still use more traditional methods of bookkeeping, and it's important for the designer to be familiar with them.

Some offices record charges and payments on patient ledger cards. Once a month the bookkeeper sends out statements. The workstation requires a lowered countertop area (or floor space if on mobile carts) for the ledger card files, which are approximately 12 inches tall and are clamped into a metal holder that permits them to move in a fanlike manner, forward or back (Figure 3-14).

These ledger files can also be kept on a mobile cart, which is moved up to the desk as needed. A flat countertop work surface is needed for the daily journal and for equipment having to do with posting charges, copying, and mailing statements. Note that ample electrical outlets are required for these office machines and for a typewriter and calculator as well.

A time-saving and widely used method of billing is the pegboard system. It is particularly well suited to the

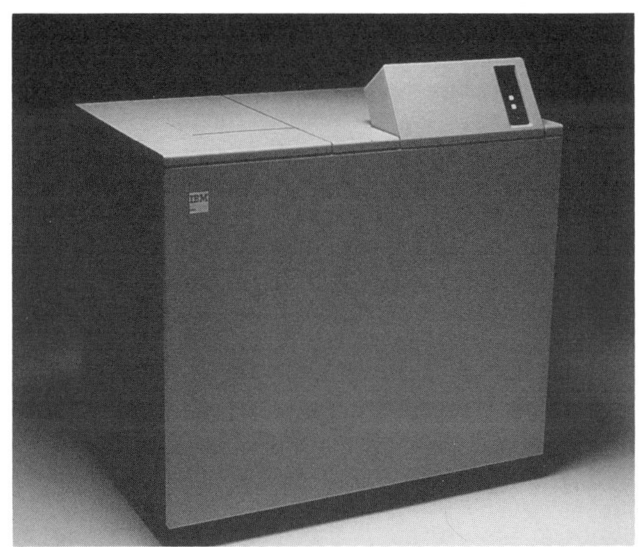

Figure 3-12. Mainframe computer. (*Courtesy IBM Corp., White Plains, NY.*)

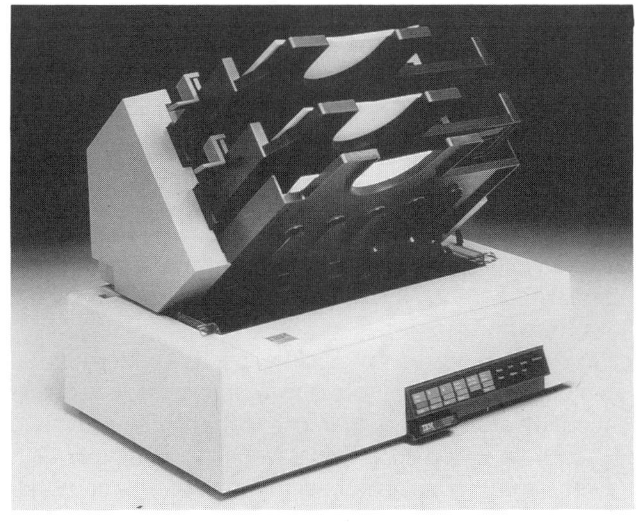

Figure 3-13. Printer. (*Courtesy IBM Corp., White Plains, NY.*)

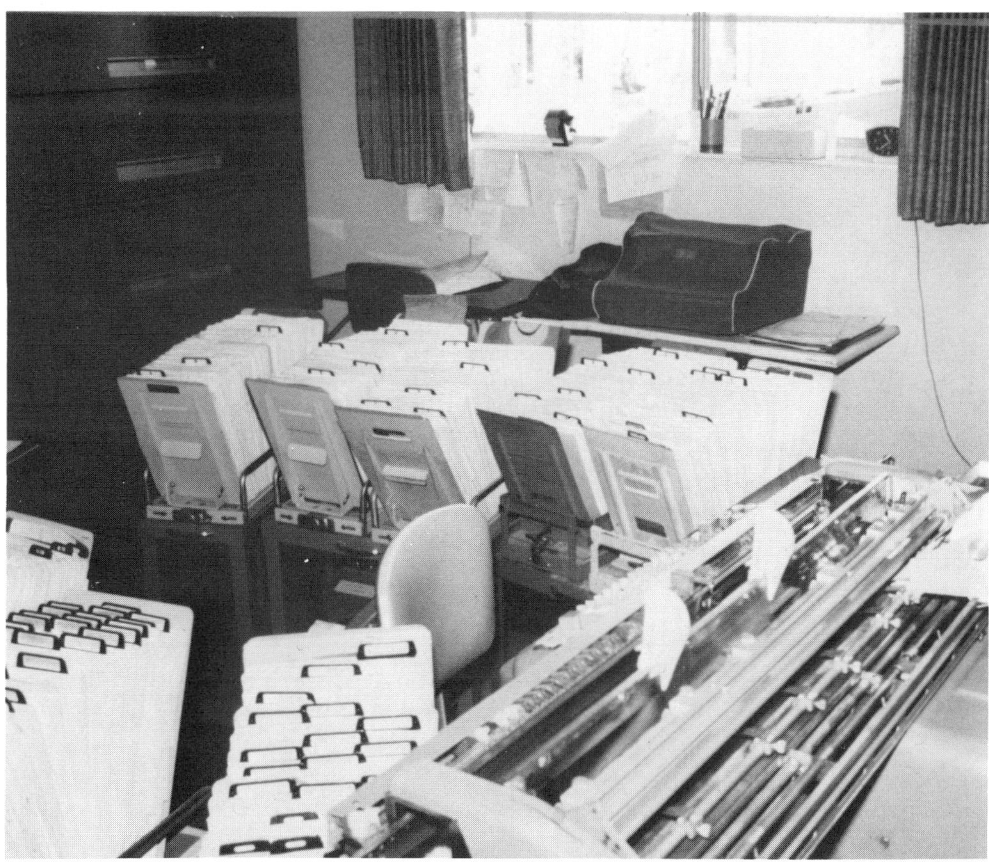

Figure 3-14. Ledger files. (*Photographer: Jain Malkin.*)

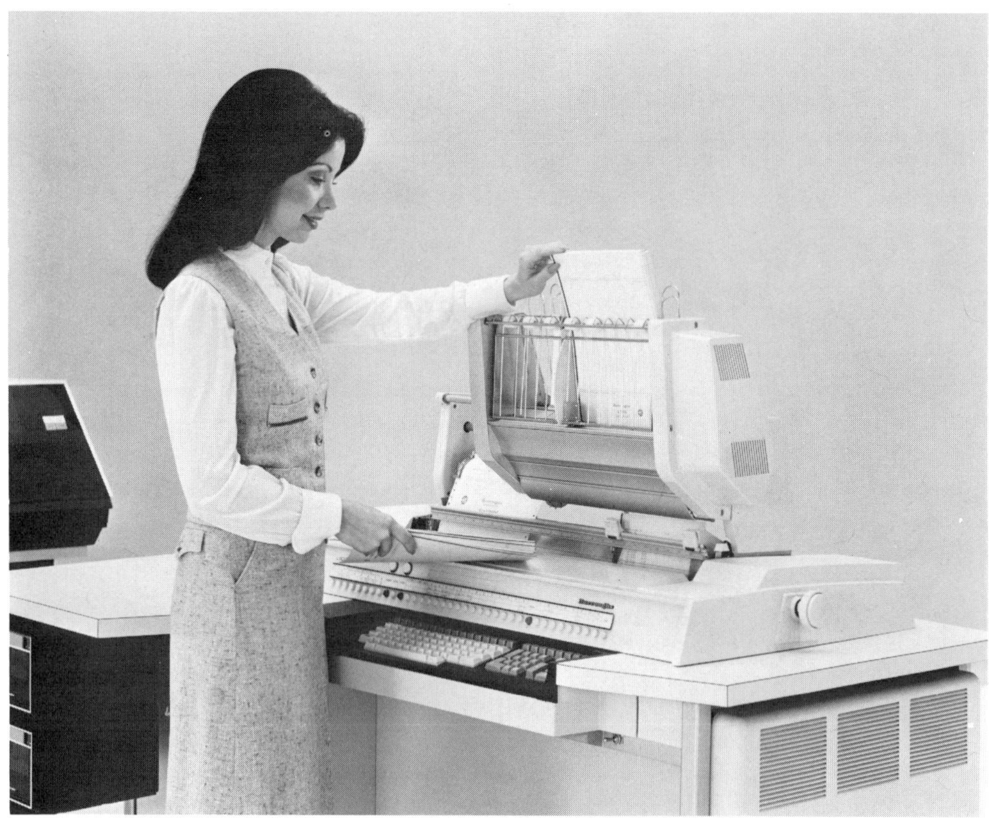

Figure 3-15. Computerized bookkeeping machine. (*Courtesy Burroughs Corp.*)

small office. The pegboard is a hard covered binder with pegs along one side, upon which one aligns a statement, ledger card, and daily journal sheet. Since the forms have carbon backing, one entry for each transaction reproduces on all forms. There are combinations of pegboard and photocopy billing. Medium-volume practices, which send more than 500 statements per month, may post and bill by a computerized bookkeeping machine that uses ledger cards (Figure 3-15).

Practices that do not have computers may use a combination of old-style posting machine and photocopy. If the machine posts one entry per minute, and it takes another minute to photocopy the ledger sheet for use as a statement (eliminating the need to address the statements each month), then one bookkeeper can prepare approximately 200 statements per day, or 4000 per month. An envelope stuffer and postage meter can further increase output.

Some practices use an outside bookkeeping service. The daily charges for service and payments received are recorded in a log and forwarded to the service, which transfers the information to a journal and mails the statements. These bookkeeping services use a computer to process the work for their clients. A monthly computer statement of all transactions would then be sent to the physician. These large computer printouts do not fit on standard 12-inch-deep shelves. The designer must provide space for these and determine whether they are to fit in large binders, on a shelf, or to hang.

In many offices, the bookkeeper is in a separate room adjacent to, but not part of, the business office/reception area. The insurance secretary may also have a separate office to provide working conditions with fewer interruptions. The designer must remember that the business office of a busy practice is an extremely hectic place. Phones ring continually; people are rushing around. It is not a good place for people who work with figures. If space permits, it is always better to protect the bookkeeper and insurance secretary by giving them separate offices. Sometimes, a space-saving pod of workstations (Figure 3-16) is used to provide privacy when private offices are not feasible.

The physician may wish to have a safe for storage of cash and the ledger files. Most medical offices take in little cash, so that is not much of a problem, but ledger cards should be locked up each night and put in a fire-resistive safe. Since the cards are stacked so tightly together when in the closed position they offer a good deal of resistance to fire, but a safe should be considered. In addition, most offices have fire extinguishers mounted on the wall where they are easily accessible. The carbon dioxide or dry powder type is preferred.

Insurance

Most medical treatment is paid by third-party payers — the insurance companies. This amounts to a great deal of paperwork, and a medical office of any size usually has a full-time employee doing nothing but insurance forms. He or she requires a desk with a typing return, a calculator, access to medical records, access to the copy machine, and proximity to the patients' ledger cards (if used). File cabinets are needed, as well as open-shelf storage, for a multitude of business forms and stationery. A guest chair should be provided for a patient. As government control increases, more and more procedures are covered by third-party payers, and the personnel required to process these forms has steadily increased.

It should be noted that it is now possible to process claims electronically (paperless) with many of the large insurance companies, providing one has the required computer software.

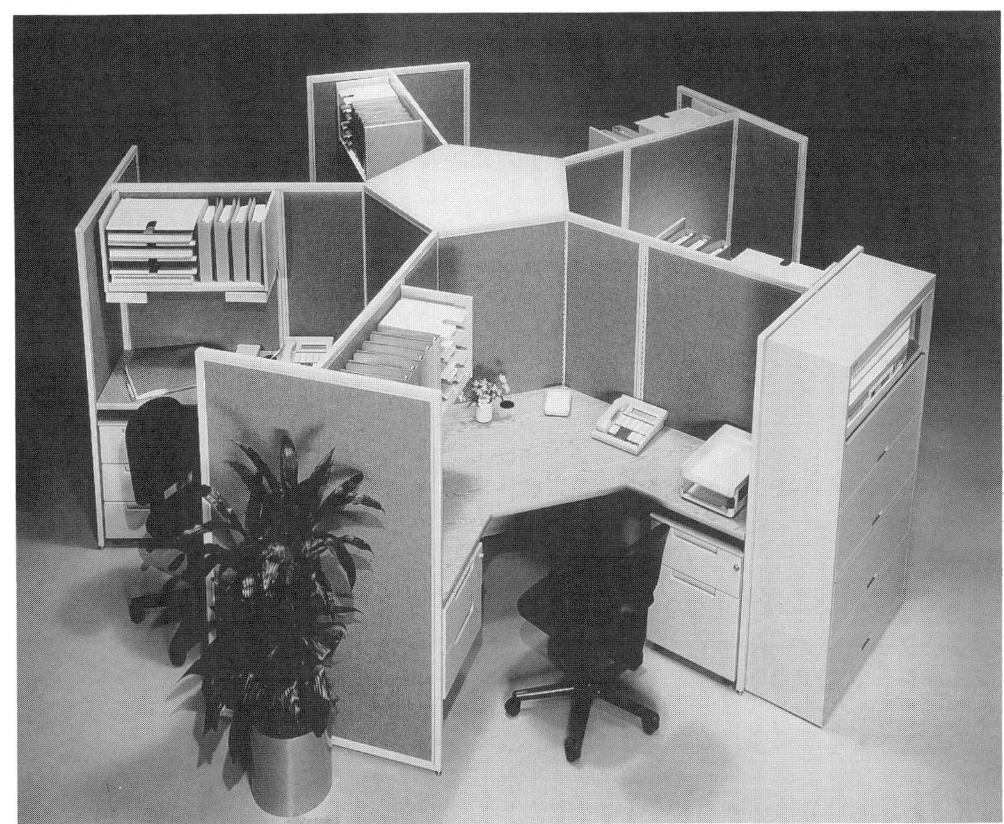

Figure 3-16. *Cluster* workstation. (*Courtesy Tab Products, Palo Alto, CA.*)

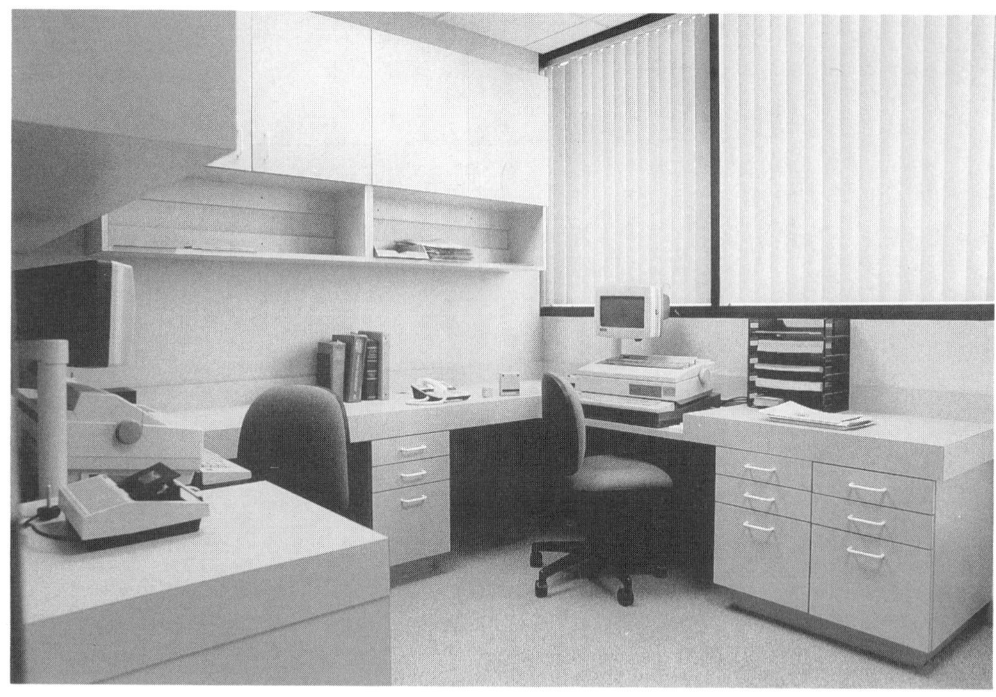

Figure 3-17. Transcription office. (*Design: Jain Malkin Inc.; Photographer: John Christian.*)

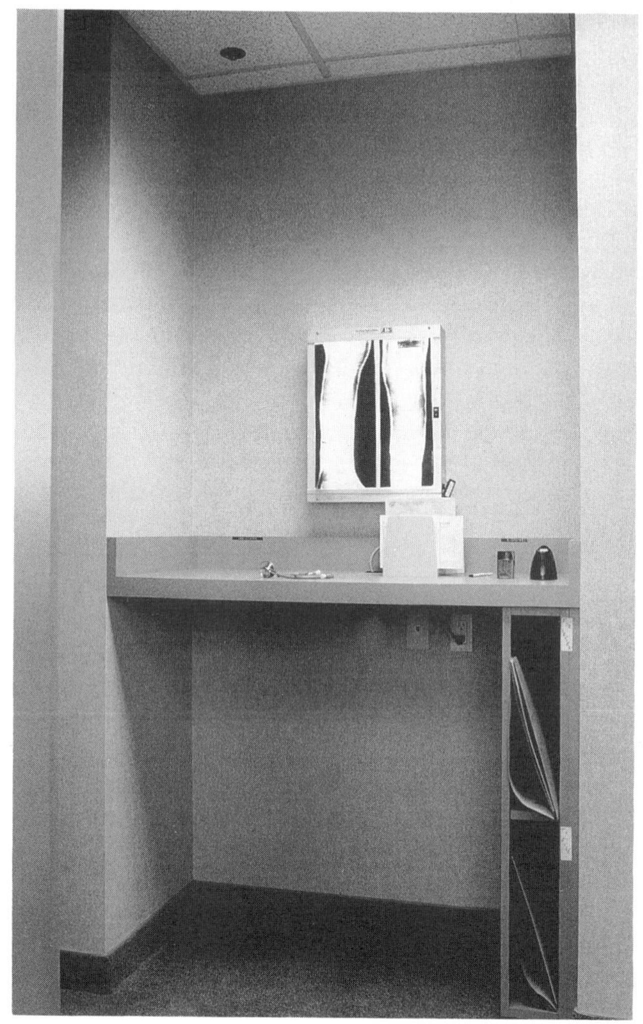

Figure 3-18. Dictation niche. (*Design: Jain Malkin Inc.; Photographer: John Christian.*)

Medical Transcription

Medium-volume to large-volume practices often have a part-time or full-time medical transcriptionist who works from dictation tapes and transcribes the physician's notes. This task is best accommodated in a separate room since the printer (unless it is a laser printer) is noisy. This arrangement also assures less distraction for the typist. Only a countertop work surface is required. It should be at 26-inch height for comfortable typing (Figure 3-17).

Some physicians send their tapes out of the office for transcription, or a physician may have a dictation line to a word processing unit on the telephone. The notes would be recorded, and the typed manuscript would be delivered, to the physician's office. Some medical offices have a dictation niche or kiosk (Figures 3-18 and 13-4) outside each bank of exam rooms so that a physician may dictate notes after examining each patient, rather than at the end of the day.

Dictation

Some physicians like to dictate at a niche in the corridor central to the exam rooms. This is also a good place to locate a wall-mounted telephone so that the doctor can take a quick call without returning to the consultation room. An X-ray view box and an open storage compartment for X-ray films would be essential features for many, but not for all, physicians (Figure 3-18).

Office Manager

Large offices frequently have an office manager or a business manager (Figure 3-19) who hires personnel, orders supplies and drugs, and assists the physicians

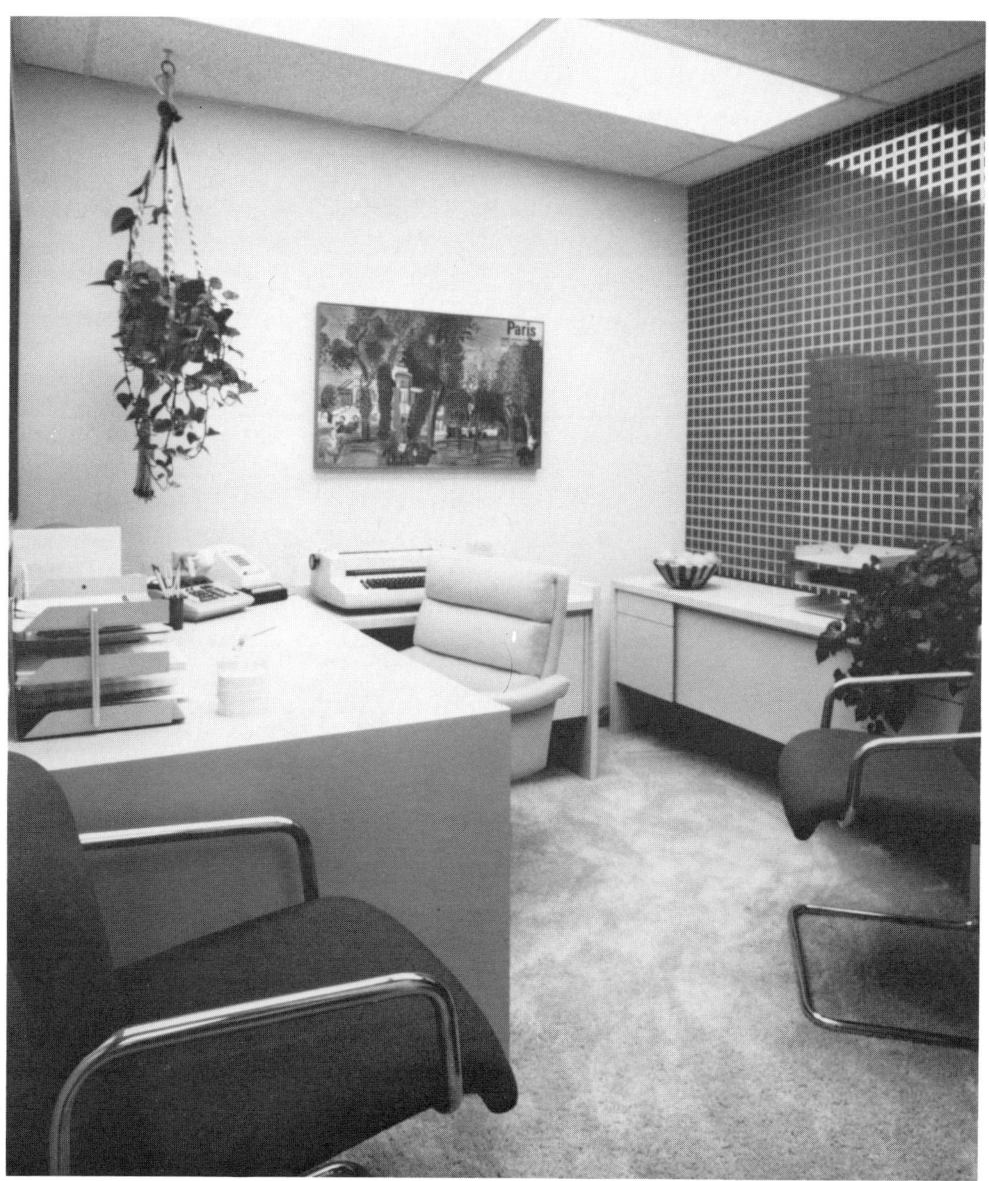

Figure 3-19. Office manager. (*Design: Jain Malkin Inc.; Photographer: Michael Denny.*)

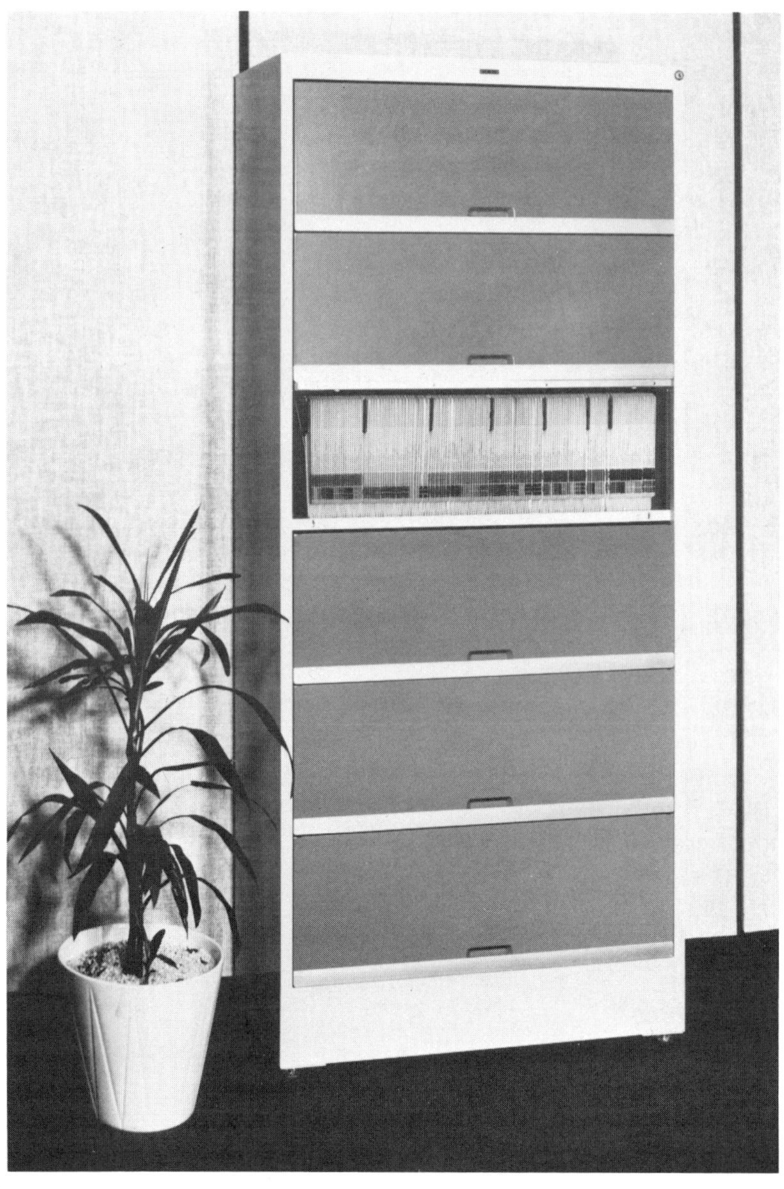

Figure 3-20. Lateral file cabinet. (*Courtesy Tab Products, Palo Alto, CA.*)

in secretarial or business matters in the capacity of executive assistant. The office manager should have a private office. It need not be large — 10 × 10 feet is adequate — and it should be located so that it faces the business office. In fact, the walls facing the business office should have glass, starting 48 inches off the floor, so that the manager can oversee the staff at all times (see Figure 3-51).

Medical Records

An important function of the business office is the storing of medical records. In order to protect the physician from legal complications as well as to provide continuity of care for patients, accurate records must be maintained where they are easy to retrieve. Primary physicians keep more extensive and more detailed records than urologists or radiologists, for example, who see patients on a referral basis.

The preferred method of record storage is the lateral file cabinet (Figure 3-20). This may be a cabinet without doors (Figure 3-21), or with retractable doors that store in the top of each shelf opening. The shelves may be stationary, or they may pull out for easier access. When filing is done laterally, the file folder tab must be on the side so that it sticks out of the file cabinet.

Color-coded file jackets are the most efficient system for medical offices (Figure 3-22). The standard file jacket accepts 8½ × 11 inch papers, but radiology files require jumbo file jackets, which are 14½ × 17½ inches. The patient's name may be encoded alphabetically, by color, and/or number. Thus a misfiled folder immediately becomes obvious, as the colors do not conform to the surrounding file jackets.

Additionally, one can encode by color special features such as the sex of the patient, certain unusual medical disorders, or the date the patient initially sought consultation. This facilitates pruning the files for inactive charts or selecting case studies of patients with various medical disorders for follow-up study. Various companies manufacture these specialized file jackets with the color-coding system. Ames Color-File (Somerville, MA) publishes a particularly good brochure explaining the details and refinements available with this system of medical record storage.

Group practices frequently utilize a large room for medical records with a mechanical retrieval system. This eliminates the need for aisles in front of all shelves, since the files move to the operator, and the access aisle is in front of the operator. This equipment can be purchased with manual controls (Figure 3-23) or motorized controls (Figure 3-24).

It is not necessary to buy factory-fabricated file cabinets. They may be custom-built on the job, particularly if the space allotted to medical chart storage does not accommodate standard file cabinet widths. These job-built file storage units would consist of open shelves with a clear height of 12 inches. However, steel file cabinets have the advantage of being able to be moved to another office, they provide greater fire resistance, and can be locked for security.

Prefabricated file units without retractable doors are less expensive and offer open-shelf easy access to charts (see Figure 3-21). Small-to-medium-sized offices may use space-saving files that are two cabinets deep with the front one sliding on a track (Figure 3-25).

It is important for the designer to project the physician's future needs for medical chart storage in the new office. The designer must ascertain, from the client interview, the number of new patients added to the practice each week or month. That number would be projected for three to five years (the length of most medical leases) and added to the existing number of medical charts. Charts should be pruned each year to eliminate patients who have not been seen in three years. These "aged" charts can be placed in storage

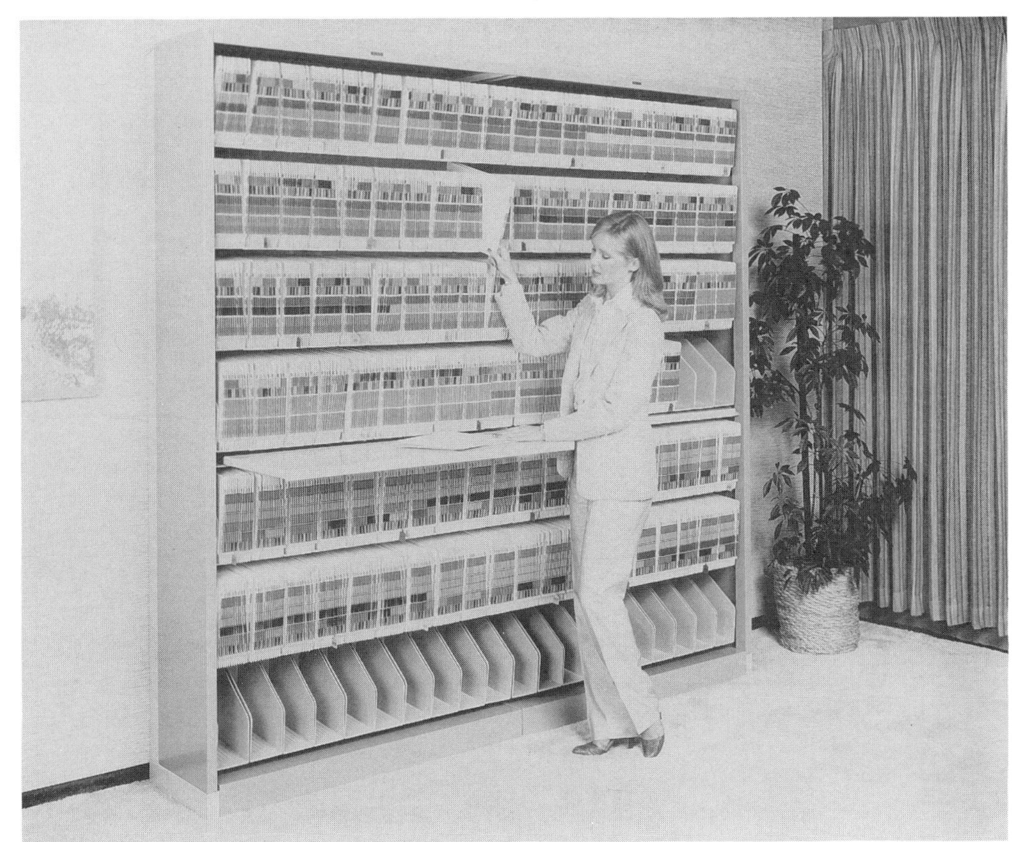

Figure 3-21. Open-shelf filing cabinet. (*Courtesy Tab Products, Palo Alto, CA.*)

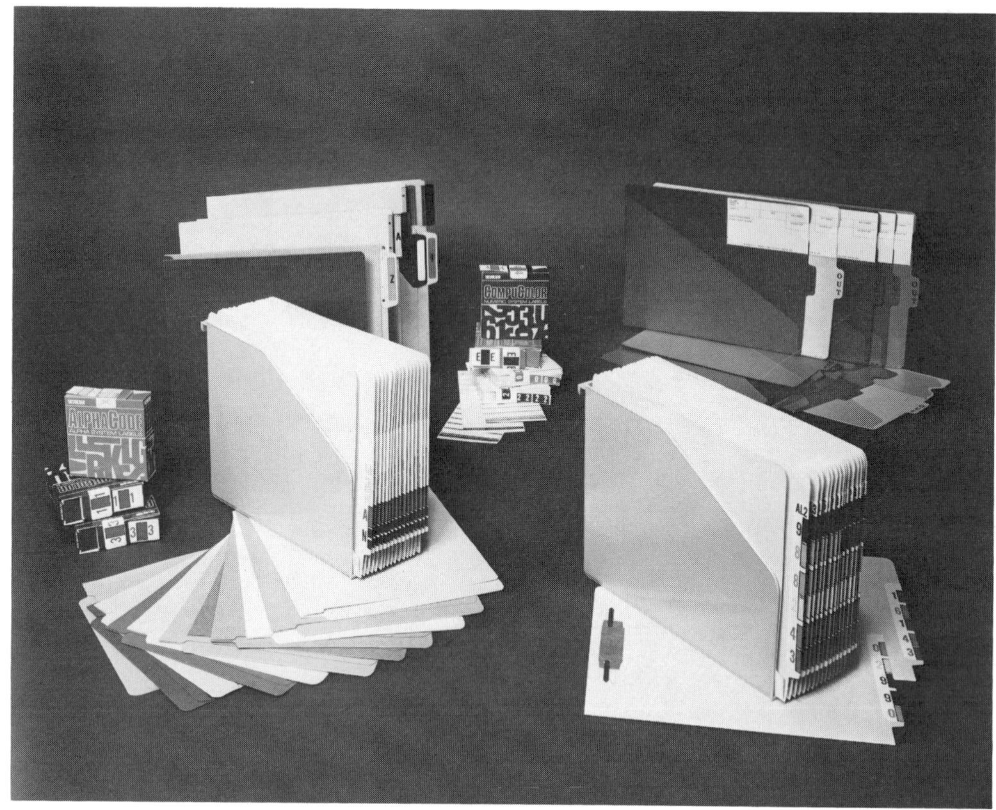

Figure 3-22. Color-coded file jackets and accessories. (*Courtesy Tab Products, Palo Alto, CA.*)

at a local warehouse that offers a quick retrieval system for physicians.

Medical records should be located so that they are convenient to the receptionists, nurses, and bookkeeper. Charts are usually pulled in the morning for patients to be seen that day. The only other time staff would need access to charts would be primarily for phone calls or prescription refills. Medical records would normally be located in the business office, but could be placed elsewhere in the suite. The bookkeeper needs convenient access to medical records for billing patients and filing insurance claims.

Private Entrance

A medical office, regardless of size, must have two entrances — one for patients, and a private one for the doctor, so that he or she can enter the office without meeting patients in the waiting room. In large suites, usually over 3000 square feet, local building codes may require two exits (separated by a distance equal to one-half the length of the maximum overall diagonal dimension of the area served, measured in a straight line between exits).

The Examination Room

Good traffic flow is imperative for the efficiency of a medical office. Several factors influence the location of the exam rooms:

1. Nurses are responsible for controlling traffic to and from the exam rooms, so the nurse station and the exam rooms should be clustered together. This enables nurses to prepare the patients in each room quickly, while traveling back and forth to the nurse station to clean instruments, or obtain items needed for the examination.

2. Exam rooms must be close to the consultation room to save the physician unnecessary steps, but it is preferable that patients not pass the consultation room when making their way to the exam room.

3. The exam room corridor(s) should be arranged so that patients must pass the business office when exiting the suite. This provides control so that future appointments may be booked, medications explained, and payment for services discussed.

The exam room is the background for diagnosis. As such, it should be designed very functionally, with an understanding of the equipment that needs to be provided and the psychological needs of the patient (refer to Chapter 1). If the amenities of the room can help the patient to relax (wallcovering, flooring, color, and artwork), it makes the examination easier.

It is desirable that patients' vital signs (blood pressure, pulse, etc.) be at normal levels prior to an examination. Anxiety, resulting from fear of a clinical and unfamiliar environment, elevates patients' vital signs, and may give false readings.

Size. The first functional consideration is size: 8 × 12 feet is the ideal size for exam rooms (gives a clear dimension of 7 feet 6 inches × 11 feet 6 inches inside the room) as it comfortably allows for a full-size exam table, a built-in sink cabinet with storage above, dressing area, small writing desk (usually wall mounted), a stool on casters for the doctor, a guest chair for the patient, a treatment stand (if required), and perhaps a small piece of portable medical equipment.

If the room is used for purposes other than routine examinations, such as stress testing, the room would contain an EKG unit and a treadmill, and it should be 9 × 12 feet or 10 × 12 feet in size. If a dressing area is not required, the length of the room can be shortened to 10 feet.

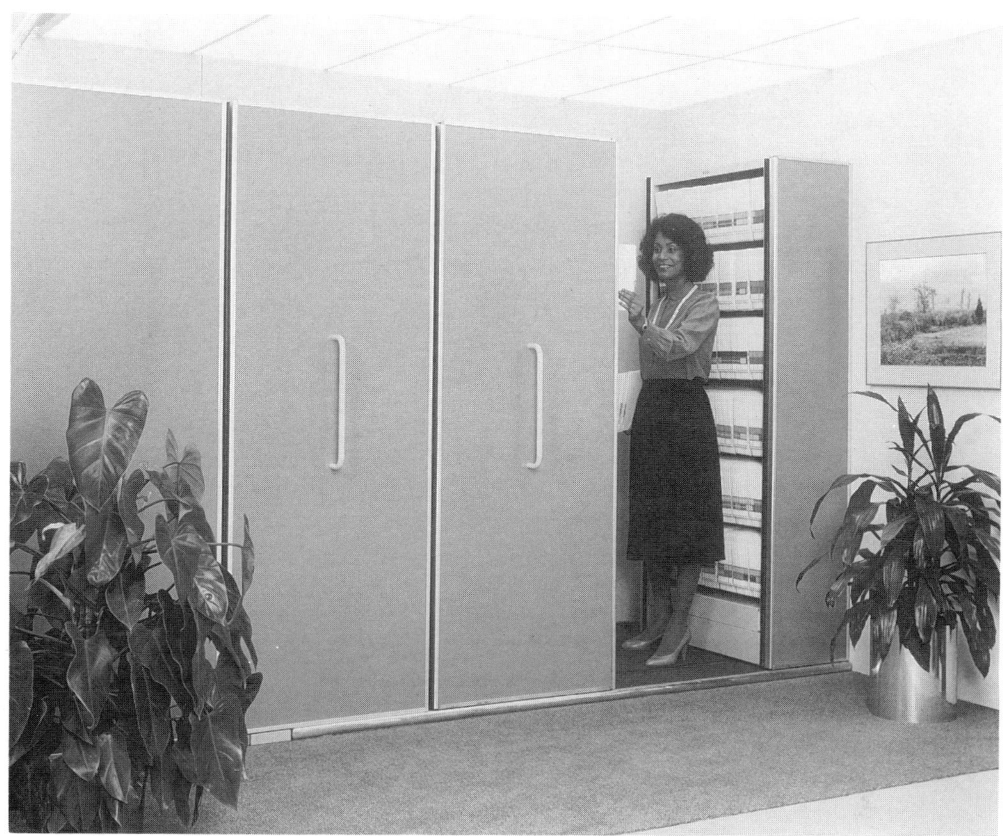

Figure 3-23. Manual *TAB-TRAC* filing system. (*Courtesy Tab Products, Palo Alto, CA.*)

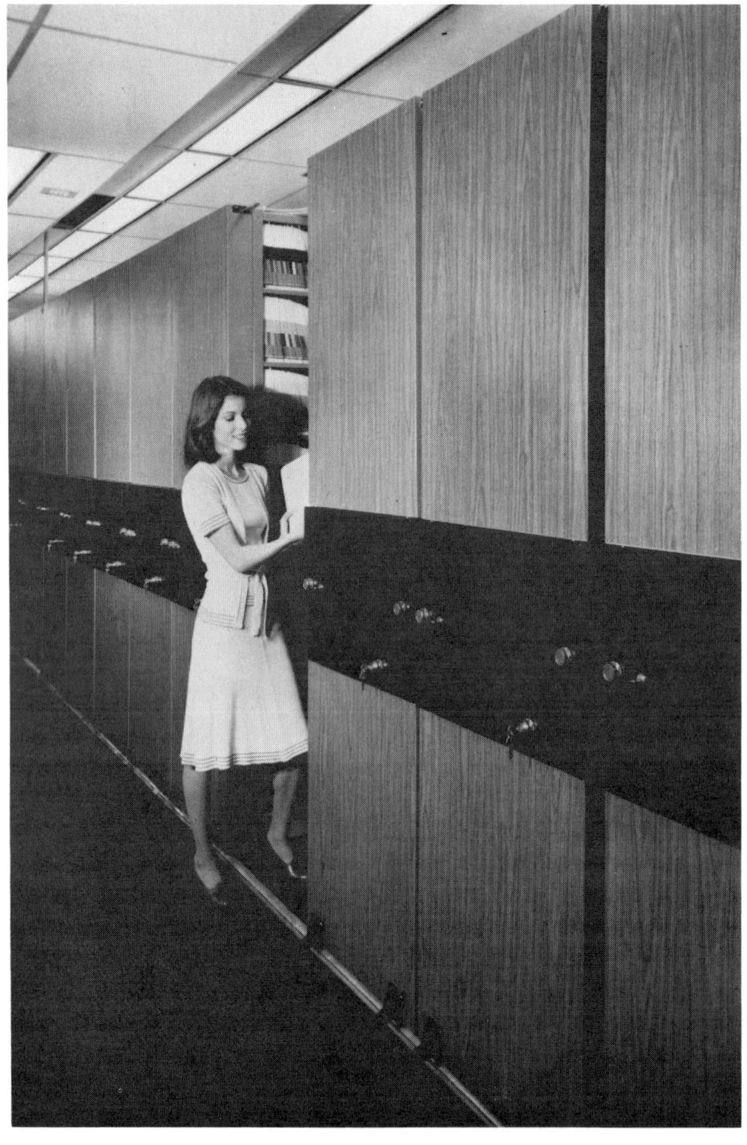

Figure 3-24. Space-efficient files, motorized operation. (*Courtesy Ames Color File Corp., Sommerville, MA.*)

Dressing Area. If space permits, it is desirable to provide a dressing area for patients. This need be no more than a 3- × 3-foot surface-mounted drapery cubicle track at the ceiling (with radius corner), with a built-in bench or a chair, clothes hooks, hangers, a mirror, and perhaps a shelf for disposable gowns. It provides patients with privacy in undressing.

The alternative is that patients must disrobe in the open exam room, with the fear that the nurse or doctor may walk in on them while they are naked, or while they are squeezing into a girdle or panty hose. Older people, and those with orthopedic girdles or braces, tend to be more sensitive about this than younger people.

There is also the possibility of creating a private dressing alcove with a 30-inch-wide door or panel hinged to the wall. It is perpendicular to the wall when in use and folds flat against the wall when not in use. The chair can be used either inside the dressing area when the hinged panel is extended, or outside, when the panel is folded flat against the wall.

With certain medical specialties, for example, ear-nose-throat (ENT) or orthopedics, patients rarely undress, or if they do so, they primarily undress just to the waist, so private dressing cubicles would not be a priority in these practices.

Position of Exam Table. The second functional consideration is the position of the examining table. The foot or stirrup end of the table should be angled away from the door (Figure 3-26) as well as the wall, so that the doctor has access to all sides of the patient, and the patient is out of view of passersby in the corridor when the door is opened.

The door to an exam room should be hinged so that it opens away from the wall (does not stack against the wall). While this might seem awkward in most rooms, it is desirable in a medical exam room because it shields the patient from corridor traffic, should the door be opened accidentally, and gives the patient more privacy when dressing, since one has to walk around the open door to enter the room.

Cabinets. Right-handed physicians (and many left-handed ones) examine patients from the patient's right side. Thus a "right-handed" exam room will have the entry door on the right side of the room with the exam table on the left, as one would face the room upon entering. The sink cabinet may be located either on the wall with the door or on the long wall, to the right, as one enters the room. The latter position is preferable in a room in which pelvic or proctologic examinations are done, so that the doctor can examine the patient with the right hand and reach for instruments with the left hand, enabling him or her to pick up and discard instruments conveniently. A sink cabinet on the long wall has another advantage: The physician, upon entering the room can, without walking around the door, quickly walk to the sink cabinet, wash hands, turn around, and be in position to examine the patient.

It is poor economy to locate sink cabinets in exam rooms back to back (mirror image) in order to reduce plumbing costs. This creates one "right-handed" room and one "left-handed" room — a most inefficient layout. For greatest efficiency, all exam rooms should be identical so that a physician can quickly move from room to room, and "with eyes closed," feel oriented.

The sink cabinet need have only a small sink (a 12- × 12-inch stainless steel bar sink works well), as instruments will be washed at the nurse station or lab. In addition, the sink should have a single-lever faucet. The sink cabinet should be a minimum of 48 inches long, 24 inches deep, and 36 inches high. If space permits, it might have a built-in compartment for trash with a hinged "trash slot" cut into the face of the cabinet door.

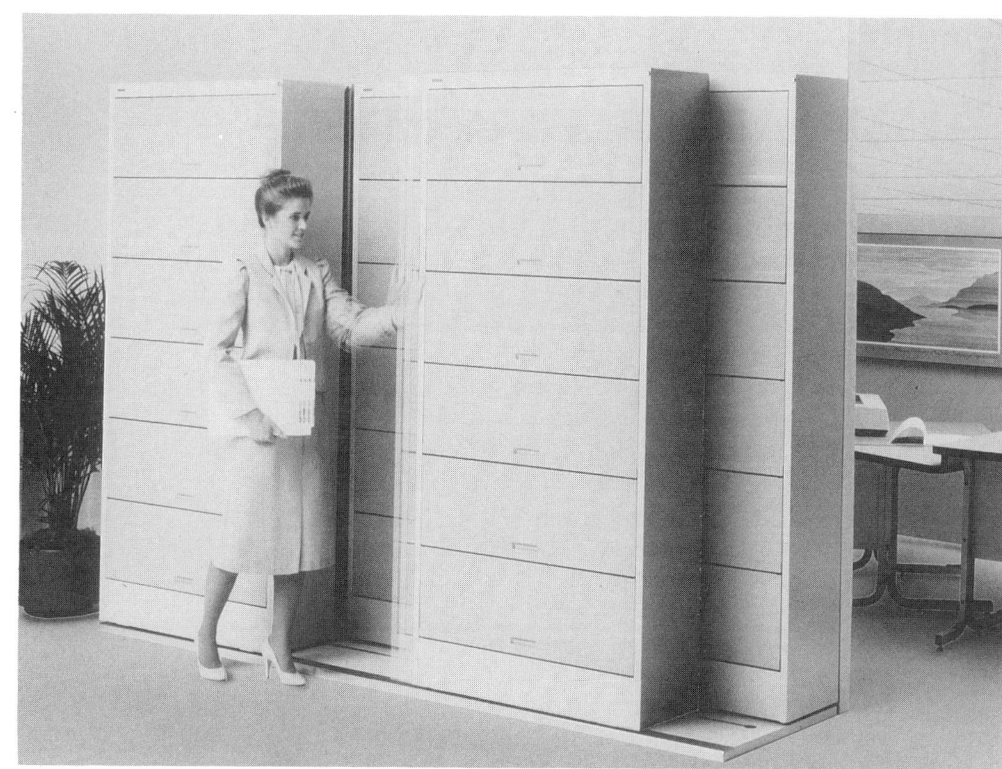

Figure 3-25. Sliding file system, *SIDE-TRAC*. (*Courtesy Tab Products, Palo Alto, CA.*)

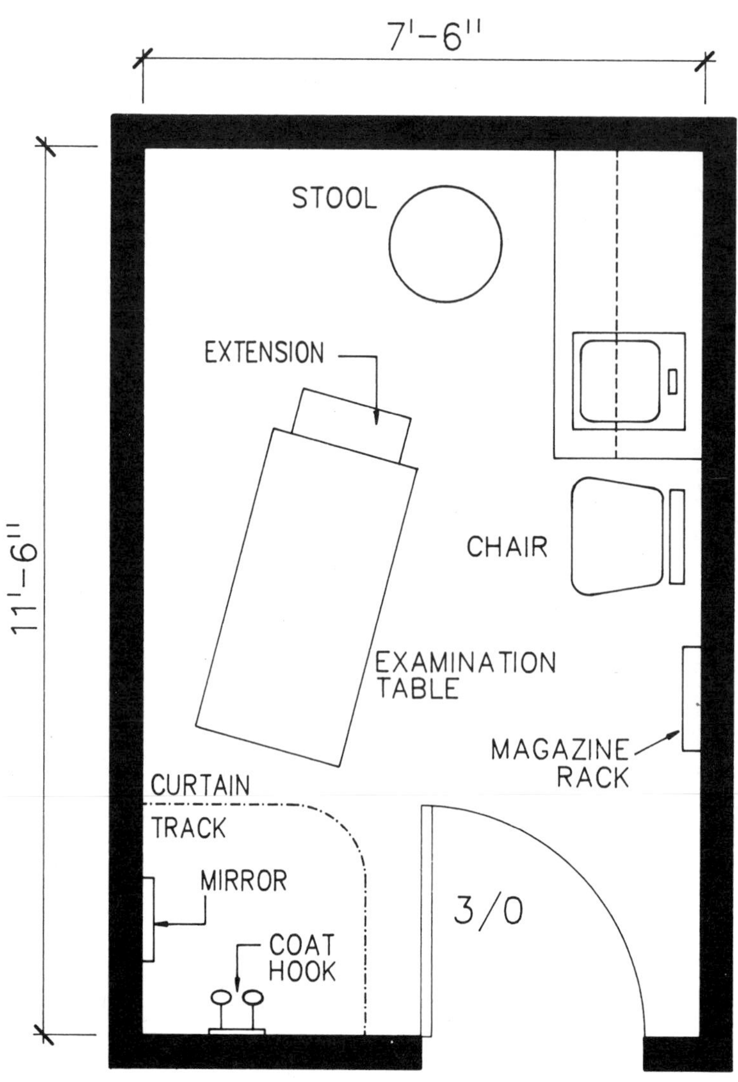

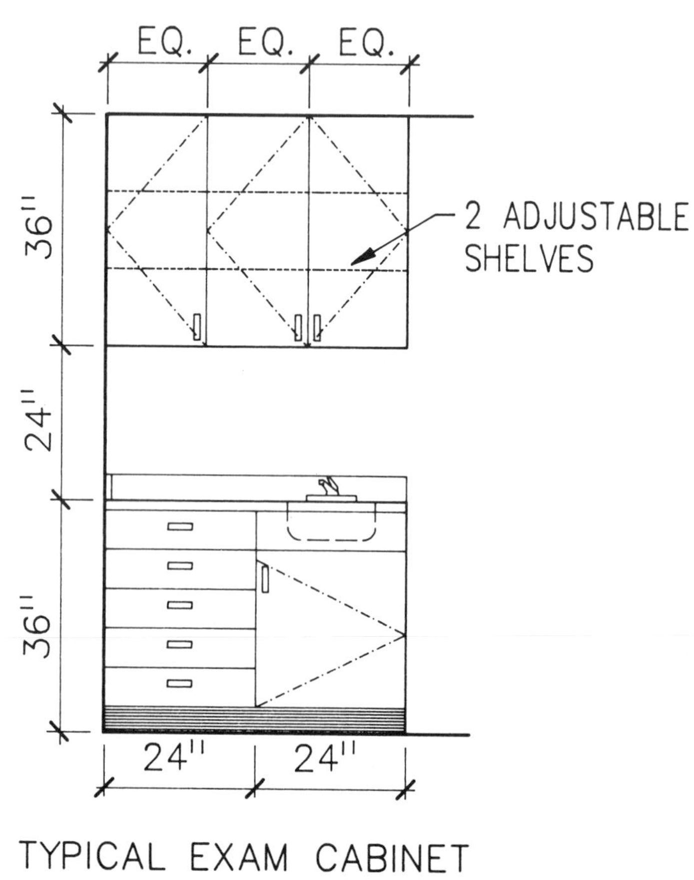

Figure 3-26. Standard examination room layout.

An upper cabinet may be provided (48 inches long, 12 inches deep, 36 inches high), over the base cabinet, for storage of disposable gowns, sheets, and other paper products (Figure 3-26). Shallow drawers in the base cabinet store instruments, syringes, surgical gloves, dressings, tongue depressors, and the like. Paper towel and liquid soap dispensers should be mounted on the wall near the sink. These items are often provided by the paper or supply vendors who service the units.

Obstetricians and gynecologists often like to warm their specula prior to examinations. For this purpose, an electrical outlet may be provided in the drawer in which the specula are stored. The more expensive pelvic examination tables have a built-in warmer.

A small wall-hung writing shelf may be provided in an exam room to enable the physician to complete most examinations in the exam room without returning to the consultation room. If the sink cabinet is located on the long wall, the countertop can be extended, and lowered, from 36 inches to 30 inches, to serve as a writing desk. A rolling stool that stores under the "desk," when not in use, should be provided for the physician.

The patient may sit on the exam table or on a guest chair while the physician is taking a patient history, or writing a diagnosis. Frequently, slots for prescription pads are built into the desk top (see Figure 4-97).

If the sink cabinet is located on the door wall, the writing desk should be placed on the long wall, perpendicular to it. The cabinetry should be clad with plastic laminate, rather than painted. The additional cost when fabricating cabinets is minimal, and well worth it, when one considers the abuse of the painted surfaces plus the inconvenience, and cost, of repainting.

Some physicians may request a connecting door between examining rooms and their consultation room. This is usually not a good idea. Considerable space is lost in the exam room by installing an extra door; there is loss of privacy in the consultation room; and there is then the tendency of the physician to bring each patient into the consultation room, which greatly reduces the number of patients the physician can see in a day.

Windows. There is controversy over the benefit of windows in exam rooms. There is no need for natural light in an exam room for most specialties (it is recommended for dermatology exam rooms however), so the inclusion of windows would be either a matter of the physician's preference or a given of the building's architecture. If present, the glass should start at a height sufficient (generally 42 inches) to afford the patient a measure of privacy.

Gray glass is superior to bronze since the latter casts an unhealthy tint on patient's skin. Narrow-slat metal window blinds or vertical blinds are particularly well suited to windows in exam rooms, for the slats can be tilted to provide privacy without cutting off the light or view entirely.

Too many windows in a medical building can make it difficult to lay out the rooms efficiently unless one wishes to have partitions that terminate in the middle of a window, instead of at a wall or a mullion. This is particularly common when the architect who designed the building was not familiar with medical space planning, and a window module was designed that is not compatible with the size of the rooms in a medical office — basically a 4-foot module.

Electrical Requirements. Three grounded duplex electrical outlets should be provided in an examination room — one above the cabinet countertop, one at the foot of the table, and one near the head of the table. Except for the outlet over the countertop, which would be at a height of 44 inches, the other outlets may be at a standard 12-inch height. Some physicians use a wall-

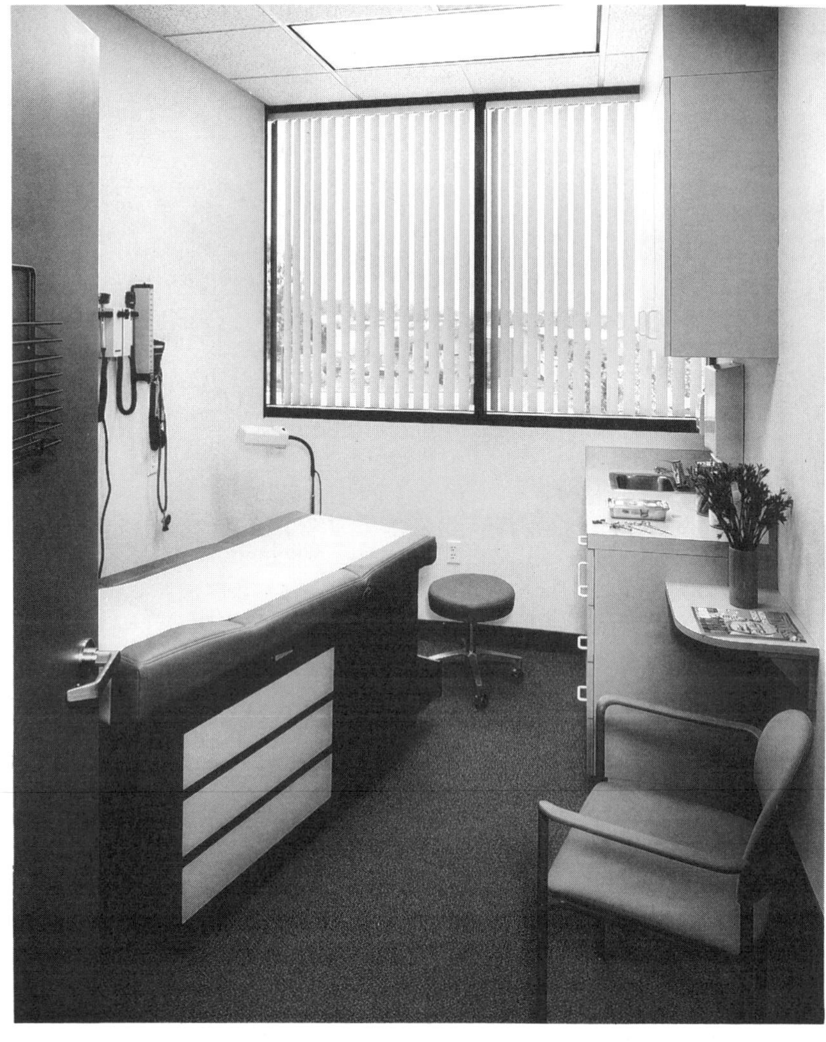

Figure 3-27. Standard examination room. (*Design: Jain Malkin Inc.; Photographer: Robinson/Ward.*)

mounted ophthalmoscope and otoscope/throat illuminator that would be positioned on the long wall, at approximately 60-inch height, near the head of the exam table (Figure 3-27). It requires an electrical outlet for the recharger. Rooms used for ophthalmic or ENT (ear-nose-throat) examinations have special electrical requirements, to be discussed in Chapter 4.

Certain exam rooms, such as pediatric or orthopedic exam rooms, often require only two electrical outlets, one over the countertop, and the other near the foot of the exam table. Outlets in a pediatric exam room must be carefully guarded and located where a child cannot reach them.

Some examinations, such as OB-GYN exams, require an additional light source, which is usually a high-intensity quartz halogen lamp on a mobile floor stand.

It may be necessary to shield a specialized exam room (one used for electrocardiograph machinery, for example) against electrical interference from surrounding medical offices or equipment, although this is increasingly rare with new equipment.

Exam Table. The standard exam table is 27 inches wide × 54 inches long with stirrups at the foot (Figure 3-29) if it is to be used for pelvic or urologic examinations, although there are specialized tables for proctoscopic (see Figure 3-52) and cystoscopic (urological) examinations (see Figure 4-91). If not used for these purposes, the table will have a pull-out foot board that extends the length of the table to about six feet.

The examining room, as described above, will be suitable for most physicians, but some medical specialties require modifications, and these are discussed in future chapters. Most notably, orthopedic surgeons use a 78-inch-long exam table, which is often placed

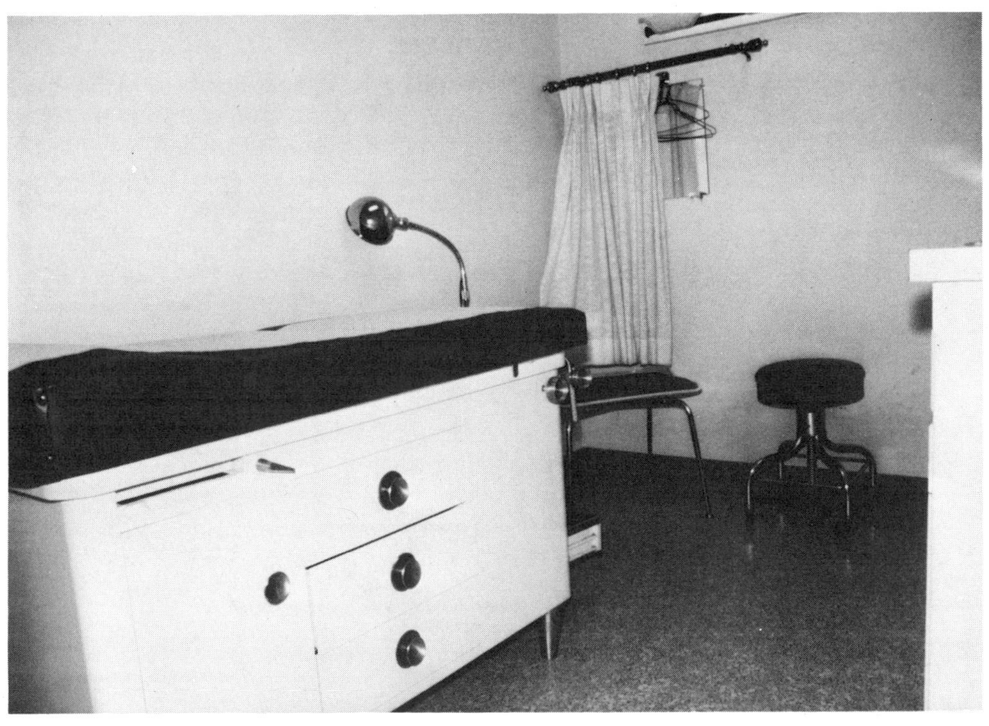

Figure 3-28. "Bad" exam room. The nonverbal messages speak loudly. (*Photographer: Jain Malkin.*)

against a wall. Pediatricians, also, place their exam tables against the wall.

The combination consultation room and examination room popularized some years ago by the Mayo Clinic is an alternative that has a place in some practices — very low-volume ones, such as neurology. Whatever the design of the exam room, the formula for a productive and efficient office is in the relationship between exam rooms, consultation rooms, nurse stations, and support areas.

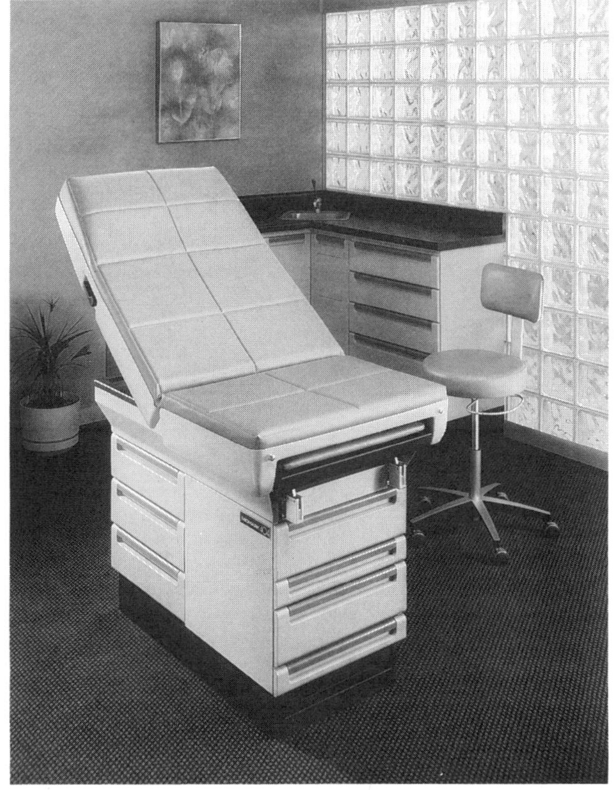

Figure 3-29. Examination table. (*Courtesy Midmark Corp., Versailles, OH.*)

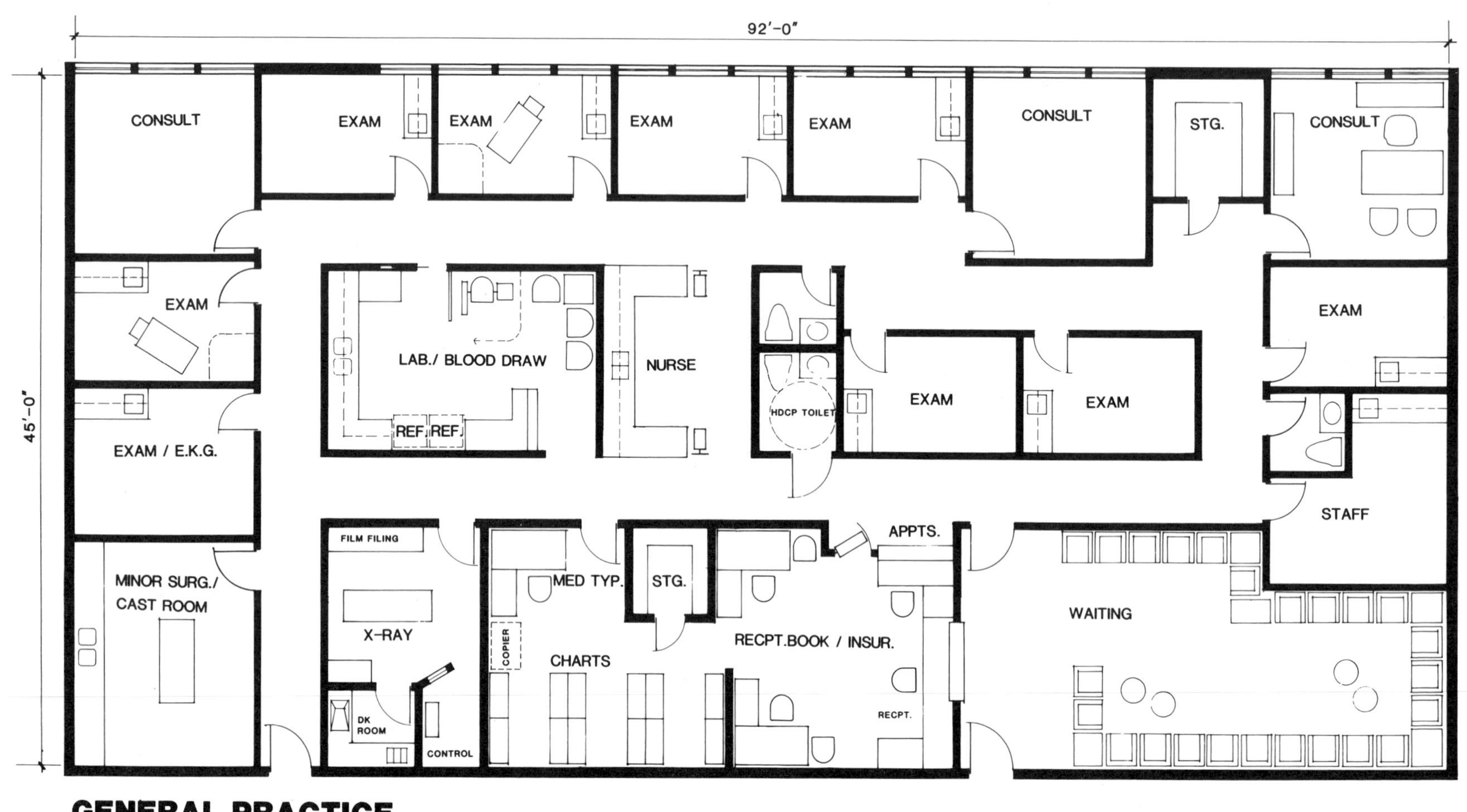

Figure 3-30. Suite plan for general practice, 4140 square feet.

Treatment/Minor Surgery

Each family practice or general practice suite will have a minor surgery room. It is sometimes called a *treatment room.* It is a large exam room (usually 12 × 12 feet) that serves a variety of purposes. It may be used as a cast room, in which case a plaster trap should be provided in the sink, and cabinets should contain a bin for plaster and for the remains of casts that have been removed (see Chapter 4, Orthopedic Surgery).

It may be used as an EKG room, an operating room for minor surgical procedures using local anesthetics, and as an emergency exam room for accident cases. In treating emergencies, the physician may need one or more aides in the room plus certain medical equipment not usually stored in the other exam rooms. Add to that the relatives who accompany the patient and frequently wish to remain in the treatment room, and the need for an oversized, multipurpose exam room becomes clear.

A minor surgery room should have a 10-foot to 12-foot length of upper and lower cabinets — one full wall of built-ins. Usually this room will have a ceiling-mounted surgical light over the treatment table, in addition to standard fluorescent lighting (Figure 3-31*a*). Proper illumination is mandatory for this room.

If the suite is so situated within the layout of the medical building as to make possible a direct entrance to the minor surgery room, it is desirable. Accident cases or those with contagious diseases do not have to walk through the waiting room if they can enter the minor surgery room directly. This would be an unmarked door in the public corridor of the medical building provided with a buzzer, or the door might simply state *Emergency Entrance — Ring Bell for Service.*

The receptionist taking the emergency call would ask the patient to go to the door marked *Emergency Entrance* and ring the bell.

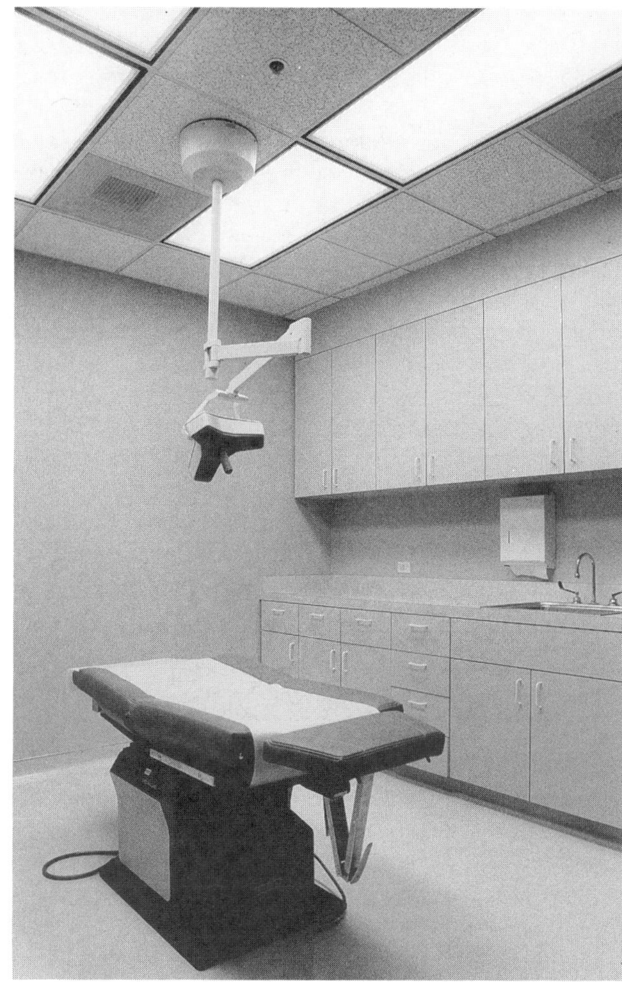

Figure 3-31a. Minor surgery room. (*Design: Jain Malkin Inc.; Photographer: John Christian.*)

The Consultation Room

This room functions as a private office for the most part, but some physicians do consult with patients here. Routine consultation can be handled in a well-designed exam room, saving the physician the trouble of continually returning to his or her private office with each patient.

Certain physicians (for example, internists and neurologists) spend a good deal of time interviewing the patient on the initial visit. In such cases, physicians may feel that the consultation room provides a more conducive atmosphere for establishing the relationship. Surgeons also tend to use their private offices for consultation with patients, but this remains a matter of individual preference for each physician.

The consultation room is also used by the physician for reading, returning phone calls, dictating notes, or just relaxing. The minimum size for this room is 10 × 12 feet, but 12 × 12 feet is better. The room must accommodate a desk, credenza, bookshelves for the doctor's library, two guest chairs, a coat closet (optional), and perhaps a private bathroom.

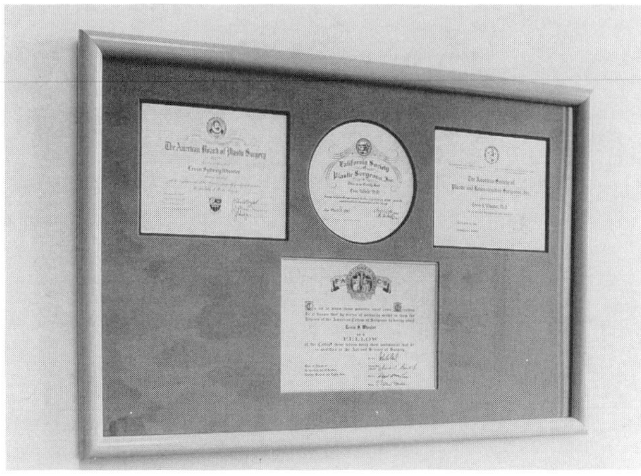

Figure 3-31. Diplomas, attractively framed. (*Photo courtesy: Jain Malkin Inc.; Photographer: Michael Denny.*)

The room should be furnished like a living room, with cut pile carpet, textured wallcoverings or wood paneling, and fabric upholstery. If the doctor has a hobby that lends itself to expression in room decor, this is the one room in the suite that can be highly personalized. Family photos, armed forces honors, and personal memorabilia humanize the doctor's image and provide a clue to him or her as a person, apart from the medical practice.

The physician's diplomas and credentials should be nicely framed and displayed in the consultation room. If grouped artistically (Figure 3-31 and Color Plate 12, Figure 4-74), they can be a handsome addition to the room's decor.

A consultation room should have natural light if possible. In addition, table lamps or indirect lighting may add to the room's homelike ambience. It is desirable to locate the consultation room at the rear of the suite to give the physician more privacy, and so that patients do not pass it on their way to the examining room. Still, some aggressive patients find their way to the consultation room uninvited and unannounced.

Frequently it is possible to locate an outdoor exit in the private office. The physician may thus enter or leave without being seen by patients. If such a door is not possible, then a private rear entrance to the suite, as previously discussed, is mandatory.

In certain suites, such as pediatrics, the consultation room is used so minimally that several physicians may share one. Their combined medical library would be stored here, and each doctor would have a small desk and telephone (see Figure 3-67).

At the other extreme, occasionally a physician will request a consultation room with a sofa large enough to sleep on, a table with reading lamp, a refrigerator, and bathroom with shower, in addition to the usual components of a private office. Such an office may serve a cardiac surgeon who, due to many emergency surgeries, may have to spend the night at the office (if it is near the hospital) or just catch up on sleep during the day between surgeries.

Nurse Station/Laboratory

The nurse station is an area where the doctor's nurses or aides perform a variety of tasks such as weighing patients, sterilizing instruments, dispensing drug samples, giving injections, taking a patient's temperature, performing routine lab tests, communicating with patients by telephone, or handling office paperwork (Figure 3-32).

The nurse station may be only a 6-foot length of countertop (with cabinets below and above) recessed in a niche in the corridor (see Figure 3-48), or it may be an 8- × 12-foot room adjacent to the exam rooms (see Figure 3-30). The size of the nurse station depends on the number of aides who will use it, the type of medical practice, and the functions to be performed by the aides.

The number of aides can be estimated on the basis of each doctor requiring one or two aides, depending on whether the practice is a high-volume specialty. The aide may assist the physician in the exam room or may actually perform certain examinations. Obstetricians and gynecologists have been using assistants in this expanded role for routine pelvic and gynecologic examinations.

Called *nurse practitioners,* these are registered nurses who take an additional course of study that prepares them to examine patients. Since OB-GYN is a very high-volume specialty, the use of nurse practitioners saves the physician time on routine examinations, and permits him or her to concentrate on patients with more demanding medical problems.

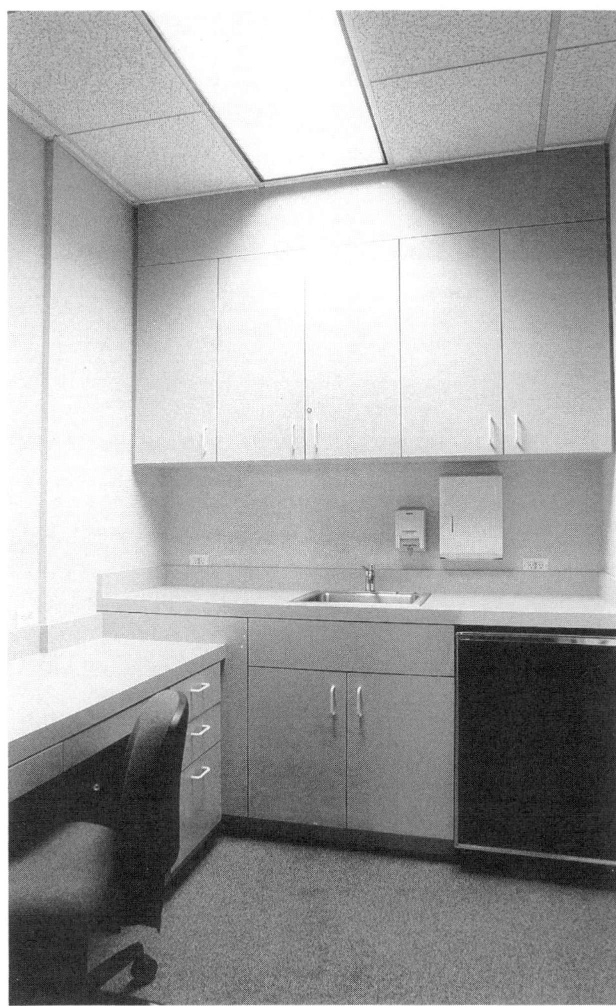

Figure 3-32. Nurse station. (*Design: Jain Malkin Inc.; Photographer: John Christian.*)

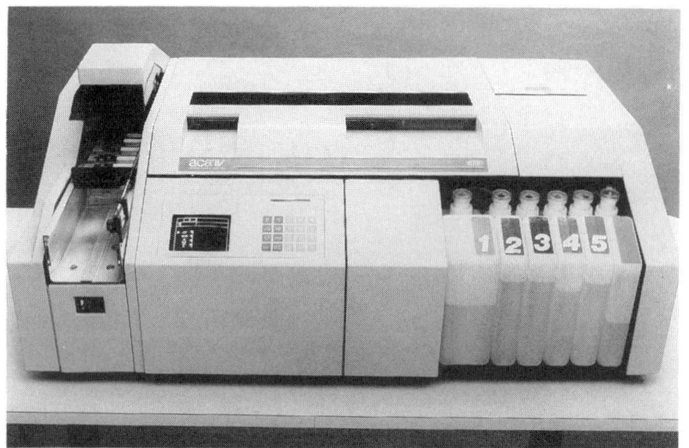

Figure 3-33. Du Pont "aca" IV discrete clinical analyzer. (*Courtesy Du Pont Corp., Wilmington, DE.*)

Therefore, the nurse station in an OB-GYN suite must be large enough to accommodate the nurse practitioners and other aides who need a kneespace for sitting down and writing notes, one or two scales (all OB-GYN patients are weighed each visit), with a writing shelf nearby. Sometimes scales are recessed into the floor, if practical, in terms of cost and construction parameters. This recess in the concrete slab can be carpeted with the adjacent floor carpet. An area of approximately 24 inches should be allowed for each scale. This is not the size of the recess but the floor space necessary to accommodate a standard medical scale with balance rod.

There is an advantage to locating the nurse station near the front of the suite in a small office (under 1500 square feet). The nurse has easy access to patients as she leads them from the waiting room to the exam room, and she can cover for the business office staff when they are momentarily away from their desks. In larger suites, each doctor may have an aide working from a nurse station convenient to his or her pod of exam rooms (see Figures 3-34 and 3-51).

In some medical offices, the nurse station is combined with the laboratory. In otolaryngology (ENT), for example, this is true since few lab tests are performed in the office. The nurse station/lab would be used for preparing throat cultures and for cleanup of instruments in the sink or for sterilizing instruments. With the widespread use of disposable syringes, gowns, sheets, and even many examination instruments, relatively few items have to be washed or sterilized.

In an OB-GYN practice, the laboratory would generally be a separate room because a good deal of lab work is processed in the suite. Each patient supplies a urine sample for analysis, which is performed in the lab, and each patient having a pelvic exam and Pap smear will have a tissue culture that will have to be prepared for sending to a cytology lab.

A number of other routine tests would be performed within the lab, plus many gynecologists do D&Cs, terminations of pregnancy, and other types of minor surgical procedures in a well-equipped minor surgery room in the office. These procedures can be messy and require an adequate area for cleanup and good-sized nurse station, plus lab support facilities.

A lab should have a double-compartment sink, a kneespace area for a microscope, a full-size refrigerator if necessary (otherwise an under-counter one), and a facility for blood draw. The blood draw area may be nothing more than a standard chair in the lab, or it may be a special prefabricated tablet-arm blood draw chair. It is advisable to shield the patient whose blood is being drawn from the sight of other patients, who often become faint upon observing the procedure.

It is desirable to have at least one toilet room adjacent to the lab so that a specimen pass-through door in the wall can give the lab technician access to urine specimens without leaving the lab (see Figure 3-12). The reader is referred to Chapter 5 for more detailed specifications of a small laboratory and to the Appendix for a diagram of a specimen pass-through.

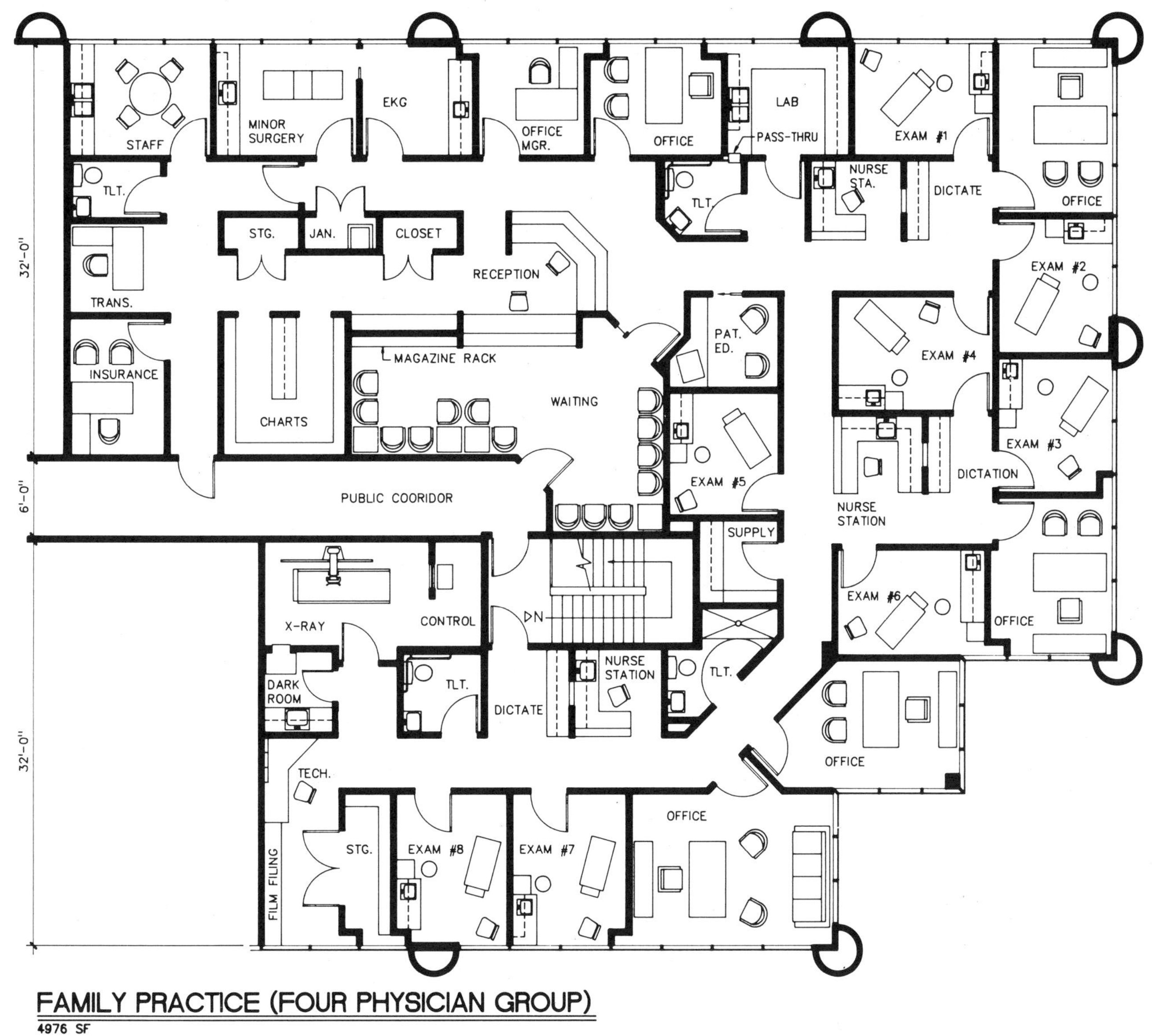

Figure 3-34. Suite plan for general practice, 4976 square feet.

The nurse station of an orthopedic surgery suite would be of minimal size since there are no lab tests performed, and no blood is drawn. The supplies needed for examinations or for making or removing casts would be stored in the respective rooms, and very little would have to be carried into a room for a procedure.

By contrast, a family practice or G.P. suite would have a large nurse station. Since such a wide variety of medical procedures are performed and there is such a wide range of patients, it would be impractical to store in each exam room all the supplies one might need. Therefore, the nurse prepares the exam room with any special supplies, injections, dressings, and instruments that she anticipates will be required. A good many of these items will be stored in the nurse station, and each nurse station might have its own autoclave for sterilization of instruments.

In addition, the nurse might give allergy or other injections at the nurse station; blood might be drawn for tests to be done in the suite's own lab or sent out for processing; patients are weighed at each visit; and many other routine duties are carried out here.

A nurse station should always have a sink and often has an under-counter refrigerator and a kneespace work area with telephone (see Figure 3-32). Most nurse stations have a scale space, with a nearby shelf, for recording the weight in the patient's chart. The reader is referred to Chapter 4 for nurse station requirements for each medical specialty.

Regarding the laboratory, the physician decides whether to do lab tests within the office or send the work out. Some do not even like to draw blood in their office, but prefer to send the patient to a lab, if one is conveniently located in the medical building. Sometimes physicians who are tenants or owners of the medical building own the lab jointly and agree to send all of their lab work there for their mutual benefit. This also generates the type of lab income that enables them to buy more sophisticated equipment lab than any of the individual physicians may wish to purchase for their own use. Automated clinical analyzers (Figure 3-33) perform more than 20 different blood chemistry tests from one blood sample in a matter of minutes.

There has been a trend towards miniaturization of this equipment. Analyzers that ten years ago occupied a large floor area have been reduced in size to sit on a countertop. Even those that remain as floor models have been considerably reduced in size.

Other Support Services

X-ray Room. This discussion will focus on the one-room X-ray unit that can be found in a G.P. or internal medicine suite. Rather simple radiographic examinations are performed here — films of extremities, chests, gallbladders, appendixes, etc. More complicated procedures will be performed in a radiologist's office. A large internal medicine practice might have a suite of radiographic rooms within its facility with a full-time radiologist on staff. But usually a patient who requires G.I. (gastrointestinal) studies, thyroid scans, Computed Tomography (CT scans), radiation oncology therapy, or other specialized or complicated radiographic procedures will be referred to a local hospital on an outpatient basis, or to a nearby radiology clinic.

A 10- × 12-foot room is adequate (not taking into account the dressing area and darkroom) for most X-ray machines used in a G.P.'s or internist's office. Usually a 9-foot ceiling height is required. The room should have a place for a patient to dress (ideally a 3- × 4-foot alcove with a drapery for privacy), a control area for the technician, and a place to process the film. Although the equipment breaks down into components, it is advisable to provide a minimum 3-foot-wide door in this room for ease in moving the equipment.

The radiography room does not need a sink or prep area unless G.I. studies are performed or contrast media are used, in which case a bathroom must be located close to the radiographic room (see Figure 5-5).

Two or more walls of an X-ray room will have to be shielded with lead to protect passersby from radiation scatter. It is necessary to obtain a radiation physicist's report, which takes into account the type of equipment and the location of the room within the suite and within the medical office building, in order to know which walls must be shielded, the thickness of the lead, and the height of the lead panels. Frequently, the door to the room must also be lead-lined. Such a door is very heavy and must have a heavy-duty door closer. The control partition, if located within the room, must also be lead-lined. It is possible to buy prefabricated, lead-lined control partitions, with glass viewing panels, from X-ray supply houses.

If the control area is located outside the X-ray room, there must be a lead-lined glass window to enable the operator to observe the patient at all times. The control area need not be large — 3 feet square is generally adequate.

There are considerable variations in size of radiology equipment, power requirements, and other specifications from one manufacturer to another. Therefore it is advisable to obtain planning guides for each piece of equipment before proceeding.

A valuable reference in designing radiology rooms is the catalog of radiology accessories marketed by each manufacturer. General Electric Co. has a particularly good one, in which thousands of items are pictured with dimensions and pertinent data. This will familiarize the designer with the many accessory items (cassette pass boxes, film illuminators, film dryers, automatic processors) that must be accommodated in a radiology room or suite.

A lead-lined cassette pass box should be located in the wall between the darkroom and the radiography room. The pass box is used for passing exposed and unexposed film back and forth between the rooms.

The manufacturer's literature will specify utility requirements and critical distances between equipment. Sometimes wood blocking is needed in the ceiling to support the tube stand. Usually the X-ray unit, if new, will be supplied by a local distributor who will assist the designer in locating the equipment in the room. Or, if the physician is relocating existing equipment to a new office, it will usually be moved and reinstalled by a skilled technician who can offer assistance as to the equipment's requirements.

Darkroom. A small darkroom must be provided and should be set up with a "wet" and a "dry" side. A 4- × 6-foot room is the minimum size. The room should have two 4- to 5-foot counters either parallel to each other or at right angles. The wet side contains the sink, automatic processor, and replenisher tanks, while the dry side is used for loading cassettes. A light-proof metal film storage bin should be located under the dry side of the counter. Ideally, the cassette pass box would be positioned in the wall close to the film storage bin.

Sometimes a rack for storage of cassettes is provided. A floor drain must be located near the processor. One outlet should be provided over the counter on both the wet and dry sides. An outlet is needed for the film storage bin as well. The processor requires only cold water if it is a recent model with an internal temperature control.

Local codes normally require a vacuum breaker on piping to darkroom tanks to prevent the chemical waste from backing up into the water supply. Also, acid-resistant pipe is recommended, since chemical waste is highly corrosive.

The room must have an exhaust fan, and some codes require that the door have a lightproof louver ventilation panel. The darkroom door need be only 24 inches wide, but it must have a light seal. It should open inward, so that if someone tries to enter while film is exposed, the technician inside the room can put a foot against the door to prevent it from opening. Some darkrooms have a red warning light that is activated when developing is in progress.

The darkroom must have two sources of light. A 75-watt incandescent fixture, surface mounted to the ceiling, will suffice for general illumination, but a safelight must be provided for working with exposed film. The safelight may be plugged into an outlet at 60 to 72 inches off the floor, and it can work by a pull chain or be wired into a wall switch. If the latter, the switch should be located away from the incandescent light switch so that the technician does not confuse them and hit the wrong one while the film is exposed. Any recessed light fixtures and the exhaust fan must have a light-sealed housing.

Counters and cabinets in a darkroom may be at a 36-inch or 42-inch height, according to personal preference. There is no need for closed storage in the darkroom. All shelves should be open shelves.

A small viewing area is required outside the procedure room, near the darkroom (Figure 3-34). This may consist of nothing more than a double-panel view box illuminator, either surface mounted to the wall, or recessed. The technician checks the films for resolution and clarity before handing them to the physician for diagnosis. If the film is not good, the patient is still at hand, with little time lost in having to take the film again. In a larger X-ray suite of rooms, the viewing area will be larger, with several banks of film illuminators and a place for two or more persons to sit down.

Today it is rare to find a medical office that does not have an automatic film processor. It is also unusual to find manual developing tanks as a backup measure in case the processor fails. The servicing of these units seems to be such that downtime is limited and infrequent. The automatic processor may be a small tabletop unit such as dentists or facial plastic surgeons use, or it may be a large piece of equipment that sits outside the darkroom with a feed tray that fits through the wall into the darkroom (see Figure 5-21). Such units are discussed in detail in Chapter 5 under Radiology.

Storage. Medical offices should have a storage room at least 6 feet square. Two or more walls should have adjustable shelves for storage of office supplies, sterile supplies, pharmaceutical items, housekeeping supplies, and cartons of toilet paper, hand towels, and facial tissue. If the office does not use a janitorial service, the vacuum cleaner and mop and pail would be stored here.

Staff Lounge. Any suite with more than three employees should have a staff lounge, if space permits. The room need not be larger than 10 $\times$ 12 feet with a built-in sink cabinet 4 to 6 feet in length, an under-counter refrigerator, microwave oven, garbage disposal, and a small table and chairs. A larger staff lounge would include a sofa where an employee may lie down. This is a private room where the staff may take coffee breaks, eat their lunch, or smoke. A staff lounge is not mandatory in a small office, but it is an amenity that pleases employees and makes their jobs a little more pleasant.

INTERNAL MEDICINE

The practice of internal medicine is broad. It encompasses subspecialties such as pulmonary disease, nephrology, oncology, hematology, gastroenterology, endocrinology, and cardiovascular disease — the major emphases. Before planning an internal medicine suite, it is important to analyze the physicians' respective specialties and practice schedules.

With such a broad range of areas of expertise, it is common for internists to practice in groups rather than as solo practitioners. A designer must also understand the structure of a physician's workday. Physicians tend to visit their hospitalized patients in the morning, before office hours. Office hours typically begin at 9 A.M. and continue to 12 noon. Medical offices are usually closed from noon to 2 P.M. and open again from 2 to 5 P.M. Surgeons try to do the bulk of their surgery in the morning and reserve the afternoon for office visits by patients.

In a five-person practice, for example, physicians' schedules will usually be arranged so that no more than three are in the office at any one time. This negates the need for each of the five to have the use of exam rooms all at the same time. By efficiently coordinating their schedules, the group can function well in less space, without sacrificing income or service to patients. One doctor may have a day off, while a second may be seeing patients at a satellite office, and a third may be seeing patients at the hospital, leaving the other two in our hypothetical group of five in the primary office. At a busier point in the day, schedules may be arranged so that three or four of the internists are in the primary office seeing patients.

Internal medicine is a medium-volume practice. It is based on diagnosis, which requires long history-taking interviews by the physician, and sometimes a complicated battery of tests. The internist, being primarily a diagnostician, spends a good deal of time with a patient. However, follow-up visits may be considerably shorter, so overall, a well-organized, efficient practice can process a fairly high number of patients each day.

Some internists prefer to do the initial interview in the consultation room, whereas others find it more efficient to do it in the exam room. If the consultation room is used, it should be large — 12 × 12 feet — with comfortable seating.

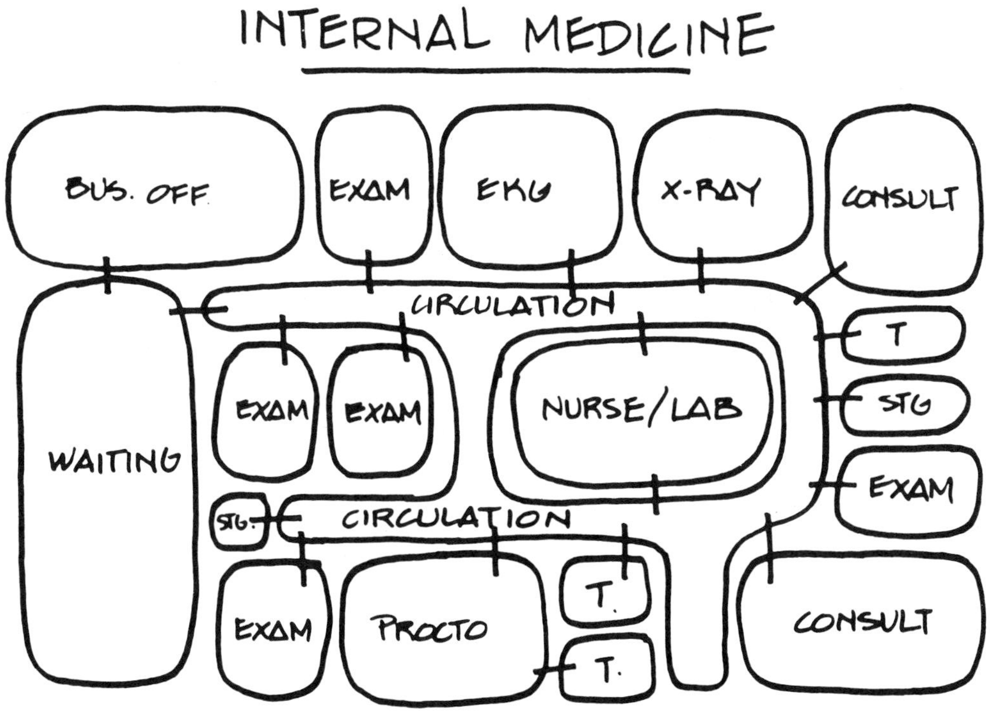

Figure 3-35. Schematic diagram of an internal medicine suite.

There is a lot of lab work associated with internal medicine, and one must determine which tests are to be done within the suite and which are to be sent out. If a substantial number of tests are to be done within the suite, a 12- × 12-foot minimum size lab should be set up. The reader is referred to Chapter 5, Small Laboratory, for further details.

An internist needs *three* exam rooms or *five* for each two physicians. Ten exam rooms should suffice for a

Table 3-2. Analysis of Program. Internal Medicine

No. of Physicians:	2		3		4	
Consultation	2 @ 12 × 12 =	288	3 @ 12 × 12 =	432	4 @ 12 × 12 =	576
Exam Rooms	5 @ 8 × 12 =	480	8 @ 8 × 12 =	768	10 @ 8 × 12 =	960
Waiting Room	14 × 18 =	252	18 × 20 =	360	23 × 24 =	552
Business Office	16 × 20 =	320	20 × 20 =	400	24 × 26 =	624
Office Manager	—		10 × 10 =	100	10 × 10 =	100
Nurse Stations	8 × 10 =	80	10 × 12 =	120	12 × 14 =	168
Toilets	2 @ 5 × 6 =	60	3 @ 5 × 6 =	90	4 @ 5 × 6 =	120
Storage	6 × 8 =	48	6 × 8 =	48	8 × 10 =	80
Proctoscopy Room[a]	12 × 15 =	180	12 × 15 =	180	12 × 15 =	180
Staff Lounge	10 × 12 =	120	10 × 12 =	120	12 × 12 =	144
Laboratory[b]	12 × 12 =	144	12 × 18 =	216	18 × 24 =	432
EKG	10 × 12 =	120	10 × 12 =	120	10 × 12 =	120
Pulmonary Function Lab	—		(optional)		14 × 16 =	224 (optional)
Radiology[c]	—		12 × 20 =	240	12 × 20 =	240
Subtotal	2092 ft²		3194 ft²		4520 ft²	
15% Circulation	314		479		678	
Total	2406 ft²		3673 ft²		5198 ft²	

[a]Includes prep area and toilet.

[b]Includes lab, lab waiting, and blood draw.

[c]Includes darkroom, control, film filing, radiology room, and viewing area.

group of five physicians, allowing that at least one person is absent at any time, and a second person may be absent for certain periods of the day.

A small X-ray room should be provided for films of the chest, gallbladder, etc. Usually the more involved gastrointestinal studies are referred to a radiologist.

A large storage room is needed for storing specialized, seldom used equipment and for storing X-ray film.

Electrocardiograph (EKG) Room

A large exam room (10 × 12 or 12 × 12 feet) may be provided for EKG studies. Some physicians dedicate a special room to this function, while others feel that dedicated rooms result in a loss of flexibility. Since the equipment is fairly portable, it can be moved from room to room as needed. A monitoring unit on a mobile cart is brought to the patient and electrodes attached to wires on the machine are placed on the patient's chest, leg, and wrist. The patient lies on a physical therapy-type table for this procedure. The instrument records the changes in electrical potential occurring during the heartbeat by photographing the vibrations and producing a printout — the electrocardiogram — which is then interpreted by the internist.

This type of EKG (where the patient lies supine) is called *static.* By contrast, a *dynamic* EKG involves an active patient whose heartbeat is monitored while walking on a motorized treadmill with remote control (Figure 3-36). The treadmill is not easy to move around, so if dynamic EKGs are done, it is better to locate the equipment in one room and leave it there.

An EKG room without a treadmill can be the size of a standard exam room (8 × 12 feet) with space for a 2- × 6-foot table for the patient to lie on, the monitoring equipment (Figure 3-37), a two-step footstool apparatus (Master's Exercise Toleration Technique — see Figure 3-38), and a 4-foot countertop area for mounting the printouts on cardboard holders. (Often the mounting area is outside of the EKG room. However, it should be noted that newer EKG units [Figure 3-37] use 8½- × 11-inch paper that does not need to be mounted.) If space permits, an alcove should be provided in which a patient can dress. A cabinet, located in the room, is used for storage of supplies associated with the procedure.

Echocardiography

Echocardiography is a noninvasive procedure that images the heart with ultrasound technology. The unit is portable and sits on a cart with a VCR and thermal video printer stored below (Figure 3-39).

This can be performed in any standard examination room, but it requires absolute quiet. The patient lies on a physical therapy-type table with the technician working from the patient's right side (Figure 3-40).

The sonographer listens to sounds as they're coming toward and away from the probe; thus, extraneous noise makes it difficult to isolate the sounds, although some sonographers wear headphones. "2-D Echo plus Doppler" means two-dimensional imaging (appears on a CRT) plus sound. It is important to be able to dim the room lights, and to be able to control light from a nearby window, in order to eliminate glare on the CRT screen. Additionally, there is a need for storage of echo tapes, which are VHS cassettes.

Holter Monitoring

Holter monitoring is a noninvasive procedure for recording cardiac activity on a 24-hour basis. Electrodes applied to the patient's chest are connected via lead

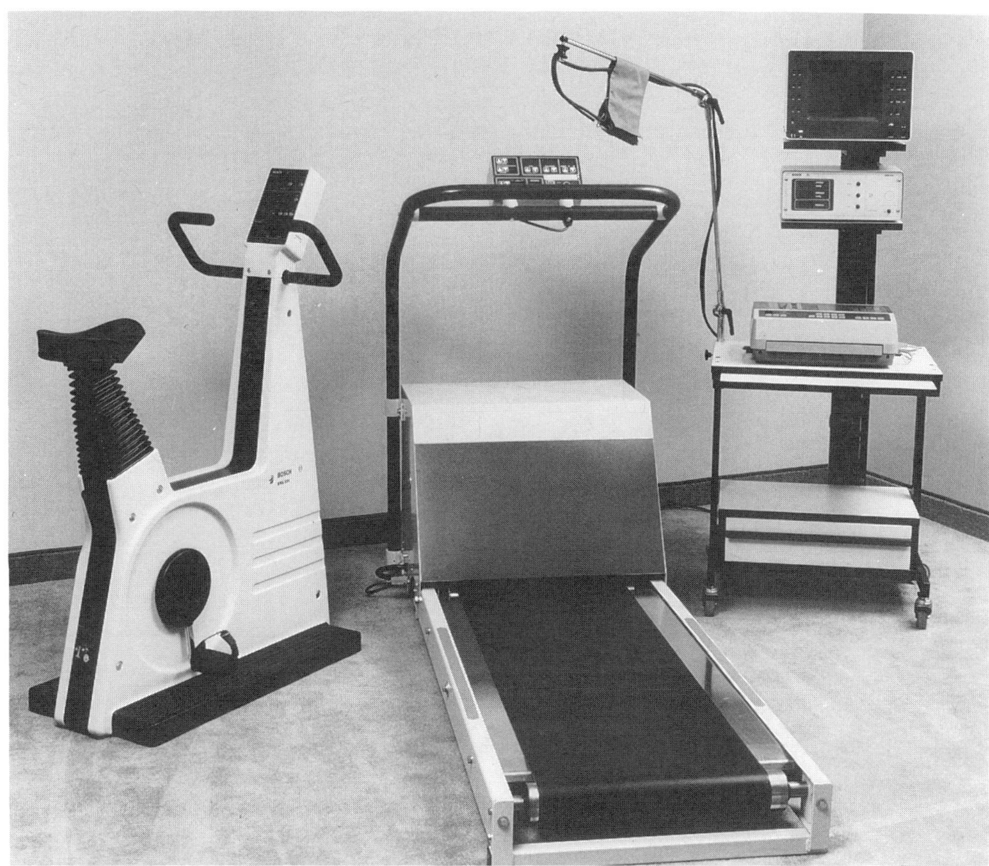

Figure 3-36. Constant Workload Stress Test system incorporating a bicycle ergometer, treadmill, and electrocardiograph unit. (*Courtesy Robert Bosch Corp., St. James, NY.*)

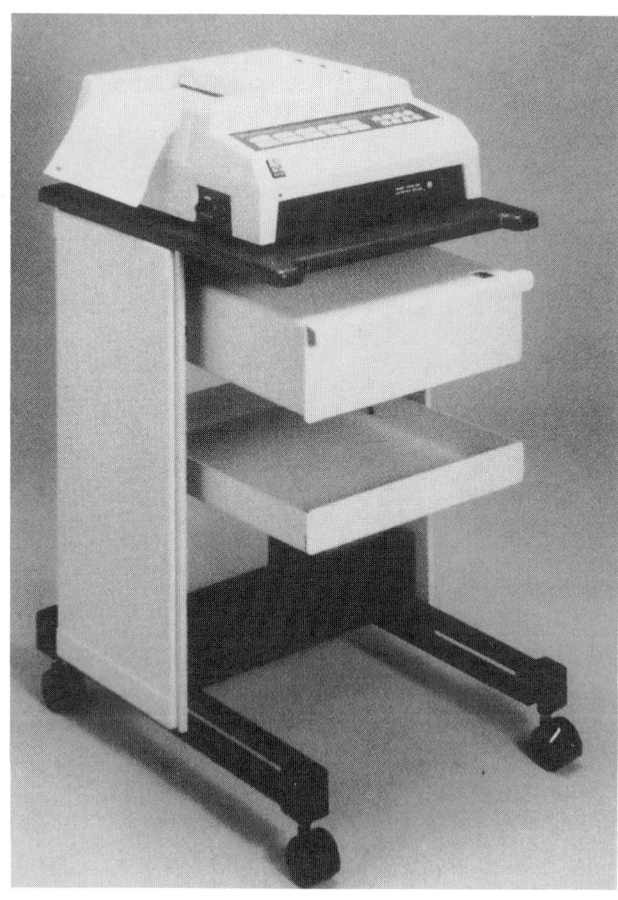

Figure 3-37. Electrocardiograph unit on cart. (*Courtesy Burdick, Milton, WI.*)

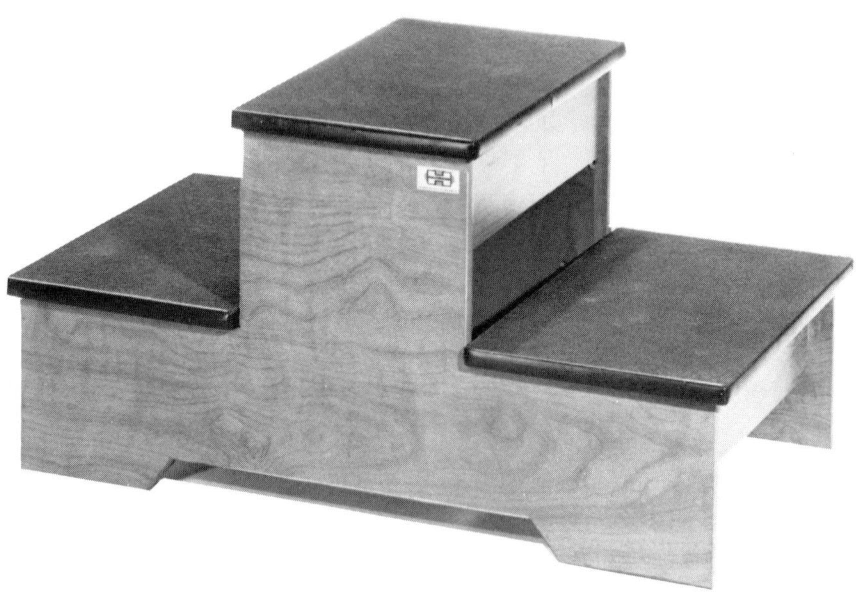

Figure 3-38. Master's two-step footstool for testing cardiac function. (*Courtesy Hausmann Industries, Inc., Northvale, NJ.*)

wires to a Holter recording unit worn on the patient's belt. The data is recorded on microcassettes or standard size audiocassettes, depending upon the individual unit. The patient returns to the office with the cassette, and the Holter tech then plays it on a Holter analyzer located at the workstation (Figure 3-41).

The patient can be fitted for the monitoring equipment in any standard exam room. A physical therapy–type table is adequate, and the room should have some cabinetry for storing supplies. The recorded cassettes can be stored in a storage room, or at the tech's workstation.

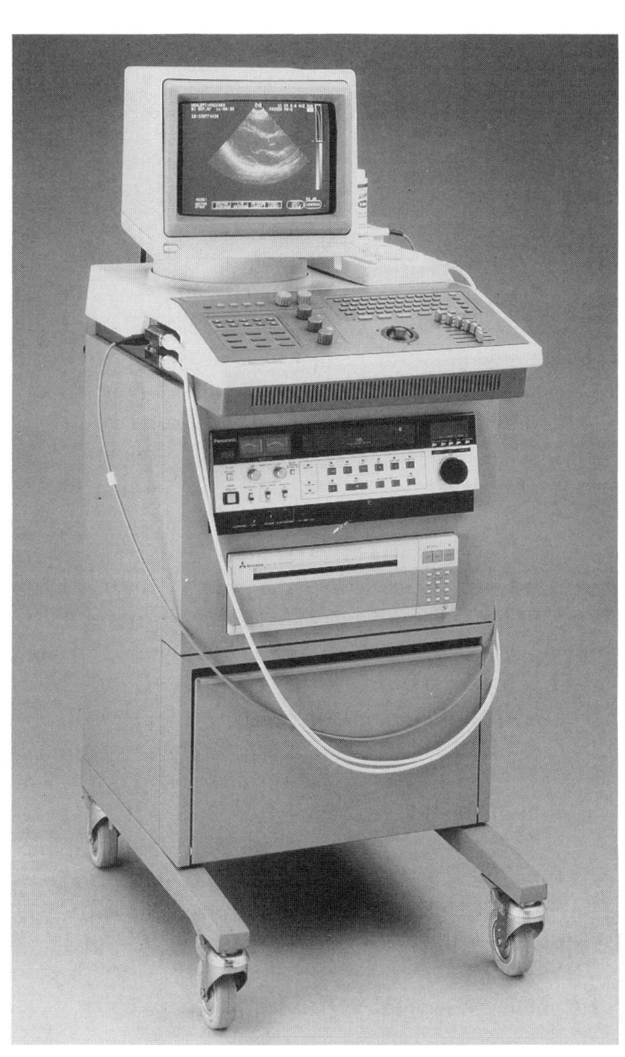

Figure 3-39. Echocardiography imaging system, *SONOS 100.* (*Courtesy Hewlett-Packard Co., Palo Alto, CA.*)

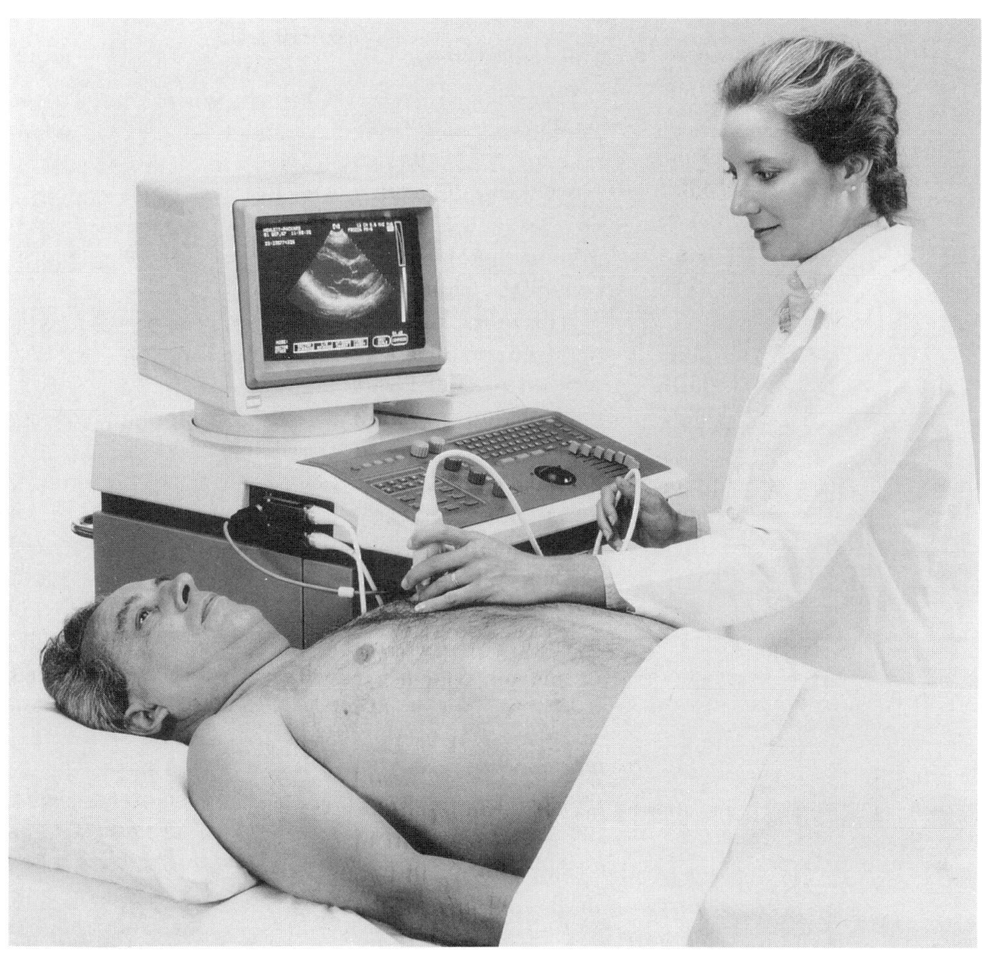

Figure 3-40. Echocardiography imaging system, *SONOS 100.* (*Courtesy Hewlett-Packard Co., Palo Alto, CA.*)

Vascular Lab

Diagnostic studies of the blood vessels are performed in a vascular lab to detect blood clots, calcium build-up, fatty deposits, and so forth. A vascular lab might be set up with two rooms, one for carotid artery studies of the neck, and one for studies of the extremities. A third room would be an office for the sonographers.

A three-room suite as described above might handle approximately 14 cases per day. The time required with each patient varies, but the norm is a 20- to 30-minute patient history-taking and 40- to 60-minute test period, followed by a 15-minute period of calculation and recording of data. Patients are usually gowned for tests, but procedures are noninvasive.

The carotid room uses a duplex Doppler ultrasonic imaging system (Figure 3-42). The room also needs a desk for the sonographer and a sink cabinet, with storage above, for supplies and for linen.

The extremities room generally utilizes a hospital-type bed that can tilt patients into various positions. There would be a treadmill alongside the tech's desk, with the treadmill telemetry unit on the desk. The duplex Doppler imaging scanner would be on one side of the bed. A resuscitation cart would be nearby. Other equipment would be a plethysmograph (records the volume changes of the limb) and a CRT to analyze the plethysmographic data. A printer is also required. The room needs to be large enough to accommodate all this equipment (Figure 3-43). The same consideration with respect to dimming of room lights, quiet, and control of glare, hold true in a vascular lab, as they do for echocardiography.

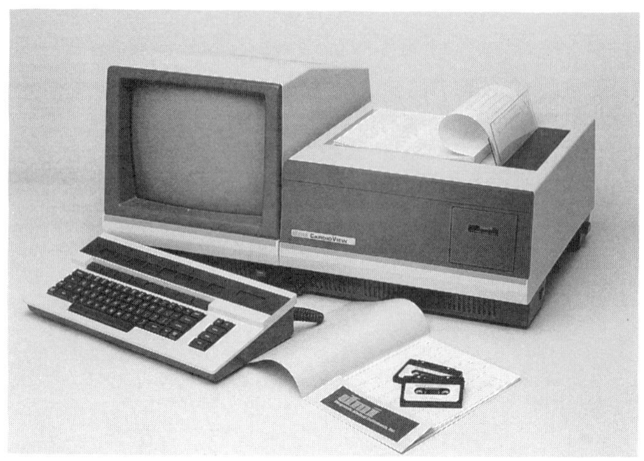

Figure 3-41. Holter analyzer, *CardioView* system. (*Courtesy DMI, Syracuse, NY; Photo layout: Paul J. Cowley & Associates, Inc.; Photography: David Revette Studios.*)

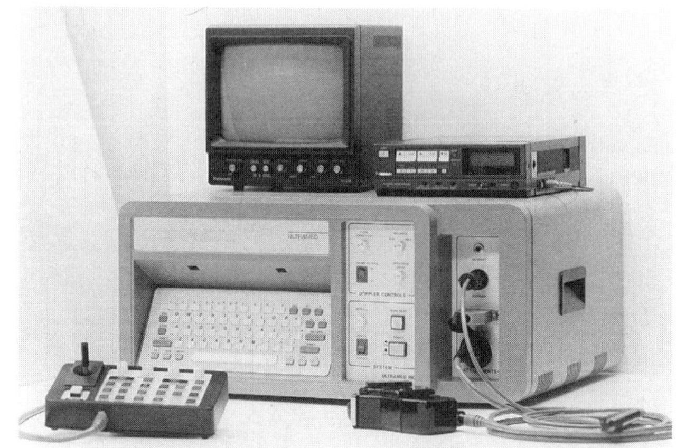

Figure 3-42. *Ultraplex II,* ultrasound imaging system for carotid bifurcation. (*Courtesy Ultramed, Inc., North Brunswick, NJ.*)

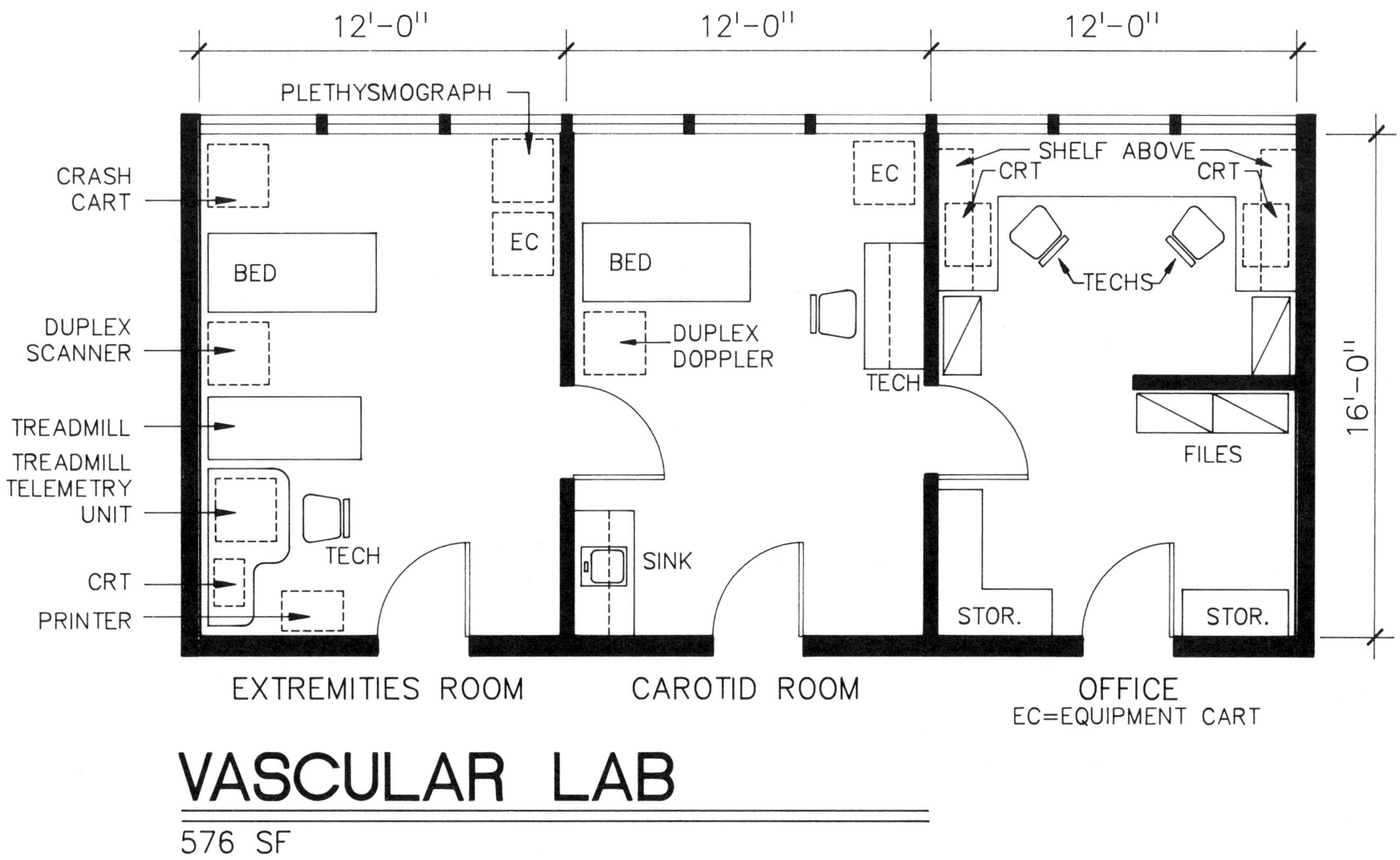

Figure 3-43. Layout of vascular lab.

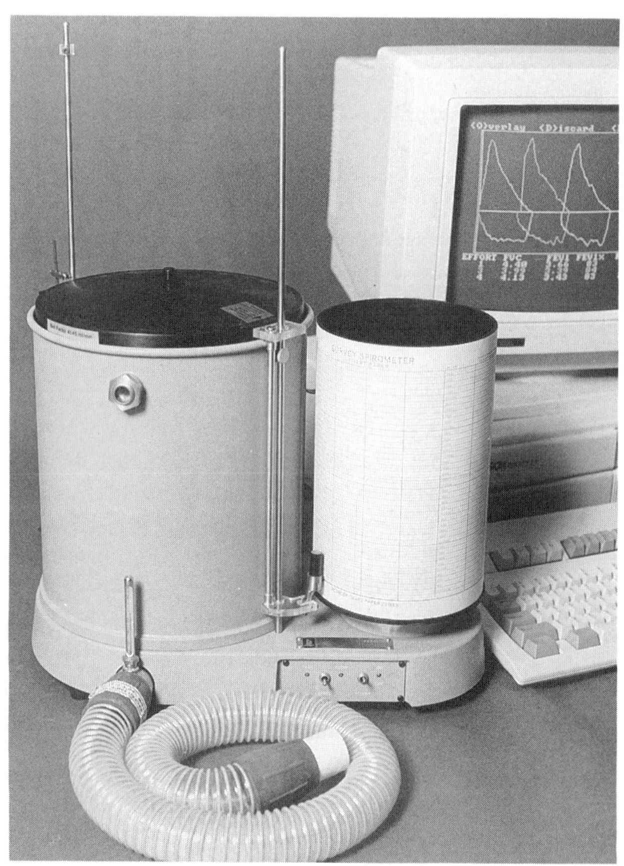

Figure 3-44. Spirometer with microcomputer to record and analyze data. (*Courtesy Warren E. Collins Inc., Braintree, MA.*)

Pulmonary Function Testing

People with impaired lung functions are diagnosed in the pulmonary function lab. The spirometer, an instrument for measuring the vital capacity of the lungs (Figure 3-44), is the basic tool for pulmonary function studies. It, along with an analysis of blood gases and other clinical tests, helps the physician to evaluate the extent and nature of lung damage. Often a bronchodilator medication is administered when spirometer studies are performed.

Pulmonary function studies are noninvasive and can be performed quickly and inexpensively with computer calculations and comparisons to predicted normal values. These studies allow the physician to monitor the course of disease and to measure the effects of therapeutic intervention.

Those seeking treatment may complain of shortness of breath, chronic cough, allergic manifestations, dizziness, or they may suffer from exposure to noxious dusts or fumes. Spirometry is generally included in annual routine health examinations, and it is required by law as part of the mandated screening program for people who are occupationally exposed to hazardous fumes. Pulmonary function tests (also called *PFT*) provide a quantitative estimation of lung impairment.

In addition to the *spirometer,* which measures *lung volume,* the microprocessor-controlled *pneumotachometer* (Figure 3-45) measures the *flow of expired air* from the lungs. Diagnostic instruments may be combined in a microprocessor-based system (Figure 3-46) that measures lung volume, residual volume, and diffusion (how gases pass into the blood).

The body *plethysmograph* (Figure 3-47) measures residual volumes, airway resistance and specific airway conductance. The technician sits outside to observe and coach the patient who is seated inside the pressure-type "body box." The unit is approximately 30 × 42 inches in size.

Once the patient has been screened, the treatment phase would be called *inhalation* or *respiratory ther-*

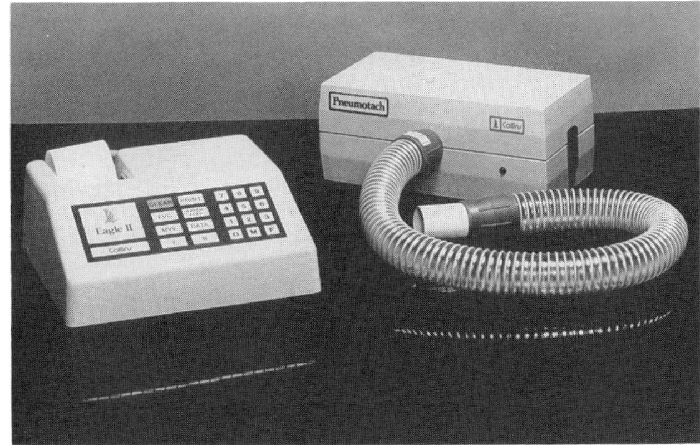

Figure 3-45. Microprocessor-controlled pneumotachometer measures flow of expired air from lungs. (*Courtesy Warren E. Collins Inc., Braintree, MA.*)

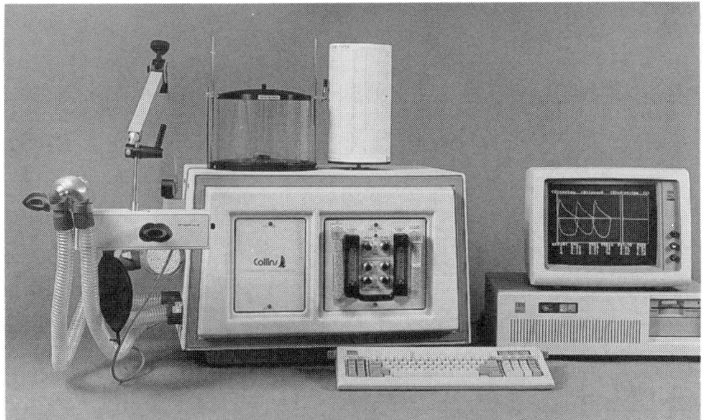

Figure 3-46. Pulmonary function testing system measures lung volume, residual volume, and diffusion. (*Courtesy Warren E. Collins Inc., Braintree, MA.*)

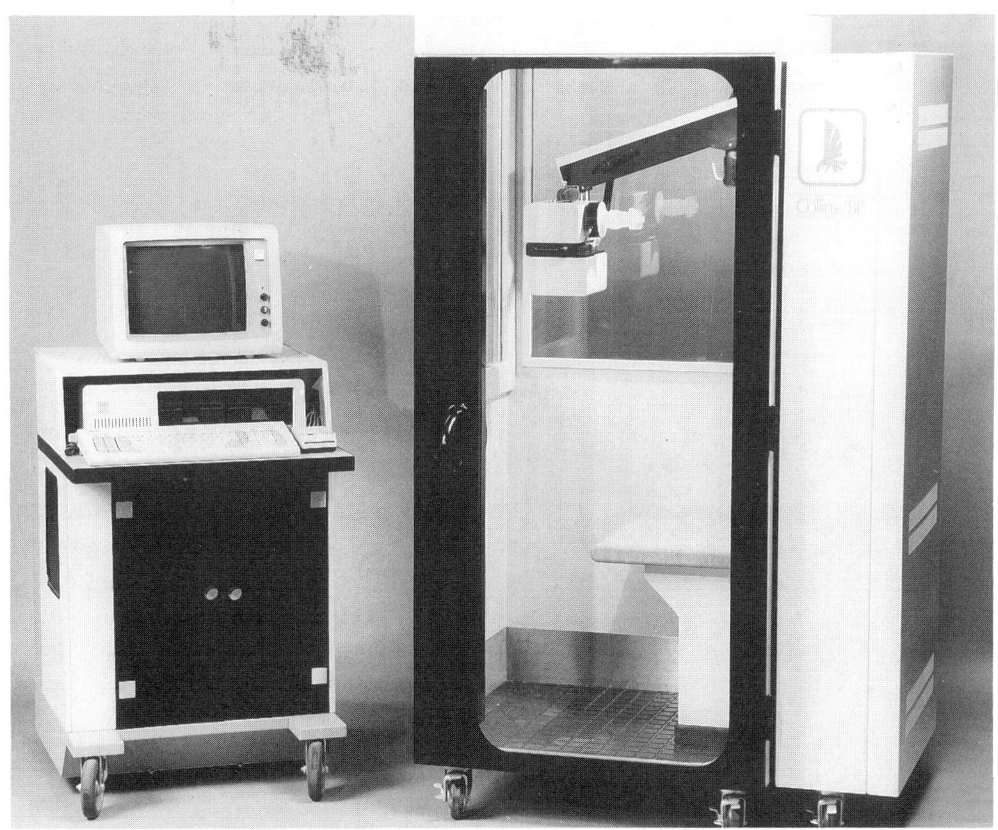

Figure 3-47. *PB/Plus* pressure plethysomograph measures residual volumes, airway conductance and specific airway conductance. (*Courtesy Warren E. Collins Inc., Braintree, MA.*)

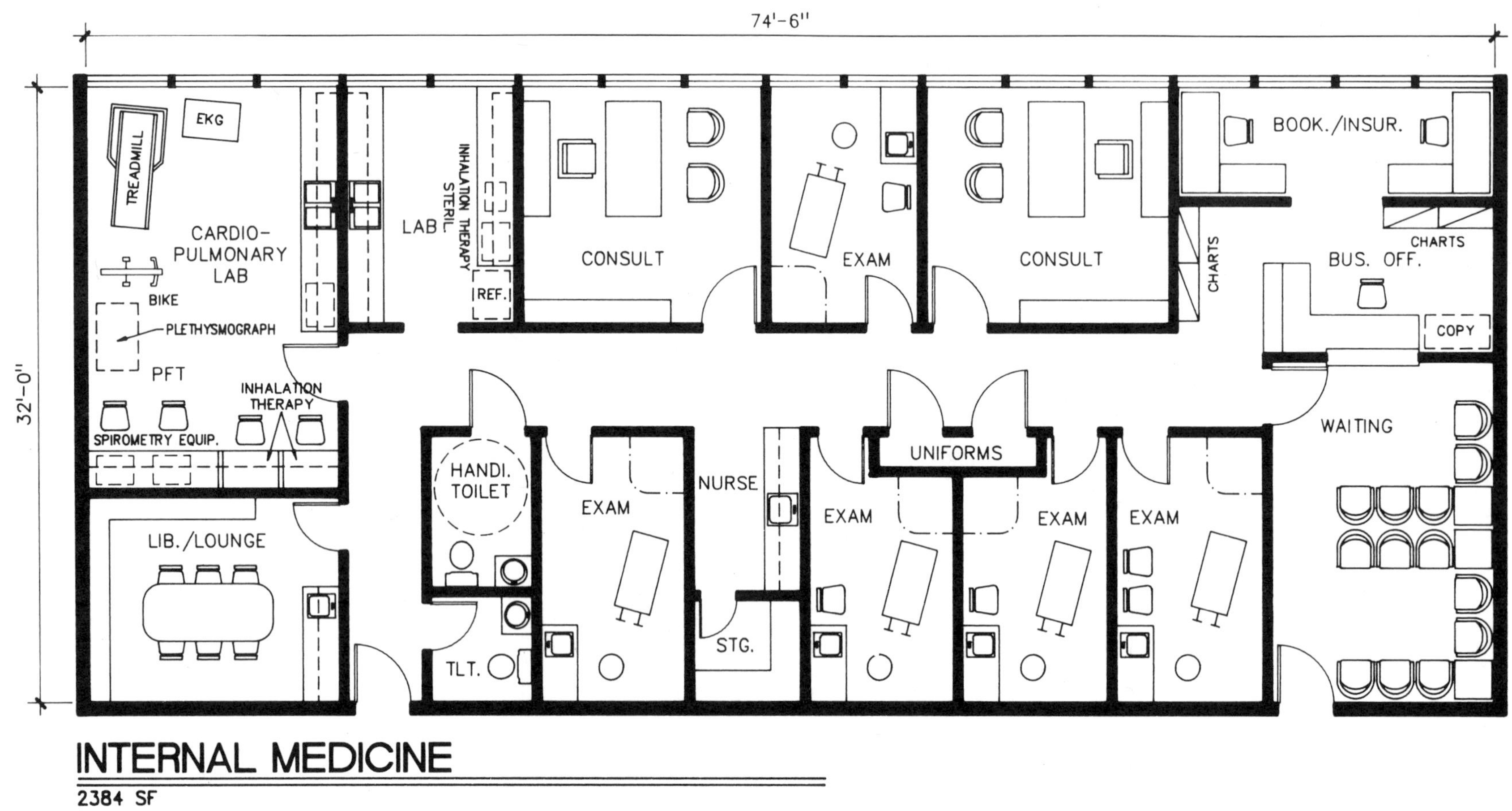

Figure 3-48. Suite plan for internal medicine, 2384 square feet.

apy. The treatment generally consists of breathing mechanically pressurized air with medication. The Bird inter-positive pressure breathing machine (see Figure 3-50) is a basic piece of equipment used in this type of therapy. The treatment might also consist of chest physiotherapy, in which a patient lies on an angled bed and gravity flow drains different lobes of the lung. The therapist, after administering bronchodilator medication, cups the patient's back, and the patient coughs up the mucus.

Layout of Rooms. There is not a generally accepted standard layout for a pulmonary function lab because it depends largely upon the specific pieces of equipment the practitioner has, whether inhalation therapy will be part of the lab, and whether cardiovascular screening will be included. In the last instance, it is called a cardiopulmonary lab. Figure 3-48 shows a layout in which PFT, respiratory therapy, and cardiopulmonary screening are done.

Typically, in such a combined usage, one might have two ergometric exercise bicycles, a treadmill with telemetry, one or two physical therapy–type tables, Holter, EKG, and PFT equipment, a crash cart with defibrillator and oxygen, desks for the respective techs, and a separate, quiet room for echocardiography. One may also find a computerized metabolic testing unit, (Figure 3-49) used primarily with an exercise bike, occasionally with a treadmill. It measures the cardiopulmonary stress response to a graduated workload.

Sometimes pulmonary function screening is separated from respiratory therapy. Pulmonologists may elect to do only the diagnostic testing in their office, and then refer the patient to a hospital or outpatient facility for the therapy. With so many variables, the pulmonologists and/or cardiologists must give the designer the parameters of their individual program before the designer can determine space requirements.

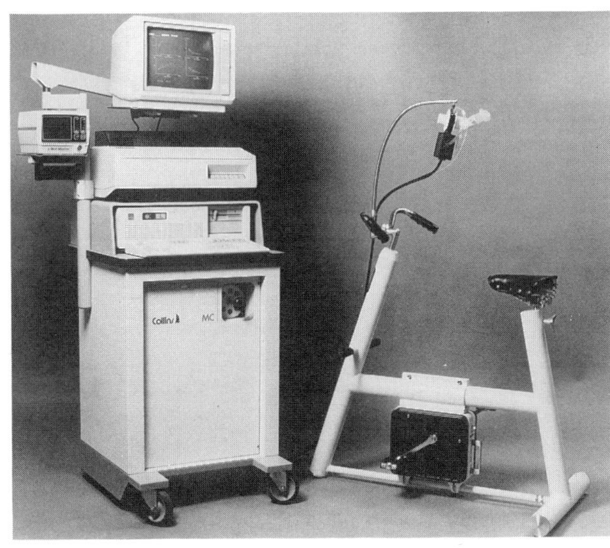

Figure 3-49. *MC/Plus* measures cardiopulmonary stress response to graduated workload challenge. (*Courtesy Warren E. Collins Inc., Braintree, MA.*)

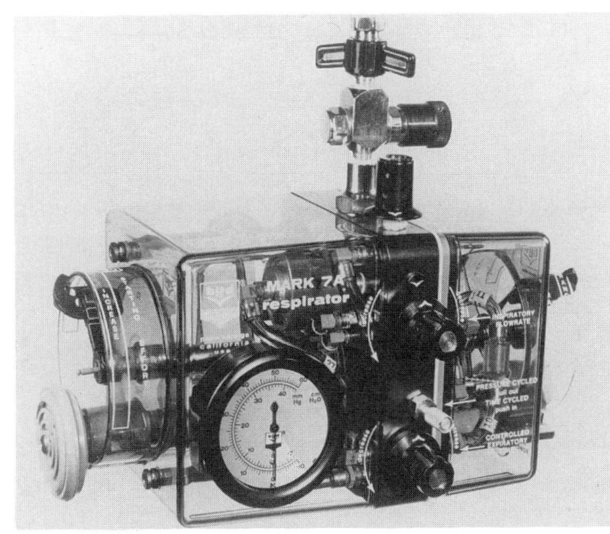

Figure 3-50. IPPB respirator. (*Courtesy Bird Corp., Palm Springs, CA.*)

If all the equipment is located in one large, common room, privacy curtains or partitions are desirable. Sometimes a cardiopulmonary lab is part of an executive health screening unit and, if so, a high-tech, high profile image is appropriate. Windows are not essential to this room, but would certainly be worthwhile. Carpeted floors and wallcoverings would soften the clinical appearance of the equipment.

Tech Work Areas

The technologists are specific to each type of diagnostic testing, and there isn't much cross-over. For the program described above, there would be four technologists: EKG, Holter, echocardiography, and pulmonary. They often have workstations or desks in the room with the equipment so they can monitor the patient while doing desk work. Their work areas need to have space for supplies used in the procedures, a place to store microcassettes or tapes of patients' test results, and file cabinets for computer printouts of test results.

Physicians' Consults

Physicians are always present when stress testing is done. Therefore, consultation rooms for the cardiologists and pulmonologists associated with the testing should be adjacent to the test area.

Inhalation Therapy

Pulmonary dysfunction may be acute or chronic. A patient recovering from pneumonia, for example, may need treatment once or twice for an acute problem, or a patient with lung cancer may need therapy twice a week for the remainder of his or her life. The composition of a pulmonary specialist's practice (age of patients, volume of patients, proximity to a hospital's outpatient respiratory therapy unit) will determine the number of individual therapy stations required. Only one spirometer is necessary even in a multistation facility, and it requires 2 to 3 feet of counter or tabletop space along with its related apparatus, or it can be on a mobile stand.

The individual IPPB (Inter-Positive Pressure Breathing) unit, a small metering device pressurized by a mechanical compressor or an oxygen tank (Figure 3-50), can be a mobile unit or can be set up at individual patient stations — a countertop area with the respirator mounted at eye level for the tech who has to adjust it. It can sit on a shelf or can be mounted on an arm. It is totally pneumatic and requires no electrical outlet. It cannot be built into a compartment because access is needed on all sides. A patient may be seated or lying down. If seated at a counter, there should be a waste receptacle and a tissue box dispenser, and surfaces (countertop and walls) should be easy to clean.

A large facility may process 2000 inhalation therapy patients in a month, with eight or ten individual stations. Or the facility may consist of just one room in an internist's office (Figure 3-48). Regardless of size, a separate sterilization area must be provided. Cold sterilization is used for mouthpieces, valves, fittings, and other apparatus. The items are first washed in soap and water, then put in a disinfectant solution, rinsed, and air dried on a towel or a drying rack alongside the sink.

A standard double-compartment sink is adequate. A small gas sterilizer unit may also be used. Today, labs use disposable supplies whenever possible, negating the need for sterilization. This volume of disposable "setups" (mouthpieces, hoses, etc.) demands a large well-designed storage/prep room with shelves and cabinets sized to accommodate the cartons in which the disposables are packed.

As with any clinical laboratory contained within an internist's suite, if it is large enough to process a high volume of patients daily, it should have its own waiting area, bathroom, supervisor's office, and storage room.

Proctology Room

Most internal medicine suites will have a proctology room for rectal and intestinal examinations, approximately 10 × 12 feet, adjacent to a toilet room, and with a small area (4 × 4 feet) for preparation nearby (Figure 3-51). The examination table used for a proctoscopy procedure is larger than a standard exam table and is motorized to adjust to Trendelenberg position (Figure 3-52). These procedures are called sigmoidoscopy.

Some physicians think that procto rooms are an outdated concept, preferring to do sigmoidoscopies in an endoscopy suite. Others feel that procto rooms are still necessary, because a patient need not be prepped or "clean" for that procedure. By contrast, a patient must be totally prepped — give a medication that totally cleans out the colon — prior to endoscopy. In a procto exam, the scope only enters the colon 15 cm., whereas in full colonoscopy, the scope can penetrate 6 feet.

Some internists will do procto exams in a minor treatment room. A patient suspected of having intestinal amoebas, for example, could be readily examined and diagnosed that same day with a procto examination, and not have to be rescheduled for a more complicated endoscopic examination, after the colon has been prepped. Therefore many internists will still want to be able to do proctoscopic exams in their office.

In summary, a large internal medicine suite (5000 to 7000 square feet) will have a proctoscopy room, an EKG room, a large lab with its own waiting room, blood draw, toilet with specimen pass-through, and storage. Certain types of X-rays may be done in the office and, if so, an X-ray room with adjoining darkroom and film viewing area will be included in the suite. The business office in a suite of this size will be composed of separate rooms for transcription, business manager, insurance, medical records, bookkeeper, and receptionist. A staff lounge should also be included. The reader is referred to Chapter 6, Group Practice, for guidance in designing suites of this size.

Endoscopy

The development of fiber optics has made possible the examination of the colon, the lungs (bronchoscopy), and the upper gastrointestinal tract with an endoscope. These are 4- to 5-foot long flexible "tubes" with an eyepiece and powerful fiber optic light at one end that transmits light down the tube to enable the internist to examine the colon, for example, in search of tumors or polyps.

These procedures are often done in an internist's office or in an ambulatory surgical center. Flexible sigmoidoscopies (examinations of the lower portion of the colon) do not require sedation, and they are often performed as part of a comprehensive physical examination for people over the age of 45. With an endoscope, as opposed to a proctoscope, the physician can enter the colon much farther and see a great deal more. However, to examine the full colon, called colonoscopy, the patient is sedated. A recovery room would be needed only when patients have been sedated.

Components of an Endoscopy Suite. An endoscopy suite would include:

- procedure rooms
- dressing area with lockers for M/F staff
- dressing area with lockers for patients
- bathrooms
- workroom between procedure rooms

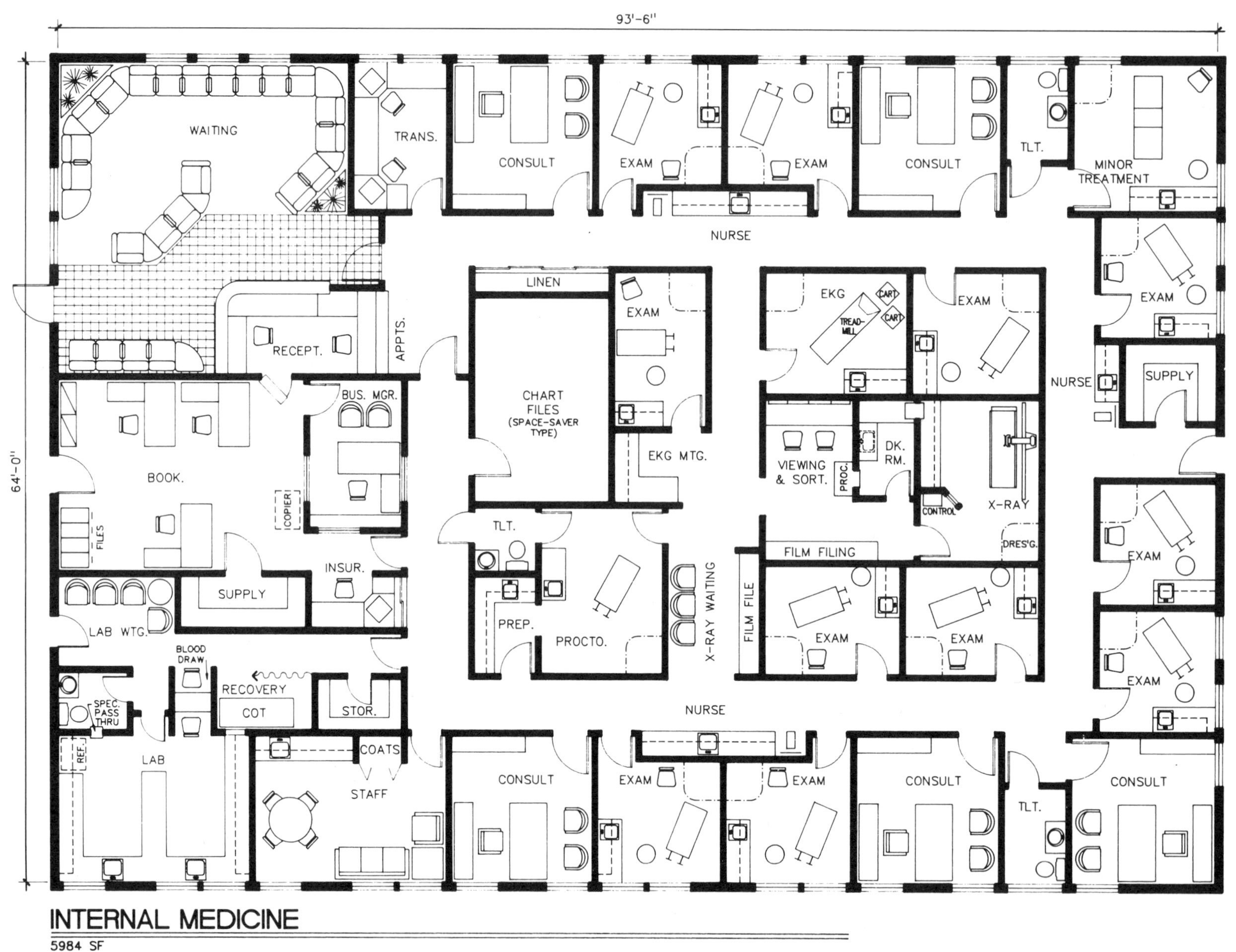

Figure 3-51. Suite plan for internal medicine, 5984 square feet.

- recovery area
- physicians' dictation/charting
- reception/administration/waiting
- linen storage

In a large outpatient clinic, one might find a layout of rooms similar to that shown in Figure 3-53. Yet an internist could perform certain procedures, not requiring sedation, in a 12- × 12-foot special procedures room with an adjacent 8- × 10-foot cleanup/workroom.

The number of procedure rooms is related to the projected volume of cases. Some pulmonary physicians prefer a dedicated room for bronchoscopy, not wanting to do these procedures in the same room where lower GIs are performed. This seems to be an emotional issue, as informed sources have told the author they know of no clinical studies showing that patients were compromised by performing both types of procedures in the same room. This is especially true since the colon is always prepped and "clean" prior to the examination. (As a point of information, endoscopy procedure rooms are not considered sterile.) However, there is a benefit to having dedicated rooms when a high volume of physicians use the facility, and a high volume of cases exists. Many hospitals, in fact, separate rooms by function in order to do more procedures simultaneously and to facilitate scheduling with physicians.

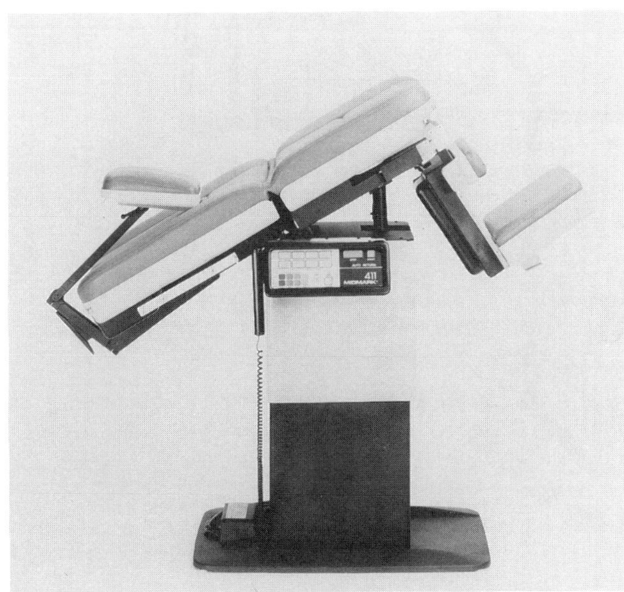

Figure 3-52. Proctoscopy table. (*Courtesy Midmark Corp., Versailles, OH.*)

Room lighting is darkened during the procedure. A combination of indirect perimeter lighting, that could be dimmed, combined with standard 2 × 4 fluorescents overhead, when more light is required, would be ideal. A ceiling-mounted surgical light may or may not be required. An adjustable table is used, and a patient would generally be transferred onto the table from a gurney. An under-cabinet "valance" light, which doesn't shine in the physician's eyes, is desirable over the sink cabinet.

Procedure rooms (Figure 3-54) must be large enough to accommodate a resuscitation cart, an endoscopy cart, and storage of clean and soiled linen (the soiled linen hamper could be a hinged bin built into the base of the fixed cabinet). X-ray view boxes and a clock with second hand are required. The floor should be sheet vinyl or vinyl composition tile. The door to the room must be wide enough to accommodate a gurney. Depending upon the procedures being performed, the rooms may need compressed air, oxygen, and suction.

There will usually be one large procedure room equipped with a C-arm X-ray unit (Figure 3-55) for doing fluoroscopy. This room would need lead shielding.

Workroom. This is one of the most important rooms in the suite. All equipment is cleaned and readied for use in this room. Supplies are stored here, as are the cleaned scopes, which are typically hung in a long cab-

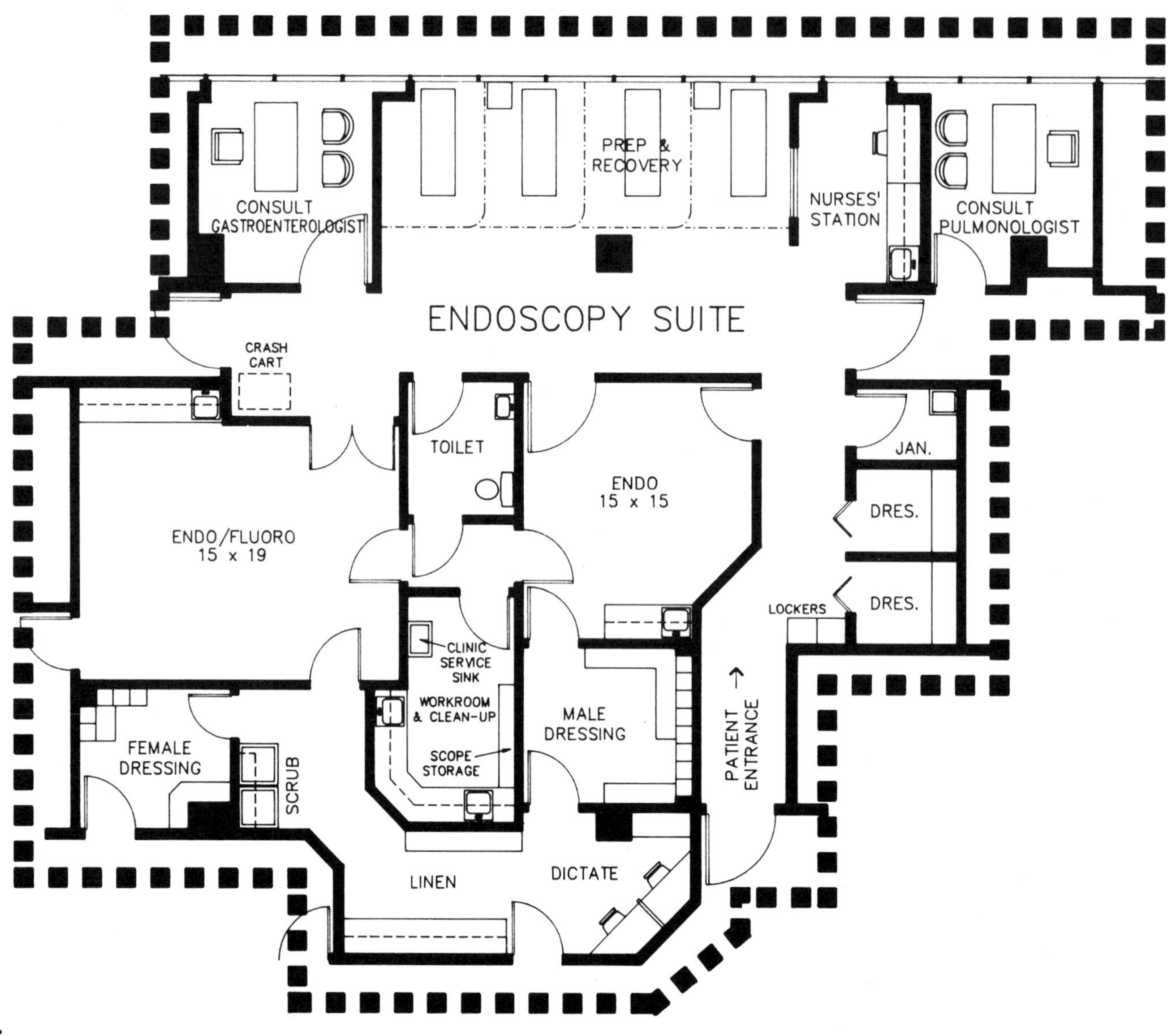

ENDOSCOPY SUITE

2170 SF

Figure 3-53. Layout of endoscopy suite, 2170 square feet.

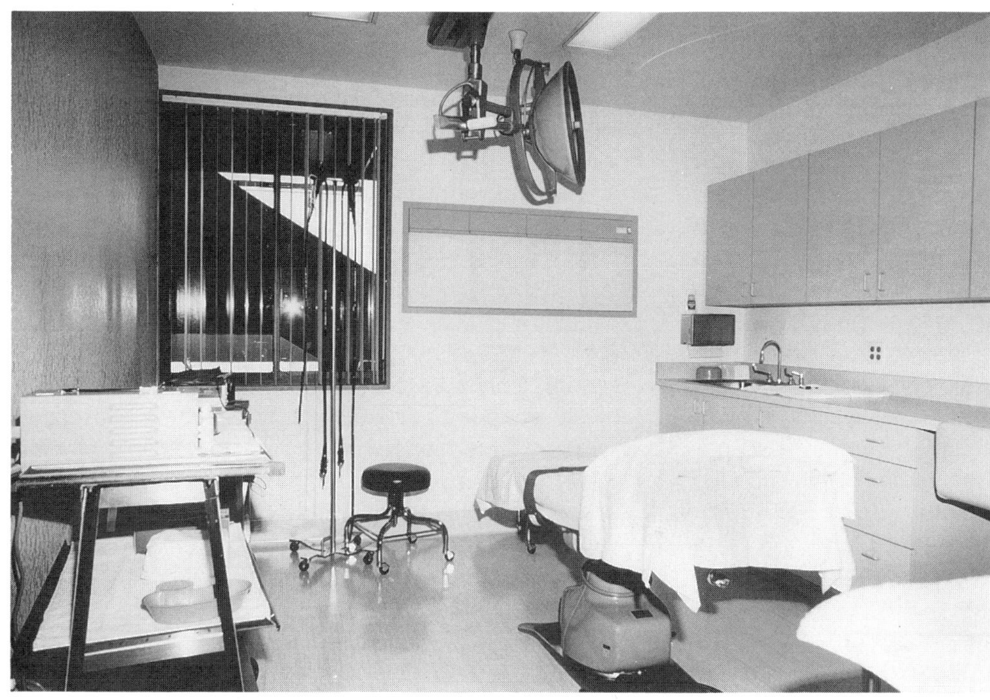

Figure 3-54. Endoscopy procedure room. (*Design: Jain Malkin Inc.; Photographer: Jain Malkin.*)

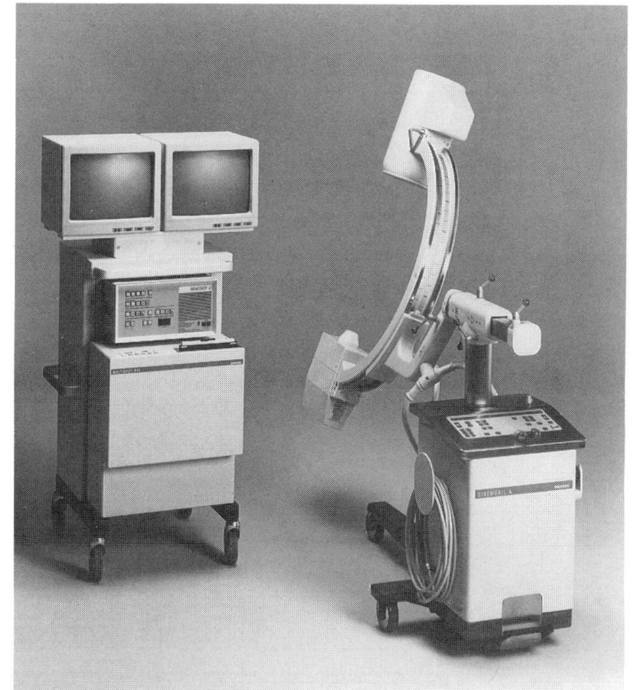

Figure 3-55. Multiformat "spot" camera with TV monitors (left) and C-arm X-ray imaging unit (right). (*Courtesy Siemens Medical Systems, Inc., Iselin, NJ.*)

inet with glass doors. Scopes are very expensive, and are handled with great care.

Some technicians like two double sinks, one for cleaning scopes used on upper G.I. and bronchoscopy procedures, and the other for lower G.I.s. The sinks would be set into countertops at right angles to each other. The sinks need to be deep and should be *lower* than the standard 36-inch high countertop. For most people, a 30-inch height is fine. As the scopes are long and require quite a bit of handling to properly clean, the lowered sink is more comfortable. Sometimes the workroom has a flush-type clinic service sink.

The nurse spends about 20 minutes washing scopes after each procedure. The nurse also preps each patient. Therefore, it is unlikely the same person can also keep an eye on recovering patients.

The workroom needs compressed air for drying scopes and suction. Somewhere in the suite, if not in the workroom, there need to be deep cabinets for storing disposables, room for the scope transport cases (these look like hard-shell briefcases), and shelves for large binders for storing the forceps used in biopsies. Each forceps is specific to each size scope, and these are often color-coded by the staff into binders, for easy retrieval.

The workroom is a busy area, packed with instruments, sterilization equipment, bottles of solutions, racks, and more. It can easily become cluttered, and therefore the room size should not be underestimated.

Recovery Room. The recovery room is standard in all respects, with oxygen and suction at each bed, and privacy curtains separating each patient. Recovery time is normally an hour, and recovering patients should be in view of nursing staff.

Interior Design

The interior design of an internal medicine suite should be tailored to the functional needs of the patient population. If the internist is a cardiologist, for example, or a pulmonologist, those patients will, for the most part, be elderly. Therefore, a conservative color palette and furnishings would be appropriate. An oncologist, on the other hand, would have a broad age range of patients and a more upbeat design might be in order. Color Plate 2, Figure 3-56, is a waiting room of a cardiac surgeon's office. Patients visit the office preoperatively and postoperatively, on two or three afternoons a week. The remainder of the time, the office is a home away from home for the surgeons — a place to relax, sleep, prepare slides for lectures, and to meet with colleagues to discuss cases.

Specific interior design requirements for this specialty are given in Chapter 4.

PEDIATRICS

A pediatrician treats children from birth through adolescence. The office visits are frequent and of relatively short duration in the exam room, but frequently involve a protracted period of time in the waiting room. This is a high-volume specialty, and the practice is almost always composed of two or more physicians. It is rare to find more than three pediatricians working in the same office, although a busy practice may staff a second or third office.

Waiting Room

Waiting rooms must be larger than for other specialties, as parents often bring all their children and sometimes a grandparent, when one child has to visit the doctor. Pediatric offices often have a *sick-baby,* or contagious, waiting room and a *well-baby* waiting room. The basis for this is to limit contagion. Since physicians rarely make house calls, children with infectious disease are brought into the office, where well children who are waiting for a routine checkup or an injection are vulnerable to contracting it.

If space is limited, a sick-baby waiting room can be devised by direct entry into an exam room (Figure 3-58). One exam room would have a door to the outside or building corridor, as the case may be, and would have a buzzer or bell to summon the nurse for entry. The nurse would tell the mother, over the phone, to come to that door and buzz. The door would be marked *Contagious Entrance.* The sick-baby exam should be near a toilet, and the room must have a sink.

If the suite is large enough to have a contagious waiting room, one exam room in close proximity to the waiting room should be designed as a sick-baby exam room, with a sink cabinet and a toilet nearby. The other exam rooms should be clustered around the nurse station (Figure 3-59).

In this specialty, it is a good idea to have a toilet accessible from the waiting room so that parents may change diapers in advance of entering the exam room, and the staff is not continually interrupted in order to direct children to the bathroom (Figure 3-60). The bathroom should have a sink countertop large enough to change diapers on, a shelf for disposable diapers, talcum and paper towels, and a large trash receptacle.

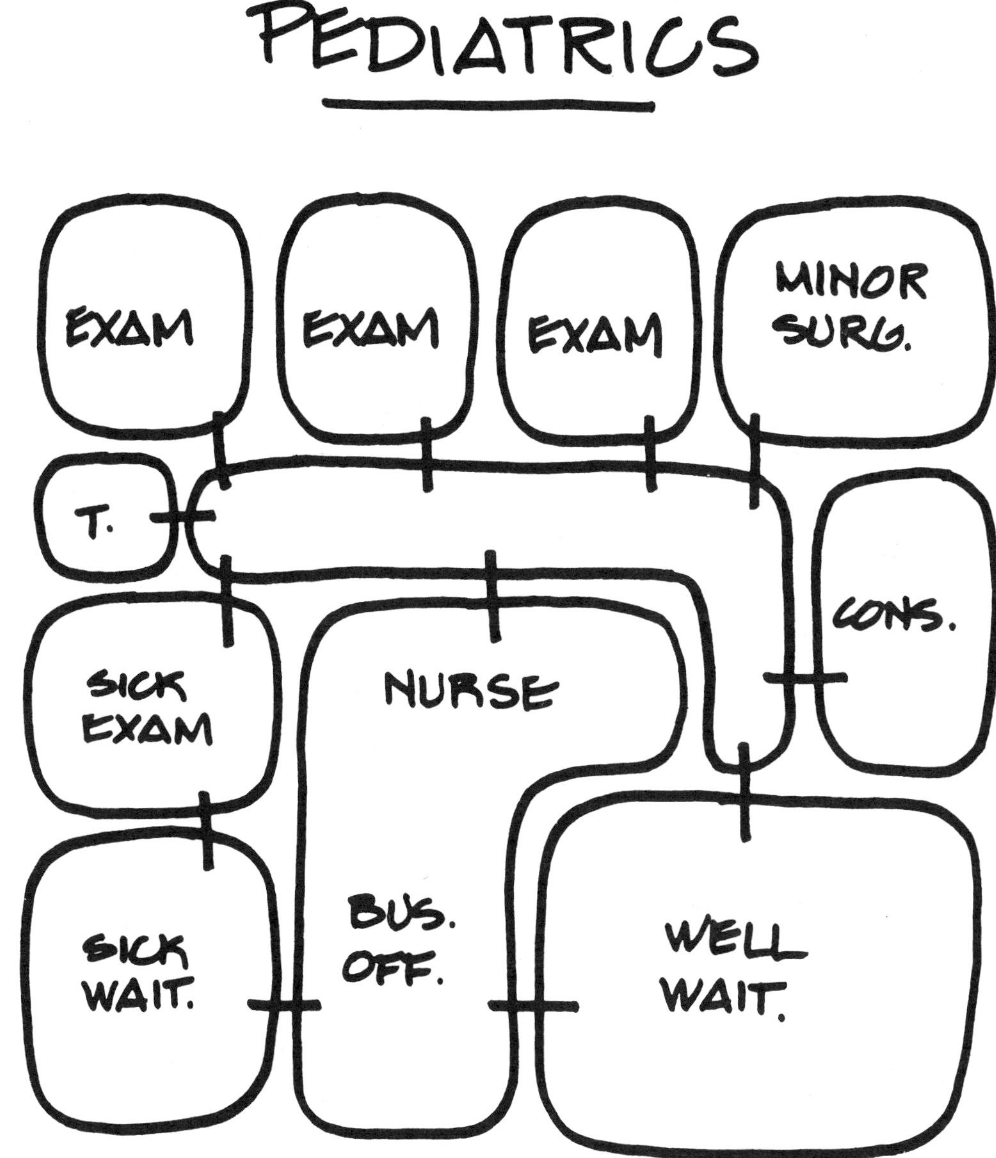

Figure 3-57. Schematic diagram of a pediatrics suite.

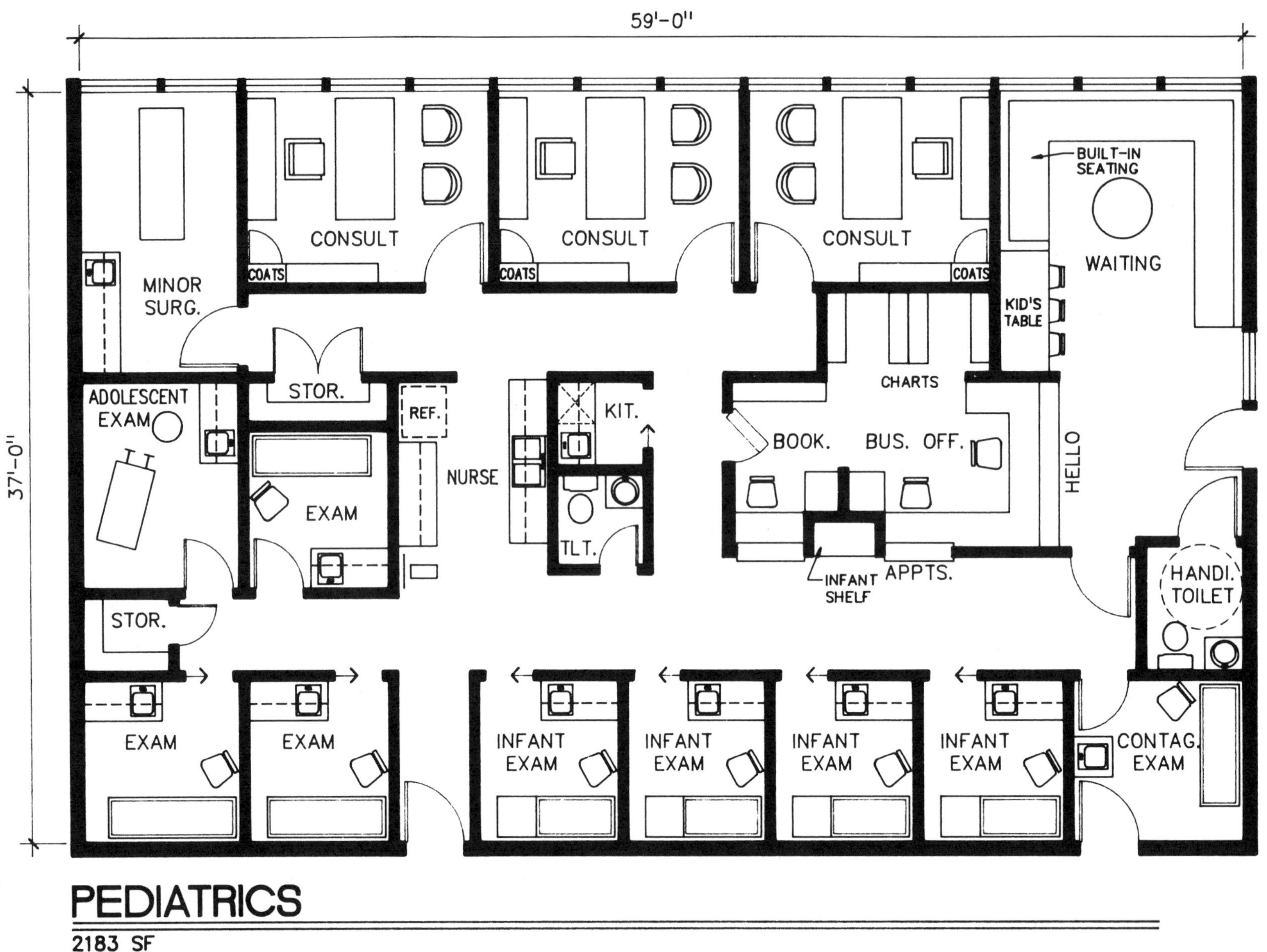

Figure 3-58. Suite plan for pediatrics, 2183 square feet.

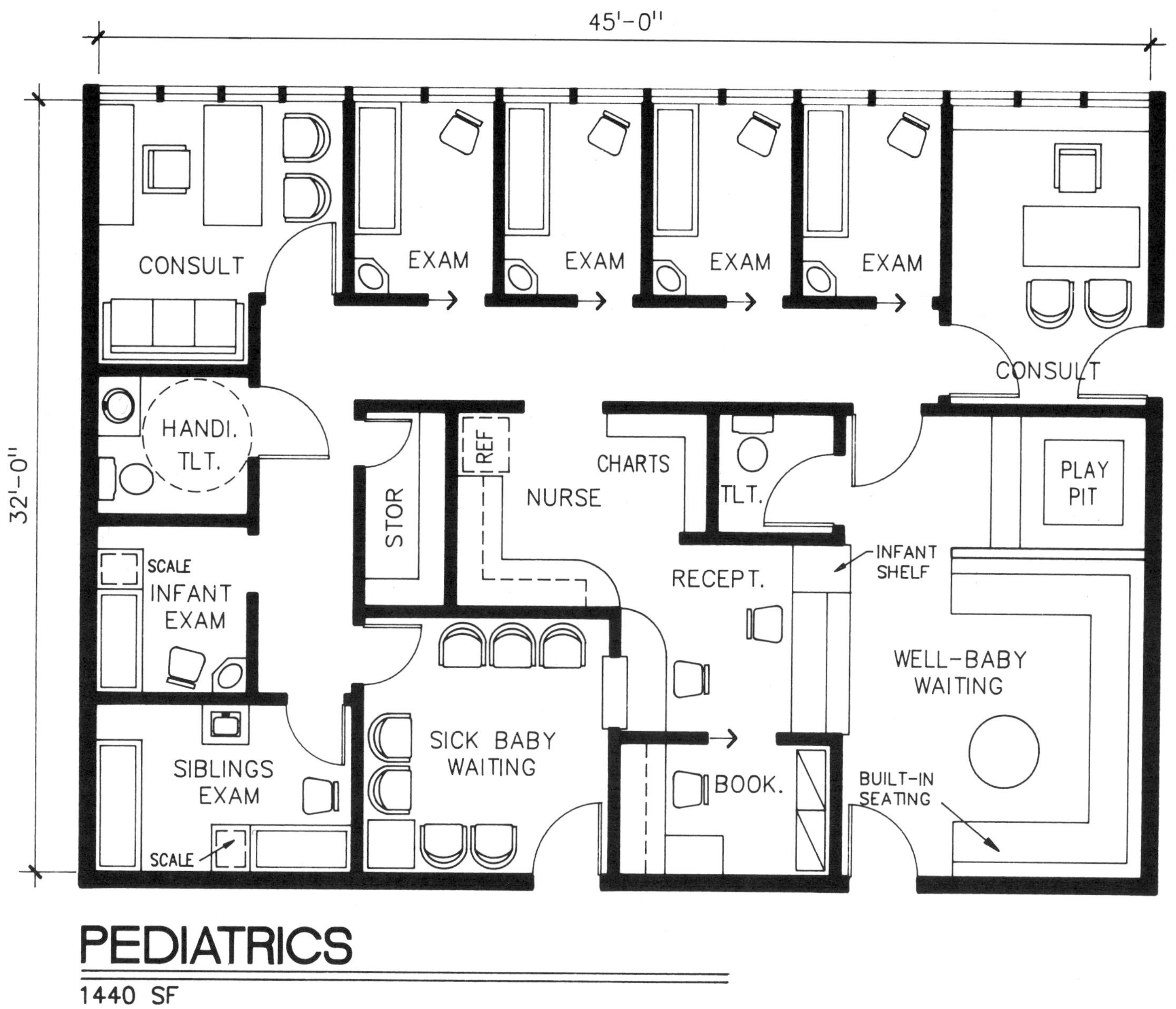

Figure 3-59. Suite plan for pediatrics, 1440 square feet.

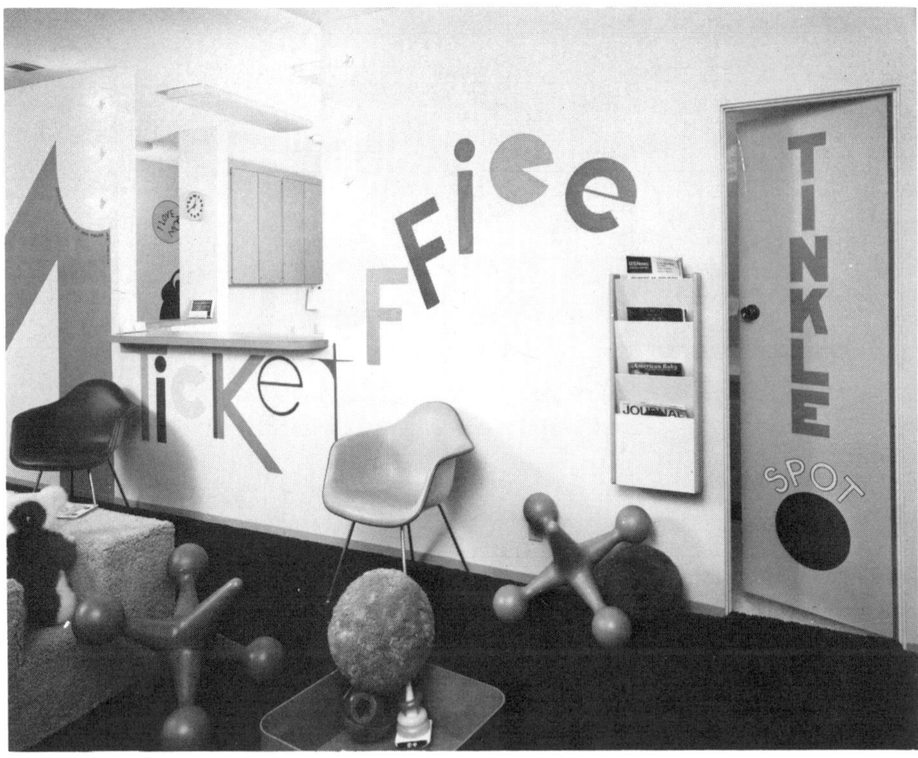

Figure 3-60. Pediatric reception area. (*Design: Jain Malkin Inc.; Photographer: John Waggaman.*)

Table 3-3. Analysis of Program. Pediatrics

No. of Physicians:	2		3	
Business Office	12 × 16 =	192	14 × 18 =	252
Examining Rooms[a]	6 @ 6 × 8 =	288	9 @ 6 × 8 =	432
Adolescent Exam	8 × 12 =	96	8 × 12 =	96
Toilets	2 @ 5 × 6 =	60	2 @ 5 × 6 =	60
Consultation Room	2 @ 10 × 12 =	240	3 @ 10 × 12 =	360
Nurse Station	8 × 12 =	96	12 × 12 =	144
Waiting Room/Sick-Baby	12 × 12 =	144	12 × 14 =	168
Well-Baby	18 × 20 =	360	22 × 26 =	572
Storage	6 × 6 =	36	6 × 6 =	36
Subtotal		1512 ft²		2120 ft²
15% Circulation		227		318
Total		1739 ft²		2438 ft²

[a]Note: Designer may wish to make one exam room 10 × 12 feet for use as a minor surgery room, as well as provide a staff lounge, if space permits.

Doctors disagree on the practicality of having a child's-height drinking fountain in the waiting room. If the room is not well supervised, it can lead to problems.

The waiting room should contain some tables or flat areas built into the seating where parents can put down an infant in a carrier without occupying an adult's seat (Figure 3-61). A pediatric waiting room may be as large as space and budget permit. Each patient is accompanied by one to three people. Children can get pretty rowdy playing in a pediatrician's waiting room, so an effort should be made to occupy them with something unique. A special seating unit or climbing play structure (see Color Plate 4, Figure 4-3, and Figures 3-62 and 3-64) can be designed.

Built of plywood, and padded and upholstered with carpet, these custom-built units appeal to children's need for physical movement. Their pent-up energy can be released while climbing through tunnels and hiding in "secret" compartments (Figure 3-63). In fact, a waiting room that is designed imaginatively can be so appealing to children that it results in tantrums when it is time to leave! Custom play furniture must be designed to eliminate sharp corners and edges against which a toddler may fall and become injured.

The waiting room should also contain bins for toys, and magazine racks, at a height accessible to children. Pediatricians disagree in their choice of toys for this room. More conservative physicians tend to feel that toys spread infection (drooling on toys, fingers in mouth, etc.) and will limit the type of amusements they condone. Younger pediatricians seem to be more relaxed and iconoclastic (many refuse to wear white coats, which may frighten children) and feel that germs are everywhere and inevitable. If a child is not exposed to germs in the office, he or she will surely be exposed to infection from playmates.

In a pediatric waiting room, one may break the rule about providing individual chairs. One may take liberties in furnishings here, since it is a homogeneous population — mostly parents from the same neighborhood, approximately the same age, and sharing a common interest — their children. Thus parents do not seem to mind sitting next to each other in continuous (common seat and back) seating. Figure 3-65 shows the author's solution for adult seating, which saves space and accommodates a maximum number of people in a small waiting room. Whatever the type of seating provided, one may wish to provide a few standard-height chairs, with arms, for pregnant women, who often find it difficult to get out of low, lounge-type seating.

Other design ideas for the waiting area include a large tackboard for display of patients' artwork, or for display of baby photos. Colorful wall murals of fanciful characters would be appropriate (Figures 3-68 and 3-71). A magnetized tic-tac-toe board or a chalkboard may be considered. But even with dustless chalk, the erasers make quite a mess. There is no end to the fanciful design ideas that can be implemented in a pediatric office. (See Figures 3-69 through 3-73.) The reader is referred to Chapter 12 for additional information on furnishings and interior finish specifications.

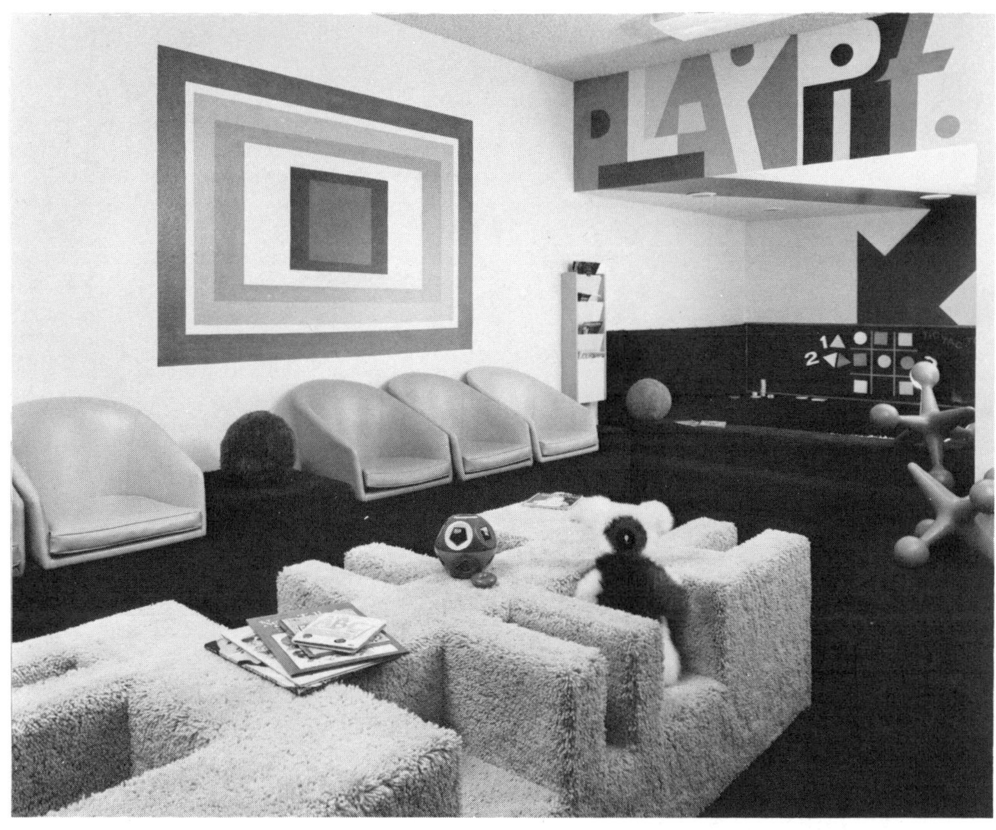

Figure 3-61. Pediatric waiting room: Note magnetized tic-tac-toe board at rear of playpit. (*Design: Jain Malkin Inc.; Photographer: John Waggaman.*)

Examination Rooms

Number of Exam Rooms. Each pediatrician should have a minimum of three exam rooms, but four is better. It is important to plan for growth. A pediatric practice grows rapidly, and before long, a two-physician practice with five or six exam rooms will be able to use eight. Thus the designer should guide the client at the outset to lease a large enough space. Since examinations are short, the physician can quickly move on to

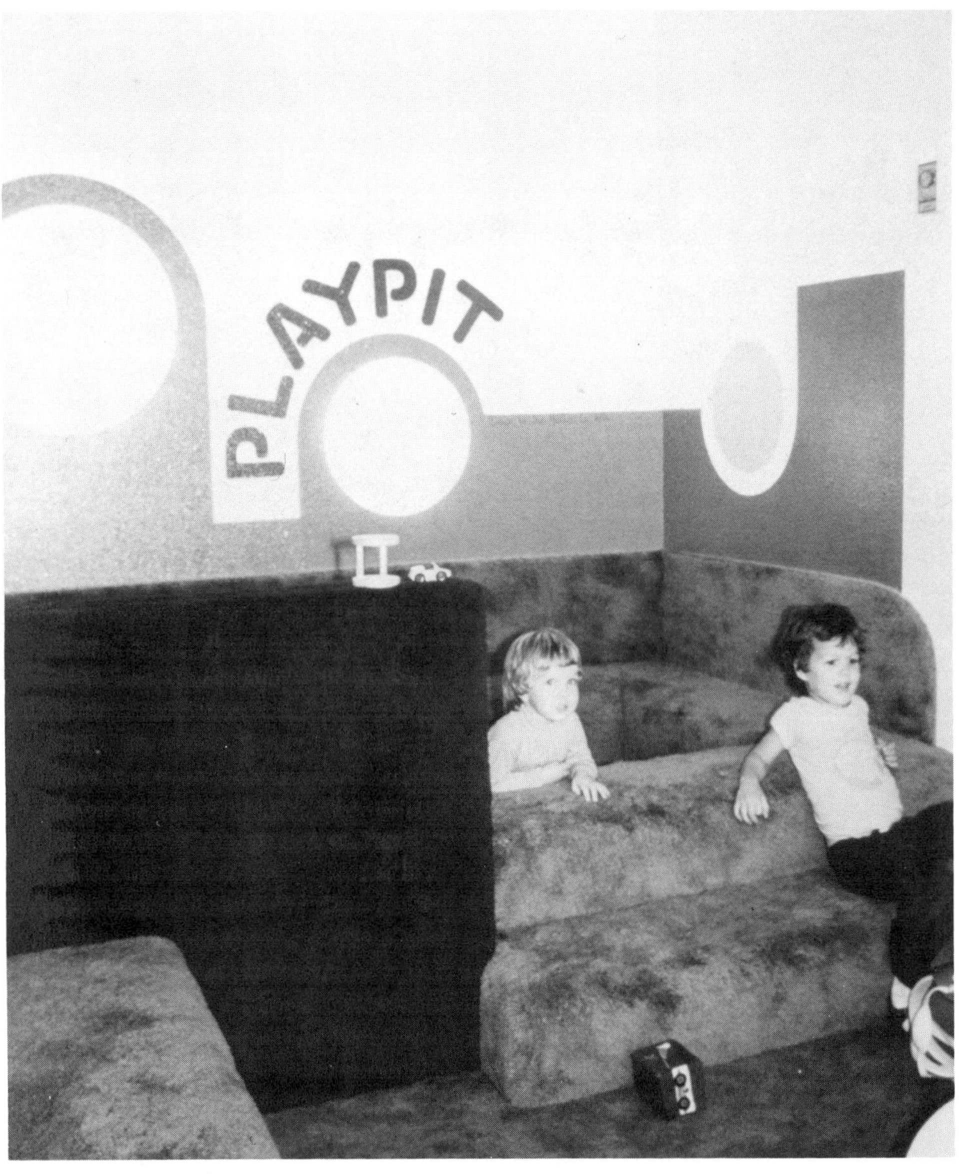

Figure 3-62. Children's play area. (*Design: Jain Malkin Inc.; Photographer: Michael Denny.*)

the next patient while the mother is dressing the child and the nurse cleaning up the last exam room.

It is a good idea to make one exam room large enough to accommodate an infant exam table and a child's table, since it is more efficient to examine two siblings in the same room (see Figure 3-59).

Adolescent Patients. Most pediatric practices (particularly true with older physicians who have been in practice a number of years) must accommodate a number of adolescent patients. A standard-size adult exam room (8 × 12 feet) should be provided, with a standard-size pelvic exam table and decor suitable to a teenager. Care must be taken in the interior design of the office not to gear it too much to infants and toddlers, as it may offend the older patients, who are quite sensitive about being considered children. Rooms designed to accommodate older children should have a floor scale. Since the children may be shy or modest about being weighed at the nurse station, it is best to have a scale in the exam room.

Location of Sinks. Some physicians consider it unnecessary to have a sink in every exam room if a sink is available nearby in the corridor. However, it is more efficient to have a sink in each exam room, since children may vomit or urinate during an examination and having a sink in the room saves time, by eliminating the need to leave the room in order to clean it up or wash hands. Today, with extreme concern about infection control and the threat of AIDS, a sink in the exam room seems mandatory.

Size of Rooms. Pediatric exam rooms may be very small, particularly an infant room. They need not have a door that opens to shield the patient. In fact, frequently exam rooms are so small that a pocket door is the most practical solution. The room may be no more than 6 × 7 feet (see Figure 3-66). If space permits, a small writing desk for the doctor and a guest chair for the parent should be included. A 6- × 8-foot or 8- × 9-foot room is not as cramped, but it is preferable to make the exam rooms minimum size in order to squeeze in an extra exam room.

It is a good idea to make one exam room large enough to accommodate an infant exam table and a child's table, since it is more efficient to examine two siblings in the same room (see Figure 3-59).

Exam Tables. Pediatric exam tables are available as manufactured items (Figure 3-74), but often are custom built with storage underneath (Figure 3-75). The size is 2 × 4 feet for an infant table (this increases to 6 feet if a lowered portion for a baby scale is included) or 2 × 6 feet for a child's table. The table is always placed against a wall to minimize the hazard of a child falling off. It should be positioned so that the doctor can examine from the right side of the patient, unless the doctor is left-handed and examines with the left hand. If a lowered area for a baby scale is not incorporated into the table, a portion of the sink cabinet countertop should be lowered for this purpose. It is better, however, to reserve this lowered portion of the sink cabinet for a doctor's writing desk.

It is possible to design an exam table that wraps around the corner to incorporate a bench for the parent, a scale space, and a sink cabinet (see Figures 3-67 and 3-76). It should be noted that any storage that is accessible to children in an exam room should be locked. Otherwise, they will empty the cabinets regularly, or catch their fingers in the doors or drawers.

Some method by which one may measure an infant's length may be incorporated into the exam table. Some pediatricians are very relaxed about this sort of measurement, and others require a fairly elaborate device. The length of the table on one side can be routed

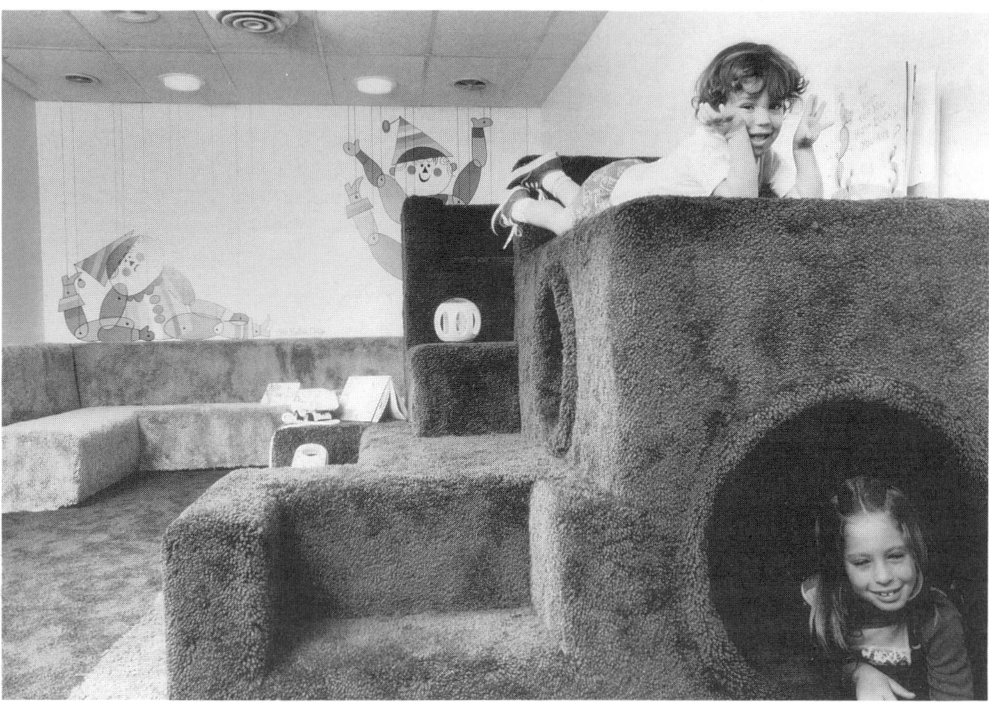

Figure 3-63. Children's play structure. (*Design: Jain Malkin Inc.; Photographer: Michael Denny.*)

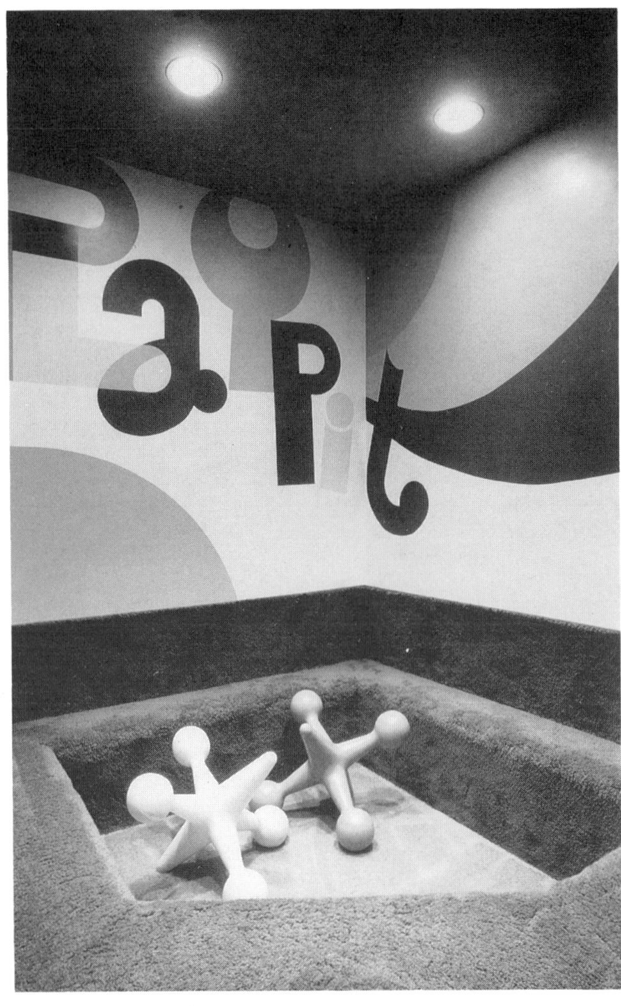

Figure 3-64. Children's playpit. (*Design: Jain Malkin Inc.; Photographer: Michael Denny.*)

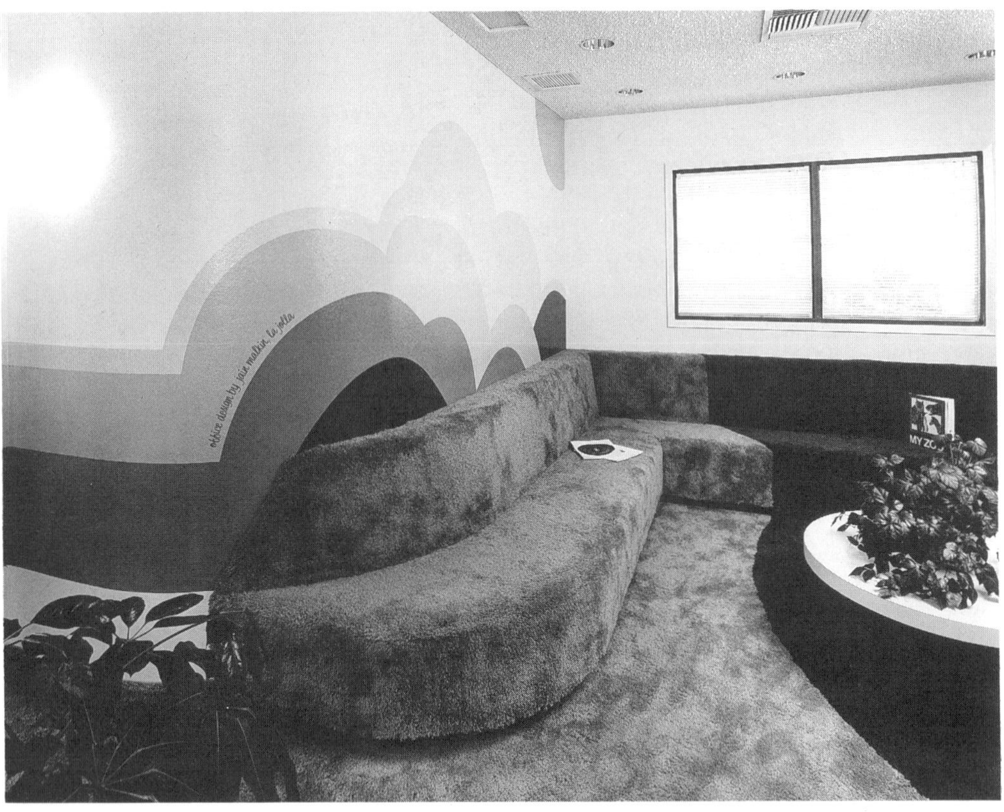

Figure 3-65. Pediatric waiting room. (*Design: Jain Malkin Inc.; Photographer: Michael Denny.*)

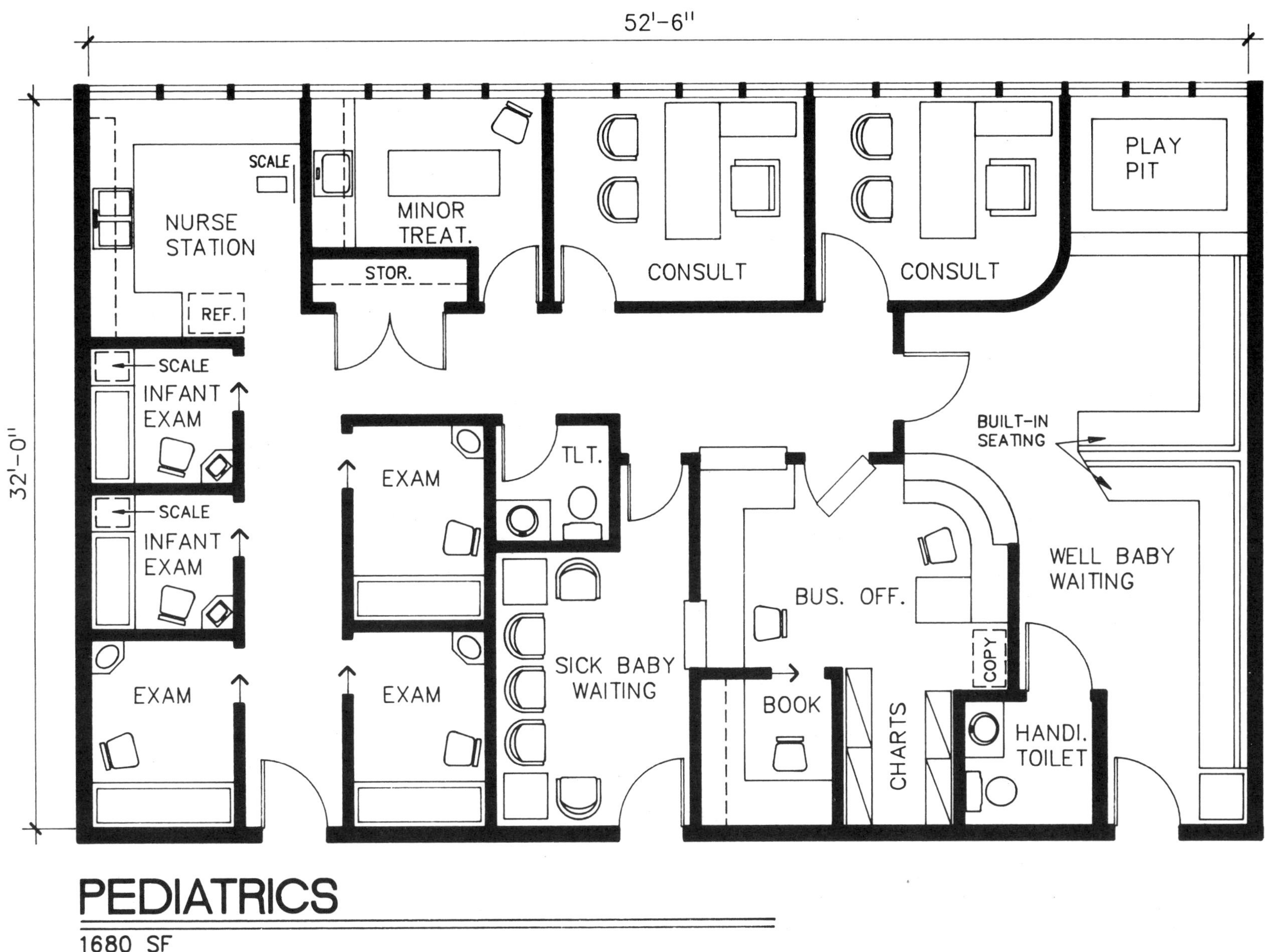

Figure 3-66. Suite plan for pediatrics, 1680 square feet.

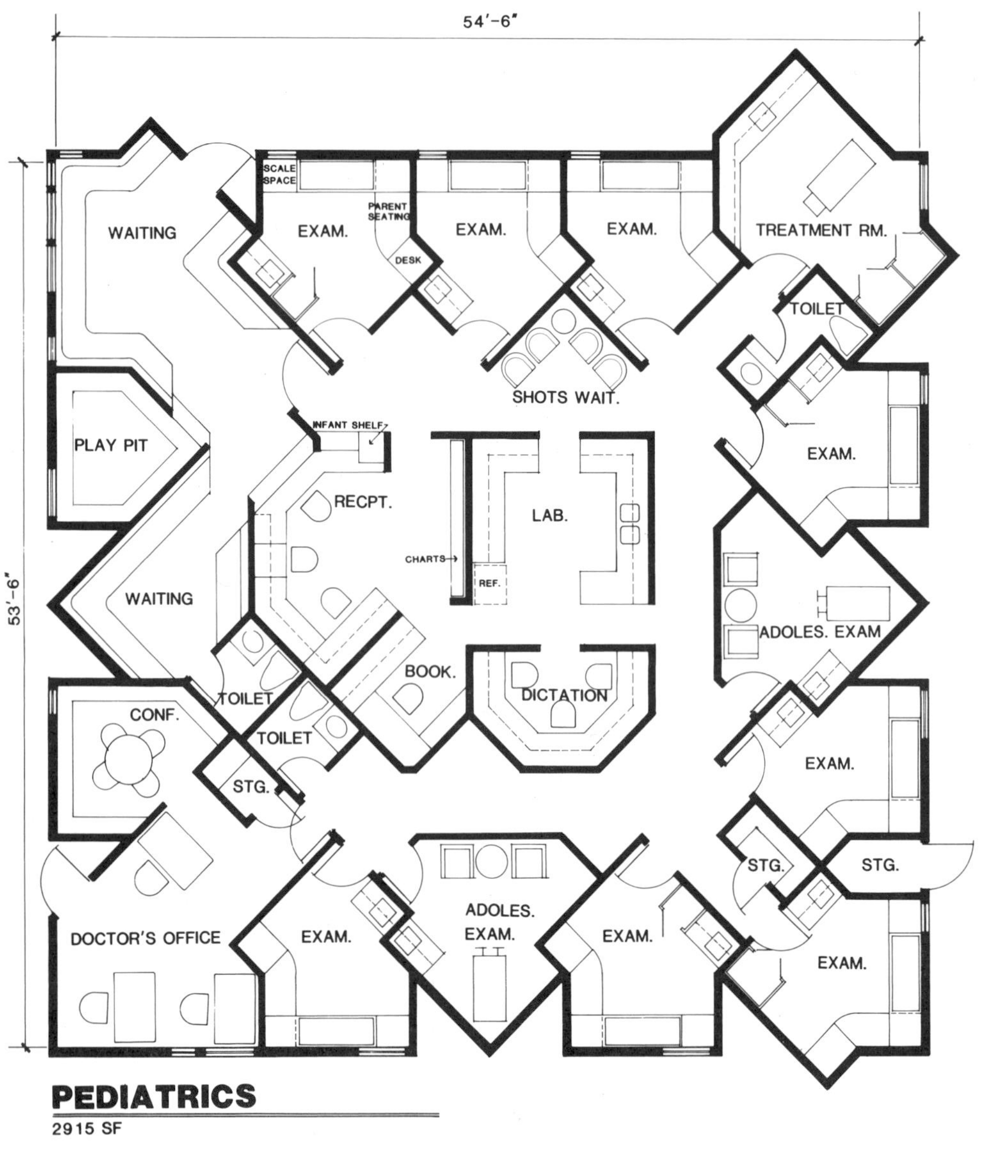

Figure 3-67. Suite plan for pediatrics, 2915 square feet.

with a slot for a tape measure, and a sliding wooden arm may be pushed up to the baby's feet to hold the child steady and at the same time indicate on the tape the child's length.

The table must also have a paper roll holder inside the cabinet with a slot in the table top so that a continuous roll of paper can be pulled over the vinyl-covered exam table pad and quickly changed between patients.

Interior Design. Exam rooms should be gaily decorated with one or two walls of colorful patterned wallcovering, perhaps a patterned tile floor (Color Plate 3, Figure 3-77), and some artwork of interest to children. Wallcovering even catches the attention of infants and serves to distract them, thus making the doctor's examination that much easier. One of the papered walls should be the long wall behind the exam table so that the children can see it while lying down.

Pediatric exam rooms should never be carpeted. Sheet vinyl or vinyl composition tile are recommended.

Nurse Station

Pediatric suites require large nurse stations because the nurses administer many injections. After an injection, a patient must be observed for 10 to 15 minutes in order to note any negative reaction to the drug. A few chairs or a bench must be provided either in the corridor adjacent to the nurse station, or perhaps within the nurse station. The nurse can attend to other business, but still keep a watchful eye on the patient. A full-size refrigerator must be accommodated in the nurse station. Pediatricians who administer allergy shots should have a nurse station located near the front of the suite, so that patients coming just for injections can enter and leave without adding to the congestion in the examination area of the suite. The nurse station should have a kneespace area with telephone, space for a microscope, and a double sink.

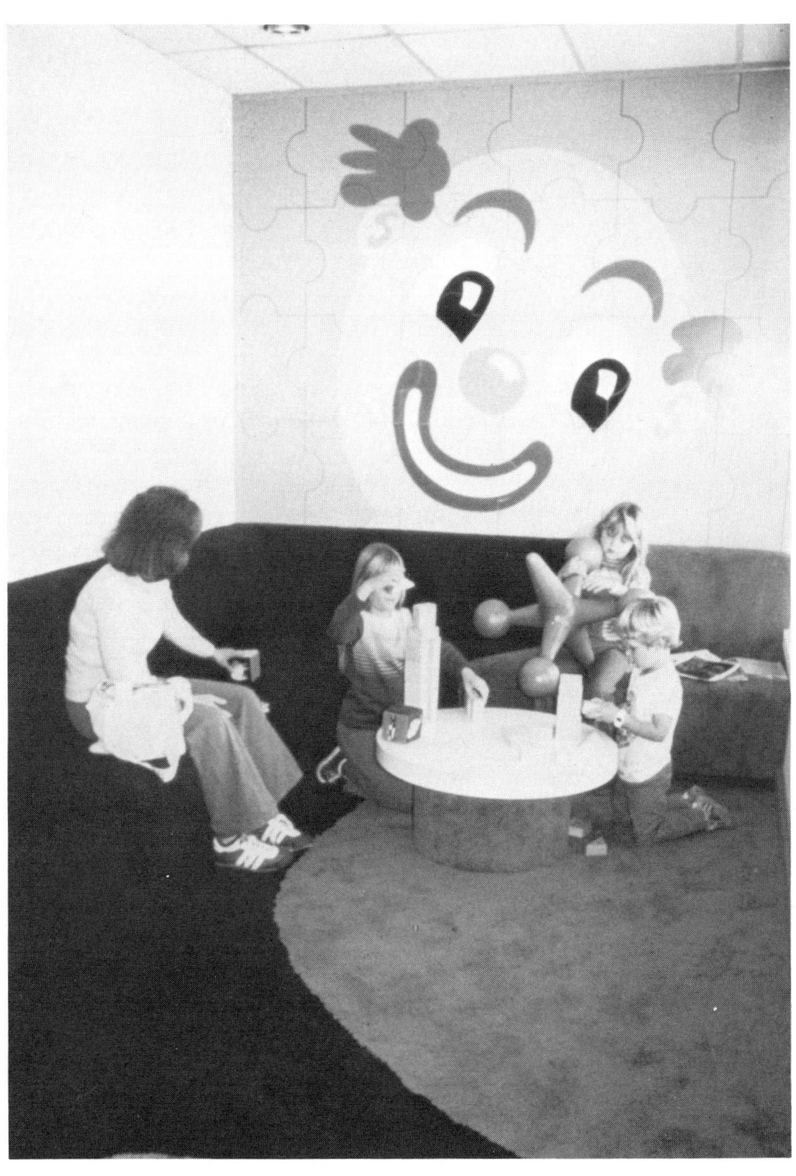

Figure 3-68. Clown puzzle wallgraphic. (*Design: Jain Malkin Inc.; Photographer: Michael Denny.*)

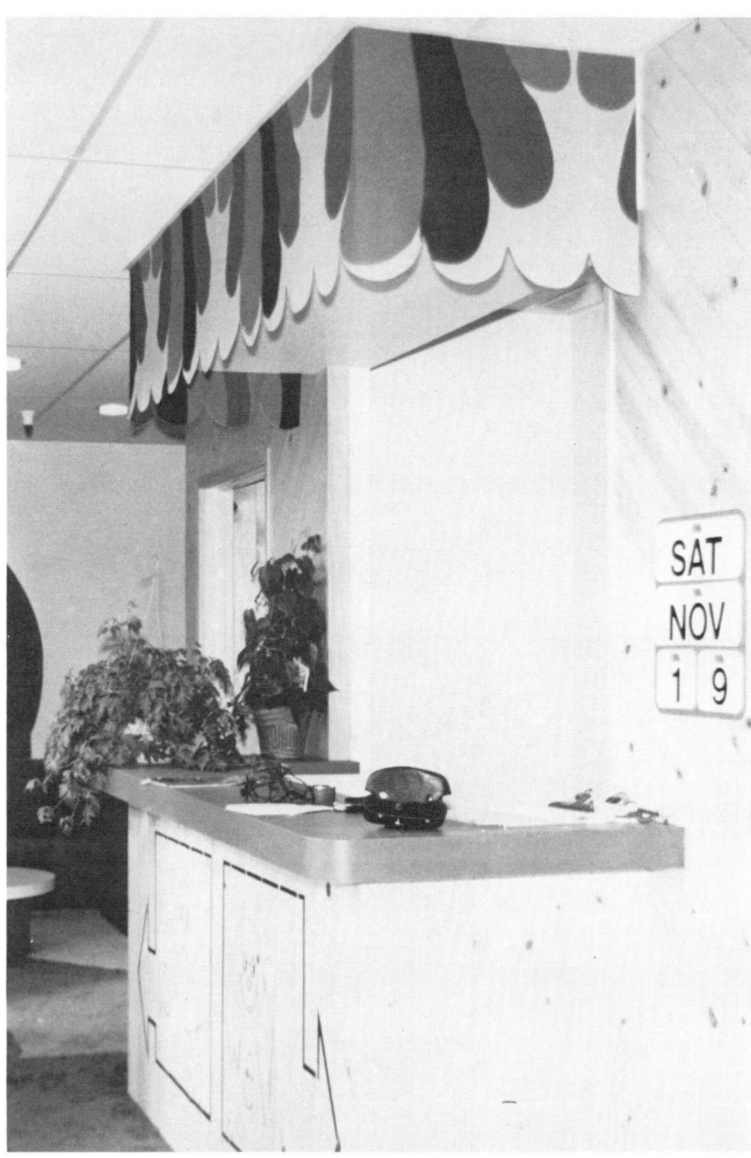

Figure 3-69. Fabric canopy makes a reception desk festive. (*Design: Jain Malkin Inc.; Photographer: Jain Malkin.*)

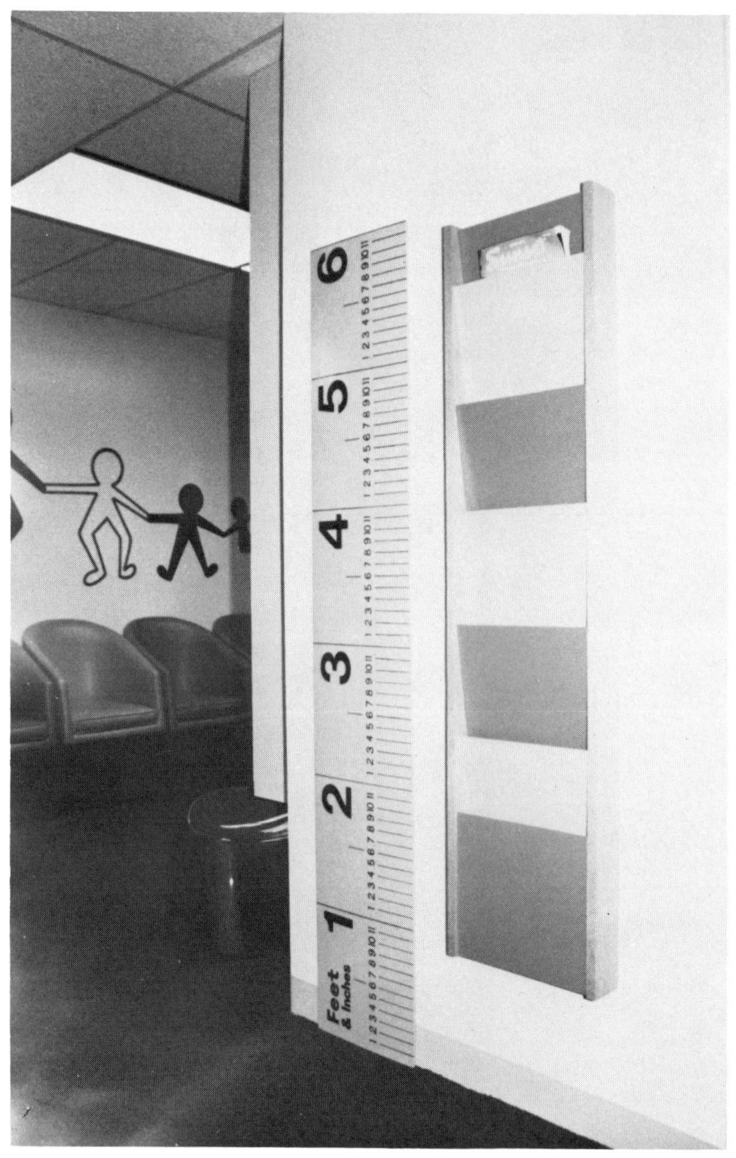

Figure 3-70. Custom yardstick lets children measure one another. (*Design: Jain Malkin Inc.; Photographer: Jain Malkin.*)

Business Office

The business office is as described in *General Practice,* although sometimes the nurse station can be combined with the business office (see Figure 3-59). This is efficient in a small office, as the staff can substitute for one another at critical periods of the day.

The pediatric business office should have a reception window facing both the sick and the well waiting rooms (see Figure 3-59). The appointment/cashier counter needs to have a wide shelf or a secure niche in the wall where a parent may put an infant in a carrier while he or she is writing a check or chatting with the staff (see Figure 3-67).

The reception window should be designed in such a manner as to appear "friendly" and nonclinical. That shown in Color Plate 3, Figure 3-79 incorporates French windows, ivory painted trim, and a fanciful carpet inset — all very residential in character. The reception window in Figure 3-80 and the adjacent wallgraphic are bright and playful, executed in primary colors.

A busy practice, with perhaps three physicians seeing patients simultaneously, benefits greatly from a separation of incoming and outgoing traffic. Figure 3-78 is designed for patients to enter through one door and leave through another, without exiting through the waiting room. This greatly enhances productivity, and reduces crowding and stress. Note that both the reception and cashier counters are very wide, to accommodate a number of transactions simultaneously. *The electrical plan and reflected ceiling plan for this suite (Figure 3-78) can be found in Chapter 13.*

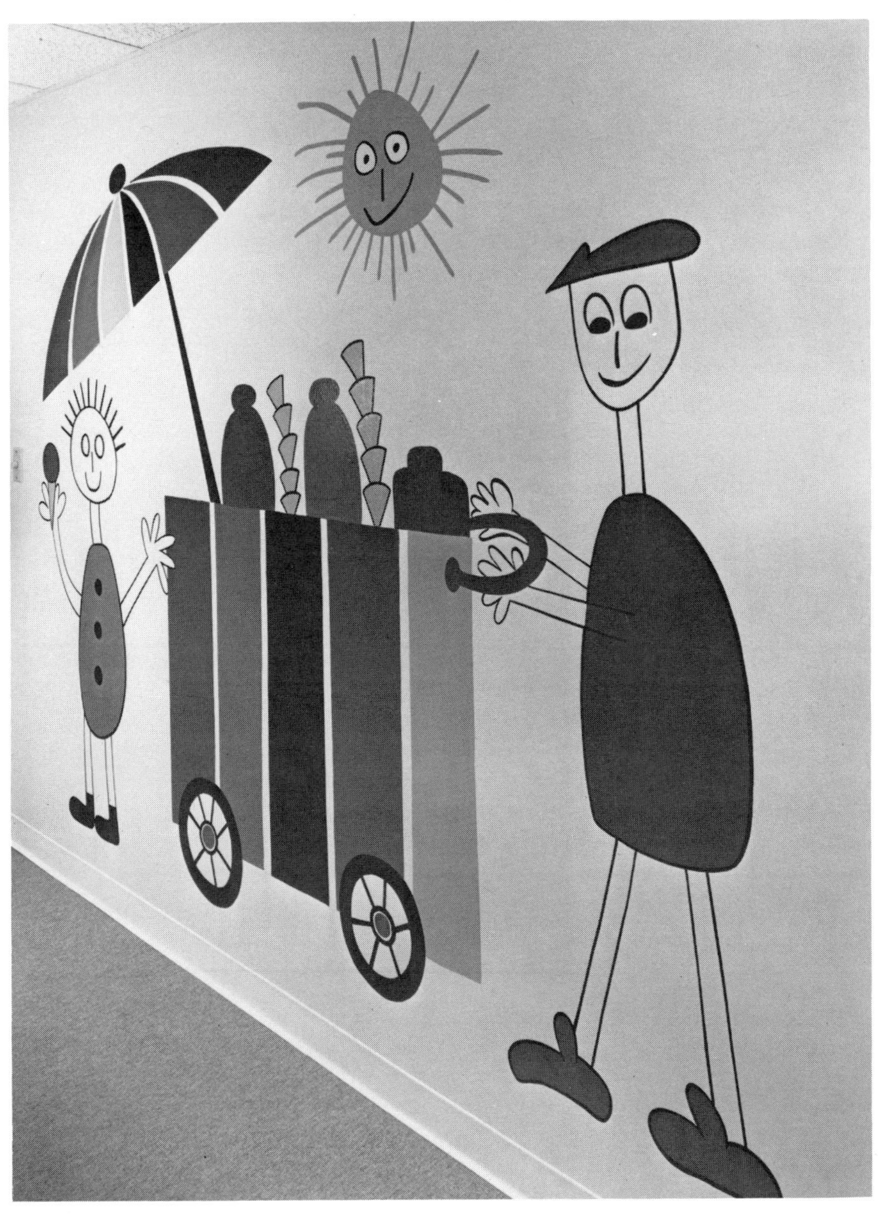

Figure 3-71. Children's art makes wonderful wallgraphics. (*Design: Jain Malkin Inc.; Photographer: John Waggaman.*)

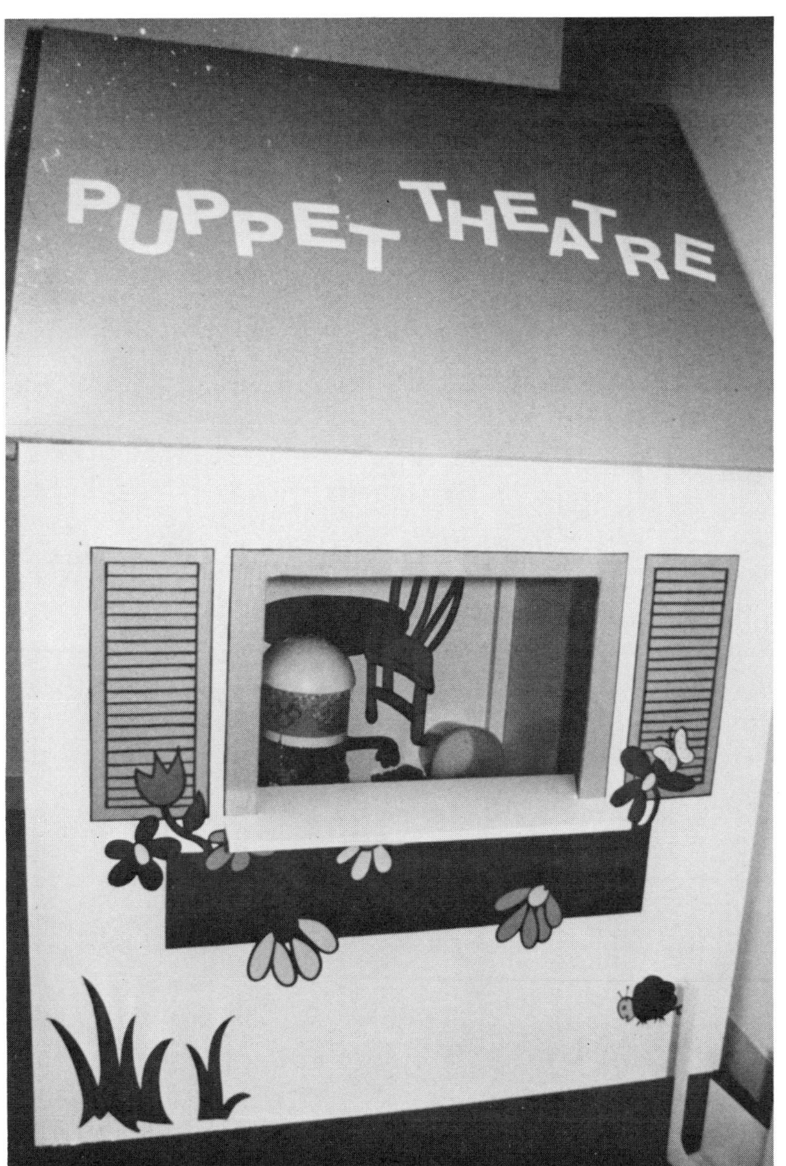

Figure 3-72. Puppet theatre in waiting room keeps children occupied. (*Design: Jain Malkin Inc.; Photographer: Jain Malkin.*)

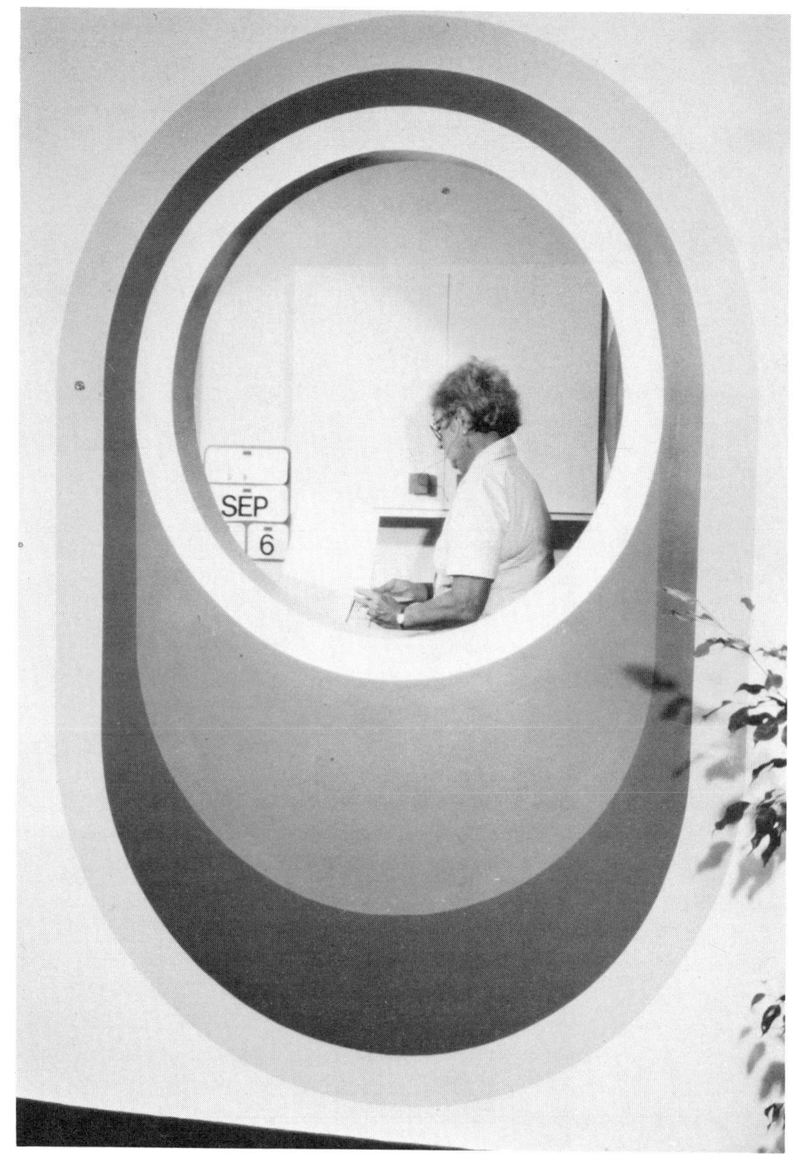

Figure 3-73. Reception window, pediatrics. (*Design: Jain Malkin Inc.; Photographer: Michael Denny.*)

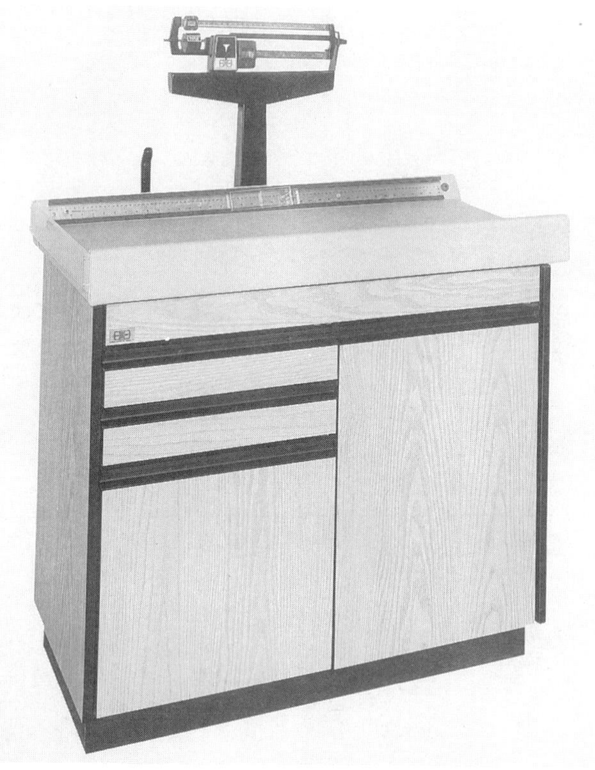

Figure 3-74. Infant examination table. (*Courtesy Hausmann Industries Inc., Northvale, NJ.*)

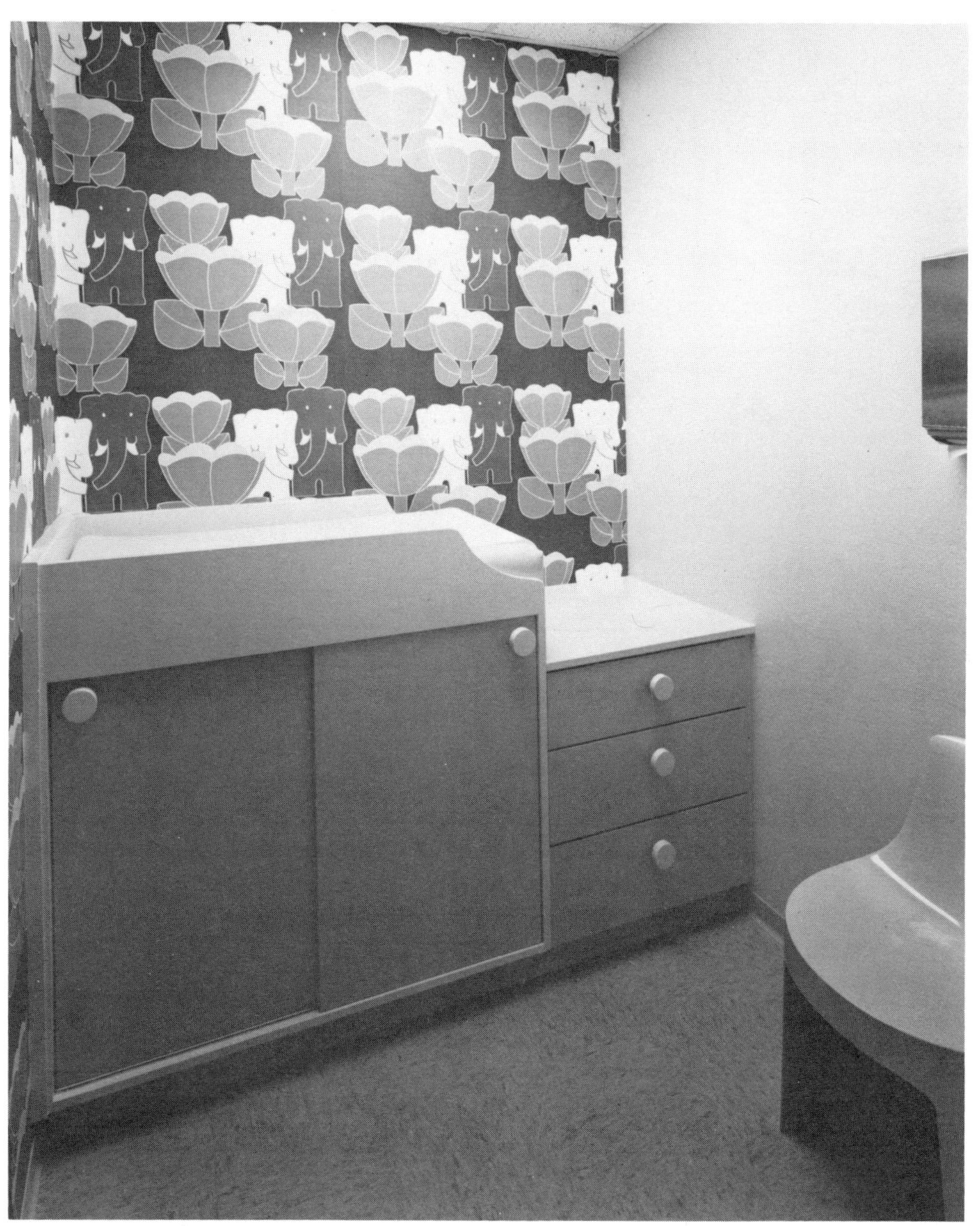

Figure 3-75. Infant exam room. (*Design: Jain Malkin Inc.; Photographer: Michael Denny.*)

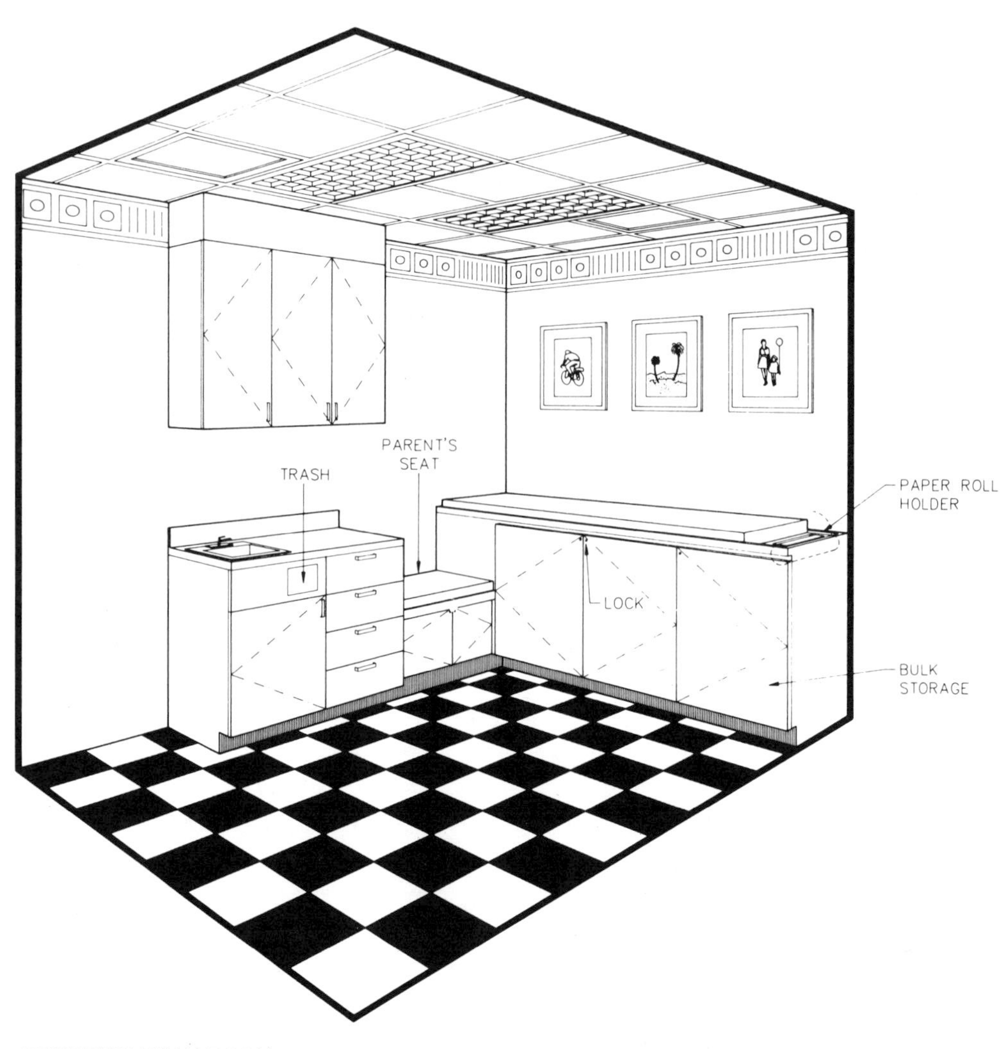

Figure 3-76. Pediatric examination table with wrap-around bench for parent, and sink cabinet. (*Design: Jain Malkin Inc.*)

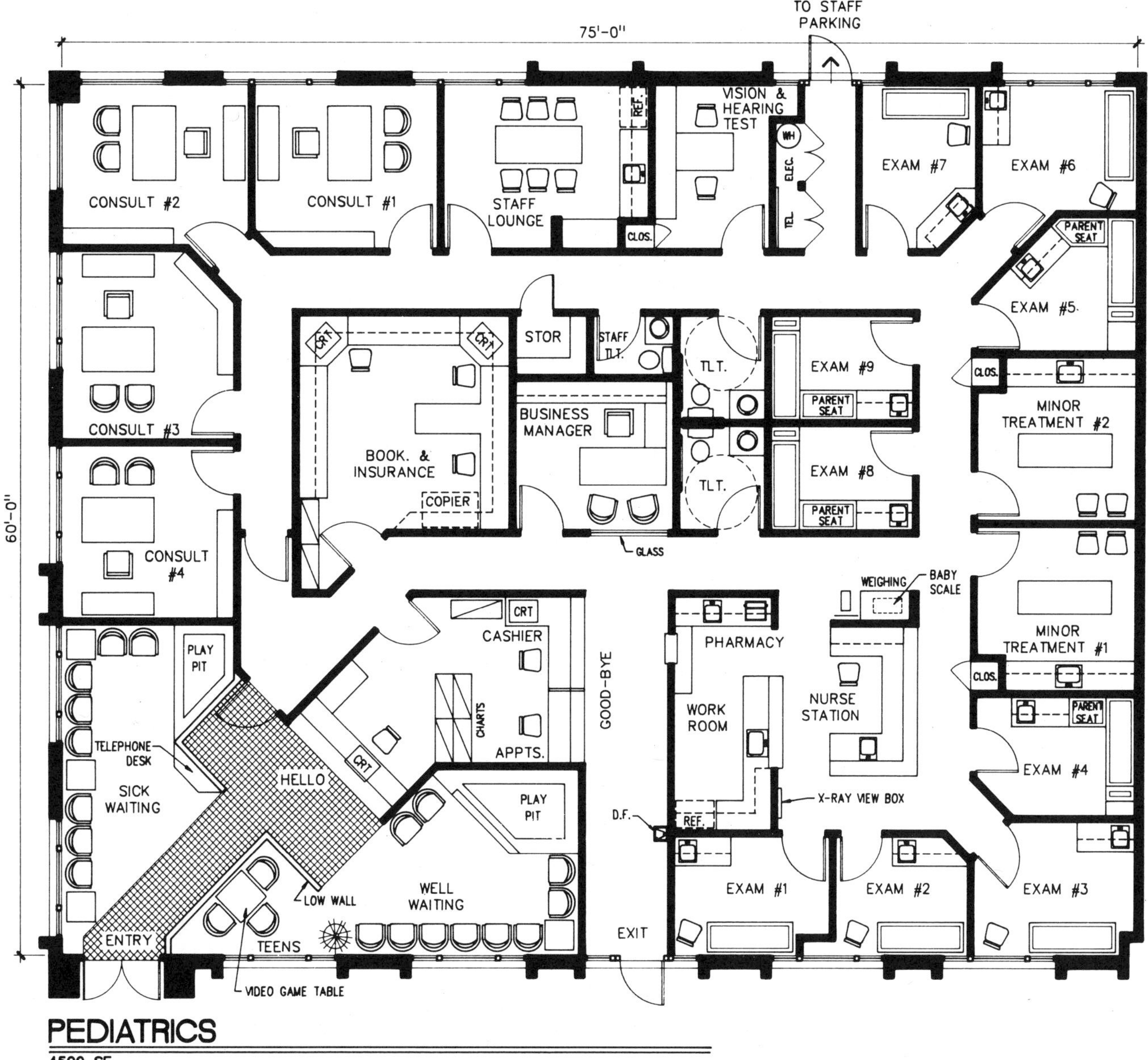

Figure 3-78. Suite plan for pediatrics, 4500 square feet.

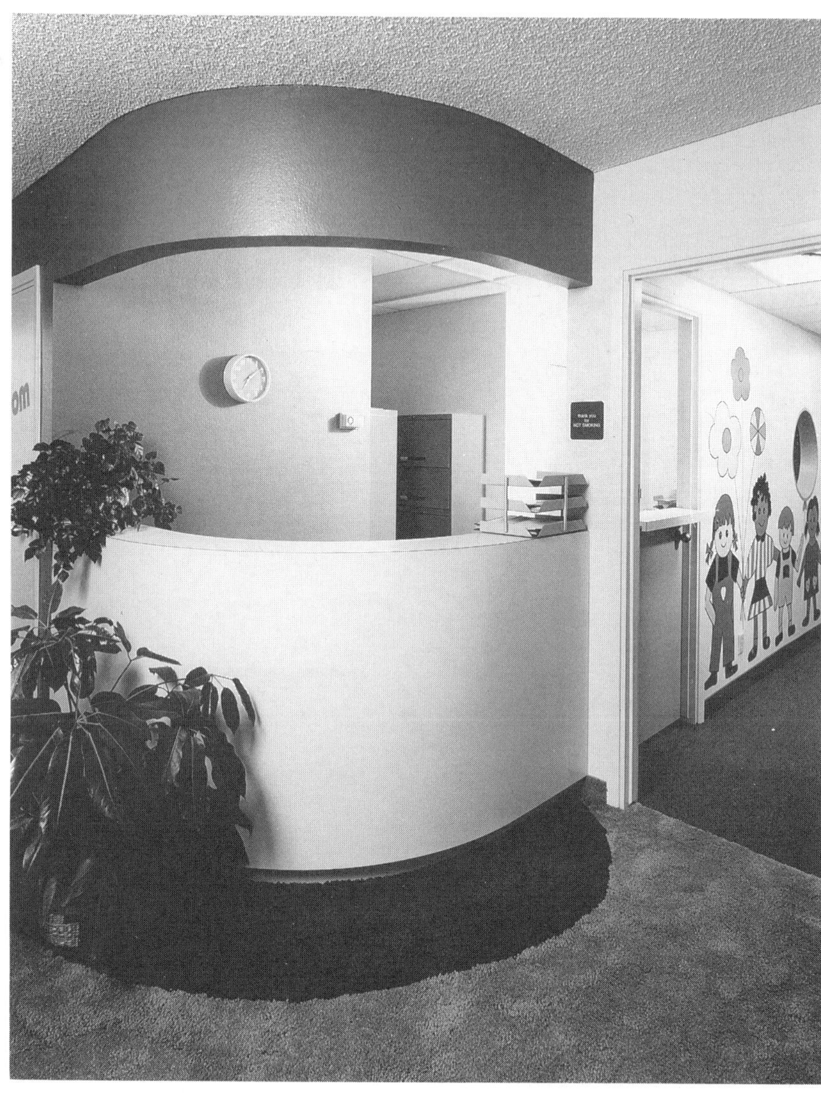

Figure 3-80. Reception desk, pediatrics. (*Design: Jain Malkin Inc.; Photographer: Michael Denny.*)

Consultation Room

Pediatricians spend little time in a consultation room and seldom see patients there; therefore, it is not uncommon for two physicians to share a private office (see Figure 3-67). Basically, it is used for storing medical reference books and for returning phone calls. Pediatricians dispense a lot of literature and pamphlets on child care, so a wall rack should be provided for the organized storage of these materials, either in the consultation room, the nurse station, or the corridor adjacent to exam rooms.

Corridor

One corridor should be selected for a 20-foot refraction lane. An eye chart would be tacked to a door, or placed on the wall at the end of the corridor for a brief eye test. A circle inset into the carpet can mark where the child's heels should be placed to assure a distance of 20 feet. The corridors should be cheerful and may have cartoon characters or colorful supergraphics.

Hearing Test Room

Some pediatricians like to do a preliminary hearing test to screen patients who need to be referred to an ENT specialist. Sometimes this can be set up in a dual-purpose room. The hearing test can be performed in a consultation room or in a small 8- × 8-foot room dedicated to that purpose. One needs a table 24 × 48 inches on which to place the equipment, a chair for the patient, and one for the technician. Walls of the room must have sound insulation and, inside the room, walls may be covered with carpet to enhance the sound-absorbing qualities. The room should be located at the rear of the suite away from the hectic front office (see Figure 3-78).

Storage

The office needs a small storage room, 6 × 8 feet, for drug samples, disposable supplies, office forms and stationery, and handout pamphlets.

Interior Design

The suite should be colorful and imaginatively designed to reduce the children's anxiety and make them forget any negative associations they may have had about visiting the doctor. All rooms except exam rooms may be carpeted. Some physicians even carpet exam rooms. Although carpeting does make the job of cleaning up vomit and urine that much harder, it has the advantage of making the room nicer for crawling infants. The reader is referred to Chapter 12 for additional information on furnishings and interior design.

CHAPTER 4

Medicine: Specialized Suites

The American Board of Medical Specialties recognizes, as of this writing, 23 medical specialties and about a dozen and a half subspecialties. The specialties are: Allergy and Immunology, Anesthesiology, Colon and Rectal Surgery, Dermatology, Family Practice, Internal Medicine, Neurological Surgery, Nuclear Medicine, Obstetrics and Gynecology, Ophthalmology, Orthopedic Surgery, Otolaryngology, Pathology, Pediatrics, Physical Medicine and Rehabilitation, Plastic Surgery, Preventive Medicine, Psychiatry and Neurology, Radiology, Surgery, Thoracic Surgery, Urology, and the newest specialty, Emergency Medicine.

Subspecialties under Internal Medicine are: Cardiovascular Disease, Endocrinology and Metabolism, Gastroenterology, Hematology, Infectious Disease, Medical Oncology, Nephrology, Pulmonary Disease, and Rheumatology. Subspecialties under Pediatrics are: Pediatric Cardiology, Pediatric Ophthalmology, Pediatric Endocrinology, Pediatric Hematology–Oncology, Neonatal-Perinatal Medicine, and Nephrology. There are a few other subspecialties under Psychiatry and Neurology, such as Child Psychiatry and Child Neurology.

Although Family Practice, Pediatrics, and Internal Medicine are primary medical practices, they are also listed as specialties by the American Board of Medical Specialties, since physicians in these specialties must take and pass specialty boards that certify their competence in their respective fields. These three "specialities," then, are primary practice physicians, whereas many of the other specialties listed above tend to be referral specialties — patients are referred by their primary care physicians.

This chapter will discuss the requirements of the medical specialties the designer or architect is most likely to encounter in a medical office building.

OBSTETRICS AND GYNECOLOGY

This is a high-volume practice, so patient flow must be carefully analyzed. Obstetrical patients usually make monthly visits, which entail weighing and a brief examination. Gynecology patients require a more lengthy pelvic examination. This type of practice requires a large staff as each physician needs one or two nurses, and often two physicians share three nurses or aides in addition to the front office staff. It is customary for a nurse to be present during pelvic examinations, necessitating more staff per doctor than required with many other medical specialties.

Nurse Practitioner

A recent trend in this field is the use of a nurse practitioner to perform routine patient examinations. An R.N. with additional training in OB-GYN can be certified to work in this capacity. This frees physicians from routine pelvic examinations and Pap smears on healthy patients, allowing them to concentrate on diagnosis of disease. Offices using nurse practitioners will need larger nurse stations or perhaps a small private office for them (Figure 4-2).

Patient Flow

There probably would not be more than three doctors working in an office at one time even if it were a four- or five-person practice, since one or two doctors may be delivering babies, or making hospital rounds, or have the day off. There should be three to four exam rooms per physician. The patient flow is from waiting room to weighing area, to toilet (urine specimen), to exam room. A good space plan will channel patients to each area by the most direct route with no backtracking or unnecessary steps. If possible, the nurse station/sterilization/lab areas should be located toward the front of the suite (centralized) so that the staff can cover for each other, and duplication of personnel is avoided.

Waiting Room

The waiting room of an OB-GYN suite should be large and comfortable. Unexpected deliveries frequently make the doctor late and necessitate a long wait for patients. The patient is apt to be more forgiving if her wait is in a well-designed room with good lighting, current magazines, comfortable seating, and interesting artwork on the walls. A play area for children would be a practical addition to the waiting room, since many patients are young mothers, who are apt to bring their children with them (Color Plate 4, Figure 4-3).

Exam Rooms

Exam rooms should have one or two walls of attractive wallcovering, carpet, and a dressing area where patients may disrobe in privacy and hang underwear out of sight. Upon dressing, they may check makeup and hair in a mirror before leaving the exam room. This dressing area may be a 3- × 3-foot corner of a room with a ceiling-mounted cubicle drape and a chair or built-in bench. Or it can be a hinged space-saver panel which opens perpendicular to the wall. Note that in Figure 4-4, the dressing area is spacious and offers total privacy. Remember that the door to the exam room must open to shield the patient.

The position of the sink cabinet is particularly important in an OB-GYN exam room. The physician should be able to examine the patient with the right hand and reach for instruments from the cabinet with the left

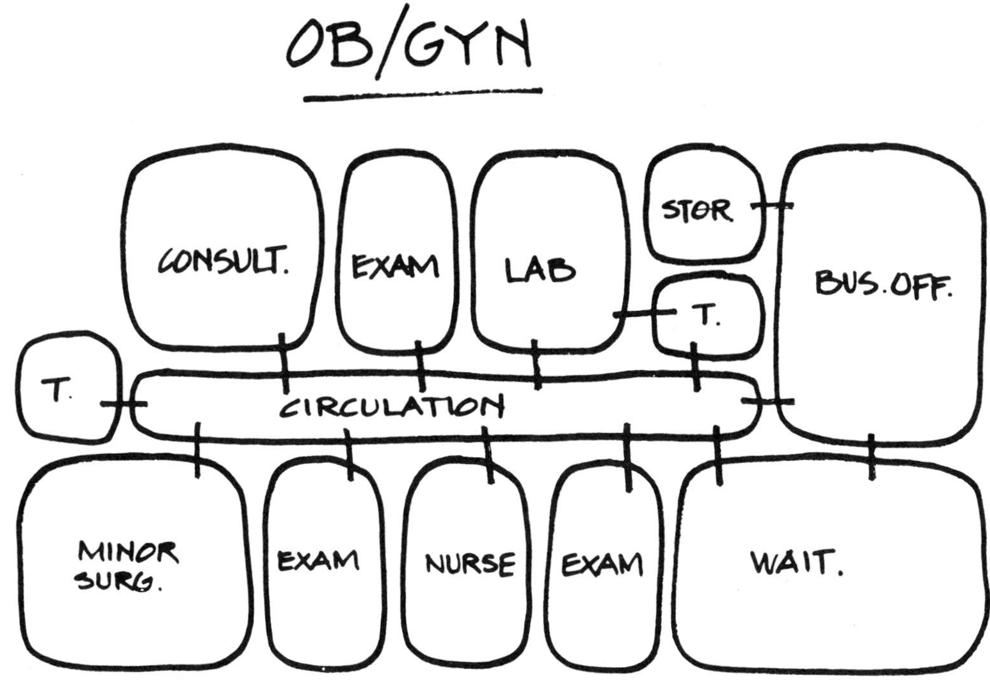

Figure 4-1. Schematic diagram of an OB-GYN suite.

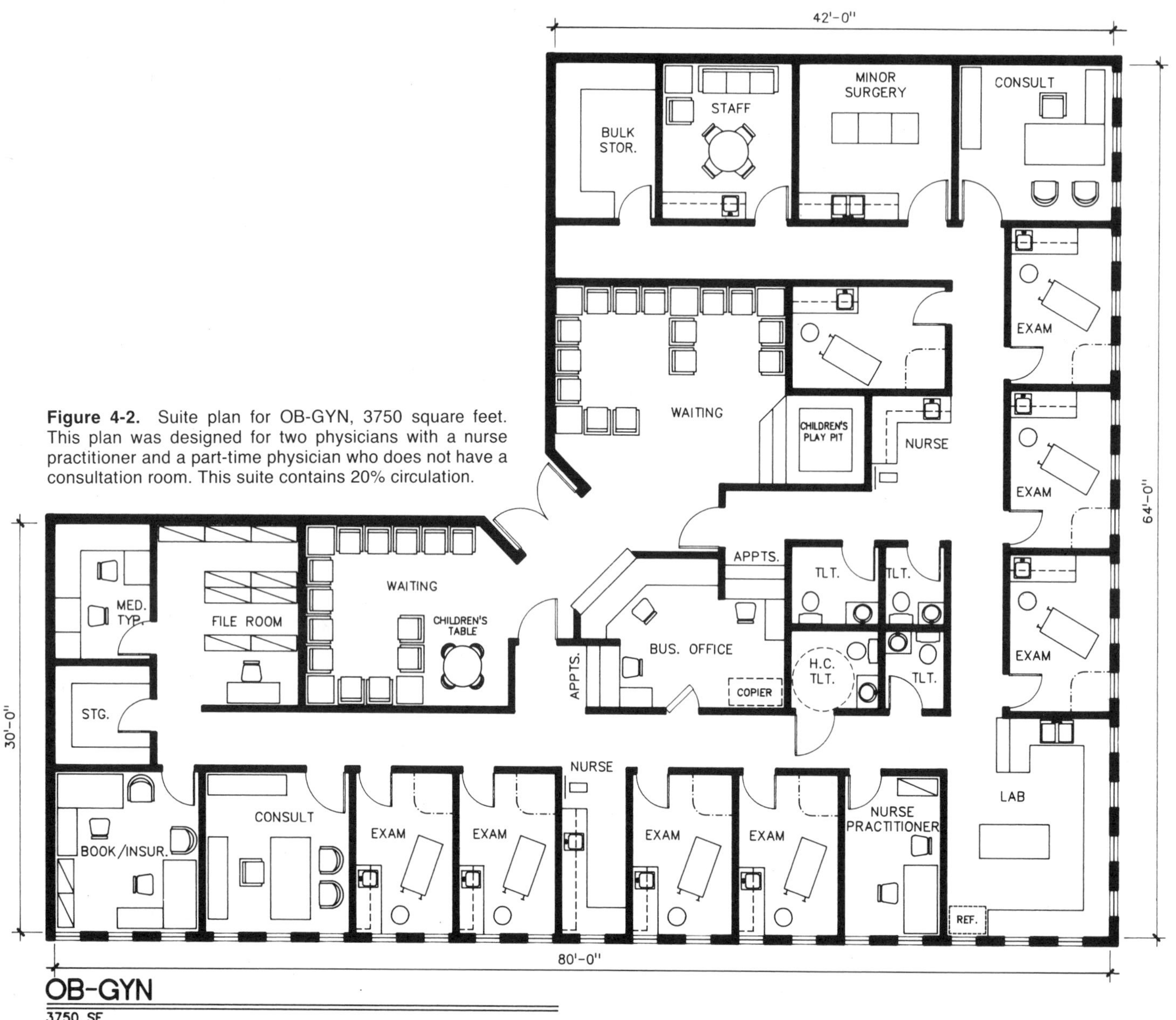

Figure 4-2. Suite plan for OB-GYN, 3750 square feet. This plan was designed for two physicians with a nurse practitioner and a part-time physician who does not have a consultation room. This suite contains 20% circulation.

hand (Figure 4-5). The exam table used here is a pelvic table with stirrups. Such tables often have a built-in speculum warmer; or one drawer of the sink cabinet may have an electrical outlet at the rear for warming instruments. Three electrical outlets are required: One must be located near the foot of the table for the examination lamp used for pelvic exams; one should be located above the sink countertop; and the third should be located on the long wall, near the head of the table.

It should be noted that some OB-GYN physicians prefer a wider examination room with a cabinet that runs along the wall at the foot of the exam table (Figure 4-6). This cabinet is at a 30-inch height so that the physician, when seated, can comfortably reach instruments and equipment. Note that patient education is handled in the exam room, with a TV monitor built into the cabinet. Monitors are wired to VCR units in the business office. The nurse selects the proper tape for the patient's viewing; thus, time spent waiting in an exam room can be productive. Figure 4-7 shows the cabinets opened. These exam rooms are carpeted, except for a 3-foot wide strip running in front of the built-in cabinet, which was done in wood parquet.

It is pleasant to have windows in an OB-GYN exam room. The wait is frequently very long and being able to look outside makes the wait a little more bearable. Narrow-slat metal window blinds serve exam rooms well since they permit light and view to enter the room while protecting the occupant's privacy.

Many physicians write a prescription in the exam room, but others ask the patient to dress and come to the consultation room. In any case, it is a good idea to provide a writing desk in the exam room so that the physician can make notations on the patient's chart and write a prescription.

Table 4-1. Analysis of Program. Obstetrics and Gynecology

No. of Physicians:	1		2 (Plus Nurse Practitioner)	
Exam Rooms	3 @ 8 × 12 =	288	8 @ 8 × 12 =	768
Consultation Rooms	12 × 12 =	144	2 @ 12 × 12 =	288
Nurse Station	8 × 10 =	80[a]	10 × 12 =	120
Laboratory	—		12 × 16 =	192
Toilets	2 @ 5 × 6 =	60	4 @ 5 × 6 =	120
Minor Surgery	12 × 12 =	144	12 × 14 =	168
Staff Lounge	—		11 × 12 =	132
Storage	4 × 6 =	24	10 × 12 =	120
Nurse Practitioner	—		8 × 10 =	80
Business Office/Book.	12 × 16 =	192	12 × 30 =	360[b]
Medical Records	—		10 × 14 =	140
Waiting Room	12 × 20 =	240	14 × 30 =	420
Subtotal		1172 ft^2		2908 ft^2
15% Circulation		176		436
Total		1348 ft^2		3344 ft^2

[a]Combined with lab.

[b]Includes transcription, reception, bookkeeping, and insurance.

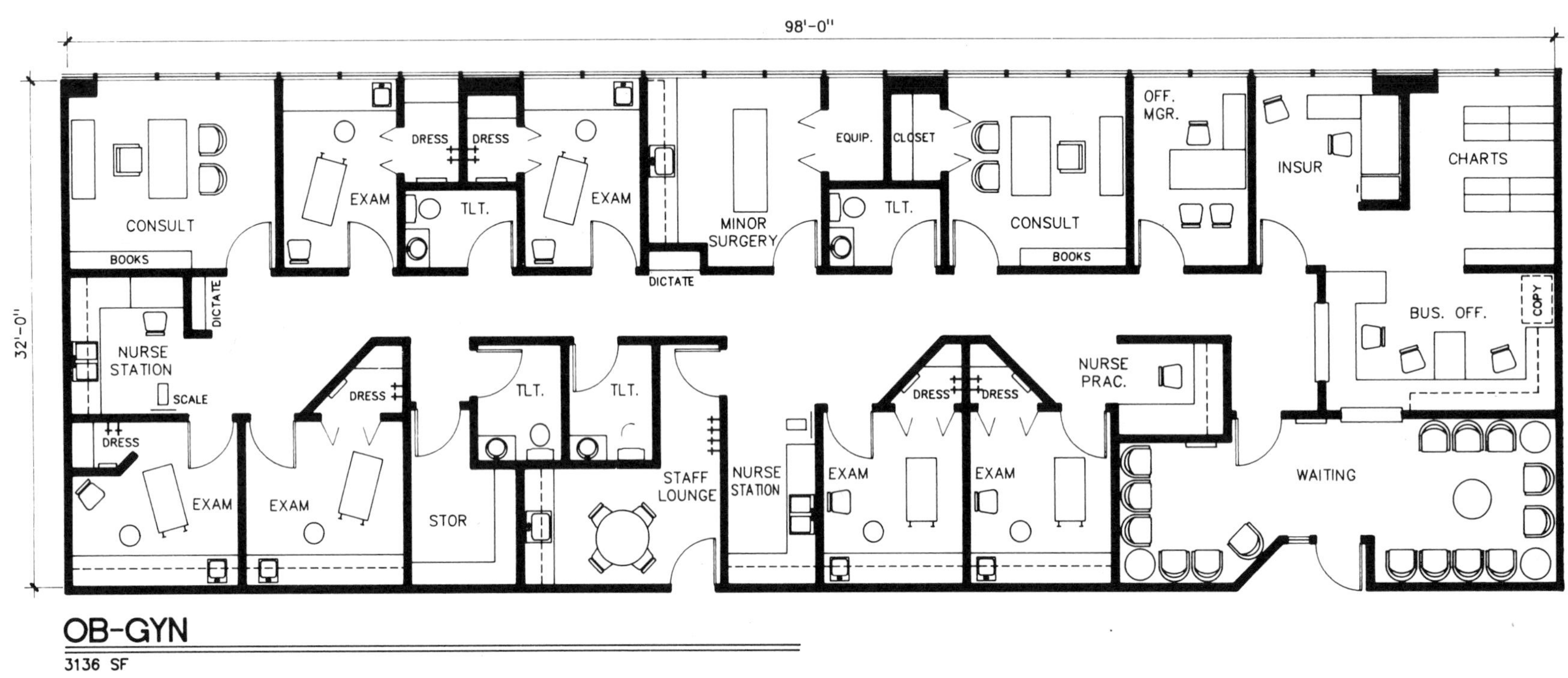

Figure 4-4. OB-GYN examination room. (*Design: Jain Malkin Inc.; Photographer: Kim Brun.*)

Minor Surgery

Most OB-GYN suites will have a minor surgery room where a variety of procedures will be performed (Figure 4-8). Although some of these procedures used to be performed in a hospital, they can safely be handled in a well-equipped minor surgery within the physician's office. The size of the room may vary from 12 × 14 feet to 14 × 16 feet depending on the number of assistants who must be in the room and the amount of medical equipment.

Patient Education

Many printed educational pamphlets are distributed, so suitable storage racks should be provided in the waiting room or in the corridor near the nurse station (Figure 4-9). A provision should be made for patient education. It might be a niche off a corridor, which would have a built-in countertop with privacy partitions, a TV monitor, and a compartment under the countertop for a VCR. Patients would wear headphones. In lieu of this, one might provide a patient education room, preferably located near the front of the suite.

Disposal of Infectious Waste

A large amount of trash is generated in this practice. A disposable gown, sheet, and exam table paper must be discarded after each patient, as well as paper hand towels and other disposable items. Each exam room should have a large trash receptacle which may be built into the cabinet or freestanding.

It should be noted that many cities have regulations for dealing with infectious waste. These used to apply only to hospitals, but with the presence of AIDS, even

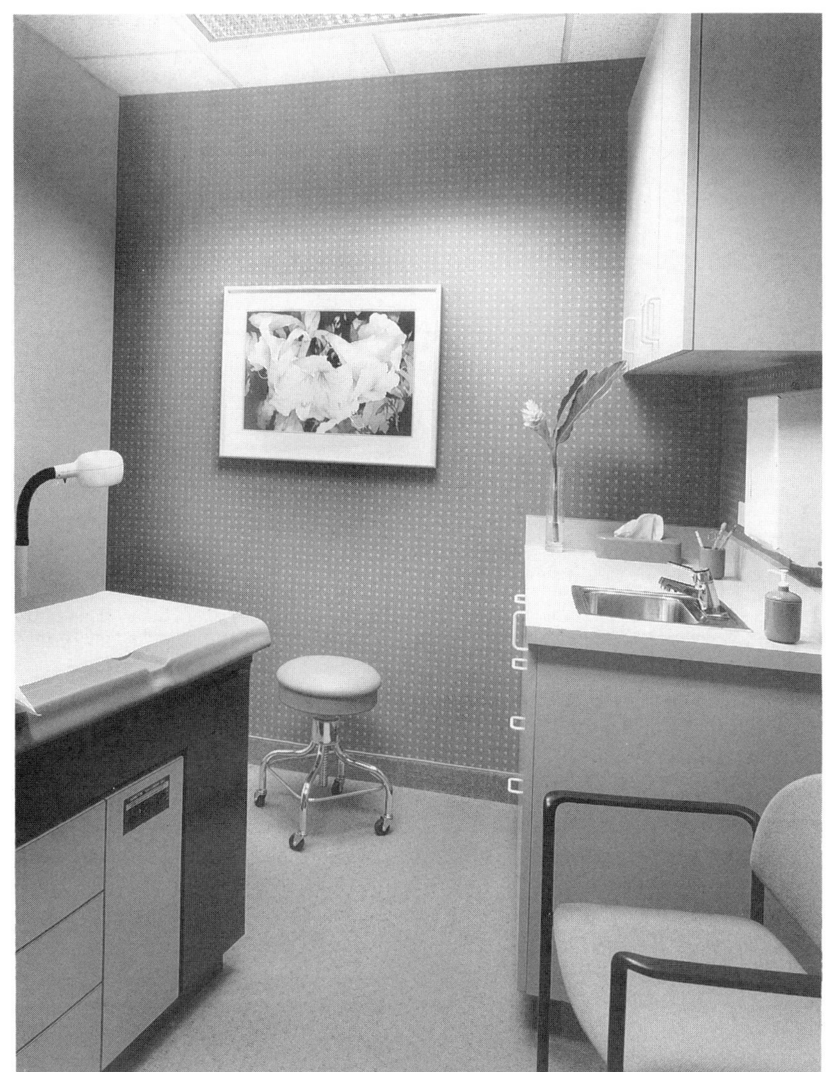

Figure 4-5. Suite plan for OB-GYN, 3136 square feet.

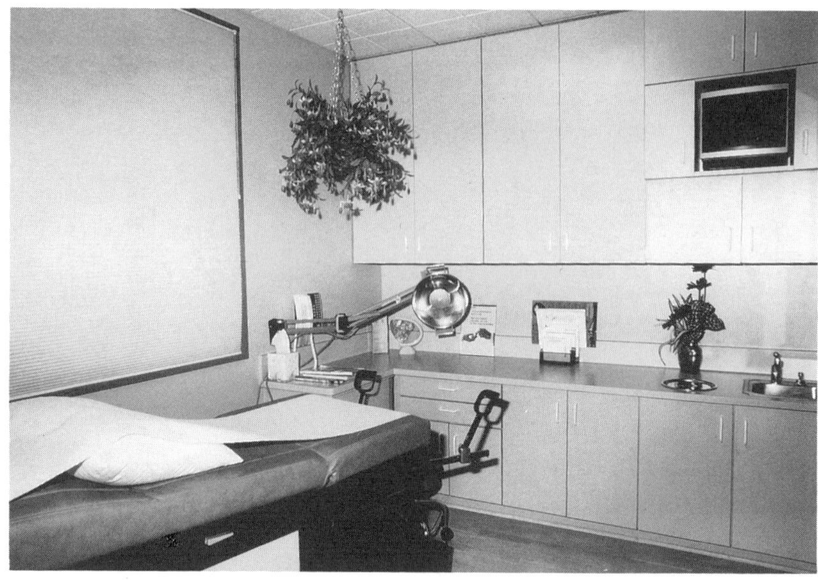

Figure 4-6. OB-GYN examination room with cabinet at foot of exam table. (*Casework Design: Ashvin Contractor, San Jose, CA; Interior Design: Jain Malkin Inc.; Photographer, Jain Malkin.*)

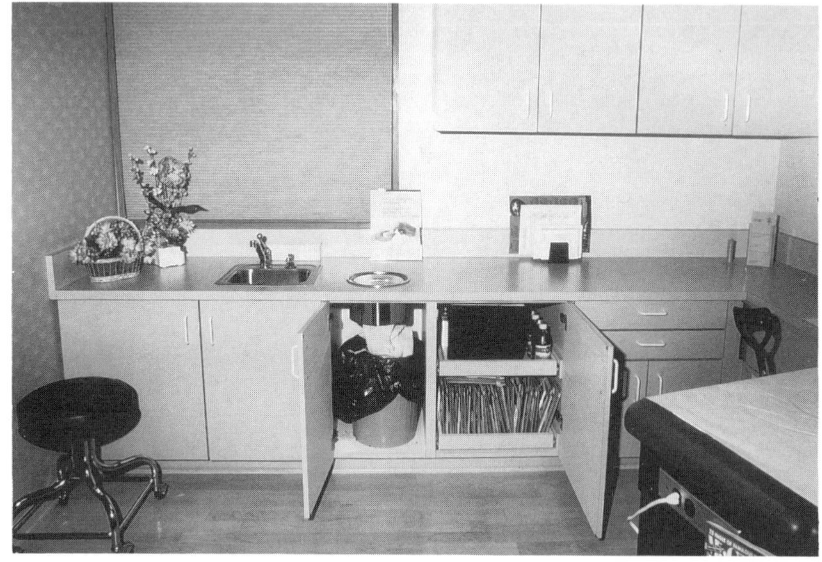

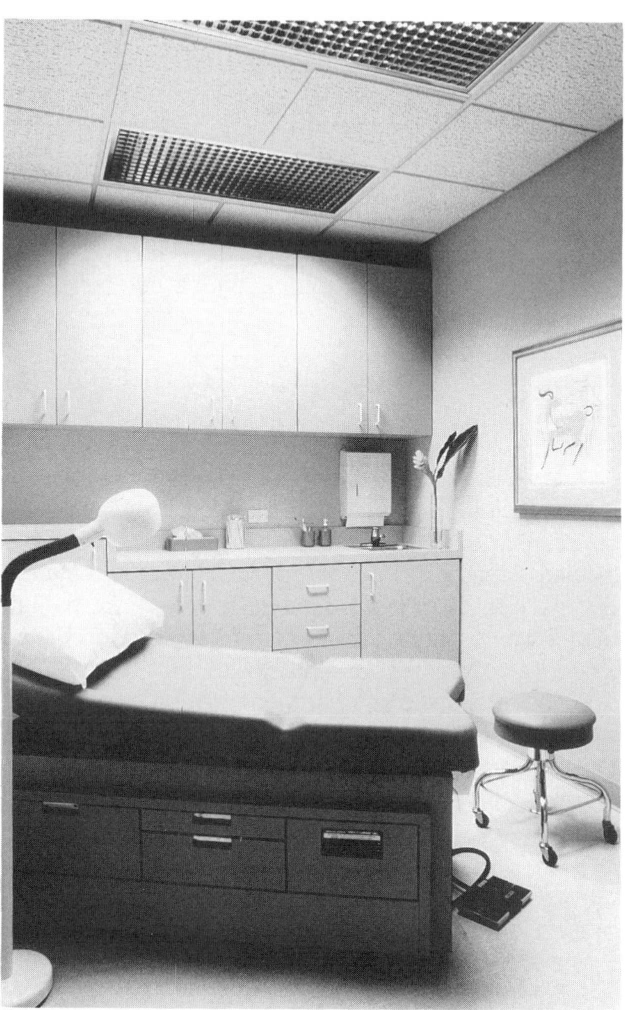

Figure 4-8. OB-GYN minor surgery room. (*Design: Jain Malkin Inc.; Photographer: Kim Brun.*)

Figure 4-7. OB-GYN exam room, interior of casework. (*Casework Design: Ashvin Contractor, San Jose, CA; Interior Design: Jain Malkin Inc.; Photographer: Jain Malkin.*)

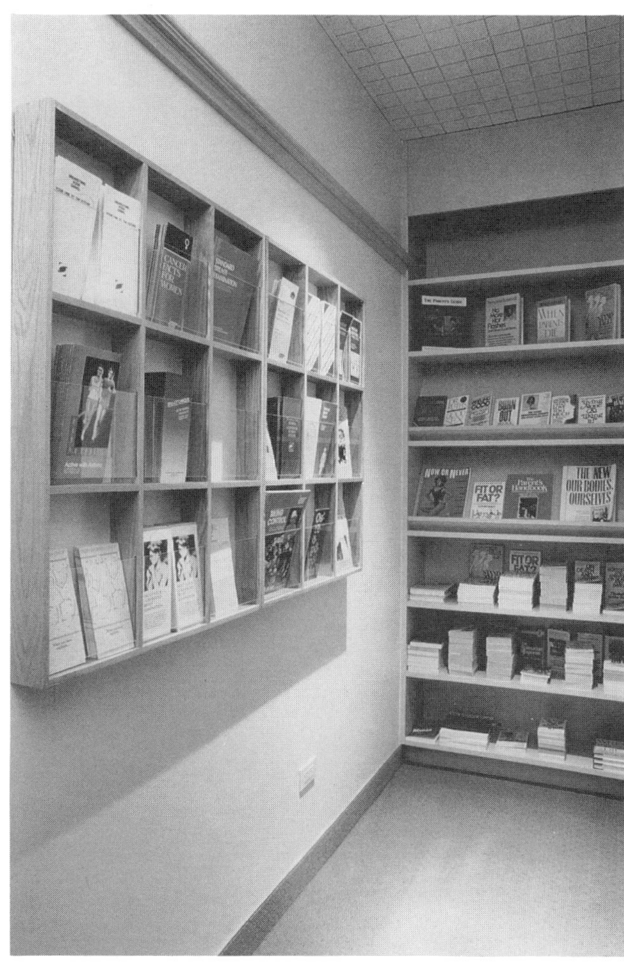

Figure 4-9. Reading nook, women's clinic. (*Design: Jain Malkin Inc.; Photographer: Kim Brun.*)

medical offices may be required to separate their trash. In this instance, provision would have to be made in the examination room for two receptacles. The paper from the exam table, paper towels, and wrappings from disposables, could go into one container and items coming into contact with patients' body fluids would be disposed of in an infectious waste receptacle. (These bags must be labeled to indicate they contain infectious waste.)

Specimen Toilets

Since each patient must empty her bladder before an examination, an OB-GYN suite needs a minimum of two toilet rooms. If it is possible to locate the toilet rooms near the nurse station or lab (Figure 4-11), a specimen pass-through (see Appendix) in the wall can eliminate the need for the patient to carry the urine specimen to the nurse station. Toilet rooms need a hook for hanging a handbag and coat, a shelf for sanitary napkins and tampons, and a receptacle for sanitary napkin disposal. It would be a nice touch to wallpaper the bathrooms.

Laboratory

The laboratory should be at least 10 × 12 feet and must include a sit-down space for a microscope and countertop space for centrifuge and an autoclave. Space should be allotted for an under-counter refrigerator. If the physicians elect to do a good deal of lab work in the suite, include a blood draw area and adequate countertop space for an automated clinical analyzer.

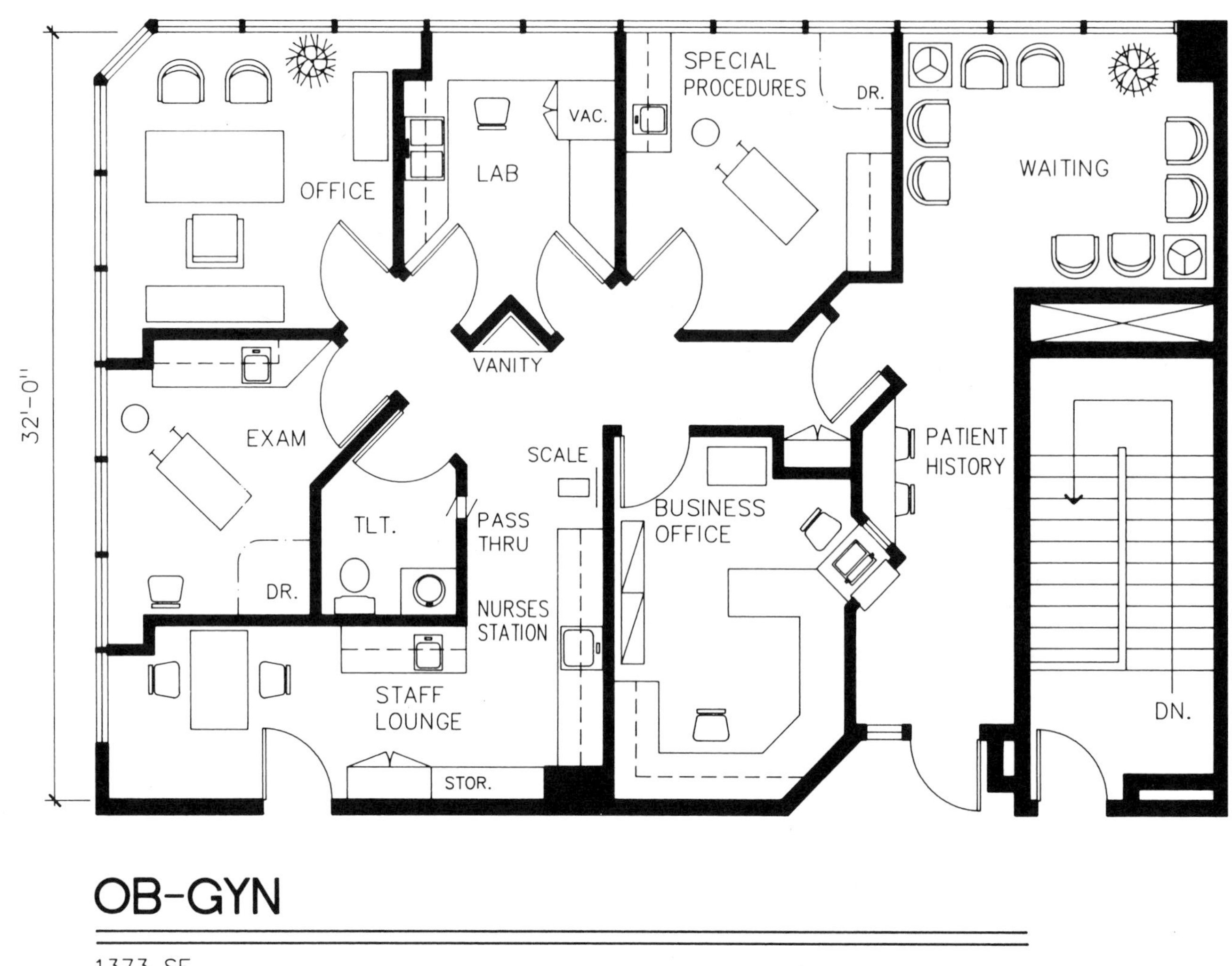

Figure 4-10. Suite plan for OB-GYN, 1373 square feet.

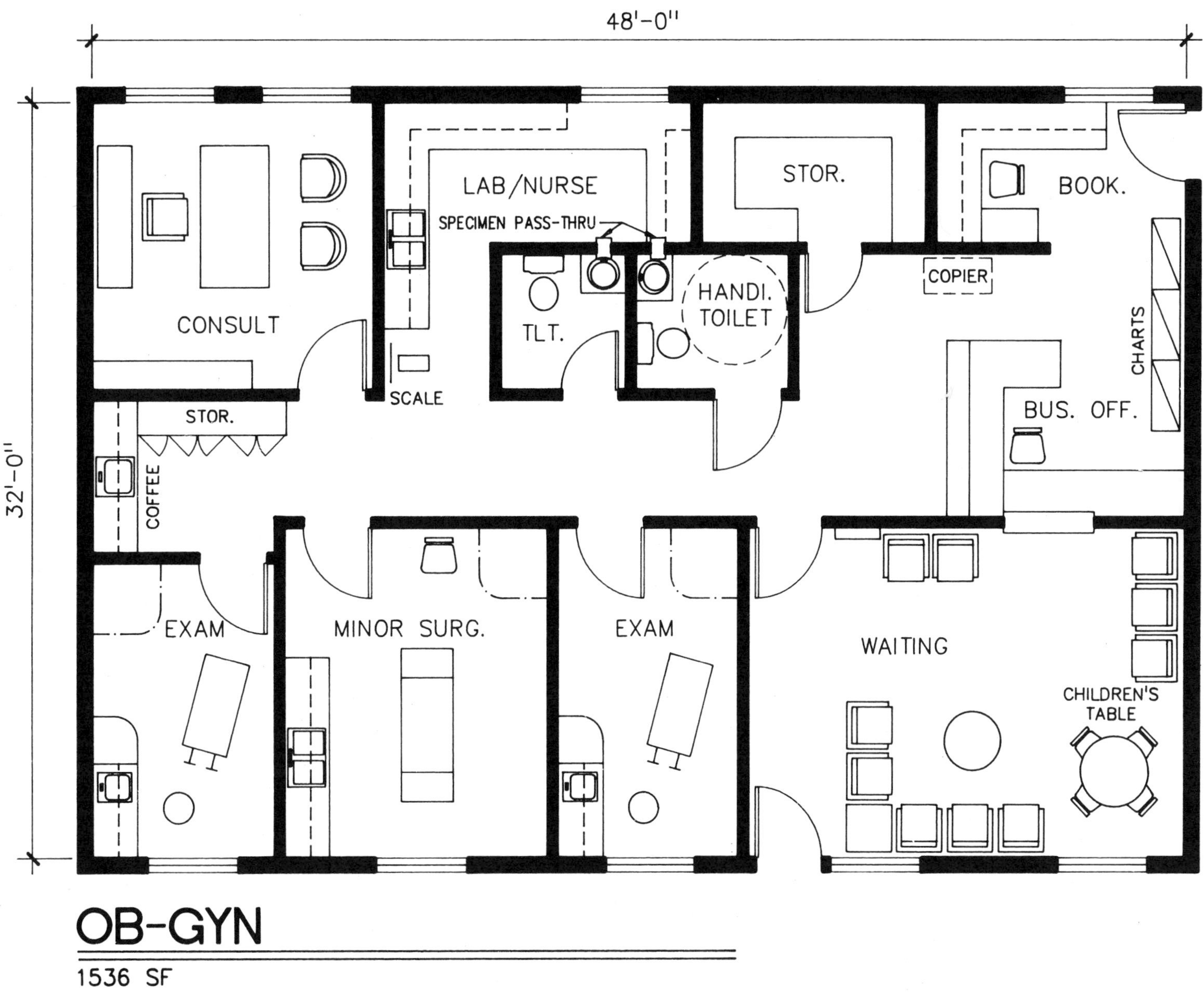

Figure 4-11. Suite plan for OB-GYN, 1536 square feet.

Interior Design

Physicians in this specialty often like a well-appointed consultation room. Furnishings are usually more elegant and refined than one might find in a consultation room of a general practice physician, for example. The room may be designed along the lines of a residential library or den, with a wood parquet floor and Oriental rug, bookshelves, fabric wallcovering, elegant upholstery fabrics, and an unusual desk. Window treatment, likewise, may be more like one would find in a residence rather than a medical office.

The waiting room, as well as the rest of the suite, ought to be designed to appeal to women (Color Plate 4, Figure 4-12). This may take the form of sunny colors — greens, pinks, yellows — and a garden design with lattice trim, white rattan chairs, flowery wallpaper, and chintz upholstery fabrics. Or, it may be elegant and sophisticated (Color Plates 5 and 6, Figures 4-13 and 4-14), perhaps a gray understated background punctuated by polished chrome and Plexiglas furniture, dramatic lighting, and an accent of violet or mauve in the upholstery.

If a physician's leanings are traditional, the style could be formal with wood moldings, Chippendale chairs with petitpoint upholstery, grasscloth or fabric wallcoverings, and Oriental rugs on a wood floor. Or, the traditional style might be less formal — country French. The options are many. This specialty allows the designer a great amount of freedom; obstetricians and gynecologists usually like to present a well-decorated office to their patients. Whatever the design style, chairs should not be so soft or so low that it is difficult for pregnant women to disengage themselves.

In summary, the patients here — due to the nature of the specialty — are generally happy, and this upbeat mood should be enhanced by the interior design. All rooms except the laboratory, minor surgery, and toilets may be carpeted. Gynecologists rarely use gentian violet anymore; therefore that argument against carpeting exam rooms is no longer valid.

WOMEN'S HEALTH CENTERS

Women's health centers arose in the mid-1980s in response to various social and economic changes. Taking responsibility for one's own health, consumer education, questioning traditional medical practices, and a more assertive population of women who work outside the home were all contributing factors. When market analysts revealed the following, the magnitude of the women's market became evident:

- Women are the decision makers on family health care.
- Women are the major users of medical and health services and, as women outnumber men in the population at large, they will continue to exert a major influence on the marketing of health care services.
- Women were often dissatisfied with the patronizing manner of some health care professionals.

Spawned by a desire to meet the demands of this "new" consumer, health care providers have been courting women with marketing incentives that differ considerably from the traditional doctor-knows-best approach of former years. Promises of no waiting, evening and Saturday office hours, convenient parking, child care, and health education seminars are attractive incentives.

These are not the only things that draw women to these facilities. The attitude of the staff is often dramatically different in a market-driven practice than in the traditional health care setting. There is an expressed respect for women and an opportunity for them to participate in their own health care. There are no secrets. Patients are not kept waiting. Prices are quoted in advance. Lab test results — even normal ones — are related to the patient. During patient/physician consultations, the patient is clothed and seated at the same level as the physician. There is a special emphasis on making the patient feel like a welcome guest.

Common to many women's centers is an all-female professional staff that may include family practitioners, internists, psychiatrists and psychologists, nurse practitioners, nutritionists, obstetrician/gynecologists, and social workers. These professionals focus their attention on gender differences in each area of specialization and thereby offer patients a measure of understanding that is sometimes lacking in health care provided by professionals outside the women's center network. This is a major issue for women who are looking for continuity of care, instead of maintaining a relationship with five or six practitioners in different offices.

Some of the newly opened centers are affiliated with a hospital, but other clinics are operated by physicians or entrepreneurial for-profit corporations. The for-profits tend to operate their facilities with an eye on the bottom line — that health care can be packaged and delivered as a product, and earn a profit at the same time. Viewing health care as a business, rather than as a community service, makes the for-profits particularly sensitive to marketing trends and customer satisfaction. This is good news for designers. A client who is aware of marketing opportunities understands that the design of the facility will attract patients and, in turn, will lead to many patient referrals.

Women find these facilities comfortable and nonclinical, with carpeted floors, wallcoverings, and residential style lighting and furniture. Clients who are attentive to these issues may actually reduce their marketing costs due to increased referrals by satisfied patients.

In order to design a women's health center properly, one has to understand the range of services offered — and this varies from facility to facility. These may include gynecology, mammography, osteoporosis screening, primary care, internal medicine, diet and exercise programs, nutrition counseling, weight loss clinics, counseling on family or social problems, and prenatal care. Great emphasis is placed on prevention and patient education. Seminars and lectures by health care experts occur regularly. Other features may include a library or reading area for information on health care topics.

Interior designers who plan women's health centers should be aware of the following considerations:

- Color and design should appeal to women, but not be overly frilly. Too often, facilities try to appear "feminine" by using inexpensive French Provincial furniture, velvet cushions, or artwork framed with ruffles and lace. This may appeal to some women, but the majority may prefer a more sophisticated treatment.

- The reception window should be wide and open so that the patient does not feel closed out and isolated.

- Patient education carrels should be located in view of one of the receptionists, but should afford privacy for the patient.

- A large multipurpose meeting room is needed for lectures and seminars. It should be furnished with tablet arm chairs and a number of small tables that can be pushed together for meetings.

- Exam rooms need dressing cubicles for patient privacy and for hanging clothing. Medical equipment and instruments should be stored out of sight so that the room appears nonthreatening to the patient. Exam rooms (except those used for minor surgery) should be carpeted. It should be noted that recent developments in commercial carpet fibers and backings as well as antimicrobial and stain-resistant properties make carpet a viable option for exam rooms. Thoughtful amenities would be a magazine rack, artwork, fresh flowers, and a mirror (see Figure 4-4).
- The physician's consultation room or private office should have — in addition to a desk — some lounge chairs or a small sofa and coffee table to provide an informal, friendly, residential setting.
- A library, if space allows, can be located in a separate room or in a nook off the entry, but within view of the receptionist or cashier. For brochures, which are meant to be handed out, a rack in the reception area or corridor would be sufficient (see Figure 4-9).
- The scale at the nurse station should be placed to afford privacy for those self-conscious about their weight. Ample storage areas for drug samples and other items must be provided in the nurse station, as well.
- One room will be a breast exam room, which means that the patient will usually lie down on a divan or high bed and watch a video describing how to do a breast self-exam. There also needs to be a chair for a nurse or aide.
- Light fixtures should not shine into patients' eyes; therefore, alternatives such as wall sconces, wall washers, indirect perimeter, or low voltage downlighting should be used. Limit the use of lay-in 2 × 4 fluorescent lighting to examination or treatment rooms.
- If the facility is to be staffed primarily by women, the height of such items as X-ray view boxes, countertops, and cabinets must be considered. The average height of a woman is 5 feet, 4 inches.
- Patients appreciate a specimen pass-through between the restroom and lab so that the patient does not have to carry the specimen into the corridor.
- Cabinets in the minor surgery room can house large pieces of equipment, such as the suction machine, the colposcope, and the emergency crash cart, which tend to be anxiety-provoking items (see Figure 4-8). More casework is needed here compared with a standard exam room. Also, the floor should be sheet vinyl or other easily cleaned material.
- For acoustical privacy, exam rooms should have solid core doors and Fiberglas insulation batting in the walls.

Women's health care centers (Figure 4-15) offer designers an opportunity to break away from conventional ideas about what medical offices should look like. It is hard to predict whether gender-specific health care for women will continue to be provided, long term, in high-profile specialized facilities, or if these programs will become integrated into primary care networks.

OTOLARYNGOLOGY

An otolaryngologist treats diseases of the ears, nose, and throat. The specialty is more commonly known as ENT (ear, nose, and throat), and its practitioners often practice facial plastic surgery as well.

A solo practitioner needs three examination rooms, a waiting room that seats 10 or 11 persons, an audio test room, a minor surgery room (or if facial plastic surgery is practiced, an outpatient surgery room and recovery room), an X-ray room and darkroom, a business office, a consultation room, and a nurse station/lab (Figure 4-17). A two-physician suite may not be much larger, but would have an additional consultation room (Figure 4-18).

The consultation room is large (12 × 14 feet) since patients are often brought into this room to discuss fees for surgery or to discuss the feasibility of a surgical procedure. The X-ray room can be as small as 8 × 12 feet (depending on the physician's equipment) since films are limited to the head and neck. The reader is referred to Chapter 3 for space planning details of an X-ray room, control area, darkroom, and lead shielding. The darkroom can be small, since the physician will probably have a tabletop model automatic film processor similar to the kind used by dentists. The designer must obtain the specs on utility requirements from the manufacturer of the unit.

Exam Rooms

Examination rooms need be only 8 × 12 feet, with the sink cabinet located on the long wall. A special motorized examination chair (see Figure 4-12) is located in the center of the room on an angle, with the patient facing the door. The physician works off of a cart along the wall, to the right of the patient. Most of the time, the physician is seated on a stool with casters. Each exam room needs an X-ray view box recessed in the wall.

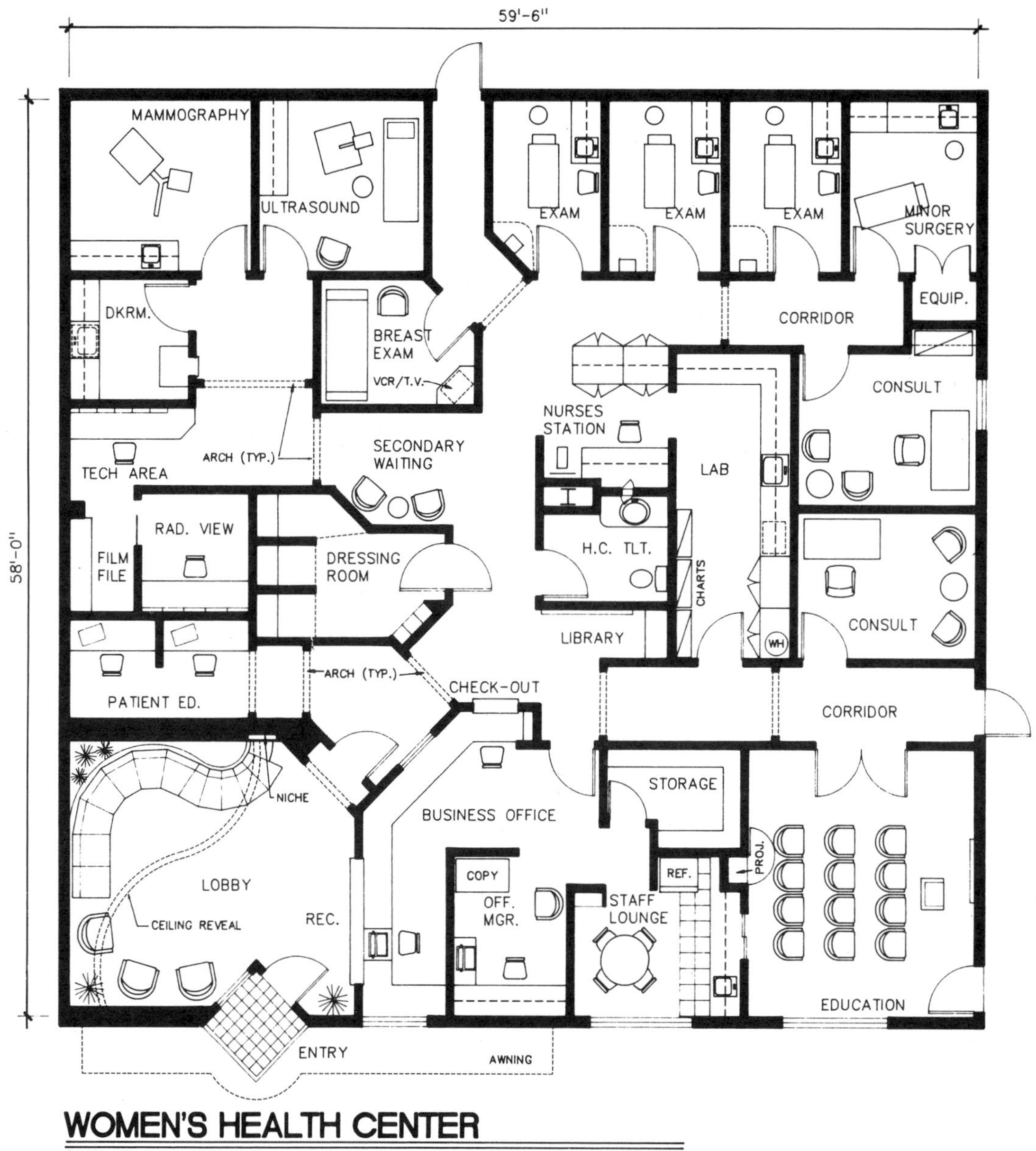

Figure 4-15. Suite plan for women's health center, 3450 square feet.

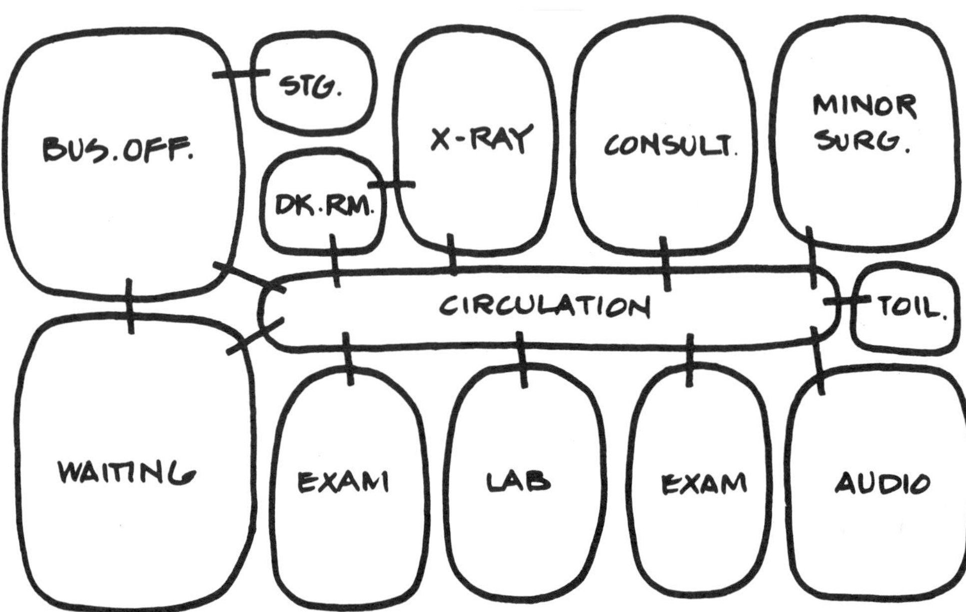

Figure 4-16. Schematic diagram of an otolaryngology suite.

Table 4-2. Analysis of Program. Otolaryngology

No. of Physicians:	1		2	
Exam Rooms	3 @ 8 × 12 =	288	5 @ 8 × 12 =	480
Consultation Rooms	12 × 14 =	168	2 @ 12 × 14 =	336
Business Office	12 × 18 =	216	12 × 18 =	216
Nurse Station/Lab	8 × 10 =	80	8 × 12 =	96
Waiting Room	14 × 16 =	224	14 × 20 =	280
Audio Room	11 × 12 =	132	11 × 12 =	132
Toilets	2 @ 5 × 6 =	60	2 @ 5 × 6 =	60
Minor Surgery	12 × 12 =	144	—	
Outpatient Surgery	—		12 × 16 =	192
Recovery	—		8 × 14 =	112
Storage	6 × 8 =	48	6 × 8 =	48
X-ray	9 × 12 =	108	9 × 12 =	108
Darkroom	4 × 6 =	24	4 × 6 =	24
Staff Lounge	8 × 10 =	80	10 × 12 =	120
Subtotal		1572 ft²		2204 ft²
15% Circulation		236		330
Total		1808 ft²		2534 ft²

Note: The one-physician suite outlined above would serve an otolaryngologist who does not practice facial plastic surgery; the two-physician suite is designed for practitioners who do.

The unit from which the physician works is usually a specialized manufactured stainless steel cabinet on casters (Figure 4-19) containing a suction unit and pump, compressed air, a cautery, an electrical panel for instruments, racks for solution bottles, and a shelf and drawers for medications, cotton jars, irrigation syringes, and atomizers. The unit also has a pull-out writing shelf. Approximately 23 inches wide × 18 inches deep × 46 inches high, it requires a grounded duplex outlet. Figure 4-20 shows a similar unit by another manufacturer.

Sometimes the medical examination cabinet is purchased without suction and air features, in which case the designer needs to provide a vacuum system within the suite. A small room, 4 feet 6 inches × 5 feet, should

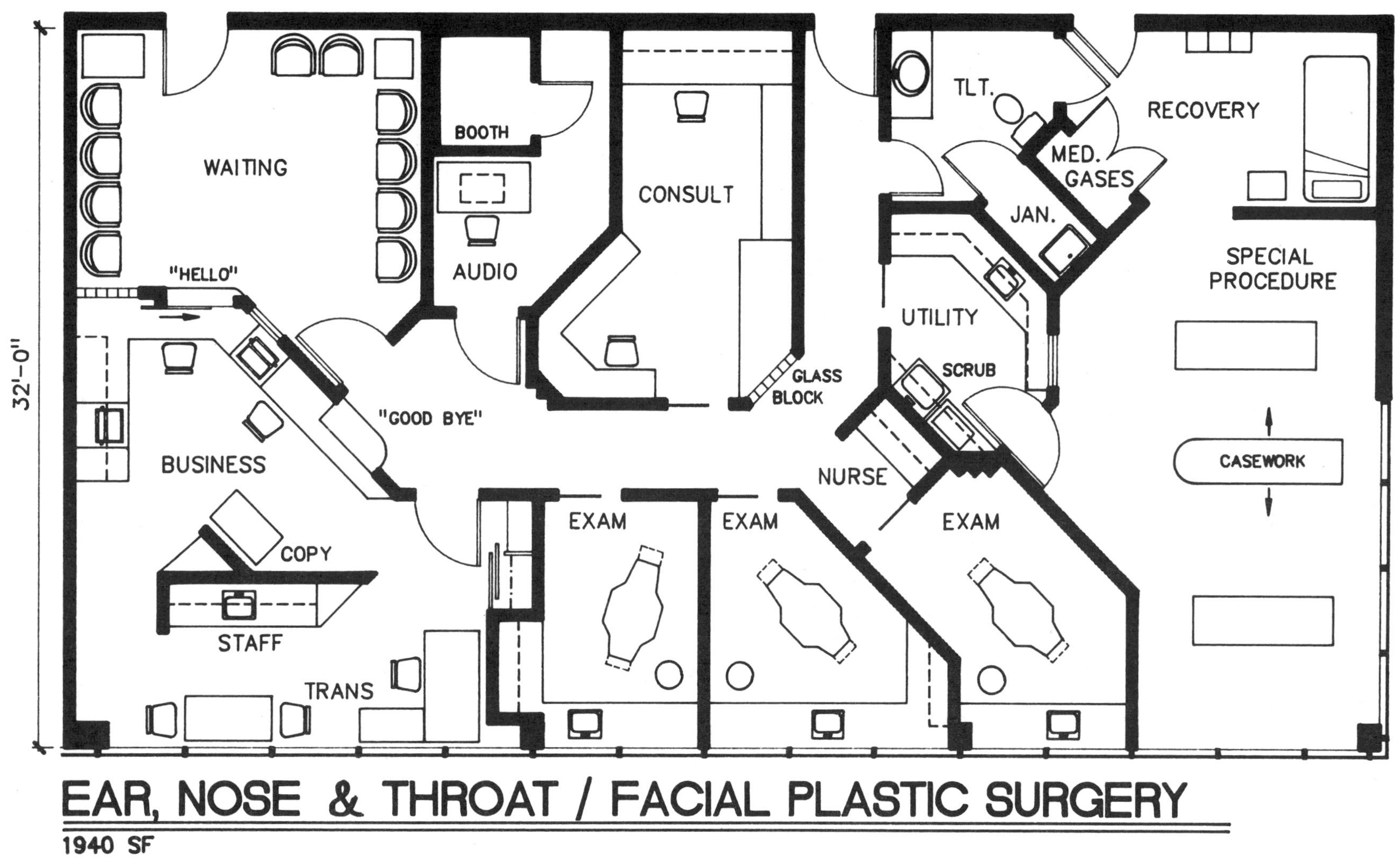

Figure 4-17. Suite plan for ear, nose and throat/facial plastic surgery, 1940 square feet.

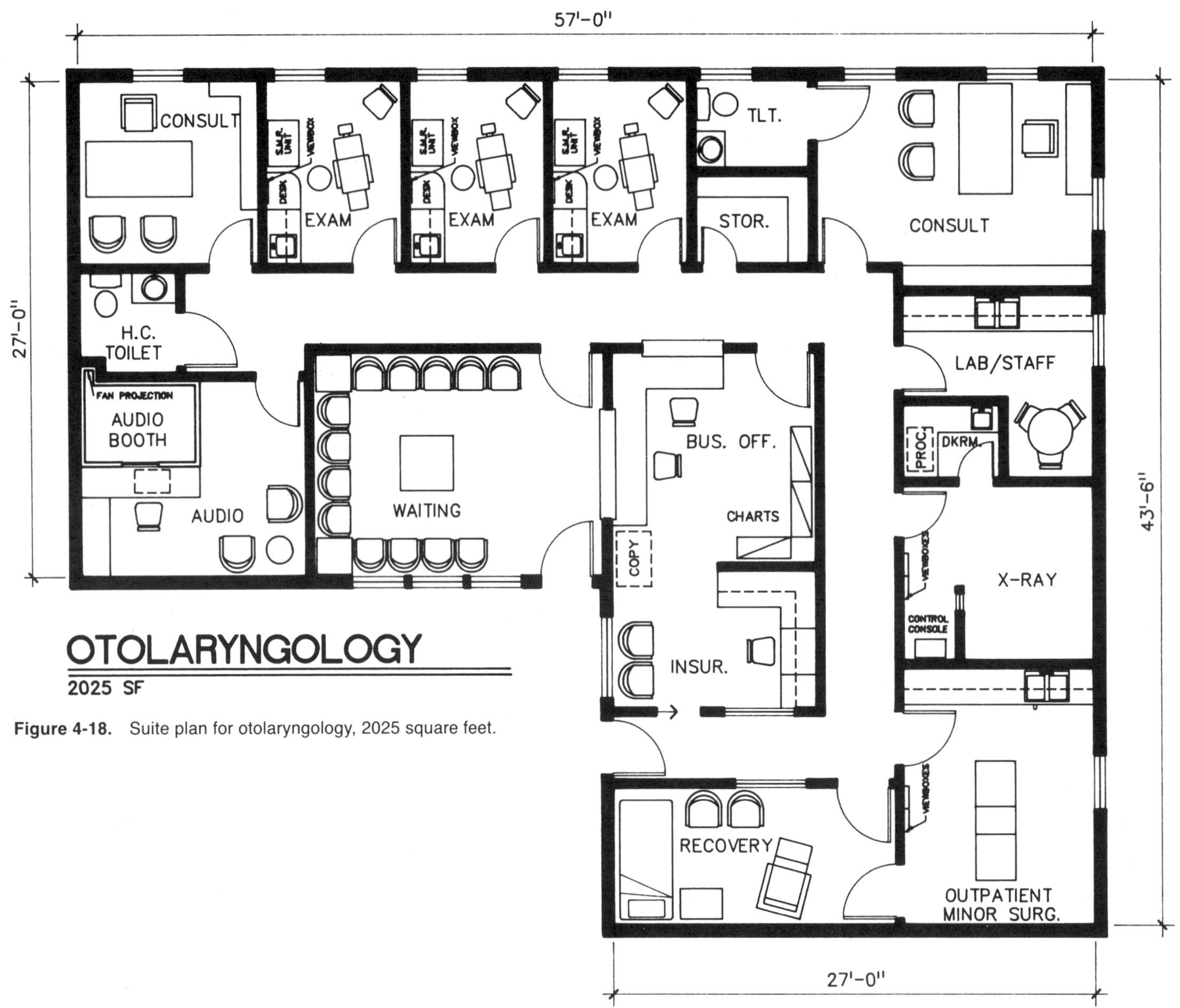

Figure 4-18. Suite plan for otolaryngology, 2025 square feet.

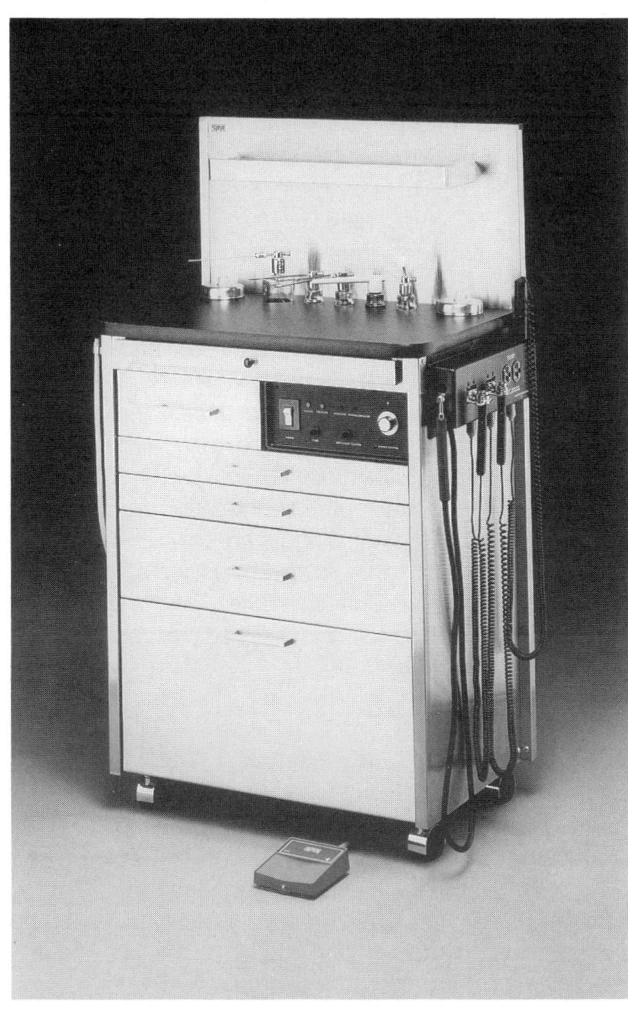

Figure 4-19. ENT cart. (*Courtesy Storz/SMR, St. Louis, MO.*)

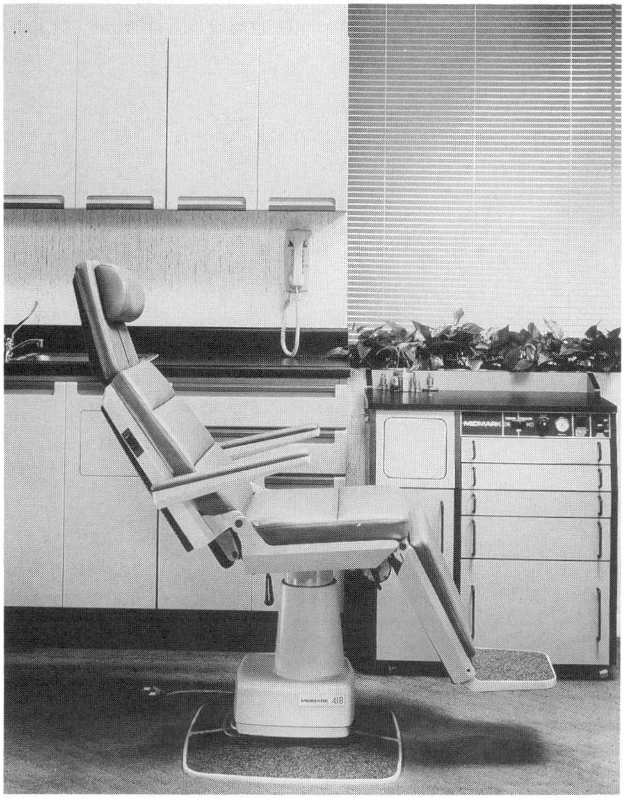

Figure 4-20. ENT cart. (*Courtesy Midmark Corp., Versailles, OH.*)

be provided close to the examination rooms to eliminate long-distance piping. Vacuum pumps and air compressors are noisy, so the walls of this room should be well insulated. Usually two 20-ampere separate circuits will be required. A local vacuum contractor will provide the designer with specs on the equipment and will install the plastic piping. The piping would be done after the HVAC (heating, ventilating, and air conditioning) has been completed, but before the partitions are closed up.

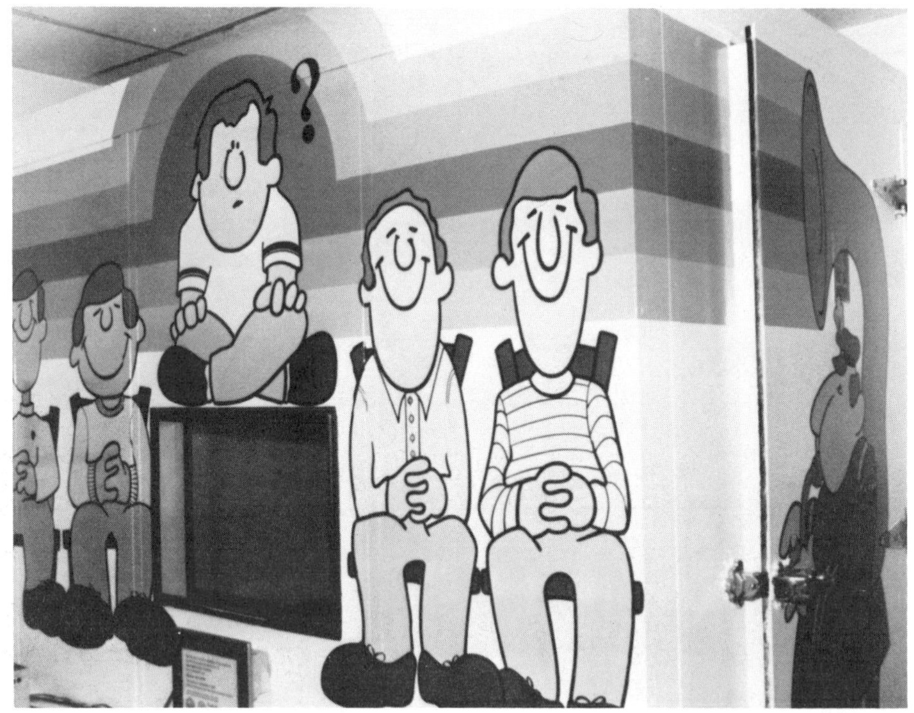

Figure 4-21. Audio booth with cartoon design. (*Design: Jain Malkin Inc.; Photographer: Jain Malkin.*)

A nice feature in exam rooms and the recovery room is a wall-mounted cosmetic mirror — perhaps a small plastic laminate cabinet with two hinged doors which, when opened, reveal a good-quality mirror and two rows of makeup lights that are electric-eye operated, so that opening the doors activates the lights. A dressing area is not required in ENT exam rooms.

Office-Based Surgery

If the physician does only ENT and no facial plastic surgery, a minor surgery room (refer to Chapter 3, General Practice) would be used for special procedures and for emergency care. As the practice matures, an otolaryngologist tends toward more cosmetic and reconstructive facial plastic surgery because it is more lucrative and, perhaps, more interesting than routine ENT procedures. Procedures such as nose reconstruction, face lifts, eye tucks, repair of cleft palate and face peels may be performed in the office in a well-equipped outpatient surgery room with ancillary recovery room, scrub, and prep areas (see Figure 4-17).

The surgery room should contain one wall of built-in cabinets, and the sink will have a plaster trap and foot lever control for hot, warm, and cold water. Scrub and prep can be done in the surgery room if the room is large enough, and if patient volume is low. An electrical outlet is required in the floor for the motorized table. Other electrical outlets and connections for suction, compressed air, and instruments should be located by the physician, since this room allows for a variety of options with respect to work habits. The reader is referred to Plastic Surgery for a detailed discussion of an outpatient surgery room.

Audio Testing

A basic part of an otolaryngologist's practice involves diagnosing and treating patients with a hearing loss. An audio booth is used for testing hearing. It is a soundproofed room approximately 5 feet wide × 6 feet 6 inches long with a door at one end. The patient sits inside and listens to sounds of different frequencies through earphones. The technician or audiologist sits outside the booth, at a counter facing the patient, and looks into the booth through a window so that the patient is always in view (see Figure 4-18). This countertop contains the audio equipment from which sounds are transmitted to the patient in the booth. The patient's responses are recorded, and a graph of hearing loss is produced for the physician to evaluate.

The audio booth is available as a prefabricated unit (Figure 4-21) that breaks down into components and is assembled in the room by an installation technician. The booth has an exhaust fan and various electrical requirements, foremost of which is connecting it to the testing equipment (an exposed low-voltage cable is commonly used). The audio testing room must be located in a quiet part of the suite, away from the heavy traffic of the waiting room and business office.

A custom audio booth can be built on the job, but rigid construction specifications must be adhered to in order to achieve a sound transmission class of 55 to 60 decibels. Double-stud walls with several layers of sound board, insulation batting, and a solid-core door with an acoustic seal on all sides would be required.

Interior Design

There are no special requirements for interior design in this suite. If the practice tends toward facial plastic surgery, the office design should reinforce the image of the surgeon as a successful, skilled professional with refined aesthetic taste. The reader is referred to the Plastic Surgery section in this chapter for additional discussion of this topic.

OPHTHALMOLOGY

This specialty is characterized by a variety of options in suite design. Therefore, the individual practitioner must make the basic decisions on preferred work habits before the designer can begin.

There seems to be an ever-increasing need for specialized eye care, which means that the ophthalmologist may attain a capacity patient load within the first two years of practice. Thus, it is important to project at the outset what the ophthalmologist's space needs will be in two or three years. Often, young ophthalmologists setting up their first offices will try to be too economical. They set up a minimally functional office based on their patient projection (usually underestimated) at that moment. Then, for the remainder of their lease (usually five years), they are handicapped by a small, poorly laid out office, which greatly inhibits the growth of their practice.

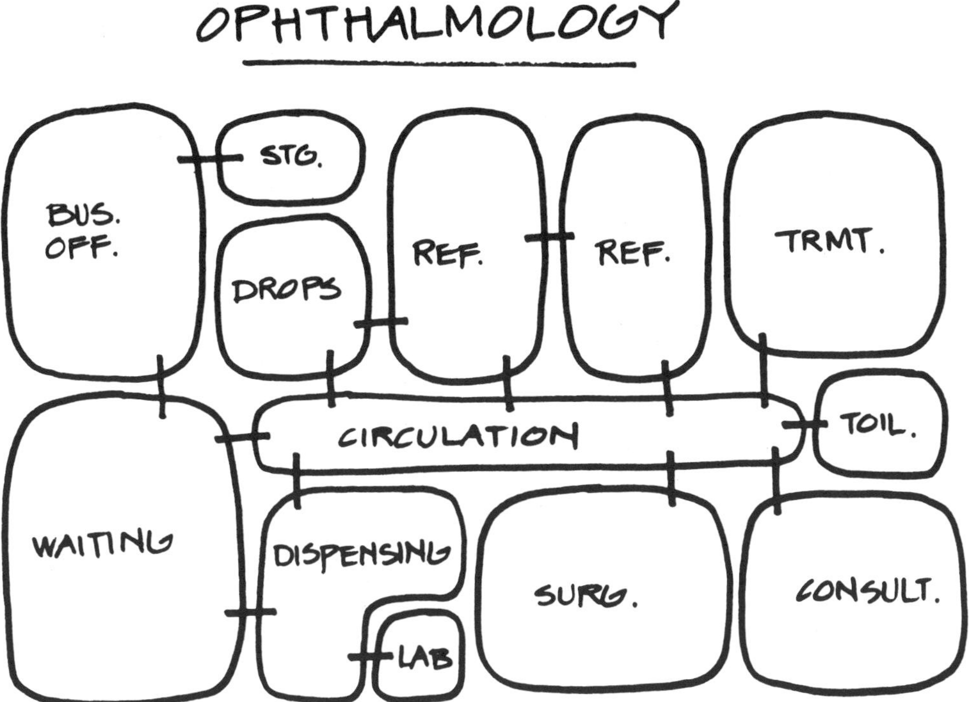

Figure 4-22. Schematic diagram of an ophthalmology suite.

Patient Volume

Many ophthalmologists schedule three patients per hour for regular eye examinations. Added to that are unscheduled patients — emergency and trauma —and post-operative patients, and it is not unusual for an ophthalmologist to see four patients an hour. Individual practice habits may differ, with some doctors spending more time informally chatting with patients than those who choose to work in a more restricted, tightly scheduled manner. The more relaxed ophthalmologist may see only two patients per hour, particularly if he or she does all the testing with little assistance from aides.

Required Rooms

A solo practitioner needs at least two refraction rooms, plus a third multipurpose or minor surgery/treatment room. While a patient whose examination has been concluded is gathering up possessions and receiving medications and instructions from the nurse or aide, the doctor has already stepped into the next refraction room and has begun to examine the patient with no loss of time. The minor surgery room can be used for removing a foreign body from the eye or for other emergency visits, or the doctor may see an unscheduled patient in this room while he or she is between patients without interrupting scheduled patients in the refraction rooms. The minor surgery room can also be utilized for photography or for visual fields testing or orthoptic evaluations.

An ophthalmologist does not need a nurse station or lab as such, but it is advisable to provide a work space in a niche off the corridor (Figure 4-23) for an assistant or aide. This is where phone calls can be received or made to reschedule patients, or prescriptions can be authorized, and medications dispensed. Ophthalmologists dispense a number of eye drops and medications, which may be stored in a rack in each examining room or at the assistant's work area.

Table 4-3. Analysis of Program. Ophthalmology

No. of Physicians:	1	2	3
Refracting Rooms	3 @ 10 × 12 = 360[a]	4 total = 700[b]	8 total = 1400[b]
Minor Surgery	11 × 12 = 132	2 @ 12 × 12 = 288	12 × 22 = 264
Consultation	10 × 12 = 120	2 @ 12 × 12 = 288	4 @ 10 × 11 = 440
Fields Room	8 × 8 = 64	—	10 × 11 = 110
Data Collection	—	11 × 12 = 132	10 × 14 = 140
Waiting Room	12 × 18 = 216	16 × 28 = 448	22 × 26 = 572
Drops	6 × 6 = 36	8 × 12 = 96	Use waiting room
Toilets	2 @ 5 × 6 = 60	2 @ 5 × 6 = 60	2 @ 5 × 6 = 60
Business Office	12 × 14 = 168	12 × 16 = 192	12 × 20 = 240
Storage	4 × 6 = 24	6 × 8 = 48	6 × 8 = 48
Optician, Lab, and Contact Lens	10 × 24 = 240	(Nondispensing physician)	18 × 30 = 540
Staff Lounge	—	8 × 10 = 80	12 × 12 = 144
Subtotal	1420 ft²	2332 ft²	3958 ft²
15% Circulation	213	350	594
Total	1633 ft²	2682 ft²	4552 ft²

[a]Using mirrors

[b]Twenty-four foot refracting rooms (two "interlocking" together occupy approximately 10 × 35 ft.)

Optical Dispensing

It is common for ophthalmologists to practice as solo practitioners with the help of an assistant or technician. An optician may also be part of the practice, in which case an area approximately 10 × 24 feet is needed, divided into a lab, a contact lens area, and a fitting area (Figures 4-23 and 4-24). The lab has walls lined with cabinets and work counters and requires shadow-free lighting.

The contact lens area requires a small fitting table 2 × 4 feet with a mirrored top. The patient sits on one side and optician on the other. The room may also have a storage cabinet and a small sink. The fitting area has a long table divided into a number of fitting stations, each with a mirror and may have panels of

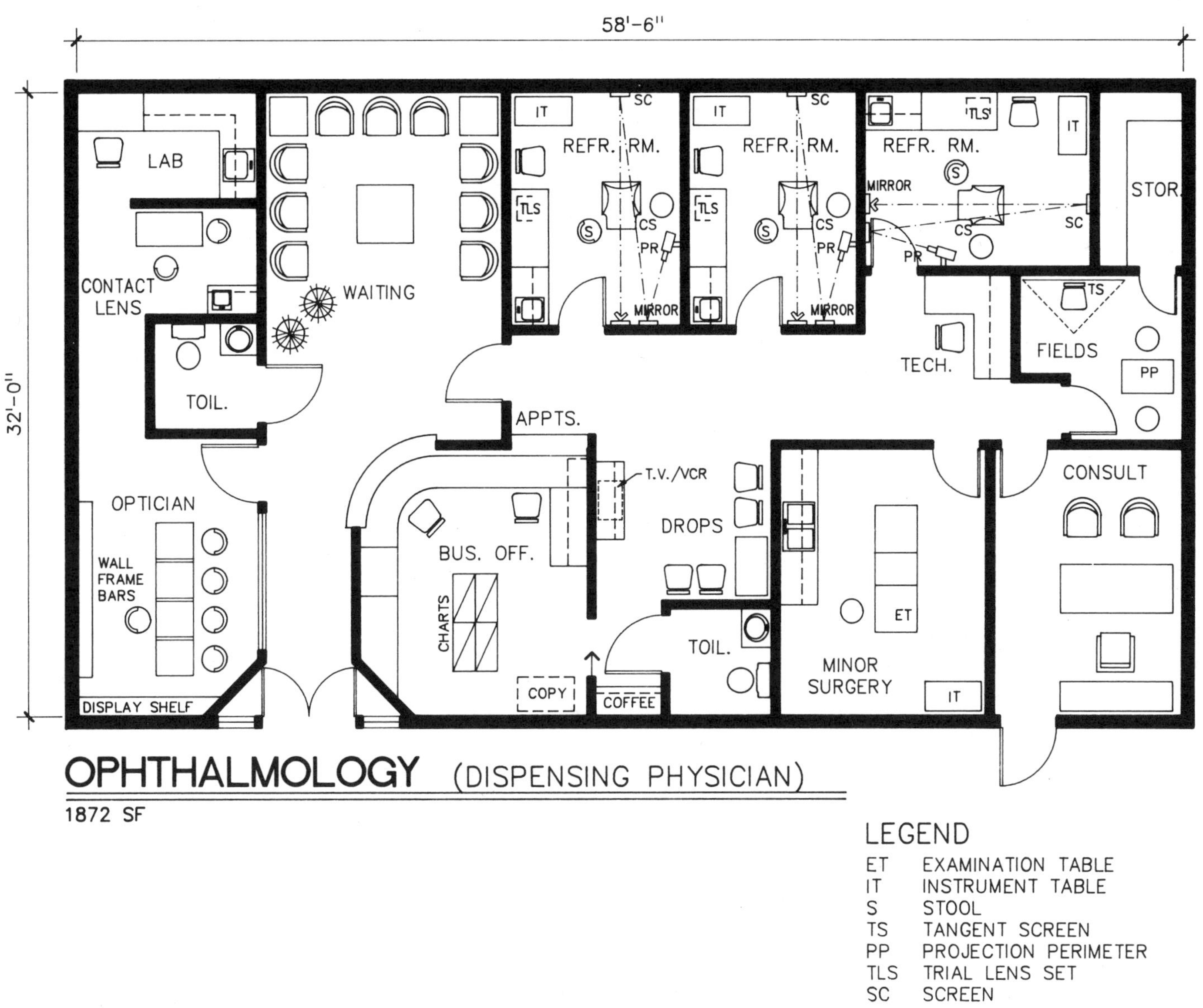

Figure 4-23. Suite plan for ophthalmology, 1872 square feet.

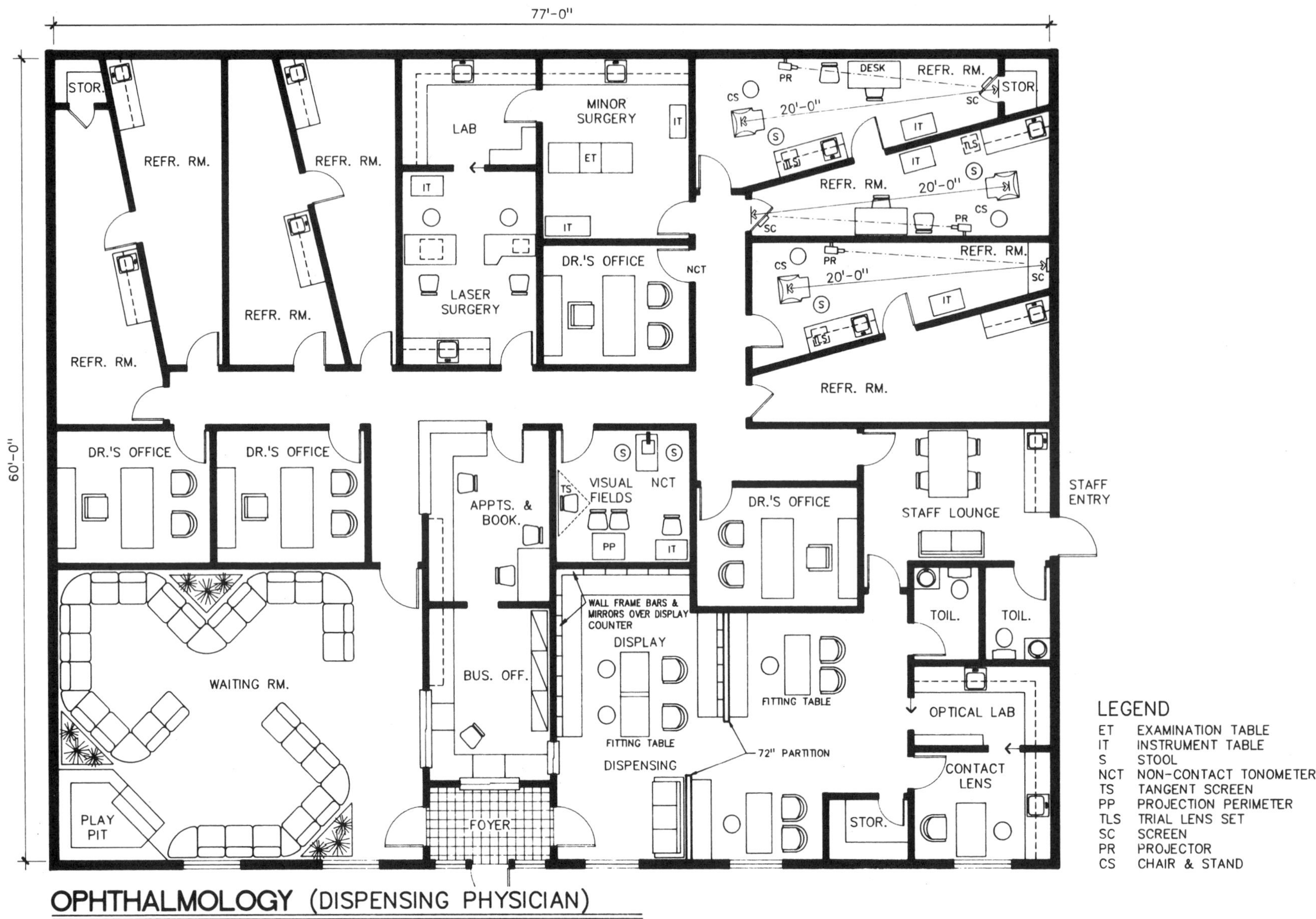

Figure 4-24. Suite plan for ophthalmology, 4620 square feet.

eyeglass frames (*frame bars*) located on either side of the patient. The optician sits on a stool behind the table and works from drawers and cabinets to the side and behind. Attractive wall frame bars can be purchased ready-made, or they may be designed and custom fabricated to hold the many eyeglass frames to be displayed.

Ophthalmologists who offer the services of an optician are called *dispensing physicians.*

Multipurpose Room

Ophthalmologists used to arrange their offices so that different tests were performed in different rooms. Some ophthalmologists may still practice that way. However, it is far more efficient for the patient to remain in one room. Each time the patient has to gather his belongings and move to another room, then again get comfortable, valuable time (and money) is lost. For most ophthalmology practices, a complete examination and treatment can be done in the same room with the patient in the same chair.

Refraction Room

The most important room is the refraction room, a multipurpose examination room with equipment and instruments grouped around the patient and the doctor sitting either in front of the patient or just to one side. Right-handed physicians will prefer to examine from the patient's right side. The dimensions of this room are crucial, and both the ophthalmologist's work habits and instruments will dictate the critical distances that must be observed.

Refraction rooms have two basic sizes. Since a standard eye chart is designed for a distance of 20 feet from chart to patient's eye, the traditional refraction room is approximately 24 feet long (20 feet for the refraction lane plus 4 feet for the examining chair and space to walk around it) as in Figures 4-24 and 4-25. However, with the aid of projectors and mirrors, the room length may be reduced to 12 or 14 feet. A 10-foot-wide × 12-foot-long room would be suitable.

To compensate for a room length of less than 24 feet, two mirrors are placed on the wall in front of the patient, and a screen is placed on the wall behind the patient (Figure 4-23). A projector (Figure 4-26) projects the text characters onto one of the front mirrors, which in turn projects it back to the screen behind the patient. The second mirror, in front of the patient, reflects the image from the rear screen. The refracting lane, in this case, is the distance measured between the second mirror and the screen plus the distance between the mirror and the patient. The letters of the eye chart can be adjusted in size by the projector so that correct visual acuities can always be maintained.

There are several types of procedures performed in the refracting room, but the primary task is to determine the refractive power of the eye. To do this, the physician selects various lenses from a partitioned rack (Figure 4-27), a *trial lens box* (approximate size 12½ × 20½ × 2½ inches), and places them in a holder through which the patient looks. The patient is asked to read the test letters to determine which lens is best. Sometimes a *refractor,* an instrument containing lenses, is used.

The interior of the eye, the fundus, is examined by an *ophthalmoscope,* a handheld light source, while the conjunctiva, lens, iris, and cornea (the front portions of the eye) are examined by a *slit lamp,* an illuminated microscope (Figure 4-28), which may be mounted on a shelf of the instrument stand (Figure 4-29) or may be on a mobile instrument table. A *keratometer* (Figure 4-30) measures the curvature of the cornea. The instrument in Figure 4-31 measures the curvature and thickness of contact lenses.

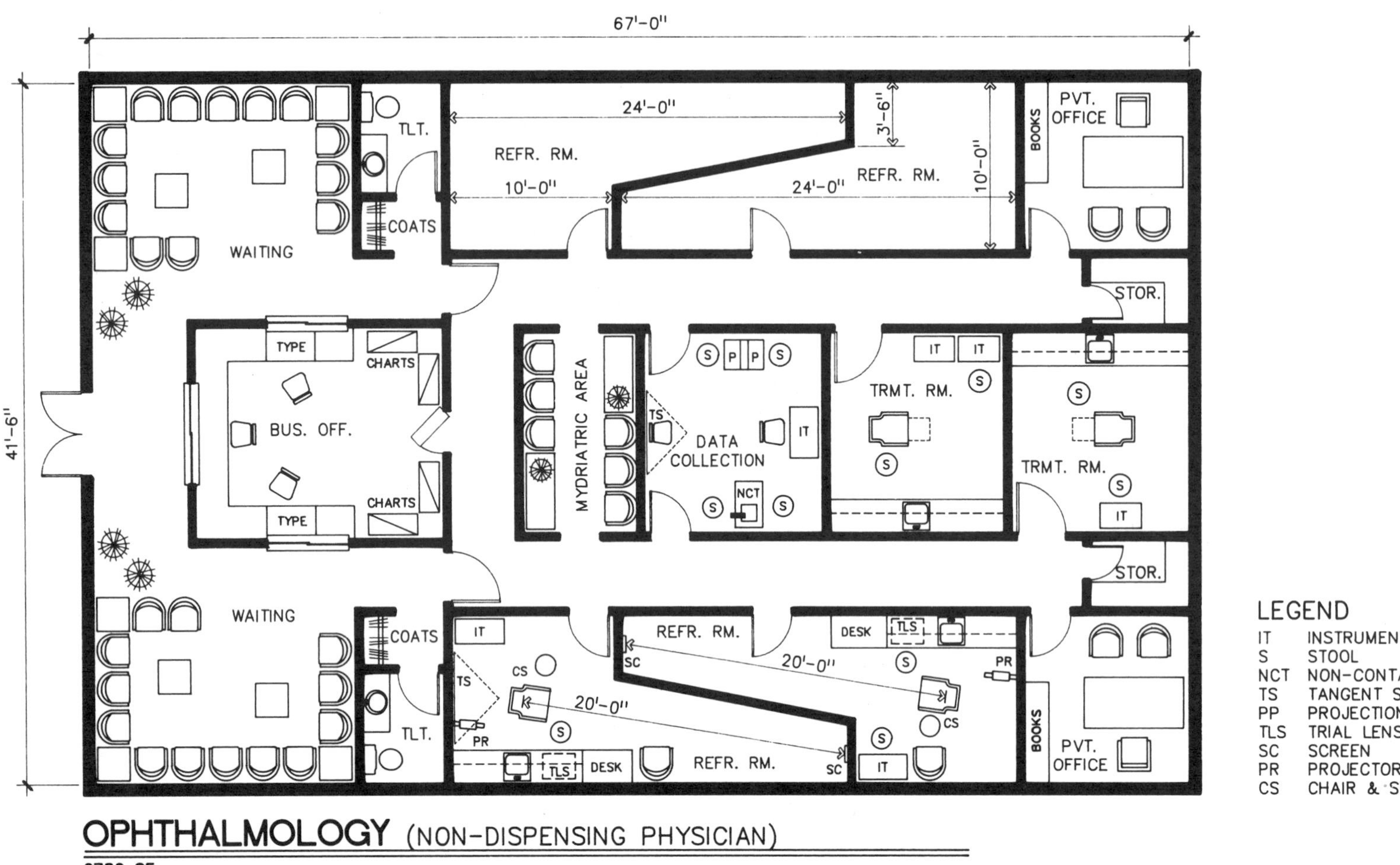

Figure 4-25. Suite plan for ophthalmology, 2780 square feet.

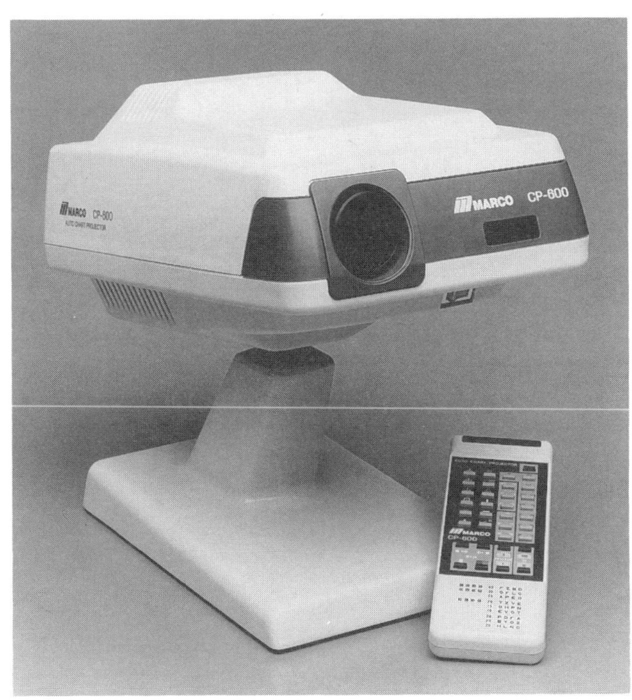

Figure 4-26. Ophthalmology chart projector. (*Courtesy Marco Ophthalmic, Jacksonville, FL.*)

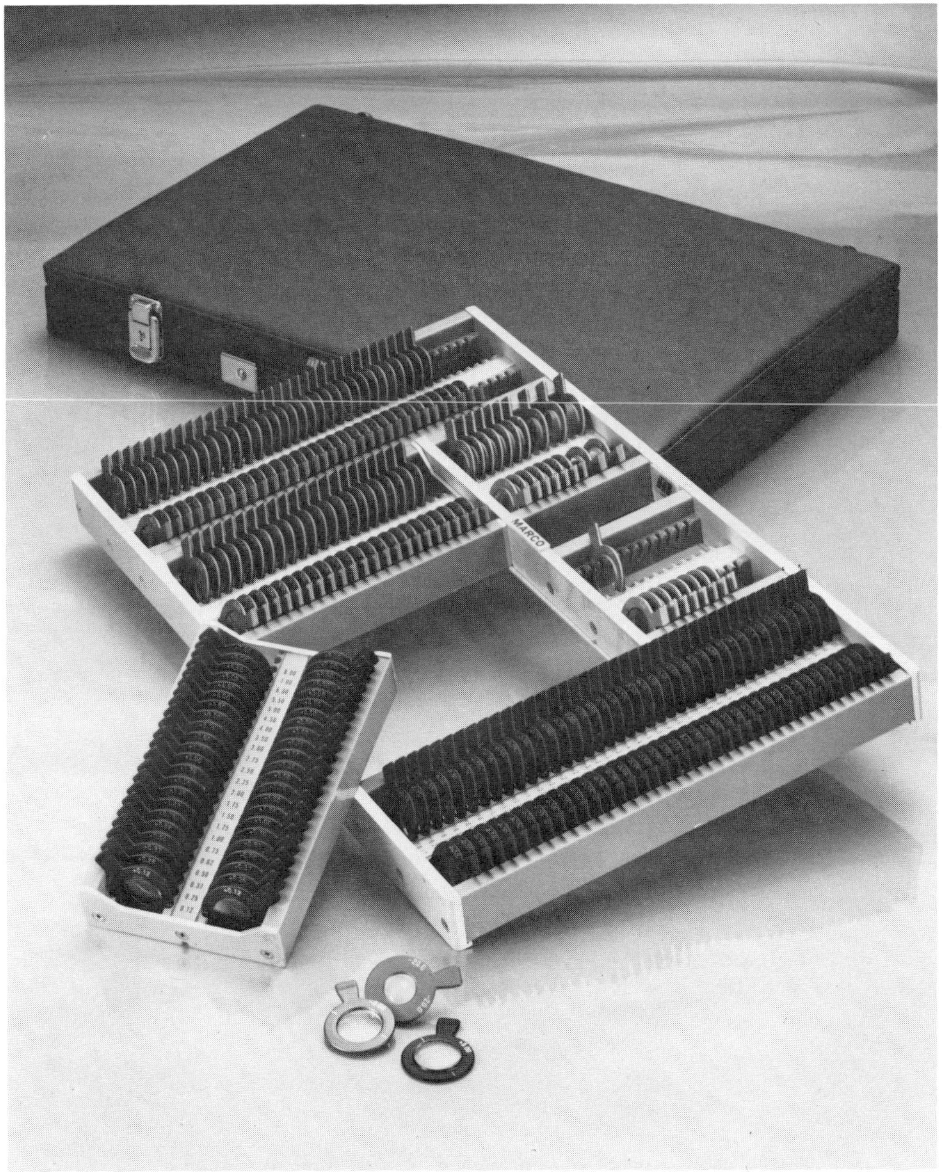

Figure 4-27. Trial lens box. (*Courtesy Marco Ophthalmic, Jacksonville, FL.*)

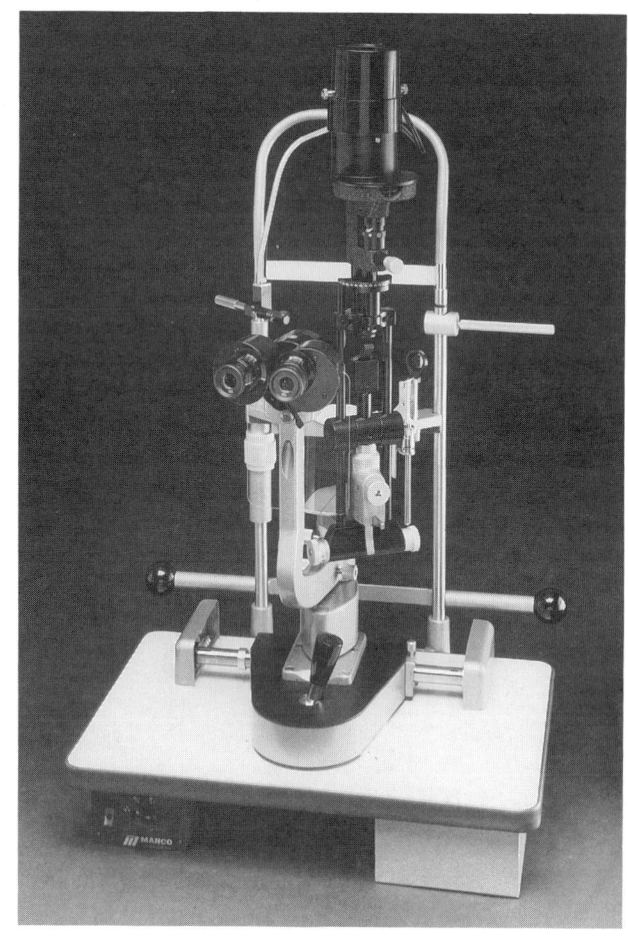

Figure 4-28. Slit lamp. (*Courtesy Marco Ophthalmic, Jacksonville, FL.*)

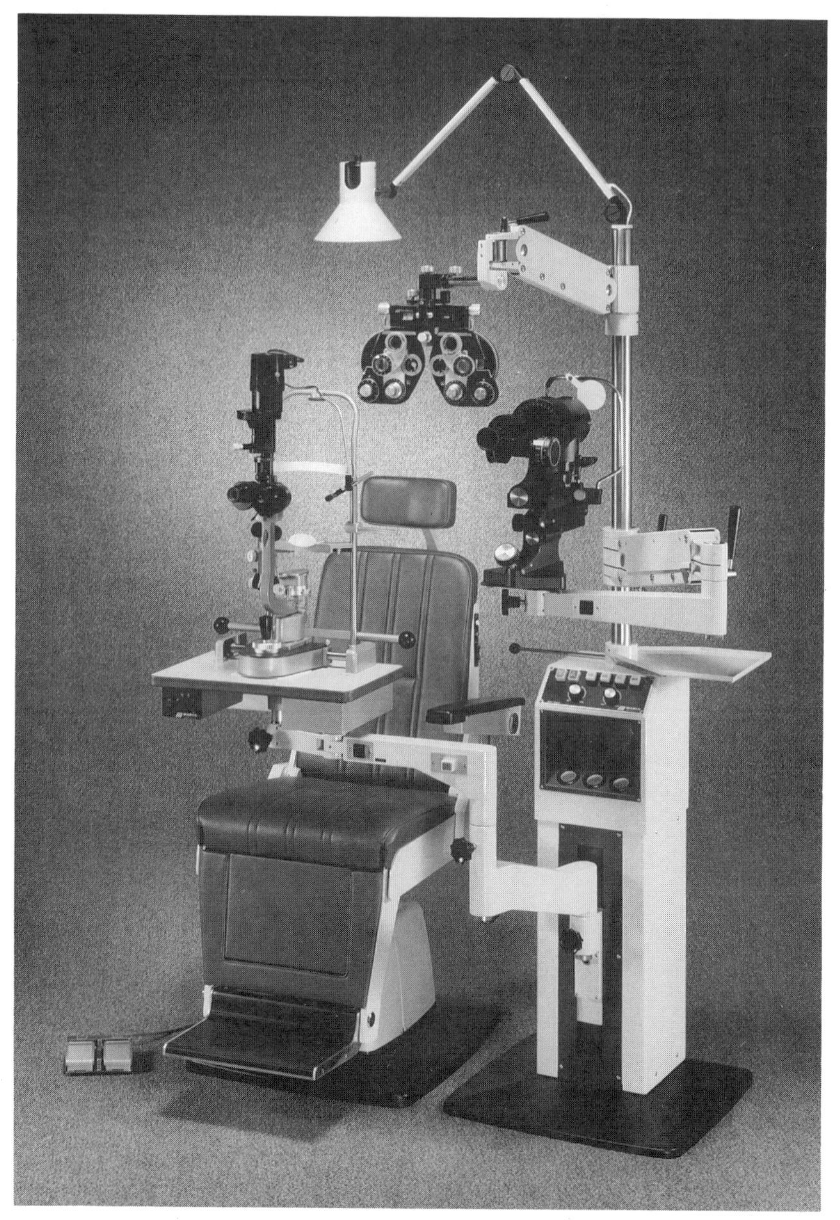

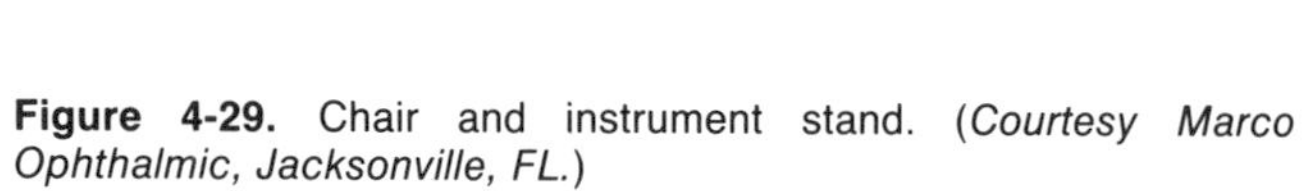
Figure 4-29. Chair and instrument stand. (*Courtesy Marco Ophthalmic, Jacksonville, FL.*)

Examining chairs are available in tilt or nontilt models. In a room for a right-handed physician, the chair is positioned with the instrument stand console to the patient's left. The chair should be positioned in the room so that the physician can walk behind it (allow 3 to 4 feet behind it) even when the chair is in reclined position. The chair and attached instrument stand console together are approximately 4 feet wide (Figure 4-29). A clear space of 24 to 30 inches to the left side of the patient (in a right-handed room) and 5 to 6 feet to the right is desirable. As with any medical equipment, the designer must verify dimensions and critical spatial relationships before designing the room. This chapter lists general dimensions, but each manufacturer's literature must be consulted for specifics.

The physician may work off of the instrument stand as well as the sink cabinet located to the right of the patient. The instrument stand console may be specially wired so that the physician can control the room lights, fixation light, projection chart, and other instruments from it. Or, the sink cabinet may be extended to include a kneespace and an electrical panel for remote control of the room's overhead lights, projector, fixation light, and nurse call buzzer. (Switches and controls may be located on the face of the cabinet or in the kneespace opening so that they are within easy reach of the ophthalmologist during the examination.) Thus the ophthalmologist, from a seated position alongside the patient, may control illumination and instrumentation from either the instrument stand or the wall cabinet, or both (Figure 4-33).

Room lights should have a three-way switch so that they can be controlled from the wall and the console, and they should have a dimmer control. (Local codes must be checked with reference to controlling room lights from the instrument stand. Low-voltage wiring is usually required.) Indirect lighting works well in an ophthalmology exam room. For example, fluorescent

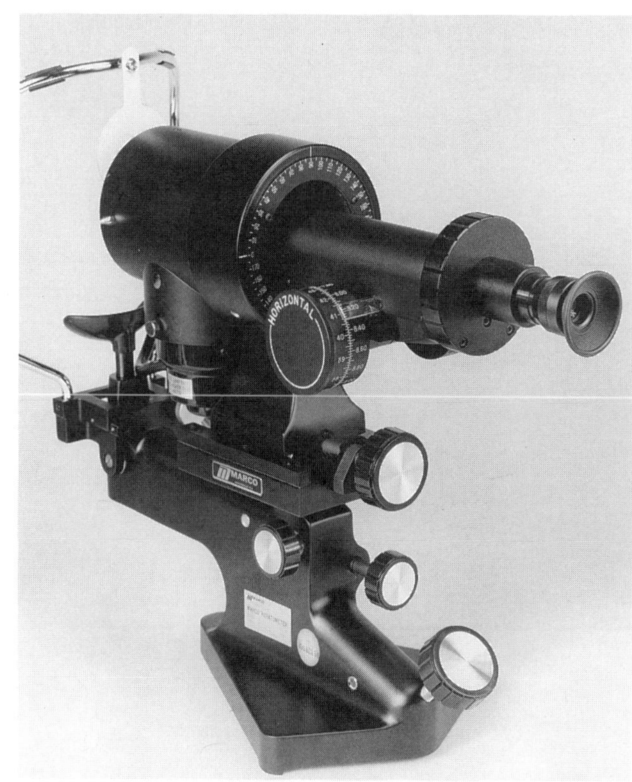

Figure 4-30. Keratometer. *(Courtesy Marco Ophthalmic, Jacksonville, FL.)*

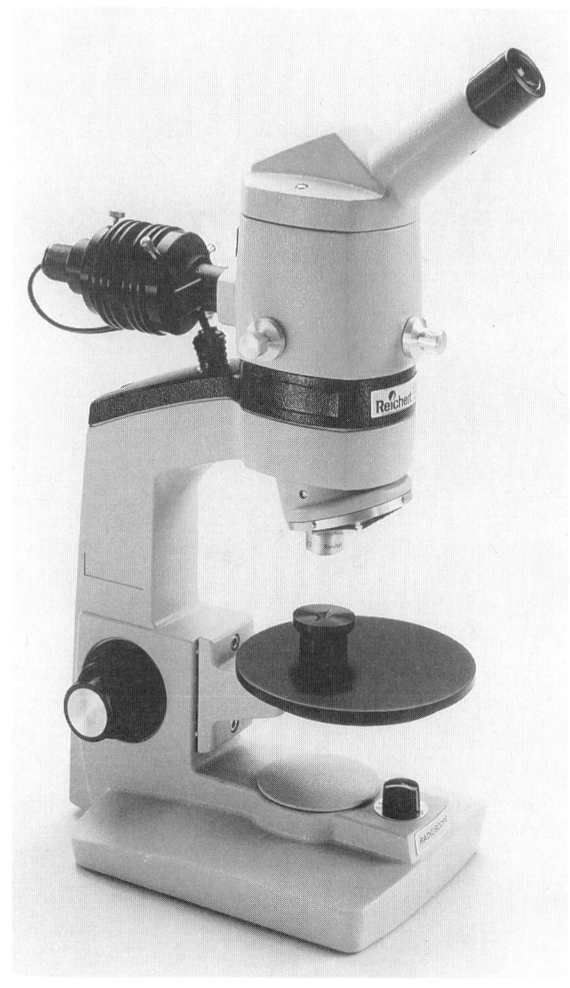

Figure 4-31. Radiuscope™. (*Courtesy Reichert Ophthalmic Instruments, Cambridge Instruments Inc., Buffalo, NY.*)

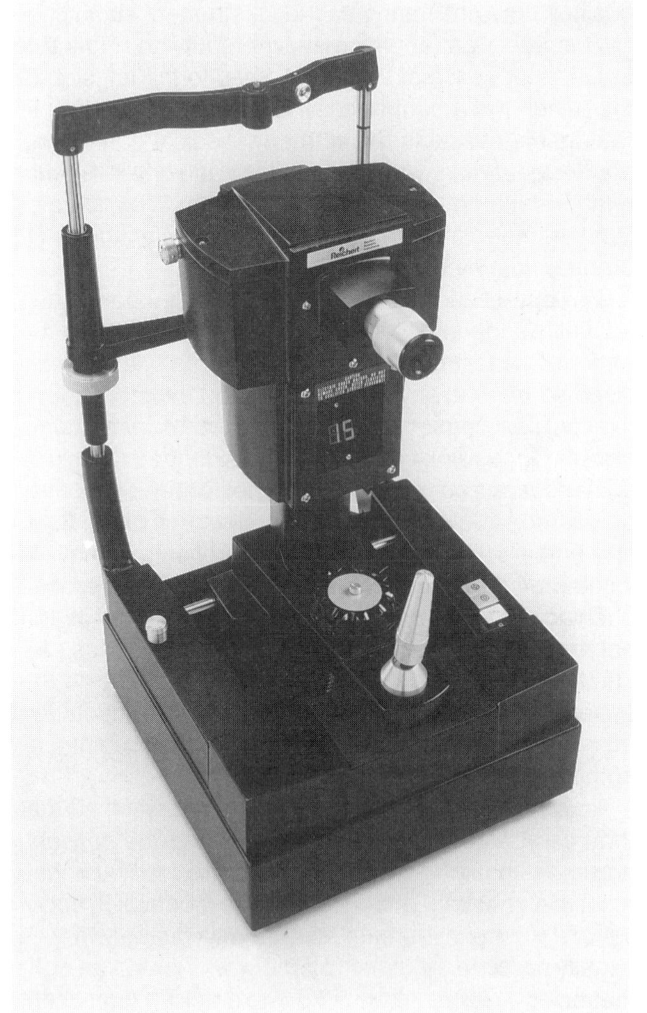

Figure 4-32. Non-Contact™ II Tonometer. (*Courtesy Reichert Ophthalmic Instruments, Cambridge Instruments Inc., Buffalo, NY.*)

lamps around the perimeter of the room, concealed by a wood valance, eliminate the brightness of overhead lights when patients' eyes are dilated.

Other electrical requirements for the room are: an outlet for a *fixation light* mounted on the wall at approximately a 72-inch height directly behind the patient; an outlet for the *projector,* usually at a 60-inch height on the wall to the left of the patient or behind the patient (the designer must specify wood blocking in the wall to support the weight of the projector); a duplex outlet above the countertop for miscellaneous instruments and recharger modules for the cordless hand instruments; and a floor outlet (15-ampere circuit) for the instrument stand console.

One duplex outlet should be located at a 12-inch height on the wall to the left of the examining chair, and all outlets should be grounded. The electrical requirements of refraction rooms are highly specialized. A thorough review of the practitioner's practice habits and specific instrumentation is necessary before planning the electrical layout.

The trial lens case may be placed on a countertop (see Figure 4-27), or it may fit in a drawer or be built into a mobile cart designed for that purpose. If it is to fit in a drawer, the designer must determine if the rack should be tilted for easier visibility, in which case the drawer must be deeper.

All refracting rooms should be exactly alike in layout, arrangement of instruments, and quality of equipment. If one room has a better slit lamp than another, the rooms will not get equal usage. Patients will be shifted around so the doctor can use favored equipment, thus defeating the basic efficiency of the suite.

The distance the doctor must walk between refraction rooms should be minimal. To this end, some ophthalmologists request connecting doors between two refraction rooms (see Figure 4-24). Although it saves steps, it creates an acoustic problem. And since

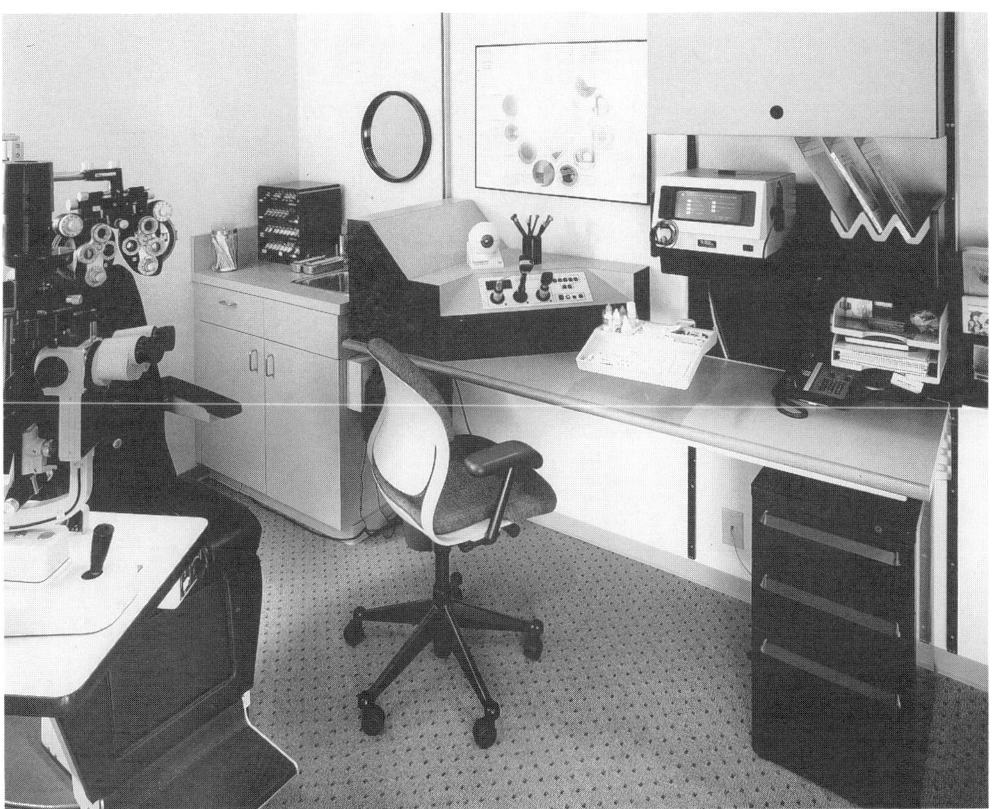

Figure 4-33. Refraction room. (*Design: Jeffrey B. Morris, M.D.; Photographer: Robinson/Ward.*)

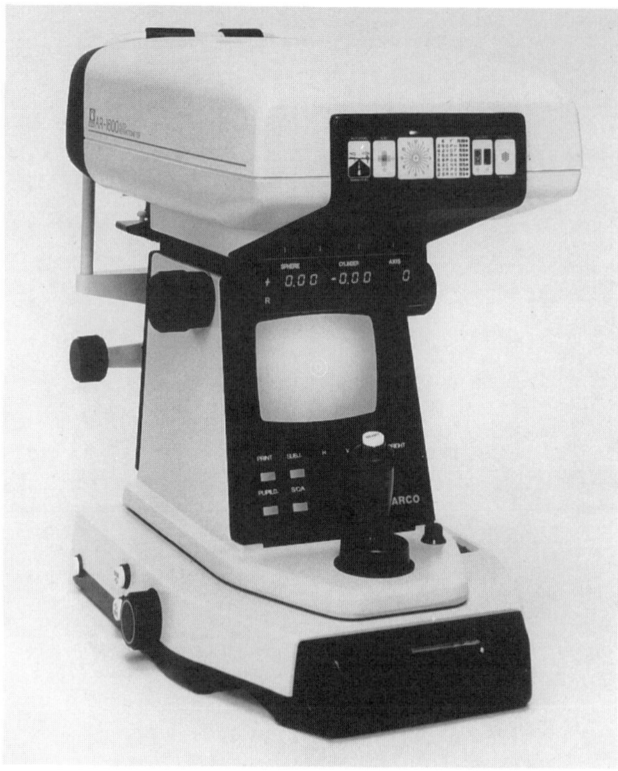

Figure 4-34. Automated refractor. (*Courtesy Marco Technologies, Jacksonville, FL.*)

many persons with poor eyesight happen to be elderly, they may also suffer from a hearing loss, which means the doctor may have to shout to be understood — all the more reason to provide good sound insulation around these rooms.

Mydriatic Area

Toward the end of an eye examination, the patient may receive eye drops to dilate the pupil. Then the patient is asked to return to the waiting room or a secondary waiting area adjacent to the refraction room called a *drop* or *mydiatric room* to wait 15 to 20 minutes before being readmitted to the refraction room to conclude the examination.

Automated Refraction

An *automated refractor* (Figure 4-34) is an electronic tabletop instrument for objectively measuring the patient's visual acuity. It is commonly used by a technician, thereby reducing the number of physician-performed refractions and streamlining those that are necessary. One of the advantages of this unit, in addition to the time it saves over the conventional method of refraction, is that it does not rely upon the patient's subjective comparison: *Is this clearer than that?* The patient looks into the viewing window of the unit and adjusts a knob until the image is in focus. The machine automatically gives a digital readout of the patient's visual acuity. It can also compare the patient's current prescription with the new one.

When used as a general screening device, this machine would be located in the *data collection room* along with other instruments used by aides (see Figure 4-25). After a patient has been refracted by this instrument, he or she moves to an examination room where the ophthalmologist would review the findings and study the patient's medical history. If the difference between the old and the new prescription is not great and the patient has no complaints, a conventional examination by the physician may not be necessary.

In spite of advantages afforded by an automated refractor, many ophthalmologists prefer the traditional method of refraction done in the examination room. It is generally performed by a technician or aide who also takes the patient history in advance of the ophthalmologist entering the room. The ophthalmologist then examines the eye with a slit lamp, and may use the *Non-Contact™ Tonometer* (Figure 4-32) to check for glaucoma or perform other procedures, as required, to diagnose the patient's problem.

Visual Fields

The charting of visual fields is commonly done with a *tangent screen,* which is a piece of black felt with meridians marked off (Figure 4-35). Tangent screens may be rigid or roll-up, the former being preferred because they permit greater accuracy. They are available in four sizes ranging from 1 to 2 meters, the smaller screen giving the smallest amount of information. A 1½-meter screen is commonly used, and if it is placed in a dedicated room, the room need be only 8 × 8 feet. A 1-meter screen needs a room only 6 × 6 feet in size.

The tangent screen may be in the data collection room, in a refracting room, or in a visual fields room, depending on the practitioner's preference and the composition of the practice. A glaucoma specialist may have one in each refracting room. Others may have only one screen in the data collection room.

The patient sits at a specified distance from the screen (which resembles a target), and pins are placed in the felt to chart the limits of the patient's visual field. If the screen is placed in the refraction room, it is con-

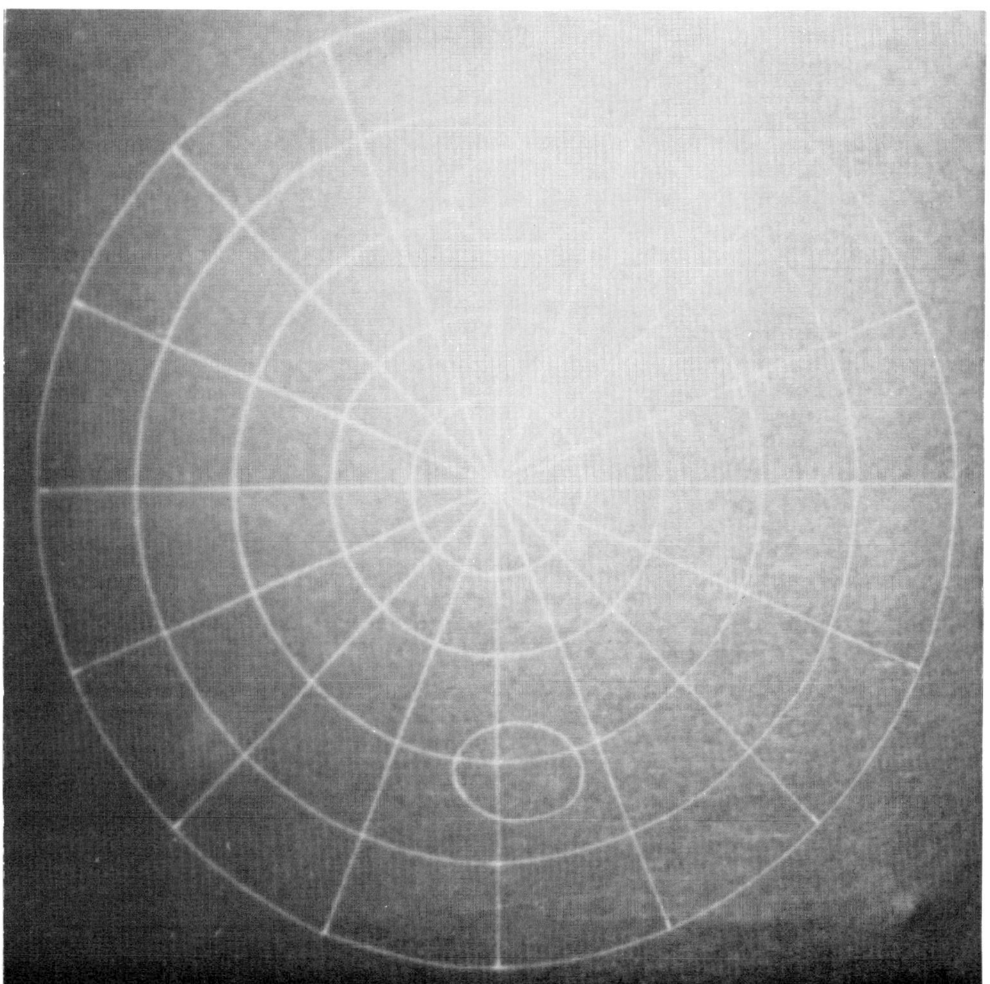

Figure 4-35. Tangent screen. (*Courtesy Richmond Products.*)

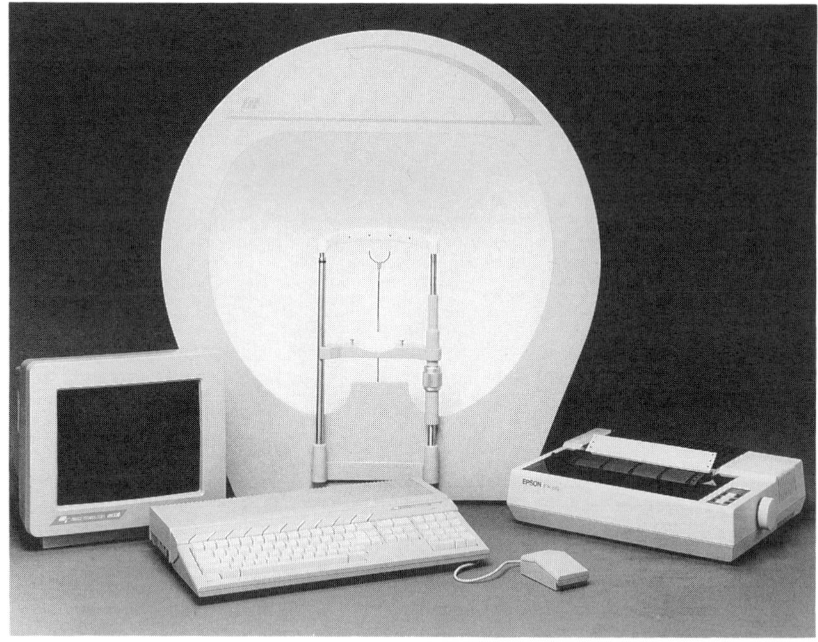

Figure 4-36. Projection perimeter. (*Courtesy Marco Technologies, Jacksonville, FL.*)

venient to locate it on the wall behind the patient. Thus the physician can spin the patient's chair around to face it. The chair must be 1½ meters (60 inches) away from the screen (with a 1½-meter screen).

However, the tangent screen is a basic screening device and not terribly accurate, since one has no control over movement of the patient's head. Perimetry is a more advanced method of doing peripheral and central fields. An *automated projection perimeter* is a computerized piece of equipment that sits on a 24 × 30-inch instrument table (Figure 4-36). The patient and technician sit on the same side of the table. The patient's visual field is charted automatically and accurately since the patient's head is firmly held. The instrument fits in a room as small as 6 × 6 feet. It may be placed in a visual fields room or in a data collection room, but the room's illumination must be controlled by a dimmer, since the procedure is done in a dark room. Not all ophthalmologists will have this piece of equipment.

Lasers

Laser surgery makes possible the correction of many vision problems on an outpatient basis in the ophthalmologist's office. Lasers are used to treat diabetic retinopathy, macular degeneration, retinal tears, glaucoma, retinal vein occlusion, and to open the clouded posterior capsule that sometimes forms following cataract surgery.

Laser light is within the normal visible spectrum, but it is coherent light of a single wavelength — all the energy works together and in one direction. This allows it to be focused precisely on a certain point.

Choosing a wavelength color that the eye tissue being treated can absorb, controlling the power and time of exposure, and varying the size of the laser beam allow the physician to use the laser to seal tears, make tiny openings, evaporate small amounts of tissue, and stop bleeding.

Ophthalmologists use four types of lasers. The color associated with each type enables it to target specific tissues without damaging others.

Argon lasers produce blue and green light. *Krypton* lasers are red. *Dye* lasers are available in a range of colors, depending on the specific need. *YAG* lasers use infrared rays in the near-visible spectrum to treat problems in the front of the eye. Argon, Krypton, and Dye lasers are called *photocoagulation lasers* that use heat (light) to spot-weld tears and leaks in the retinal vessels of the eye and to produce openings in the iris in the front of the eye. The YAG laser is called a *photodisruption laser* and it uses rapid, tiny bursts of energy to make tiny openings in the eye.

A laser room may be as small as 8 × 8 feet or 10 × 10 feet. Ophthalmic lasers come out of a slit-lamp microscope, which sits on a portable stand. The ophthalmologist sits on one side of the table and the patient on the other, resting the chin in a support to immobilize the head (Figure 4-37). A sink cabinet 6- to 8-feet long long is a general requirement for any special procedure room, and room lights must be able to be dimmed during the procedure.

As lasers are expensive, some physicians have them in their office, while others may do laser procedures in an outpatient eye clinic at a nearby hospital. As it becomes possible to do an increasing variety of procedures with lasers, they will no doubt become common in all ophthalmologists' offices. The advantages are many: The eye is not opened surgically; there is no needle or stitches, no need for hospitalization, and no risk of infection.

It should be noted that laser use requires the observance of safety precautions. The American National Standards Institute (ANSI) publishes standards for the

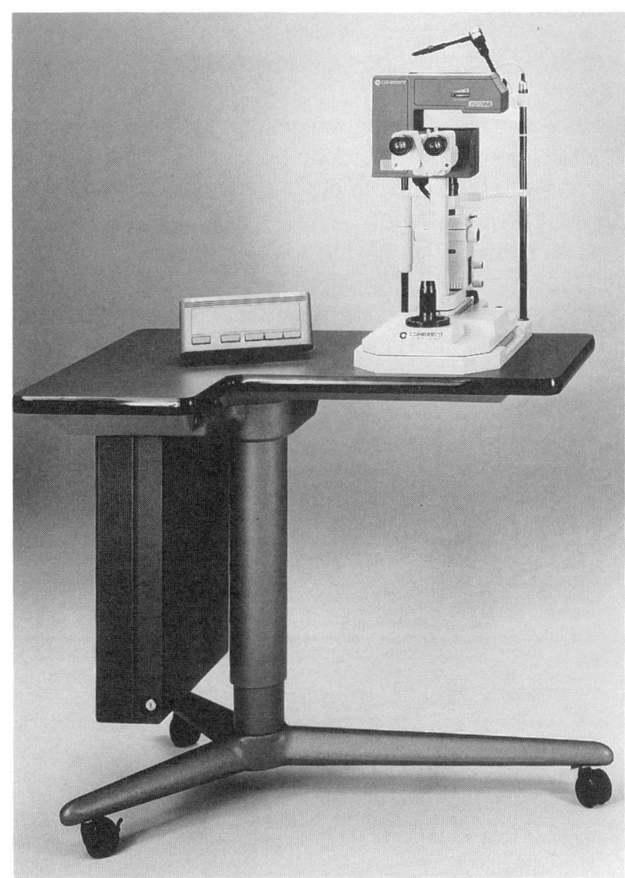

Figure 4-37. YAG laser. (*Courtesy Coherent Medical Group, Palo Alto, CA.*)

safe use of laser systems. Specific safety devices and warning labels must be used. The eyes are most susceptible to laser injury.

Rooms in which lasers are in use must have a warning sign posted on the door that reads: *DANGER — Laser Radiation — Avoid eye or skin exposure to direct or scattered radiation.* When using infrared wavelengths such as the YAG, the word "invisible" must be included in the warning sign.

It is important to have nonspecular (nonreflecting) and fire resistant material in or near the beam path. Doors must have safety latches or interlocks to prevent unexpected entry into laser controlled areas. If the door to the room has a window, it must have a window shade that can be rolled down during laser use. Everyone in the room must wear goggles to protect their eyes. (Goggles are specific to each type of laser that is used.)

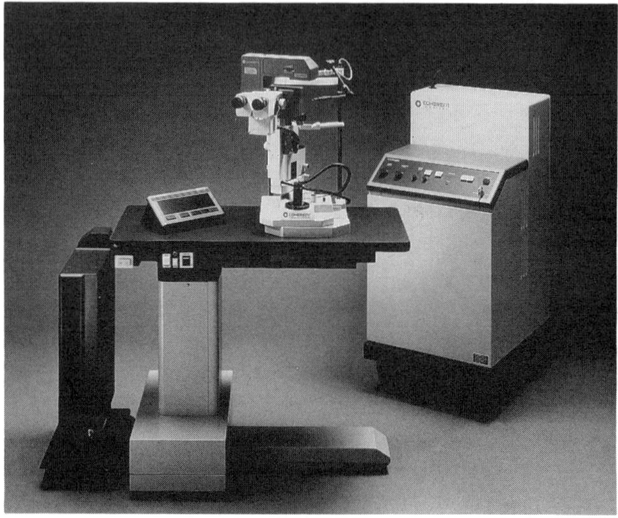

Figure 4-38. Argon/Nd: YAG Laser system. (*Courtesy Coherent Medical Group, Palo Alto, CA.*)

It should be noted that all Argon (Figure 4-38) and some YAG lasers on the market at this time require external water to cool the power plant within the laser chassis. The disconnecting and reconnecting of water hoses may cause leaks and wet floors, which become a potential physical and electrical hazard. The reader is referred to Chapter 7 for additional discussion of these issues. The YAG pictured in Figure 4-37 is cooled by air convection and does not require water.

Fluorescein Angiography

Not all ophthalmologists do fluorescein angiograms in their offices. Some refer their patients to a retinal subspecialist or to an outpatient eye clinic associated with a nearby hospital. Fluorescein dye is injected into the patient's arm. The resulting photographs of the retina show if there is leakage of fluids, edema, or poor circulation. This procedure can be done in a minor treatment or special procedures room, and it is performed by a technologist, not the physician.

No special accommodation is required in the room, as the patient sits on a standard chair on one side of an instrument table, with the tech on the other side. A small darkroom should be nearby. A workroom for the tech is optional and depends on what other rooms are close at hand. A retinal specialist would have a dedicated room for angiograms with an adjacent office for the photographer, and a mydriatic or drop room nearby. The entire procedure, including waiting time for dilation of the pupil, can take as long as 45 minutes.

Office-Based Surgery

It is a matter of personal preference whether an ophthalmologist chooses to do surgery (nonlaser) within the office. Some may elect, for a variety of reasons, to use an ambulatory surgical center located in the medical office building or one located in a nearby hospital. The advantages of performing surgery in one's office are convenience for the patient, convenience in scheduling procedures, and revenue generated for the medical practice. Disadvantages are the initial cost to create a surgery facility that meets state licensing and/or Medicare certification criteria, the cost of equipping it, additional coverage, and the risks assumed, however slight, when performing surgery outside the traditional hospital setting.

Since eye surgery is generally not elective in nature, a physician would want to be certain the office-based surgery facility meets requirements for reimbursement by third-party payers. In fact, the majority of patients needing surgery are over 65 years of age, and Medicare reimbursement would be essential to an ophthalmologist's practice.

Removal of cataracts is one of the most common types of ophthalmic surgery. It is generally done under a local anesthetic, administered by a nurse anesthetist or an anesthesiologist. An incision is made; the clouded lens (cataract) is removed; and an intraocular lens (artificial lens) is inserted. The surgical portion of the procedure takes an hour to an hour and a half. The patient recovers in a recliner chair for about 15 minutes before being released to go home.

Some ophthalmologists do all of their surgery in an ambulatory surgical center. Others do only those surgeries requiring general anesthesia in an ambulatory surgical center, and procedures done with a local anesthetic such as cataract surgery and radial keratotomy are done in the office. Some use a room no larger than a standard minor treatment or special procedures room, with an adjacent nurse station, small recovery area, and clean utility room. When general anesthesia is used, State Fire Marshal and Medicare certification requirements become strict. Many Life Safety Code regulations must be met. The reader is referred to Chapter 7, Ambulatory Surgical Centers, for a more complete discussion of this issue.

The designer should note that ophthalmic surgery is done while looking through a microscope. Therefore, vibration can be a problem. If the office is in a medical building near a railroad track or close to a major freeway, there could be some undesirable vibration, depending on the height of the building, the location of the suite within the building, and the type of structural system that supports the building.

Other Considerations

An ophthalmologist may accumulate 11 to 12 lineal feet of medical charts in a year, so the file area should accommodate about 48 lineal feet per doctor. Inactive charts can be stored in file transfer boxes in the storage room or off-site.

The consultation room functions as a private office, a place to relax between patients, to read mail, or to make phone calls. It is rarely used for consulting with patients; thus, it can be small.

Interior Design

The interior design of this suite should be cheerful, and lighting is of critical importance. The waiting room should have good reading light, as many of the patients are elderly. With age, people develop cataracts, and require bright illumination in order to read with comfort. It would be thoughtful to provide large-print magazines for patients who do not see well. The drop room needs subdued lighting, because bright light is uncomfortable to an eye that has been dilated.

In refraction rooms, the designer must be extremely careful to select wallcoverings that have absolutely no visual rhythm or figure/ground reversal. People who visit an ophthalmologist have a variety of vision problems, some of which include distortions. A person who sees a triple image or one whose vision is blurred might experience considerable discomfort in looking at a busy wallpaper or a geometric design. The waiting room in Color Plate 7, Figure 4-39, would be quite appropriate for an ophthalmologist's office if patients are predominantly elderly. Note the unusual design of the reception window in Color Plate 8, Figure 4-40, using modular furniture systems.

As the lens ages, it thickens and yellows. To know how colors might be perceived by the elderly, one can look through a pair of yellow lenses.

DERMATOLOGY

A dermatologist treats diseases of the skin. It is not uncommon to find a one-physician practice. Since dermatologists rarely make hospital rounds or emergency house calls, their appointment schedule is strictly adhered to without the sort of interruption that plagues many other physicians. A one-physician suite would be composed of three small examination or treatment rooms, a waiting room to accommodate eight to ten persons, small lab, toilet room, business office, consultation room, minor surgery, and large storage closet for drug samples (Figure 4-42). Larger practices may include a surgery facility, as well as ancillary services such as electrolysis and facials.

Table 4-4. Analysis of Program. Dermatology

No. of Physicians:	1	2
Exam Rooms	3 @ 8 × 10 = 240	6 = 8 × 10 = 480
Minor Surgery	12 × 12 = 144	12 × 12 = 144
Toilets	2 @ 6 × 7 = 84	2 @ 6 × 7 = 84
Business Office	12 × 14 = 168	16 × 18 = 288
Waiting Room	12 × 16 = 192	14 × 18 = 252
Consultation Room	12 × 12 = 144	12 × 12 = 144
Laboratory	8 × 10 = 80	10 × 10 = 100
Electrolysis/Facials	10 × 10 = 100	10 × 10 = 100
Storage	6 × 8 = 48	6 × 8 = 48
Subtotal	1200 ft²	1640 ft²
15% Circulation	180	246
Total	1380 ft²	1886 ft²

Examination Room

Exam rooms can be 8 × 10 feet instead of the standard 8 × 12 feet. The exam table used is usually a flat physical therapy table, 24 × 78 inches × 36 inches high, which is often placed against the wall. When placing the table in this room, the head of the table should be placed so that the physician can work on the patient's right side. Natural light (a window) is important in dermatology exam rooms. The room should have a sink cabinet and perhaps a dressing room, and a high level of illumination, free of shadows, supplied by full-spectrum fluorescent lamps.

Surgical Procedures

The minor surgery room is 12 × 12 feet, with a long sink cabinet along one wall. Medical equipment to be accommodated in this room would depend on the scope of the procedures. However, the equipment would include an operating table or chair that adjusts to different positions (Figure 4-44) and a ceiling-mounted surgical light over the table.

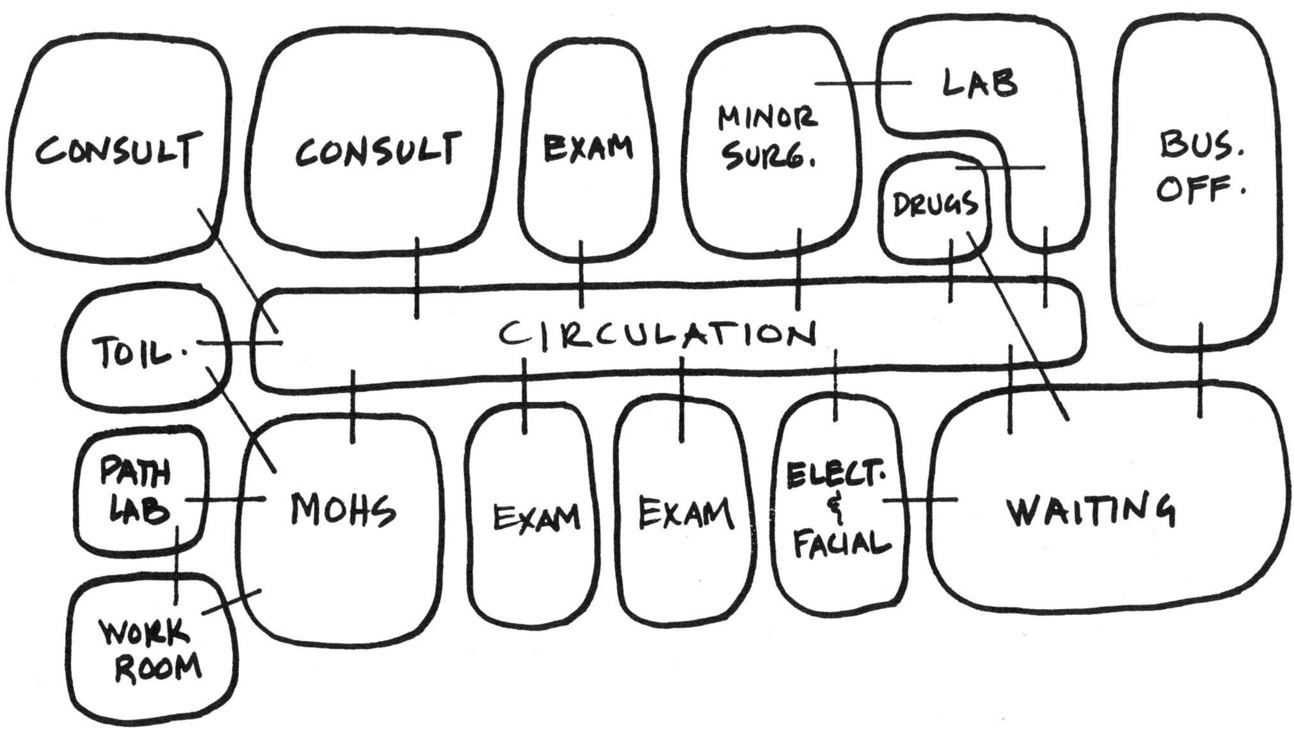

Figure 4-41. Schematic diagram of a dermatology suite.

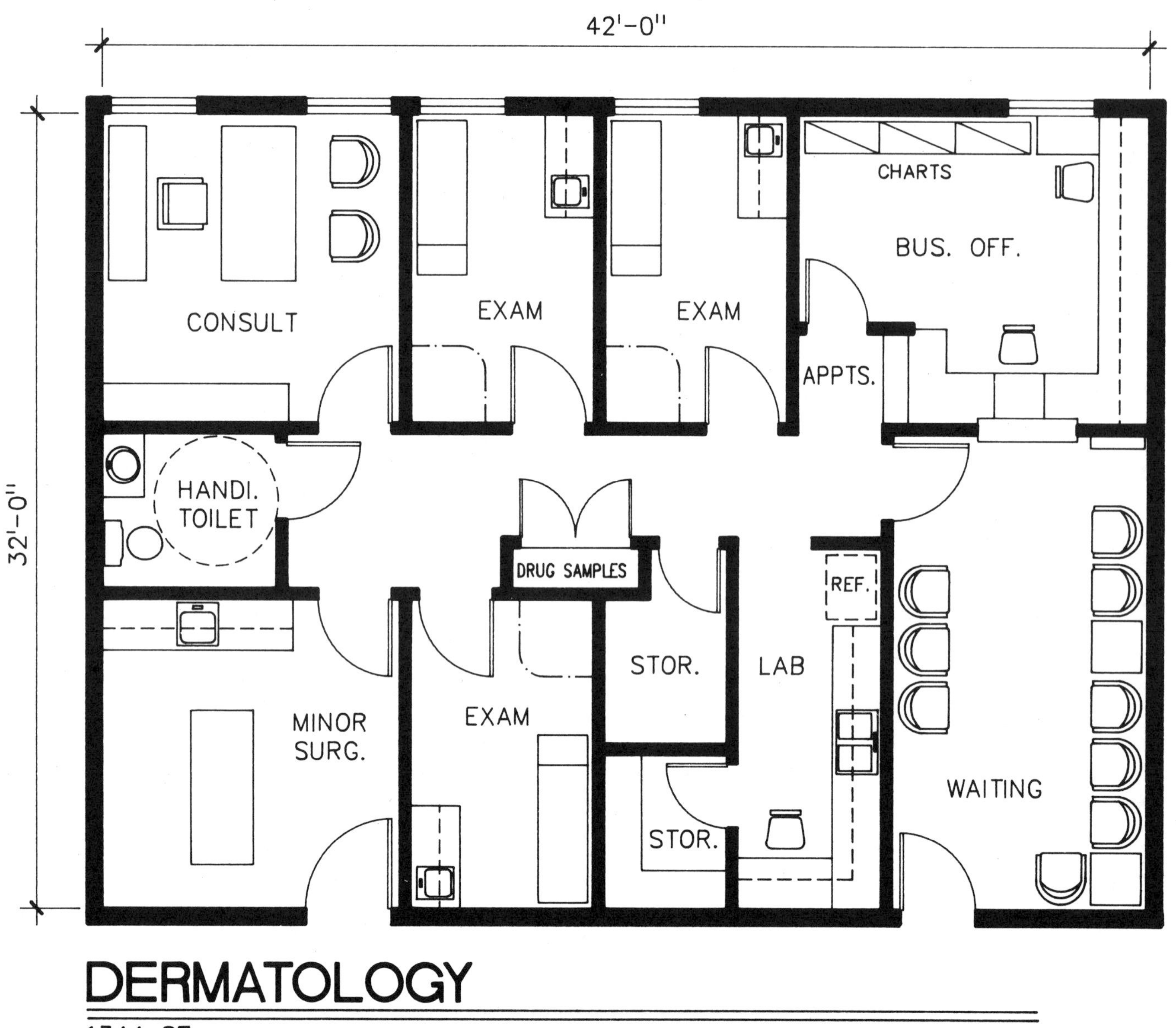

Figure 4-42. Suite plan for dermatology, 1344 square feet.

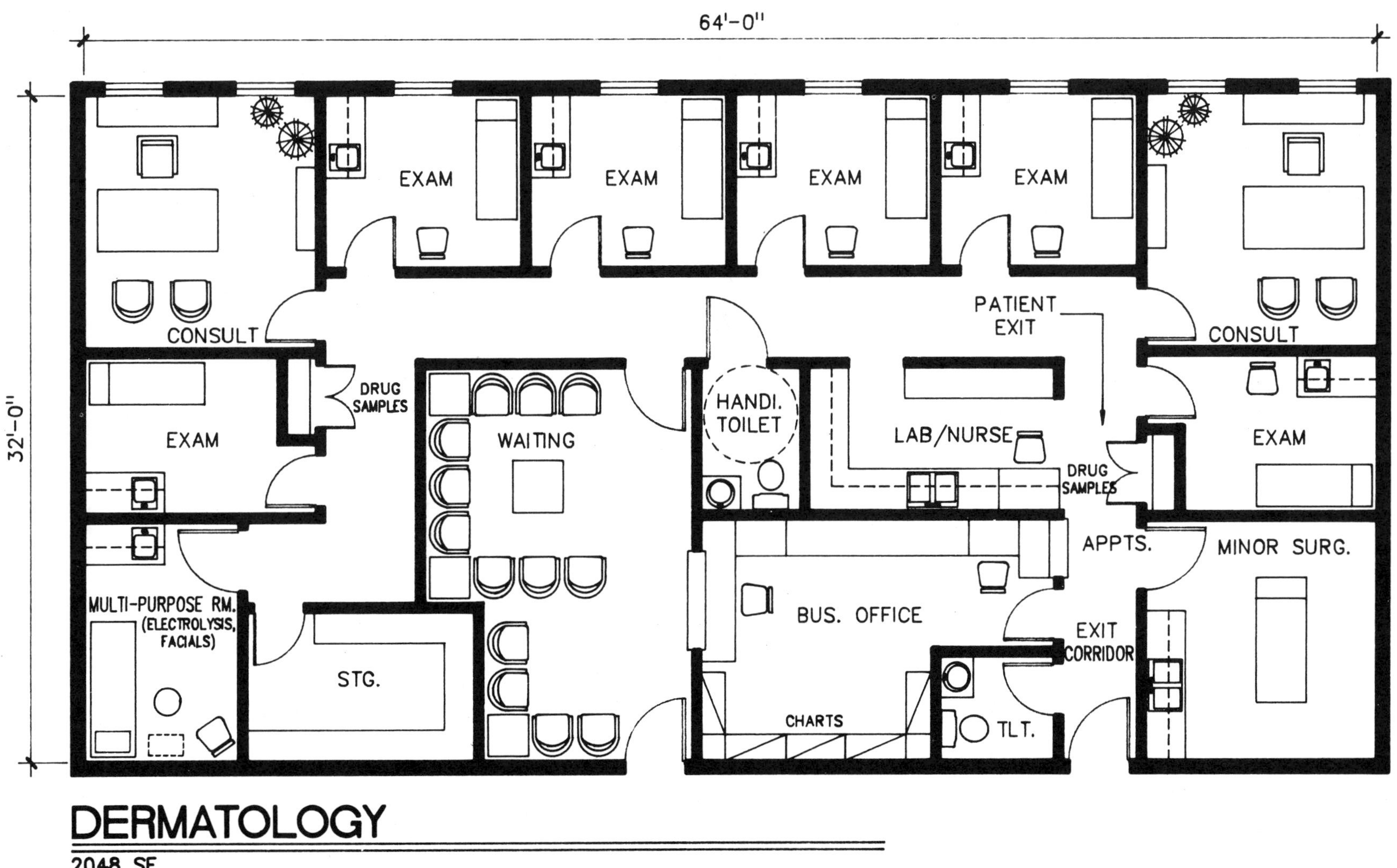

Figure 4-43. Suite plan for dermatology, 2048 square feet.

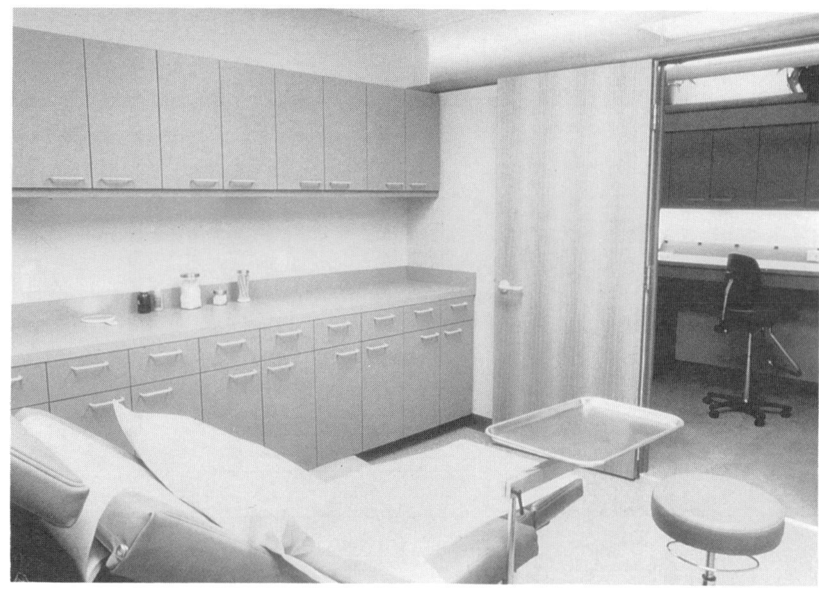

Figure 4-44. Minor surgery room, dermatology. (*Architecture/Interiors: Richard Deno, Cardiff, CA; Photographer: Kim Brun.*)

Dermatologists do many surgical procedures in the office. Surgery may be done to improve the skin's appearance, to biopsy tissue to establish a diagnosis, or to prevent or control disease. Different types of surgical procedures include:

Curettage — scraping the tissue with a sharp surgical instrument called a curette.

Excision — cutting into the skin surgically, removing the tumor or growth, then closing the wound with stitches.

Cryosurgery — using liquid nitrogen sprayed on the tissue to freeze it and thereby destroy the unwanted cells.

Dermabrasion — a "sanding" of the skin using an abrasive rotary instrument to remove scars, acne, or damage done by exposure to the sun.

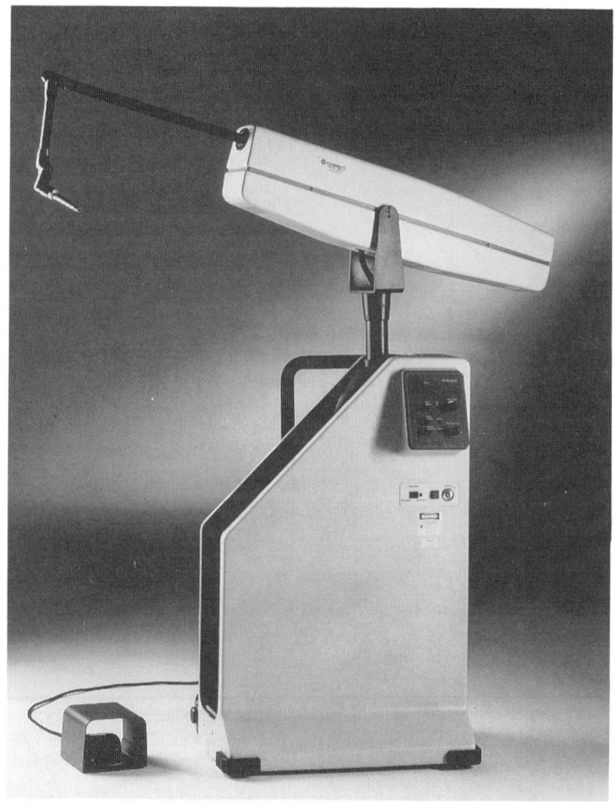

Figure 4-45. *Ambulase* CO_2 laser. (*Courtesy Coherent Medical Group, Palo Alto, CA.*)

Laser Surgery — using a highly concentrated, focused beam of light to eradicate unsightly skin abnormalities such as tattoos, portwine stains, birthmarks, and broken blood vessels. The CO_2 laser is the most common type used in dermatology practice. The unit shown in Figure 4-45 requires a standard 110/115-volt electrical outlet, and is air cooled; thus, it does not require water. (The reader is referred to a discussion of lasers under the Ophthalmology section of this chapter and also to Chapter 7, Ambulatory Surgical Centers.)

Mohs' Histographic Surgery — a specialized surgical technique developed by Frederick Mohs, M.D., some 40 years ago, it is a method of detecting the root of the tumor through the use of a sequential examination of tissue with a microscope immediately after the tissue has been excised. Because the microscope guides the physician in how much skin needs to be removed, taking "extra margins" of tissue just for safety's sake is unnecessary. This technique is used especially where cancers have occurred or where they are at high risk of recurring.

This differs from other surgical techniques because the excision of tissue is guided by the use of diagrams, dyes, microscopes, and special surgical techniques. A local anesthetic is used during this procedure. The suite plan in Figure 4-46 shows a Mohs' suite with adjacent scrub and prep area, pathology lab, and sub–waiting area. Note that surgical patients have a direct route to the surgery suite, without walking through the examination area.

Psoralen Ultraviolet Light (PUVA)

Psoralen ultraviolet light, type A (PUVA) was approved by the Food and Drug Administration in May 1982 for treatment of severe psoriasis that cannot be controlled by conventional therapies, including ultraviolet light, type B. Psoriasis is a noncontagious skin disorder characterized by elevated red patches on the skin, covered by a dry scale. The disease is the result of an excessive build-up of skin cells. PUVA reduces this cell reproduction and temporarily clears symptoms for anywhere from a few weeks to a couple of years.

PUVA involves a combination of long-wave ultraviolet light (type A) and a prescription oral medication. Patients usually require three treatments a week for a total of approximately 30 treatments.

Most dermatologists do not do PUVA treatment in their offices because PUVA equipment is fairly expensive, requires a dedicated area, and would need a high volume of patients to make the investment worthwhile. The equipment generates a great deal of heat, and a separate air conditioning unit is required for the PUVA treatment room.

Other Design Considerations

Dermatologists dispense a lot of drug samples, salves, ointments, and shampoos. A specialized closet should be provided in a convenient location in the corridor for storage of drug samples. The closet might have doors fitted with compartments or bins for sorting and making accessible frequently used products (Figure 4-47).

Interior Design

There are no special interior design considerations in a dermatology suite. Patients are all ages and in relatively good health. Exam rooms are often used for treatment; therefore, a hard surface floor is preferable to carpet.

The use of planters to provide privacy for sub–waiting areas (Figure 4-48) is an interesting space-planning device.

The reader is referred to Color Plate 9, Figure 4-49, for a dermatology suite waiting room, to Chapter 6 for a decentralized plan of a group practice dermatology suite, and to Figure 4-46 for a centralized plan.

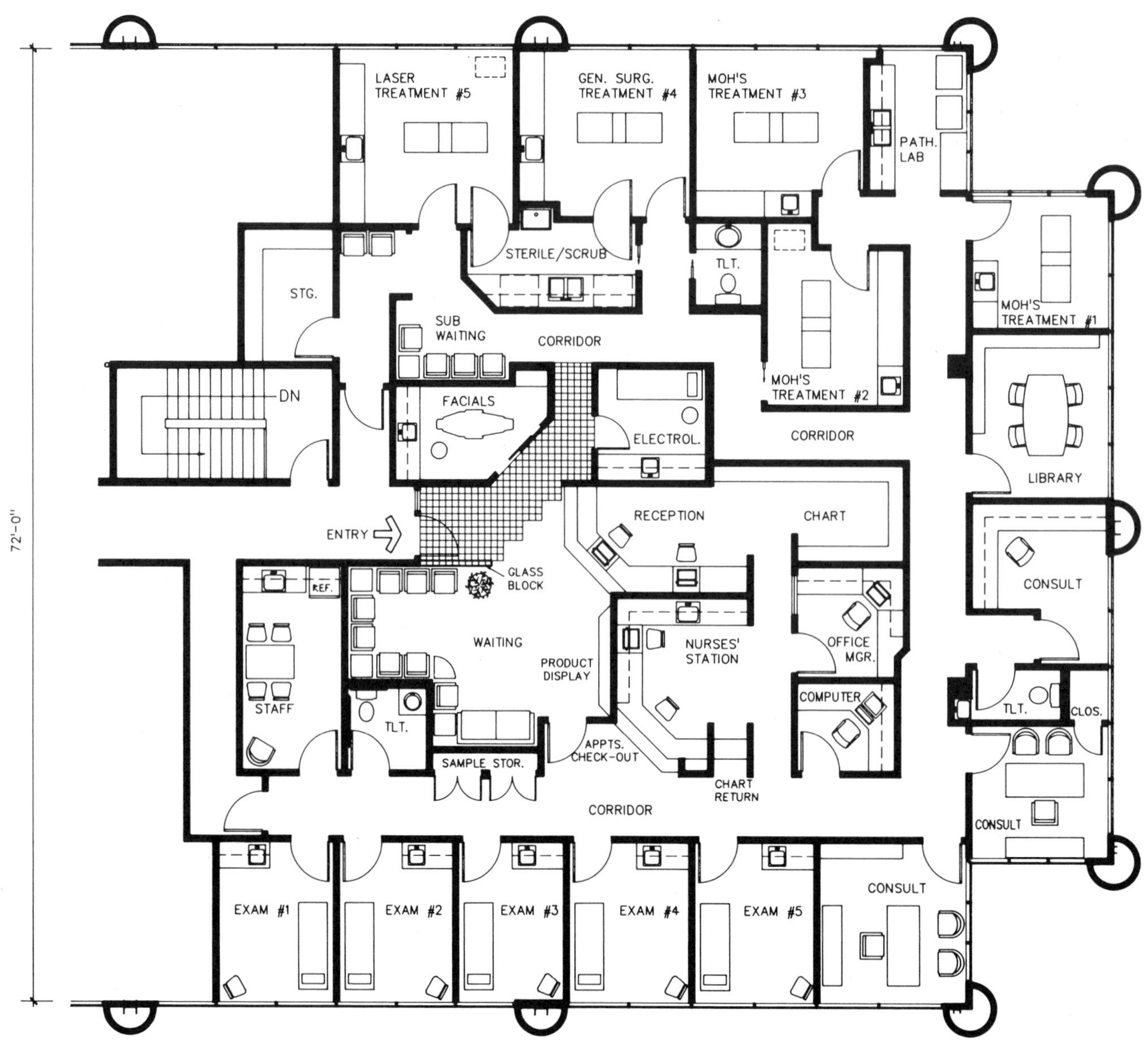

Figure 4-46. Suite plan for dermatology, 4384 square feet.

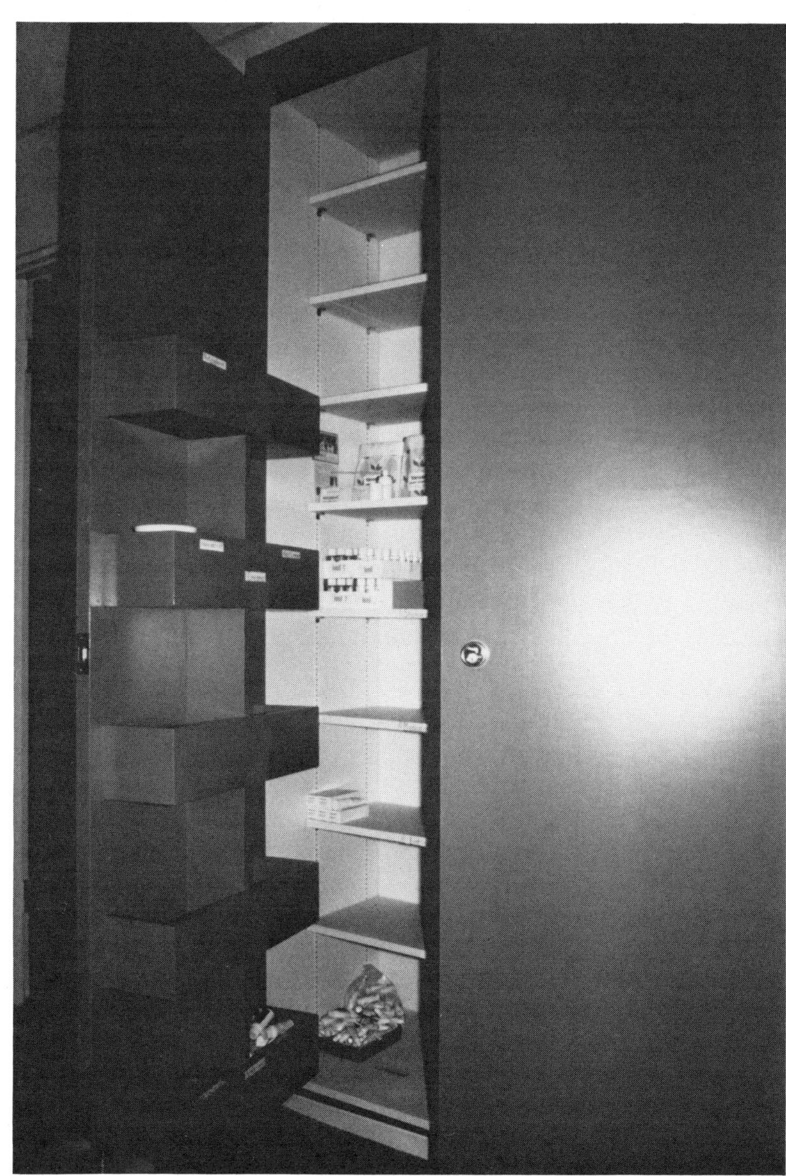

Figure 4-47. Drug sample cabinet.

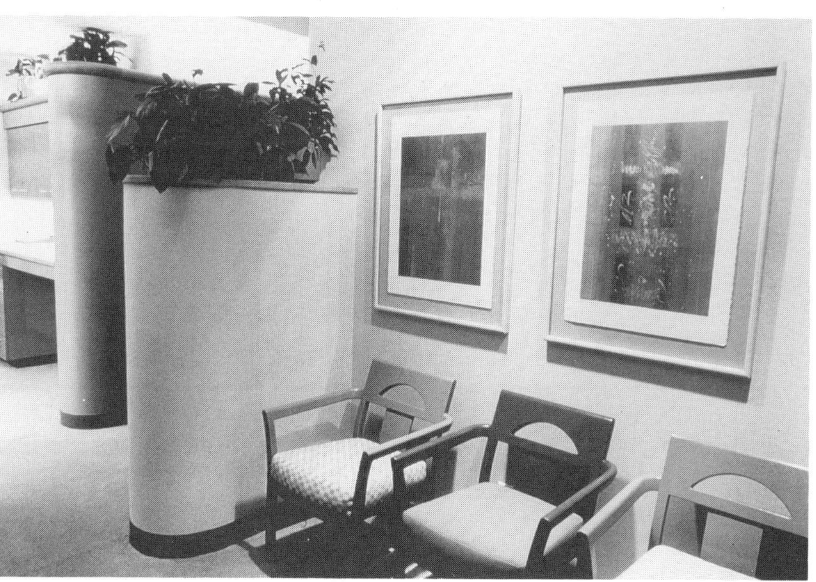

Figure 4-48. Sub-waiting area, dermatology suite. Note effect of planters used as room dividers, and to create privacy. (*Architecture/Interiors: Richard Deno, Cardiff, CA; Furniture: Kathy Burnham; Art: Richard Fitzpatrick, M.D.; Photographer: Kim Brun.*)

PLASTIC SURGERY

Plastic surgery suites are somewhat similar to a general surgery suite, except they are usually larger and often have an outpatient surgery facility in which healthy, low-risk patients might be operated on for face lifts, breast implants, liposuction, *rhinoplasty* (reconstruction of the nose), hair transplants, hand surgery, and other cosmetic or reconstructive procedures.

Liposuction has become one of the most commonly performed procedures for removing unwanted fat from the stomach, buttocks, thighs, or other areas. Briefly, in this procedure an incision is made in the skin, a *canula* (tube) is inserted, and the fat is suctioned out.

There are a number of reasons for performing plastic surgery on an outpatient basis in the surgeon's office. Principally, the patient is more comfortable in a physician's office, because it is a less clinical environment than a hospital, and it affords more privacy. Patients undergoing cosmetic procedures are often very concerned about bumping into friends and neighbors. It is not uncommon for people to visit a plastic surgeon in another city in order to safeguard their "secret."

There are other advantages to surgery outside the hospital setting. Theoretically, it lowers the cost for the patient and permits the physician to charge a fee for the use of the operating room, rather than lose that fee to the hospital. The surgeon has more control over scheduling when procedures are done in the office, and the patient avoids the generally frightening experience of being admitted to a hospital.

In some plastic surgery practices, approximately two-thirds of the surgery caseload can be performed in a properly equipped operating suite within the office.

Plastic surgeons who elect not to do surgery in their own offices often use an ambulatory surgical center, which may be located in the medical office building or in a nearby hospital. This would be an intermediate step between the physician's office and the traditional hospital setting. However, ambulatory surgical centers usually lack the comforts available in the plastic surgeon's office, which may include lavishly designed waiting rooms, private drop-off and pick-up entrances, subdued lighting, and staff who are trained to offer a lot of tender loving care.

Circulation Patterns

If a plastic surgeon is going to do office-based surgery, the optimum flow would be that shown in Figure 4-51, in which surgical patients are separated from the pre-op and post-op examination area of the suite. There are separate waiting rooms, but there is no duplication of staff required since the receptionist can monitor both rooms. Similarly, the nurse station is centrally located to serve the surgery area or the examination area.

The flow through the suite for elective cases would begin with the initial consultation, and if the patient decides to proceed, would then include two or three pre-op visits, the actual surgery, plus two or three post-op visits. Trauma cases or emergencies would generally be seen at the hospital.

The plastic surgeon takes "before" and "after" photos of patients. These photos can be taken in the examination room (where a pull-down panel of blue fabric is mounted to the wall as a background) or in a small 6- × 8-foot room designed for that purpose. A darkroom is usually not required.

With many procedures, the patient is operated on in the morning, spends two to four hours in the recovery room, and goes home that afternoon. The doctor's afternoons would be spent visiting hospitalized patients, conducting consultations in the office with prospective patients, and seeing post-operative patients to change dressings or remove sutures.

Secluded Entry

The composition of the plastic surgeon's practice will dictate the design features that need to be incorporated. A practice dedicated to cosmetic surgery may cater to an affluent clientele who expect a luxurious office. Of particular importance is a secluded entrance so that clients may park their cars and conveniently enter the office without being seen. After the procedure, they can slip out the same door and elude others in the waiting room.

For this reason, plastic surgeons who specialize in cosmetic surgery frequently prefer a ground floor location, with a private driveway or turnaround so that patients need not walk through the lobby or public areas of the medical building (Figure 4-52). This is valid even when the practice is composed of a less affluent population. Patients who elect to have cosmetic surgery tend to be sensitive about it and prefer privacy.

Examination Rooms

Exam rooms in a plastic surgeon's office are quite different from those in other types of medical offices in that they generally use a motorized chair (Figure 4-53), or one room might be designed for examining hands (Color Plate 9, Figure 4-54). Note that the last example also doubles as a recovery room when the bed that stores in the wall is pulled down and the table pushed back into the cabinet, acting as a bedside table. The room also serves for patient education, with a built-in VCR and TV monitor.

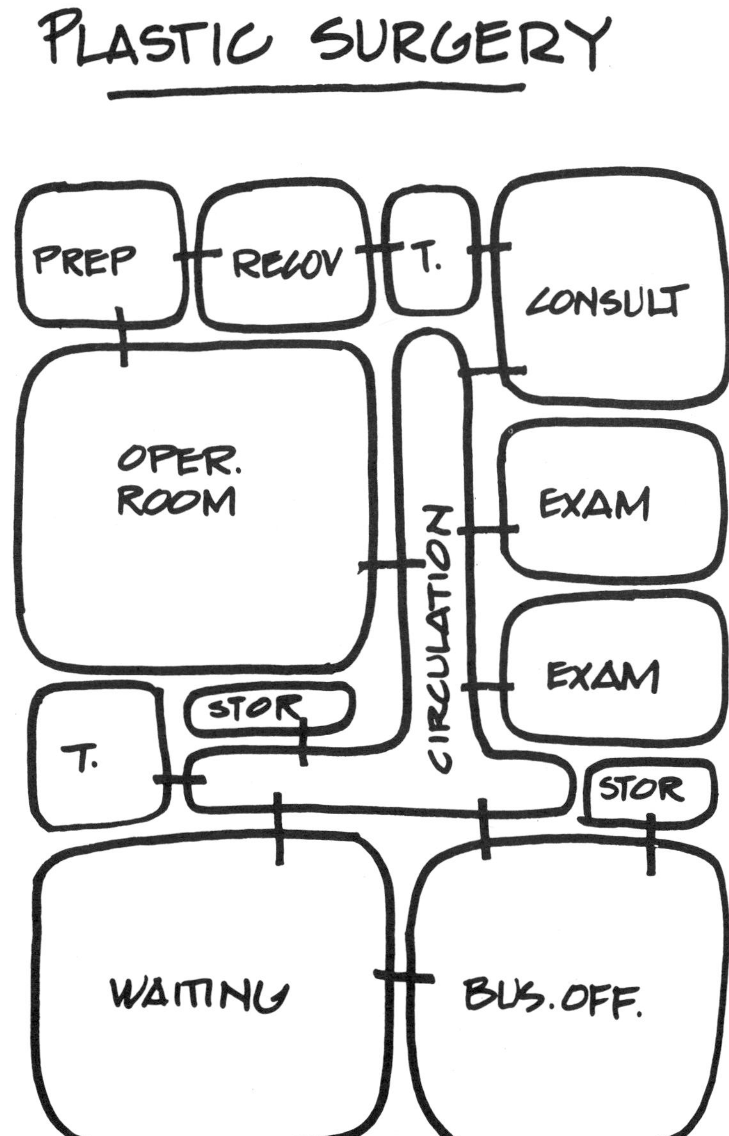

Figure 4-50. Schematic diagram of a plastic surgery suite.

Table 4-5. Analysis of Program. Plastic Surgery

No. of Physicians:	1		2	
Consultation Room	12 × 16 =	192	2 @ 12 × 16 =	384
Exam Rooms	3 @ 8 × 12 =	288	5 @ 8 × 12 =	480
Operating Suite[a]	22 × 24 =	528	22 × 30 =	680
Waiting Room	14 × 16 =	224	16 × 18 =	288
Business Office	14 × 16 =	224	16 × 16 =	256
Toilets	2 @ 6 × 8 =	96	2 @ 6 × 8 =	96
Storage	6 × 6 =	36	6 × 8 =	48
Shampoo/Makeup	—		10 × 10 =	100
Staff Lounge	10 × 12 =	120	10 × 12 =	120
Subtotal		1708 ft²		2431 ft²
15% Circulation		256		365
Total		1964 ft²		2797 ft²

[a]Includes prep room and recovery.

Note: The above is merely an approximation, since plastic surgery suites can vary considerably in size and number of rooms, depending on the physician's scope of procedures and practice philosophy.

Consultation Room

Patients considering surgery often interview more than one physician. In fact, many plastic surgeons do not charge for the initial consultation. They may spend as long as half an hour with a patient showing slides or photos of other patients who have had similar procedures, reviewing costs and the probable outcome. This initial consultation is an important element of a plastic surgeon's practice, because it is generally just this one meeting by which the patient decides whether he or she is comfortable with the surgeon's personality and qualifications.

Plastic surgeons often use their private offices (consultation rooms) to make case presentations, or a special room may be designed for this purpose (Figure 4-55). Whichever room is used, it must have X-ray view boxes conveniently located where the patient can see them, and a place to project slides.

The consultation room should convey a solid, successful image, but not be flamboyant or trendy. This room might be styled more conservatively than the remainder of the suite, although this is determined in large part by what would be appropriate for the patient population served. A plastic surgeon in Beverly Hills, to be competitive, would probably have a more lavishly designed office than one in Des Moines.

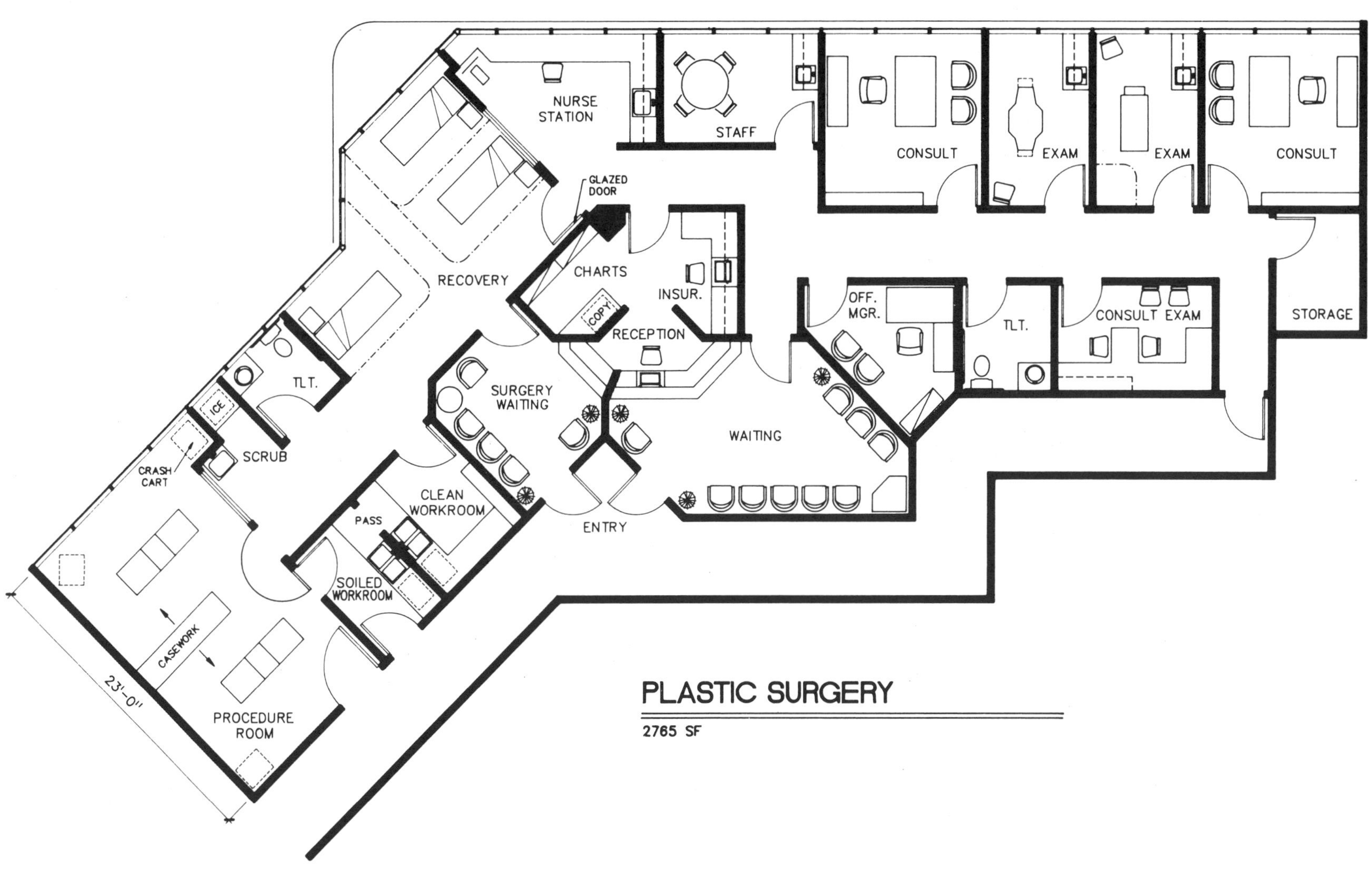

Figure 4-51. Suite plan for plastic surgery, 2765 square feet.

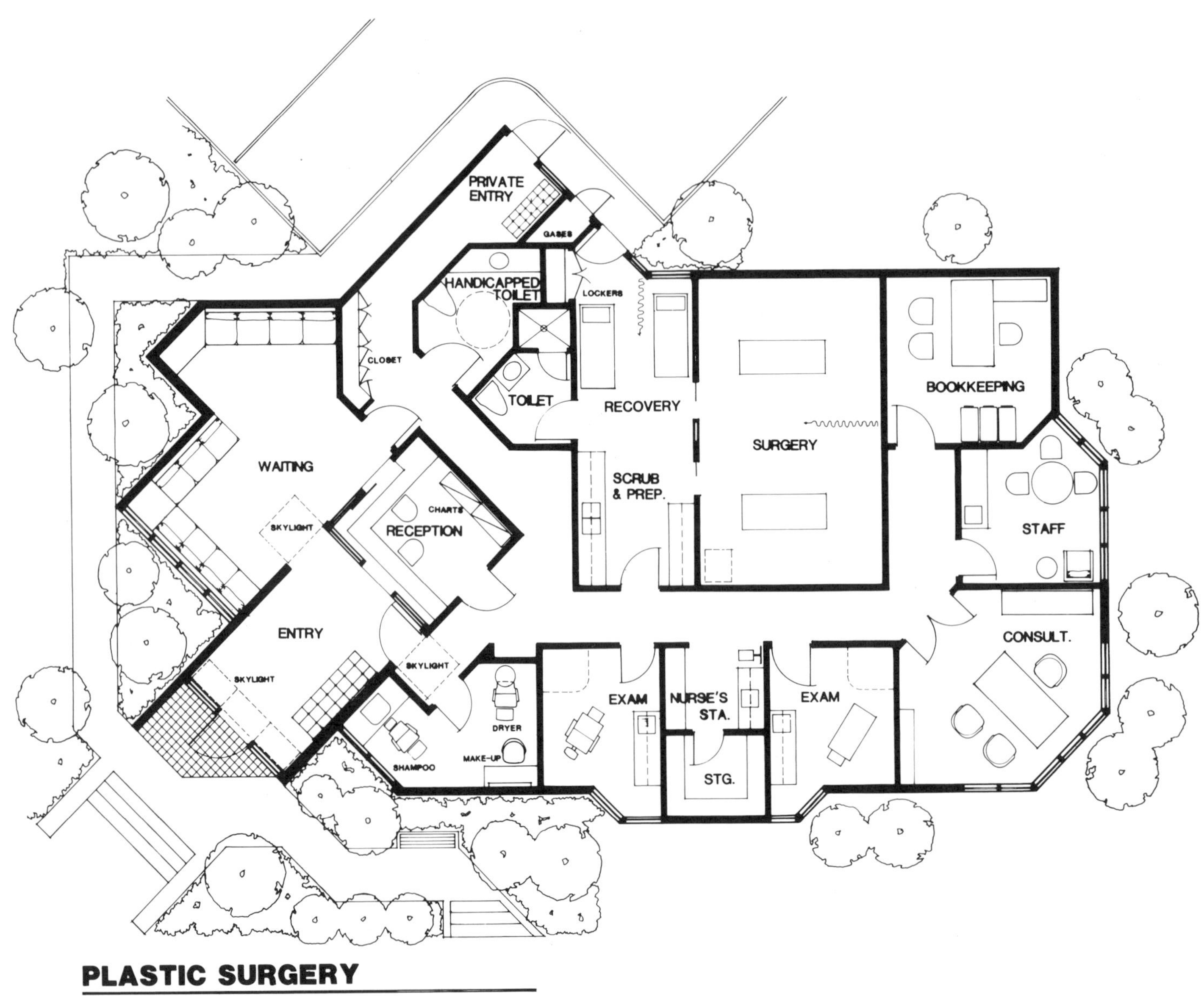

PLASTIC SURGERY

2520 SF

Figure 4-52. Suite plan for plastic surgery, 2520 square feet.

The surgeon's diplomas and awards should be prominently displayed here in elegant frames and mats. Sometimes patient education is accommodated in the consultation room (a VCR and TV would be provided), or a dedicated room is created for this purpose.

Office-Based Surgery

Surgery performed within the physician's office is called *office-based surgery,* compared with that which is performed in a *freestanding* surgical center. The latter refers to an ambulatory surgical center designed entirely for that purpose. It is called freestanding because it is not attached to or associated with a particular physician's office. The reader is referred to Chapter 7 for additional information.

Any discussion of office-based surgery begins with the issue of reimbursement. Unlike surgery performed by ophthalmologists, most plastic surgery is elective in nature and, as such, would not be covered by third-party payers. Therefore, designing the surgery suite to meet the criteria for reimbursement by third-party payers seems a moot point. Those cases that would be reimbursed (for example, reconstructive surgery to attach a severed finger, or surgery to restore a burn victim's appearance) would be done outside the office in an ambulatory surgical center or hospital.

Most insurance companies and Medicare will pay the physician's fee for any covered procedures done in the physician's office, but if the surgery suite itself does not meet certain requirements, they will not reimburse for the use of the facility.

The surgery suite in Figure 4-56 is perfectly acceptable, from the standpoint of function and size, for the type of procedures done within the office. It does not, however, incorporate all of the criteria of NFPA 101 (Life Safety Code), which would allow the facility to receive Medicare certification and would allow the phy-

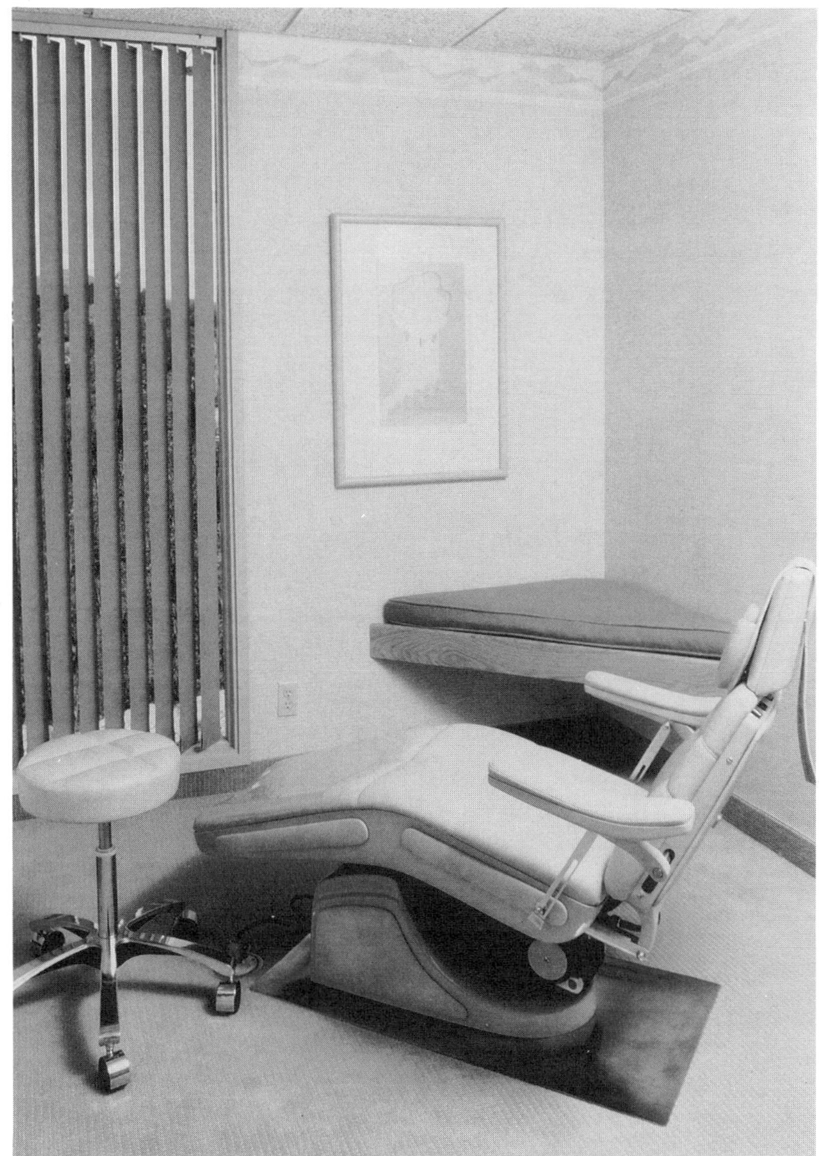

Figure 4-53. Examination room, plastic surgery. (*Design: Jain Malkin Inc.; Photographer: Michael Denny.*)

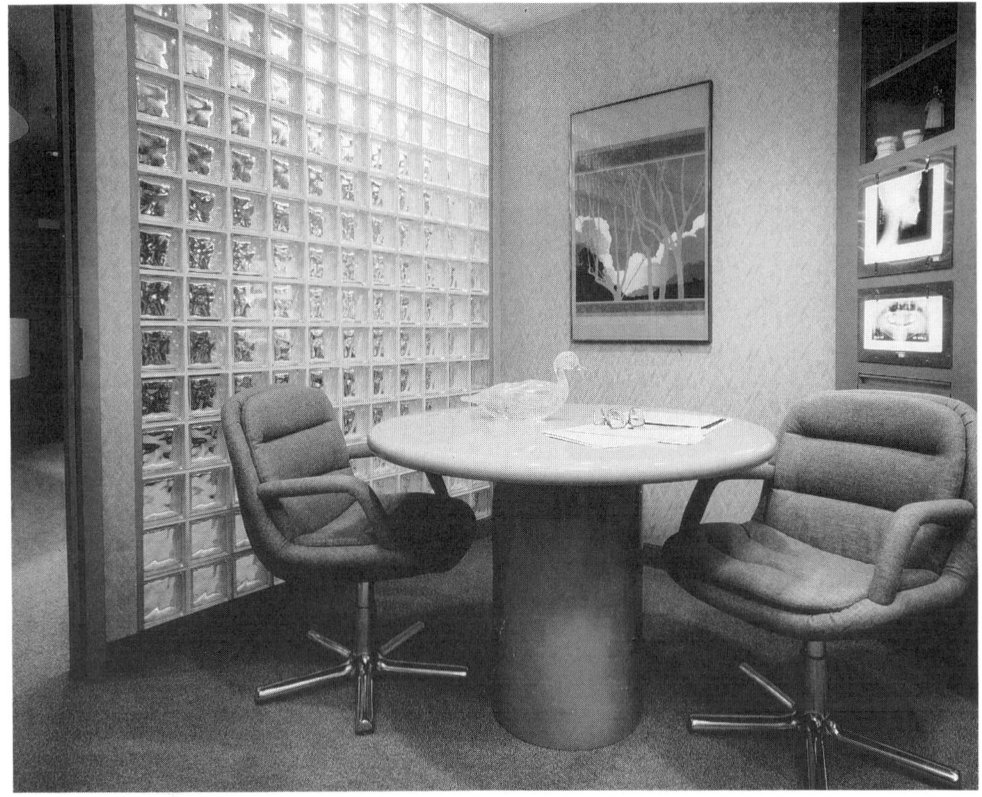

Figure 4-55. Consultation/presentation room. (*Photo courtesy Sue Walling, SW Design, Inc., Minneapolis, MN; Photographer: P.R. Siegrist.*)

sician to be reimbursed by insurers for the use of the facility. Some of these requirements are sprinklers, an air filtration system, and a washable ceiling (gypsum board or plastic-coated tile).

The American Association for Accreditation of Ambulatory Plastic Surgery Facilities (AAAAPSF), located in Mundeline, IL, publishes three booklets that will guide both the designer and the facility's staff if they wish to meet the *voluntary* accreditation standards of this organization. One booklet is an *Inspector's Manual,* another is a *Standards Manual,* and the third is a *Checklist/Questionnaire.*

The major determinant of design criteria relates to the type of anesthesia used. This in turn relates to the types of procedures that can safely be done in the office. The AAAAPSF standards classifications used in the manual are as follows:

Class A — performed under local, regional, or topical anesthesia; applies to minor plastic surgical procedures.

Class B — performed under intravenous or parenteral sedation, analgesia or dissociative drugs; applies to minor or major plastic surgical procedures.

Class C — major plastic surgery procedures performed under general anesthesia with external support of vital body functions.

The AAAAPSF standards facility classifications are:

I. Patient care standards
II. Facility standards
III. Safety standards
IV. Personnel standards
V. Quality assurance standards
VI. Administrative documentation standards

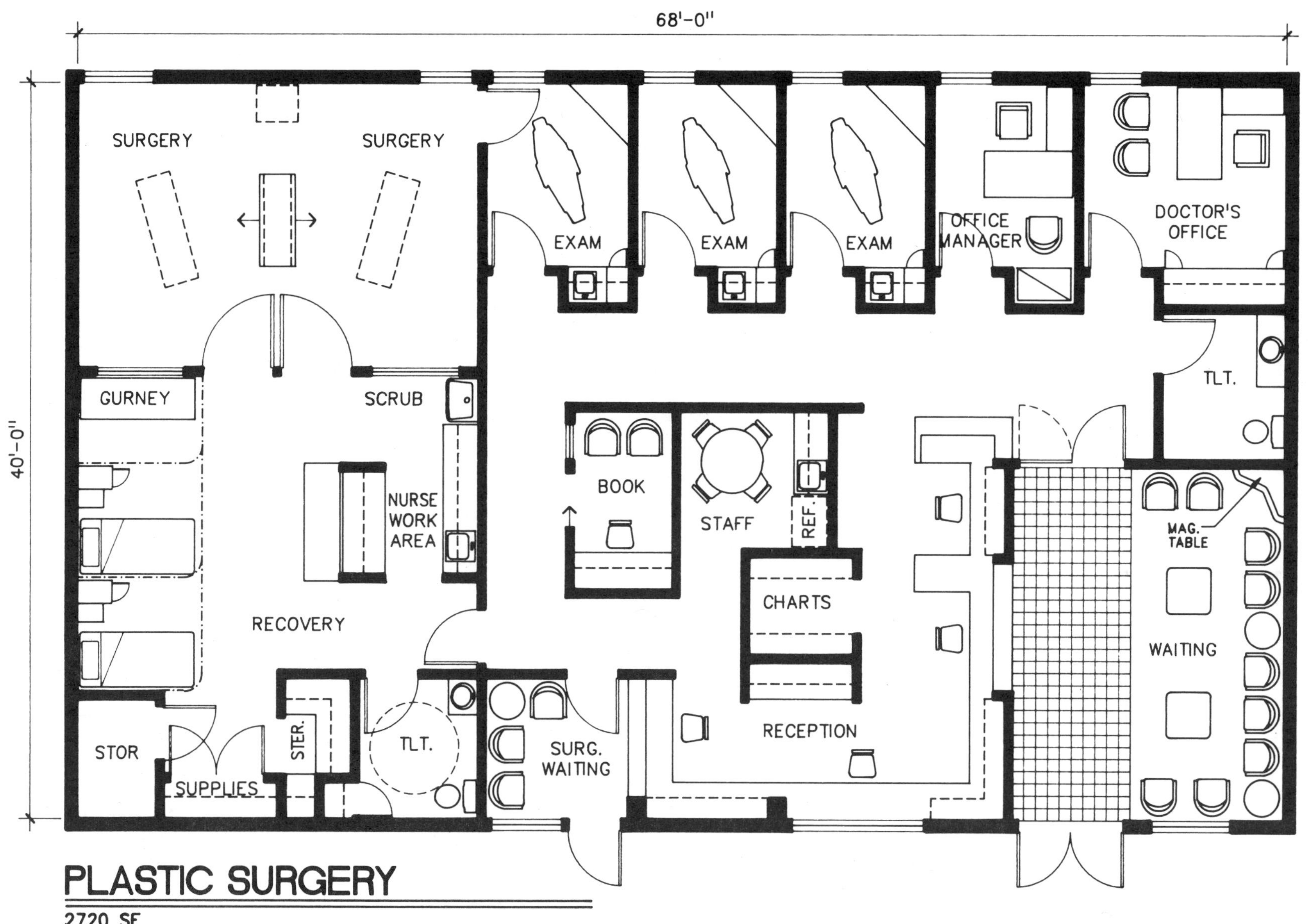

Figure 4-56. Suite plan for plastic surgery, 2720 square feet.

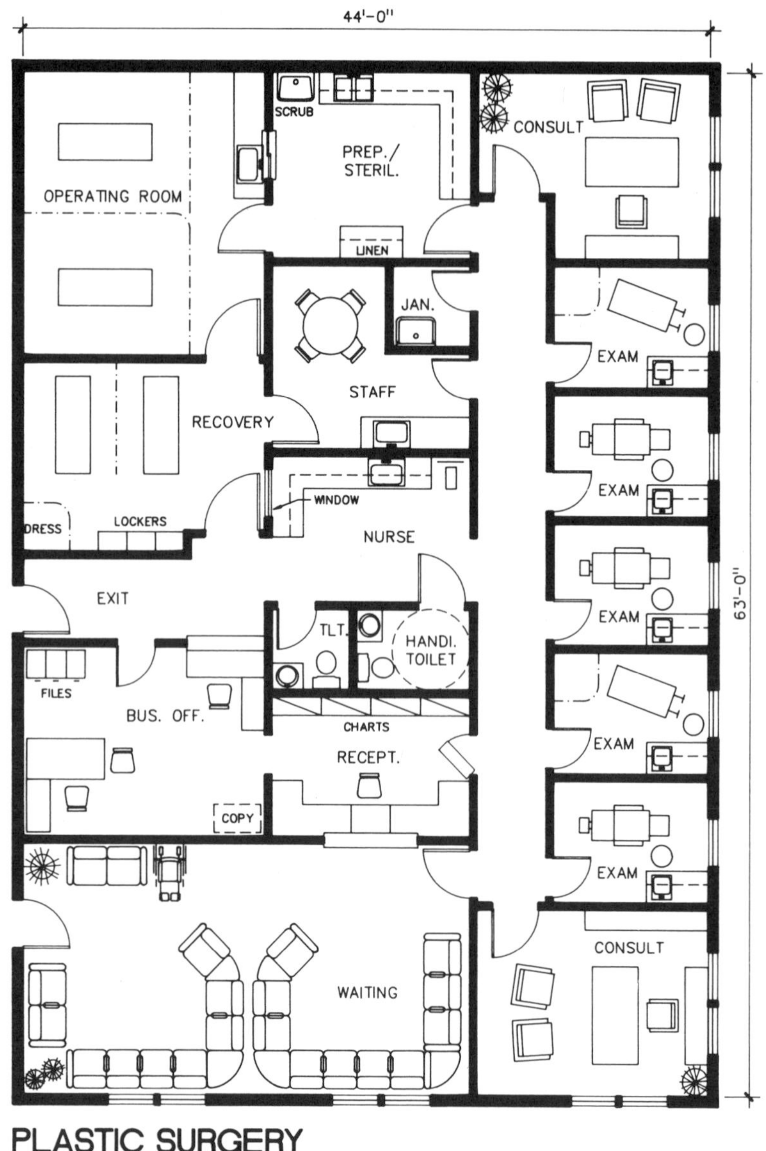

Figure 4-57. Suite plan for plastic surgery, 2772 square feet.

Although accreditation by AAAAPSF is voluntary, it does certify to the medical community and the community at large that the surgery facility meets nationally recognized standards set by members of the American Board of Plastic Surgery. Their recommendations are not considered codes, but they are guidelines for the safe handling of patients.

Operating Room Design

After a thorough discussion with the physician about goals for certification, accreditation, and/or licensing, appropriate code references must be consulted. The reader is referred to Chapter 7, Ambulatory Surgical Centers, for a discussion of these issues.

The *minimum* size of an operating room, in terms of function, number of personnel, and equipment (based on doing Class A local anesthesia procedures) is 14 × 16 feet, with one full wall of built-in cabinets containing a scrub sink with foot lever control and gooseneck spout; storage for linens, gowns, caps, disposable supplies, and surgical dressings; drawers or carts for surgical instruments, and a sterilization area.

If space permits, the scrub, prep, and cleanup room should be separate from the operating room (Figure 4-57). Similar to a large nurse station, this room should be a minimum of 8 × 12 feet lined with cabinets and work surfaces. Instruments will be sterilized and wrapped here; dressings and medications are prepared. Clinic service sinks and sinks in the prep or clean-up area should have plaster traps.

Sometimes, a practice may become known for its success with one particular procedure, such as reconstruction of the nose. In such case, a busy practice with several surgeons may perform these operations

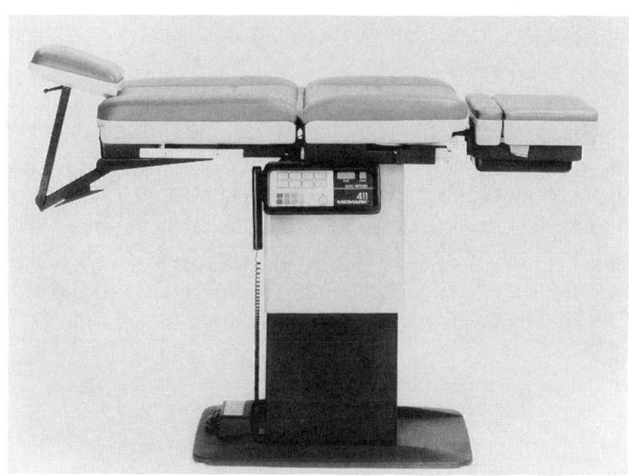

Figure 4-58. Motorized operating table. (*Courtesy Midmark Corp., Versailles, OH.*)

in such volume as to necessitate an operating room large enough to accommodate three patients simultaneously, with just a cubicle drape on a ceiling-mounted track separating the patients. While the nurse is prepping one patient, the surgeon may be completing surgery on the next, and a nurse may be applying a dressing on the third before moving the patient to a nearby recovery room. On this basis, three operating tables could be in use simultaneously, sometimes even with just one plastic surgeon working.

A power operating table (Figure 4-58) will have a ceiling-mounted surgical light (which requires support above the ceiling) centered overhead. A crash cart containing resuscitation equipment and a defibrillator (Figure 4-59) must be in the room. Oxygen and suction (vacuum) can either be piped into the room or can be portable. The designer must check local fire code requirements for storage of anesthetic gases. (See Chapters 7 and 10 for additional discussion.)

Some plastic surgeons design a large operating room that is divided into two by a wide cabinet that can be accessed from either side (Figure 4-60). If Class B and Class C type anesthetic procedures are to be done, there will be a number of pieces of monitoring equipment, plus the anesthesia machine, in the room. There will also be an anesthesiologist or nurse anesthetist, one or two nurses, and the physician. This is the reason that operating rooms are often 16 × 18 feet or 18 × 18 feet in size.

The operating room must be easy to clean. Walls should have a semi-gloss enamel paint finish or a very smooth commercial vinyl wallcovering. A floor with a minimum of joints is desirable — a commercial-quality sheet vinyl with self-coved base and heat-welded seams.

A lot of linen is used in a surgery facility, and accommodation must be made for large carts of soiled linen and storage of clean linen. It is ideal if the linen supply company can enter the soiled workroom directly, pick up the dirty linen and drop off the clean (see Figure 4-51).

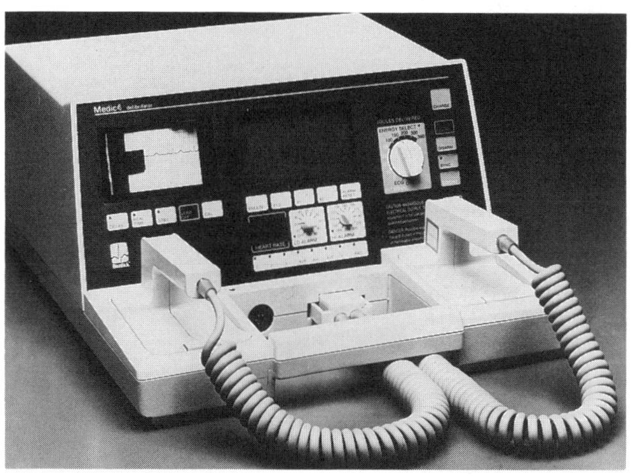

Figure 4-59. Defibrillator. (*Courtesy Burdick Corp., Milton, WI.*)

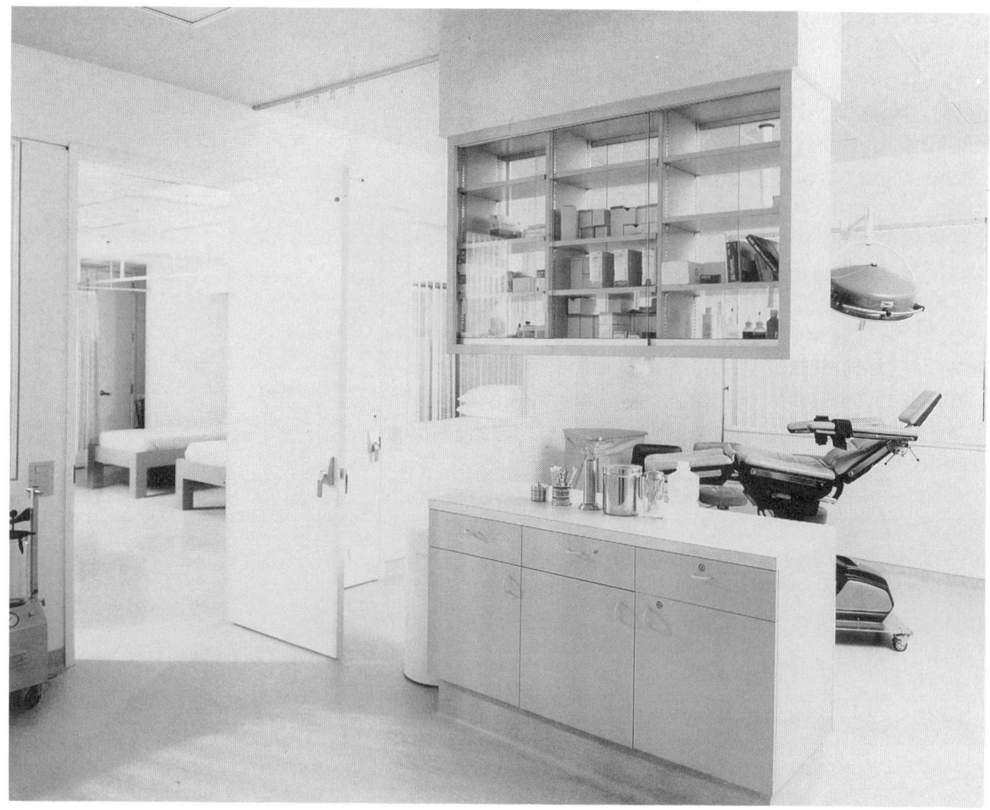

Figure 4-60. Operating room, plastic surgery suite. (*Design: Jain Malkin Inc.; Photographer: Michael Denny.*)

Dressing Area/Recovery Room

A dressing room, with lockers for valuables, should be provided for patients. Sometimes the dressing area is combined with the recovery room. The recovery area should be located near the operating room and nurse station so that staff, while readying the operating room for the next procedure, can keep a watchful eye on the recovering patient (see Figure 4-51). (Closed-circuit television, located in the nurse station, may be used for this purpose.) Each recovery bed must have suction and oxygen.

Typically, recovery beds are wheeled gurneys, 2 × 6 feet. A patient would be moved off the operating table onto a gurney and wheeled into the recovery room, so room layouts must allow for easy maneuvering of gurney carts without bumping into walls. One must be certain that all turns can be navigated. Sometimes a different type of bed (Figure 4-61) is used, but the patient should still be transported on a gurney.

Other Considerations

A busy plastic surgeon who specializes in cosmetic procedures may wish to have separate waiting rooms for male and female patients. A hair stylist may be on hand several afternoons a week to shampoo and style the hair of patients who have just had bandages removed after a face lift. Such patients may, understandably, be timid about visiting their own stylist in public until the bruises subside.

A small room should be set aside for this purpose with a standard beautician's shampoo chair, professional hairdryer, and good-quality tinted mirrors. A gray-tinted mirror will downplay bruises, yet still provide enough reflection. Attractive wallpaper and accessories will lift the patient's spirit.

A plastic surgeon may also offer the services of a professional makeup artist for patients recovering from facial plastic surgery. This could be done in the same room as hair styling (see Figure 4-52).

Plastic surgeons who specialize more in reconstructive surgery — skin grafts for burn victims, surgery of the hand, repair of cleft palate, trauma — often do not have strong sentiments about providing privacy and anonymity for their patients, and they may be less interested in the appearance or image of their office.

Interior Design

Since this is a low-volume medical practice, ease of maintenance and durability in finishes and furnishings is generally not an issue. Materials used may be residential in character (Color Plates 10 and 11, Figures 4-62 and 4-63). The plastic surgeon trades in cosmetics and vanity. The office is an expression of his or her attention to detail and an indication of aesthetic awareness; the image the surgeon projects is very important. People want to deal with a surgeon who appears to be successful — this amounts to third-party endorsement of the plastic surgeon's skills.

The plastic surgeon who spends a considerable sum on office design and furnishings will generally reap the rewards. No medical specialty benefits more from a high-profile image. Even the plastic surgeon's letterhead and business card should be striking and imaginative, and coordinated with the office design.

All rooms of this suite may be carpeted, except for the surgery suite. Office design should be stylish but comfortable, and lighting should be soft and flattering in all rooms, except the exam rooms and operating suite. Incandescent lighting is preferable to fluorescent in the waiting room (Color Plate 11, Figure 4-64), corridors, and consultation room. The waiting room especially benefits from a low level of illumination to mask bruises resulting from surgery and to keep patients out of the spotlight.

Bathroom design is important in this specialty. Large gray-tinted mirrors and interesting lighting may be incorporated into the vanity cabinet. Walls and ceiling may have an attractive wallpaper, and bathroom accessories (tissue boxes, paper towelette holders, soap dishes) should be elegant and residential in character. Other items a patient might use in light grooming before or after medical consultation ought to be provided.

Today, many people consider having plastic surgery to correct physical imperfections. Taboos about vanity have all but disappeared, and society places greater emphasis on self-expression and personal fulfillment. There is increased exposure to the benefits of plastic surgery in the media, which has given more people the confidence to obtain treatment. Plastic surgery is no longer just an option of the rich; many persons of modest income also consider it a viable option.

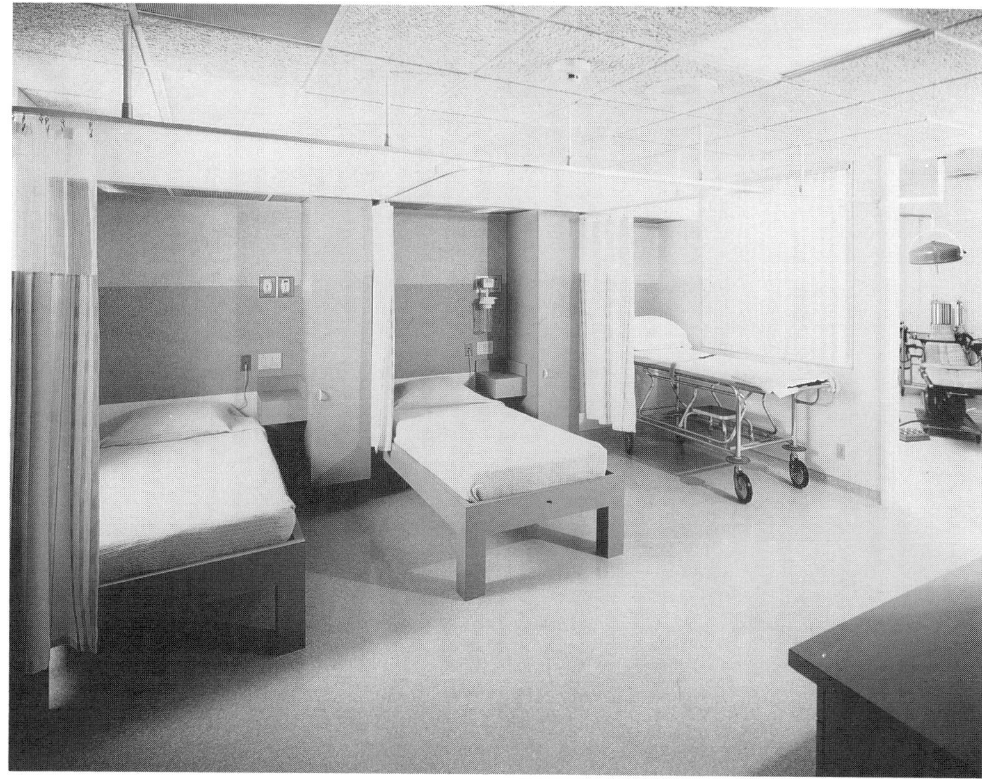

Figure 4-61. Recovery room, plastic surgery suite. (*Design: Jain Malkin Inc.; Photographer: Michael Denny.*)

Plastic surgery is a very lucrative medical specialty, and therefore its practitioners often seek to enhance their image and practice by having a luxurious office, by providing a secluded surgery and recovery facility, and by offering many patient-pleasing amenities.

ALLERGY

Allergy is defined as an altered reaction of the tissues to agents or allergens. Because these allergens cause a reaction in some persons but in similar amounts are harmless to others, allergies are often difficult to diagnose. A methodically detailed patient history is a part of any preliminary examination or interview. Some allergists use a printed questionnaire to be filled out by the patient, and in this case, several alcoves with countertop writing surface, chair, and light should be included in or near the waiting room (Figure 4-66).

Some allergists prefer that the patient history be taken by the staff, and in this case, small rooms (6 × 6 feet) should be provided with a desk (2 × 4 feet is adequate) and a chair for both the patient and interviewer, and perhaps one for a companion (Figure 4-67).

In a large practice, a combination of staff interview and printed questionnaire may be used. In this situation, an alcove may be created off the corridor for a number of tablet arm chairs. If the practice includes a large number of pediatric cases, the interview room will have to accommodate a parent, the child, and the interviewer, since the parent will usually answer questions for the child.

Pediatric Allergy

There are pediatric allergists whose entire practice focuses on children (Figure 4-68). These offices should be designed according to the needs of an allergist, but with design and color palette suitable for a pediatrician's office (Figures 4-69 and 4-70). The treatment or test rooms, instead of having number designations, may have large animals or cartoons painted alongside them, so that staff can tell the child to go to the "butterfly" or the "frog" room (Figure 4-71).

Patient Volume

An allergy practice has a high volume of patients (as high as 50 to 60 per doctor per day), which fall into two categories: short-visit (to receive an injection) and long-visit (patient interview, skin tests). Due to the high volume of patients, an efficient layout is of utmost importance. A large number of patients come two or three times a week, and others just weekly, to receive allergy shots. Thus the nurse station where injections are given should be located off the waiting room or just inside the suite near the waiting room so that these patients do not have to mingle with the long-visit patients (Figures 4-66 and 4-67).

Injection Protocol

After receiving the injection, the patient will return to the waiting room and sit for 10 to 15 minutes to check any adverse reaction he or she may have had to the desensitization shot. The waiting room must be large enough to accommodate the high volume of patients. Some offices have a small secondary waiting room within the suite where patients may wait after an injection (Figures 4-68 and 4-70). Other suites may actually have small reaction rooms furnished with a cot and chair so that a patient, after receiving an injection, may lie down for 15 to 20 minutes. If reaction rooms are provided, they should be located adjacent to the patient interview area or the injections area so that staff may observe these patients.

Skin Tests

After the minutely detailed patient history is taken, a patient will be subjected to skin tests in which he or she lies face down on a flat table, while the nurse or aide makes rows of small scratches on the patient's back, and an allergen is touched to each scratch. Intradermal tests, where a small amount of an allergen is injected just under the skin, are another type of skin test. Skin tests may be performed in small rooms, 6 × 8 or 8 × 8 feet, or in a large room that has been divided into 6- × 8-foot or 8- × 8-foot areas via a ceiling-mounted cubicle drape. The patient lies on a physical therapy table that is often placed against a wall. The technician sits alongside the patient, working off of a cabinet or a mobile cart. A rack of small vials containing allergens is carried from room to room and placed on the cart.

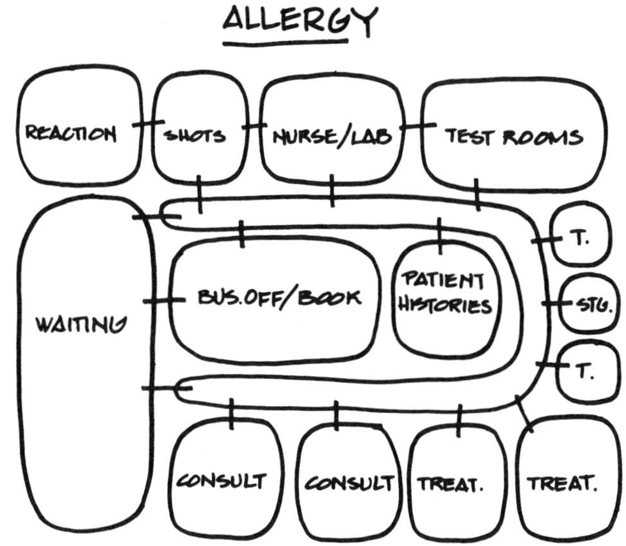

Figure 4-65. Schematic diagram of an allergy suite.

Table 4-6. Analysis of Program. Allergy

No. of Physicians:	1	2	3
Exam/Treatment Rooms	2 @ 8 × 12 = 192	4 @ 8 × 12 = 384	7 @ 8 × 12 = 672
Consultation Rooms	11 × 12 = 132	2 @ 11 × 12 = 264	3 @ 11 × 12 = 396
Waiting Room	16 × 16 = 256	16 × 26 = 416	20 × 30 = 600
Storage	6 × 8 = 48	6 × 8 = 48	8 × 8 = 64
Nurse Station/Lab	12 × 14 = 168	12 × 14 = 168	14 × 16 = 224
Toilets	2 @ 5 × 6 = 60	2 @ 5 × 6 = 60	3 @ 5 × 6 = 90
Shots	(Combine w/lab)	6 × 8 = 48	8 × 8 = 64
Recovery/Reaction	6 × 8 = 48	8 × 10 = 80	8 × 10 = 80
History Alcoves	—[a]	8 × 10 = 80	8 × 10 = 80
Test Rooms[b]	(2 persons) 96	(3 persons) 144	(4 persons) 192
Staff Lounge	8 × 10 = 80	10 × 12 = 120	12 × 14 = 168
Business Office	12 × 16 = 192	12 × 16 = 192	14 × 18 = 252
Subtotal	1272 ft^2	2004 ft^2	2882 ft^2
15% Circulation	191	300	432
Total	1463 ft^2	2304 ft^2	3314 ft^2

[a]History-taking alcoves may be worked into the circulation area or waiting room.

[b]May be one room with cubicle drape separation.

Note: The above spaces may vary greatly depending on the location of shot, test, and recovery/reaction rooms and how they are combined.

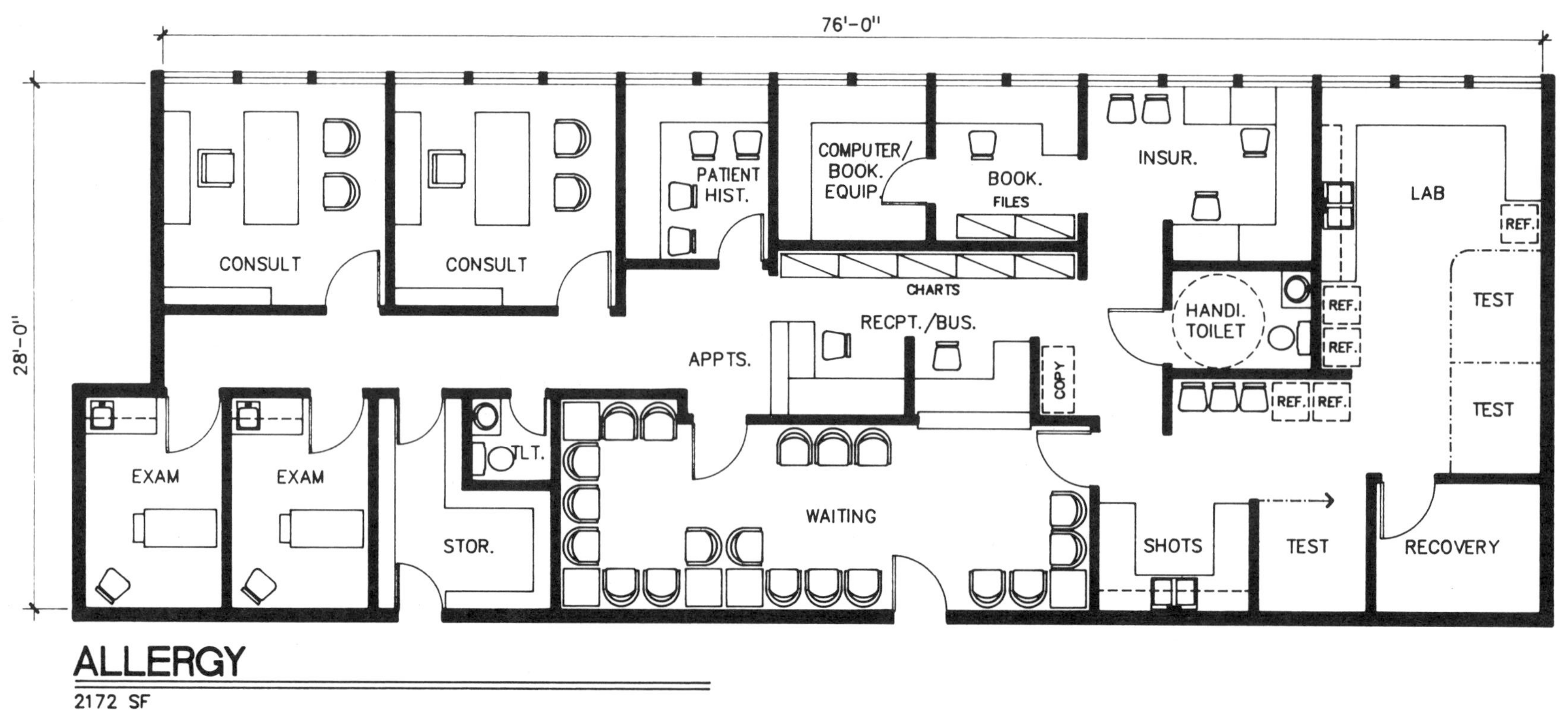

Figure 4-66. Suite plan for allergy, 2172 square feet.

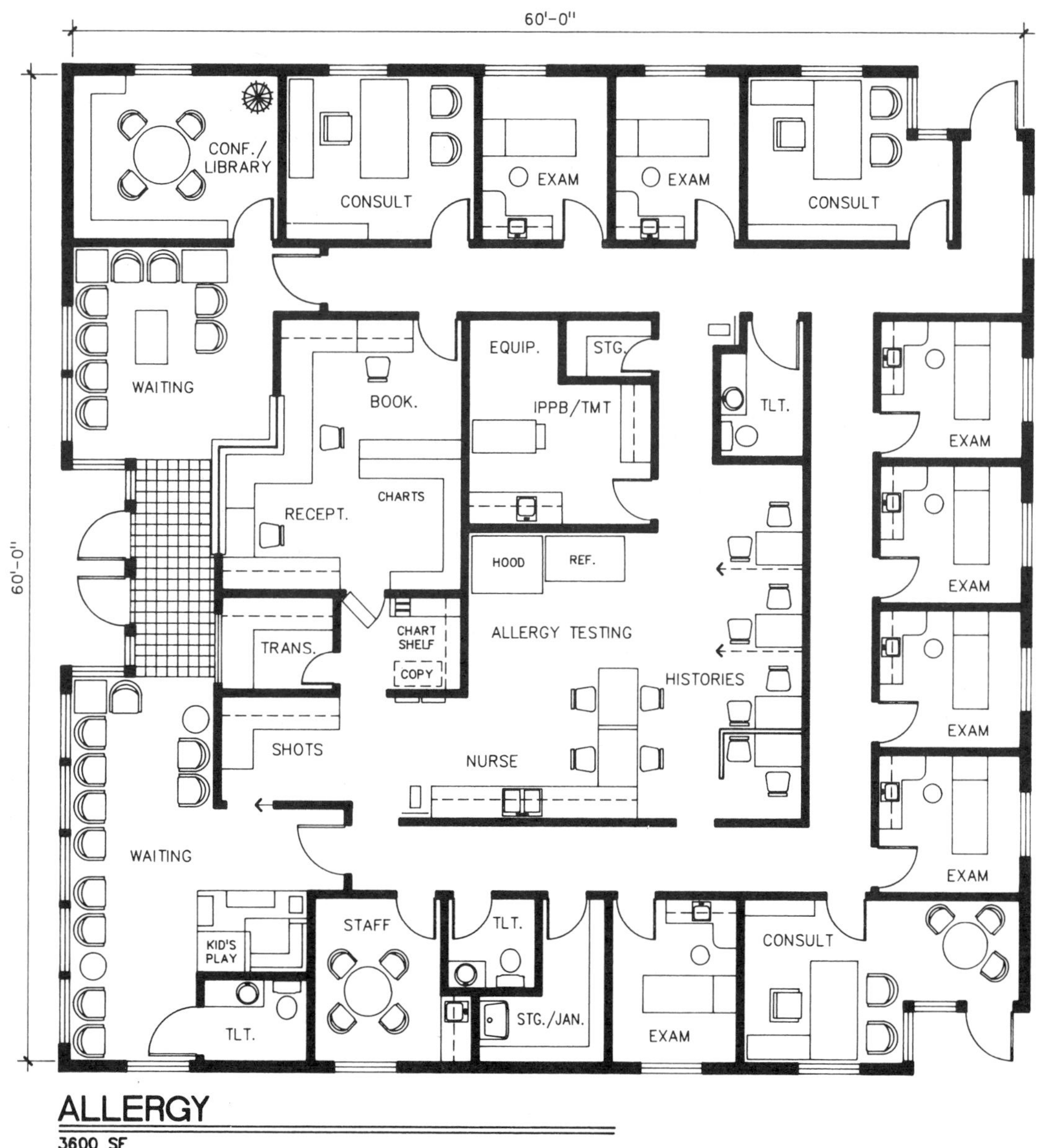

Figure 4-67. Suite plan for allergy, 3600 square feet.

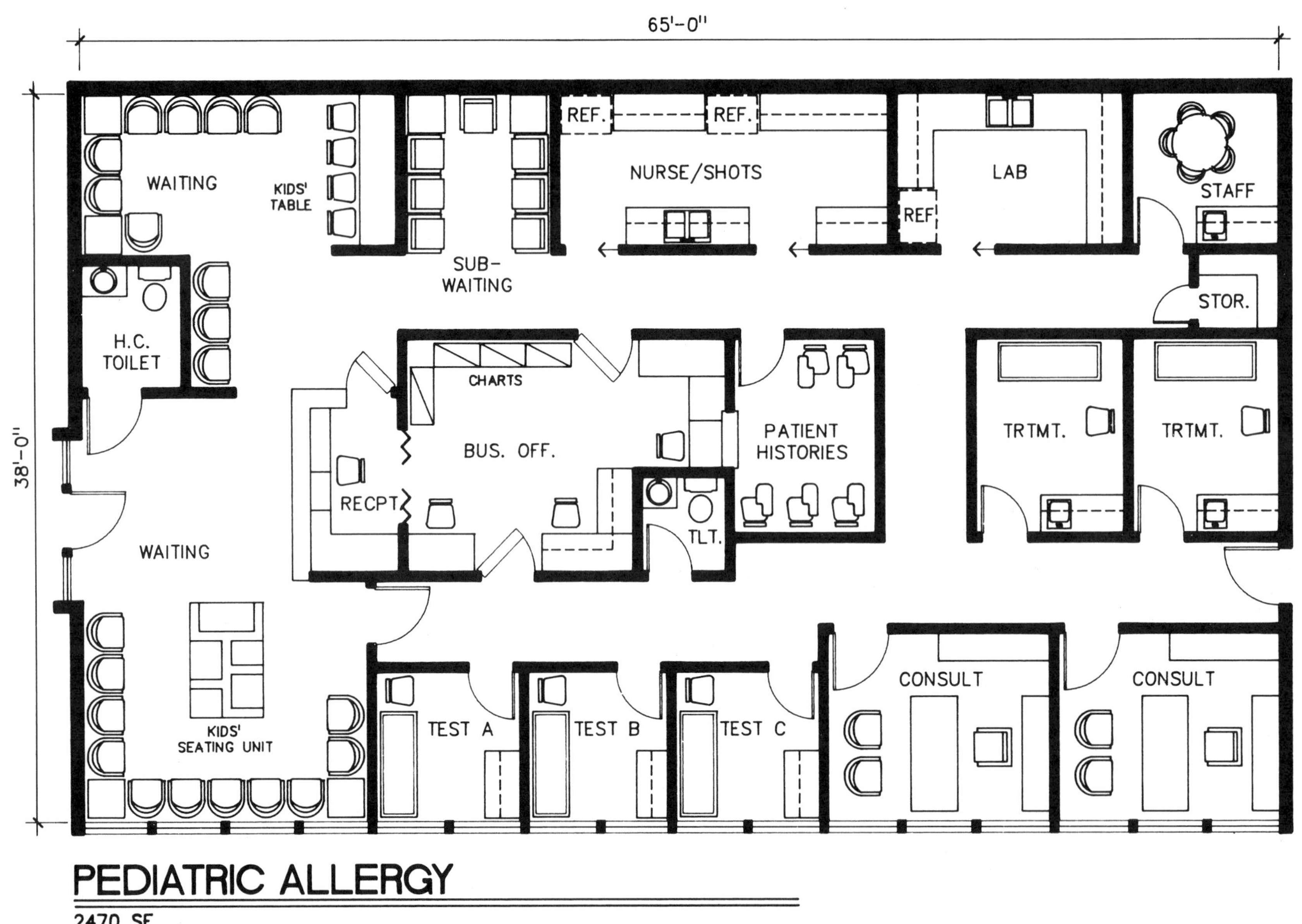

PEDIATRIC ALLERGY

2470 SF

Figure 4-68. Suite plan for pediatric allergy, 2470 square feet.

Treatment Room

Patients who are in no immediate physical danger are seen in test rooms, but patients who are experiencing severe symptoms such as asthma or vomiting will be examined in a standard exam room or a treatment room where the staff has access to water and respiratory equipment (IPPB Inter-Positive Pressure Breathing Apparatus).

After a diagnosis has determined to which agents the patient is sensitive, a desensitization treatment program is begun, in which small doses of the allergen are injected in a series of gradually increasing amounts over a period of months or, in some cases, years. The injections and tests are done by nurses and aides; therefore, one doctor may have several aides.

Other Considerations

The physician needs a large consultation room since the results of the testing and the prescribed treatment are discussed there. The nurse station/lab in this suite must be large and have space for two or more full-size refrigerators for storage of injectables.

Interior Design

Heavy textures, shag carpeting, and many fibers (wool, in particular) cause problems for those with allergies and are to be avoided in the office. Similarly, draperies, because they collect dust, are to be avoided in favor of PVC vertical blinds. All materials in this suite must be easy to sanitize and be as hypoallergenic as possible. Apart from this, there are no other special interior design considerations.

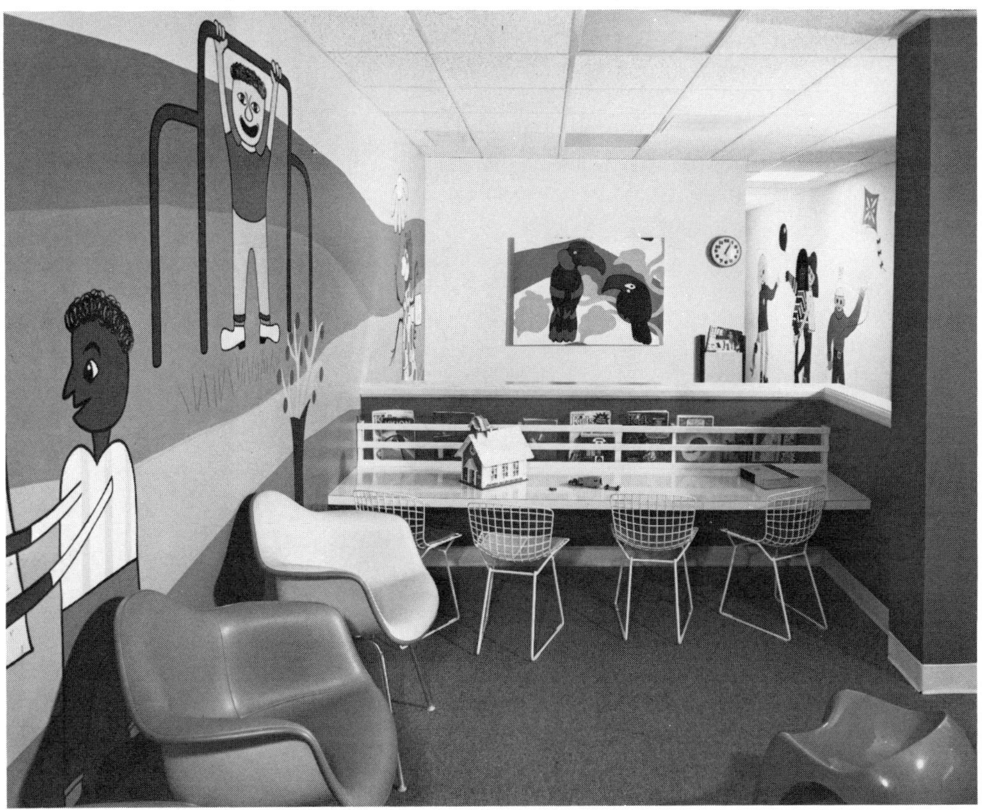

Figure 4-69. Waiting room for pediatric allergist. (*Design: Jain Malkin Inc.; Photographer: John Waggaman.*)

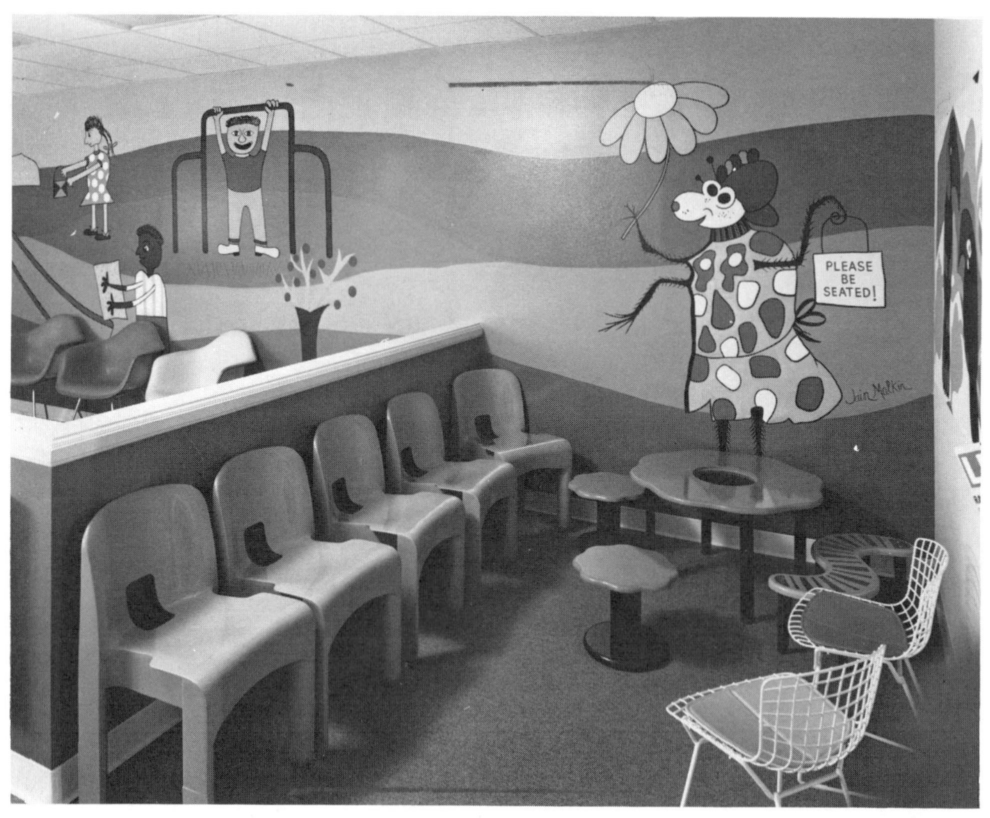

Figure 4-70. Secondary waiting room, pediatric allergy. (*Design: Jain Malkin Inc.; Photographer: John Waggaman.*)

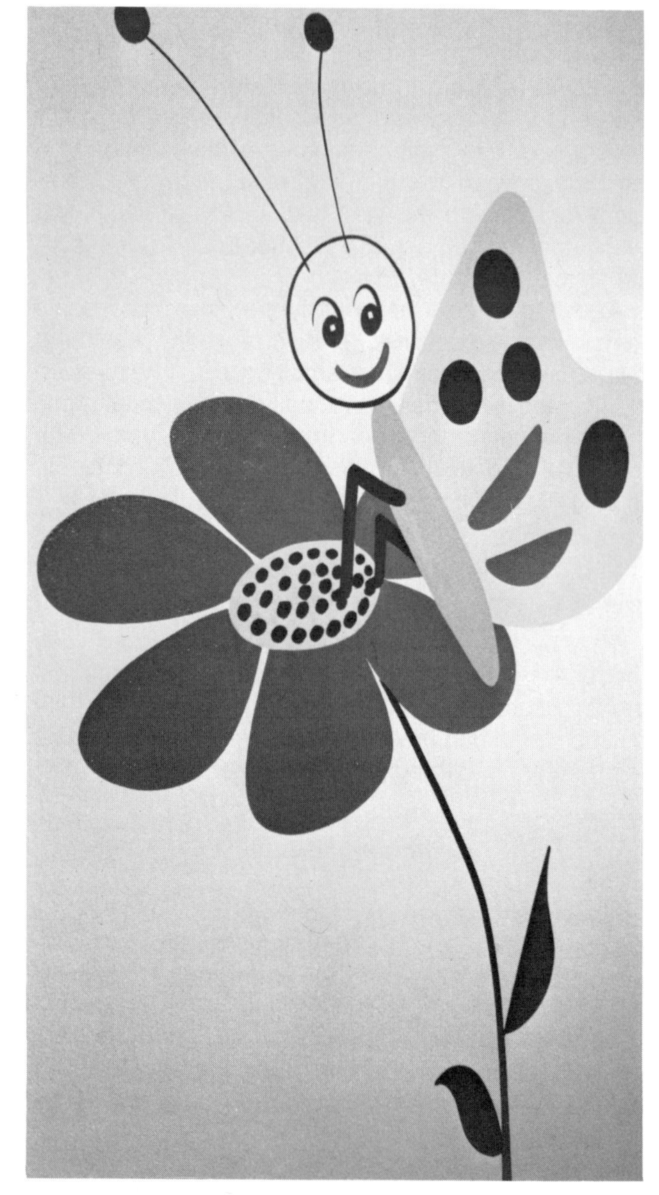

Figure 4-71. Butterfly graphic, pediatric allergy. (*Design: Jain Malkin Inc.; Photographer: John Waggaman.*)

PSYCHIATRY

This is the easiest medical suite to design. The consultation room is the key element in this suite. Each psychiatrist will have a preferred method of working, depending on his or her treatment philosophy. Some prefer a casual living room decor where doctor and patient sit next to each other in lounge chairs. Others offer the patient a sofa or chaise (Figure 4-73). Still others prefer a formal directive approach, with the doctor behind the desk and the patient across from it. Those who practice hypnosis often choose to have the patient relax in a recliner chair that rocks back to elevate the patient's feet.

Regardless of counseling style, the consultation room should be a minimum of 12 × 14 feet and preferably 14 × 16 feet. Psychiatrists usually house their professional libraries in this room, so adequate bookshelf storage should be planned. Diplomas can be framed creatively and hung as artwork in the room (Color Plate 12, Figure 4-74).

Some psychiatrists prefer a consultation room with a window; others find it distracting to the patient's concentration. Illumination should be rheostatically controlled so that it can be dimmed.

Sometimes solo practitioners share an office suite. Each would need a consultation room, but the business office, waiting room, and group therapy room would be shared. There should be two or three seats per doctor in the waiting room. Since each psychiatrist can see only one patient per hour, this is a very low-volume specialty. The group therapy room should accommodate about 12 persons. Chairs that stack are best, but they must be comfortable. The room should have a sink cabinet for preparation of coffee, and perhaps a coat closet.

Interior Design

The waiting room may be residential in character. Patients are often nervous before therapy; thus, the waiting room ought to have a relaxing color palette and feel comfortable, yet afford individuals some degree of privacy. Sound control is very important in this suite. All walls of consultation rooms and the group therapy room should have sound-attenuating construction (see Chapter 14).

The ambience of this suite is of utmost importance. Colors and design should be tranquil and serve as a background rather than be stimulating enough to be distracting. Sharp contrasts in color or pattern should be avoided in favor of mellowness (Color Plates 12 and 13, Figures 4-75 and 4-76).

Child Psychiatry

Child psychiatrists prefer to observe patients in a natural setting, necessitating a room for play therapy. Typically, this room would have a one-way glass observation window, a play table with chair or carpeted platforms, and an assortment of dolls, games, and other toys (Figure 4-77). If an easel and paints are provided, a sink should be included in the room. An attractive cabinet may be designed to house all the toys in an orderly fashion (Figure 4-78). If appropriate space is available, a secured outdoor play area can be developed to allow the psychiatrist to study children playing naturally without them realizing they are being observed.

The room in Figure 4-77 has been carefully designed for discreetly videotaping the child's activity, a necessary step for prosecuting child abuse offenders.

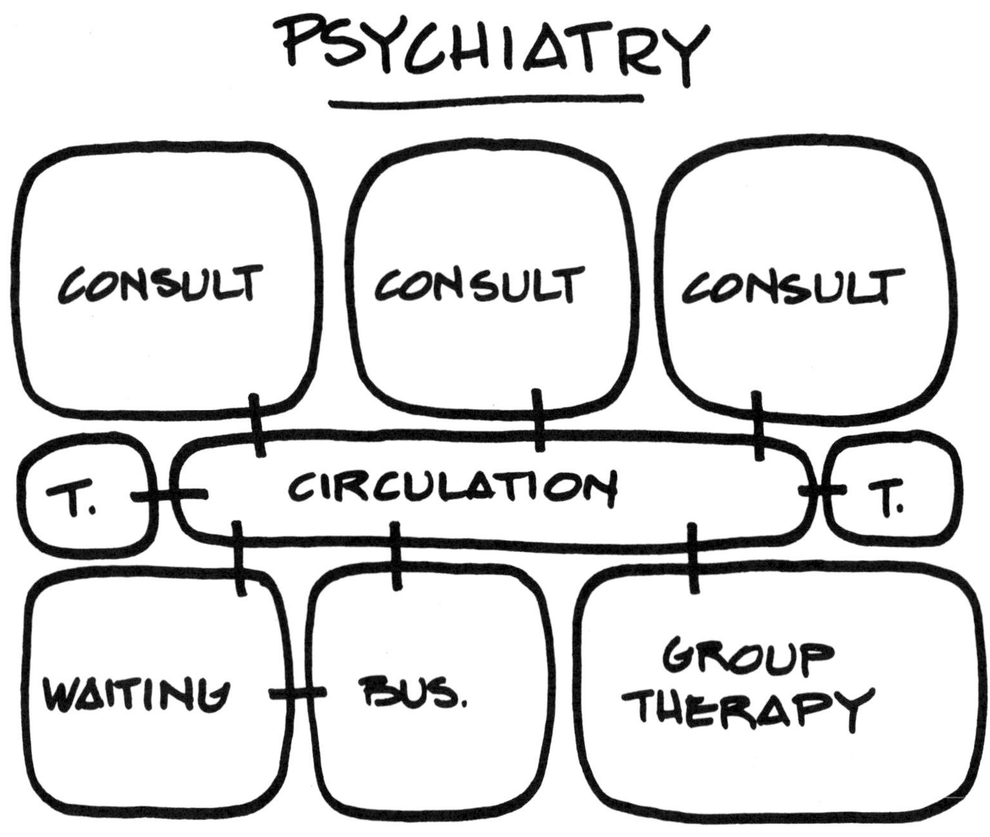

Figure 4-72. Schematic diagram of a psychiatry suite.

Table 4-7. Analysis of Program. Psychiatry

No. of Physicians:	1		2		3	
Consultation Rooms	14 × 16 =	224	2 @ 14 × 16 =	448	3 @ 14 × 16 =	672
Toilets	5 × 6 =	30	5 × 6 =	30	2 @ 5 × 6 =	60
Group Therapy	16 × 18 =	288	16 × 18 =	288	16 × 18 =	288
Business Office	12 × 14 =	168	12 × 14 =	168	14 × 16 =	224
Waiting Room	12 × 10 =	120	12 × 10 =	120	12 × 16 =	192
Storage	4 × 6 =	24	4 × 6 =	24	6 × 8 =	48
Subtotal		854 ft^2		1078 ft^2		1564 ft^2
15% Circulation		128		161		234
Total		982 ft^2		1239 ft^2		1798 ft^2

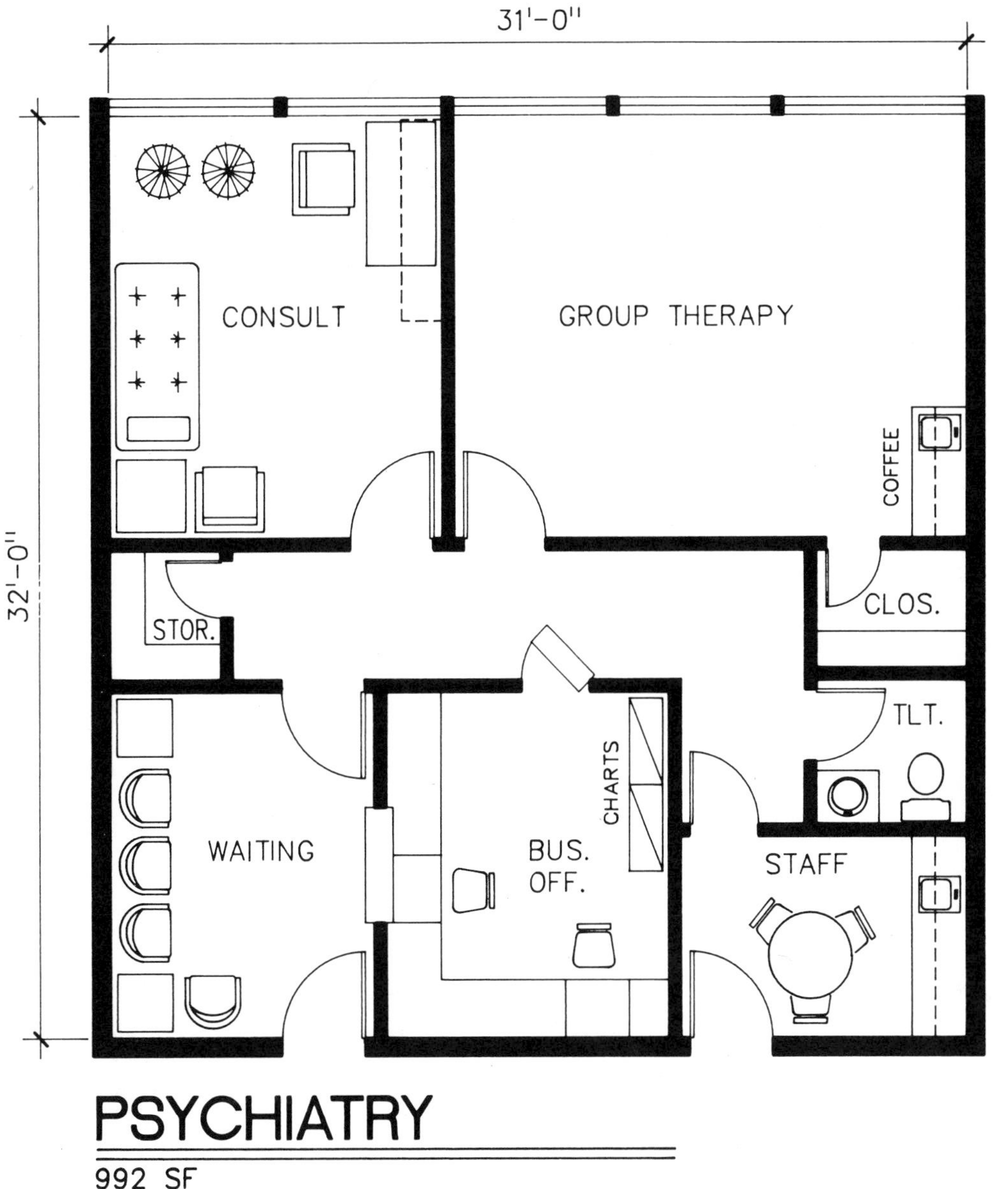

Figure 4-73. Suite plan for psychiatry, 992 square feet.

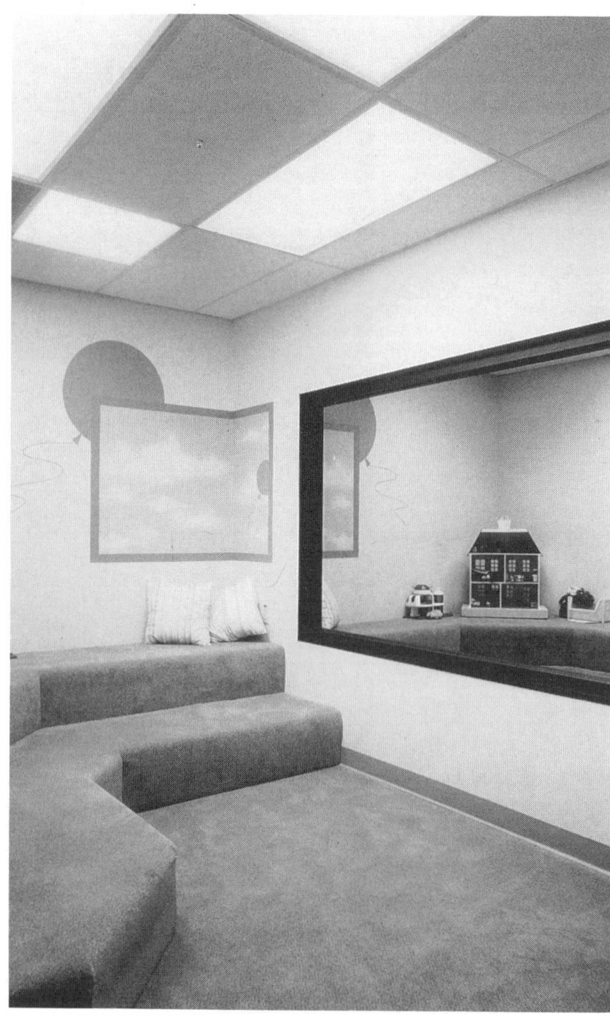

Figure 4-77. Examination/observation room, child psychiatry. (*Design: Jain Malkin Inc.; Photographer: John Christian.*)

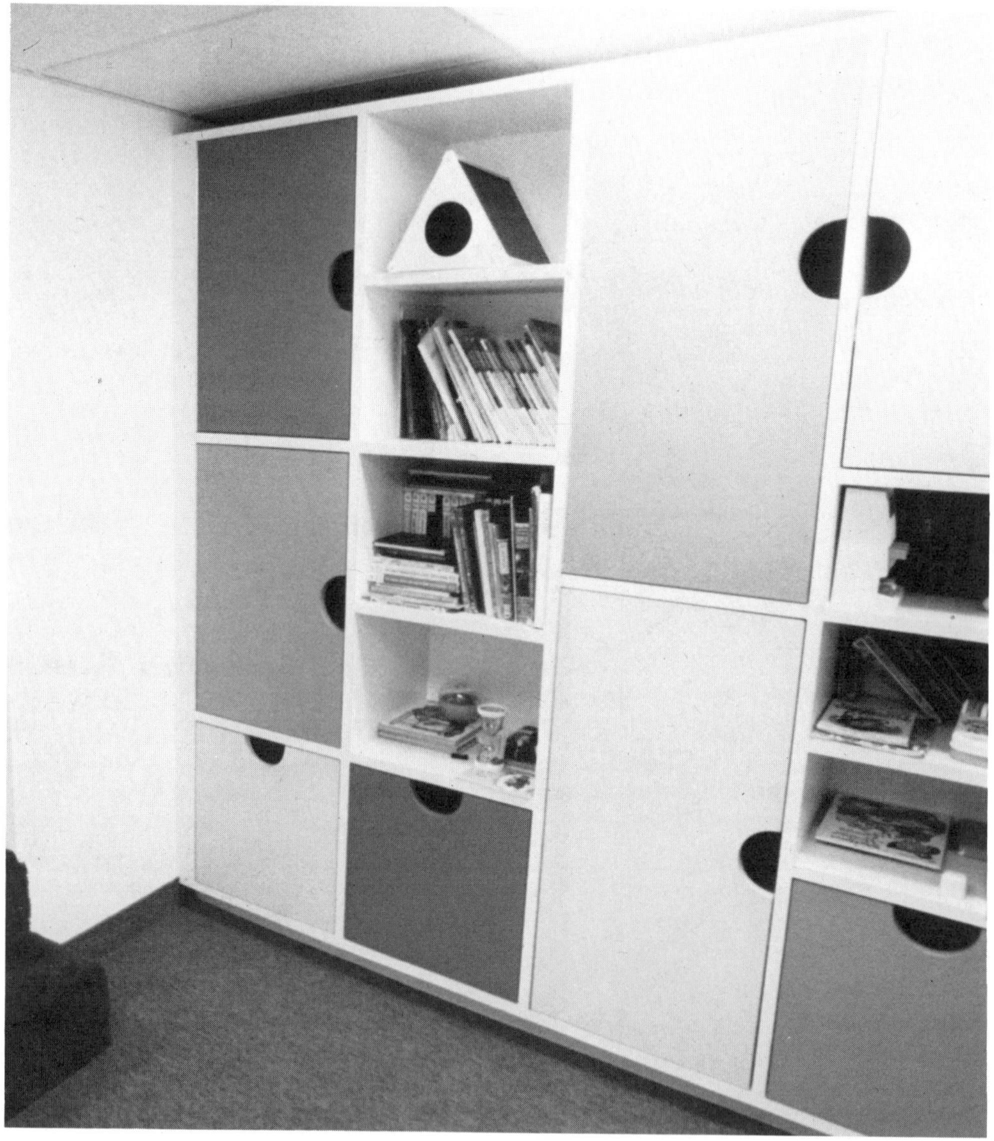

Figure 4-78. Toy storage cabinet. (*Design: Jain Malkin Inc.; Photographer: Jain Malkin.*)

NEUROLOGY

Neurologists diagnose diseases of the nervous system and brain. Their patients are always referred by other physicians. Patients may complain of headaches, epileptic seizures, damage suffered as a result of a stroke, or perhaps a cerebral palsy condition that has resulted in facial distortion — a distended jaw or a drooping mouth.

This is a low-volume specialty, with the taking of a preliminary history and an interview in the physician's consultation room requiring about 45 to 50 minutes. It is not uncommon in this specialty to have a small exam room opening off of the consultation room (Figure 4-80).

Diagnostic Procedures

After the interview, a series of tests is performed. The most common test is the *electroencephalogram* (charting of brain waves), commonly known as EEG (Figure 4-81). This can be performed in a room as small as 8 × 10 feet if the technician does not remain in the room with the patient, but sits in an adjoining control room.

There are two schools of thought on this point. Some neurologists feel that the patient is comforted by the technician being in the same room, and others feel that it is distracting to the patient. However, most prefer to have the tech in the room with the patient. In either case, the patient usually sits in a comfortable recliner chair, since this seems to make the patient less apprehensive and more relaxed. It is not essential but it is helpful to have a sink in the EEG room for hand washing.

There are three ways to administer the EEG. One way requires the application of conductive paste at the temples before the leads are attached. The paste is

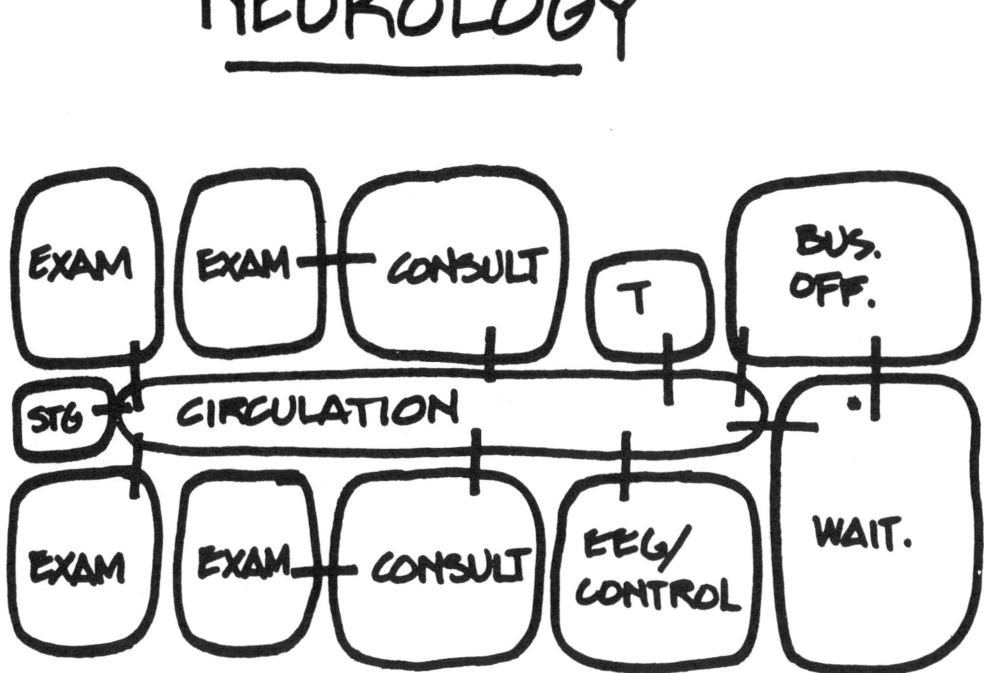

Figure 4-79. Schematic design of a neurology suite.

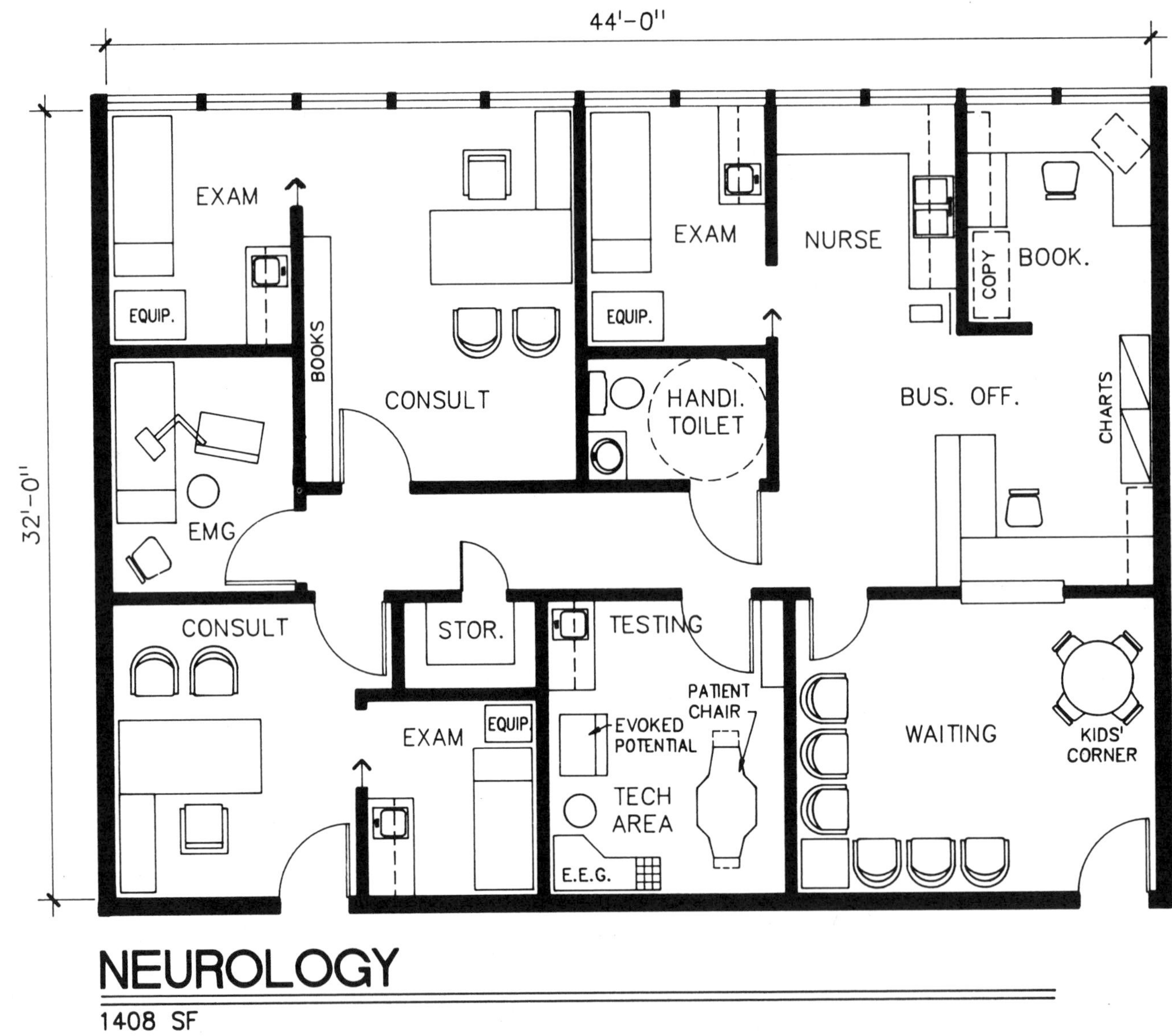

Figure 4-80. Suite plan for neurology, 1408 square feet.

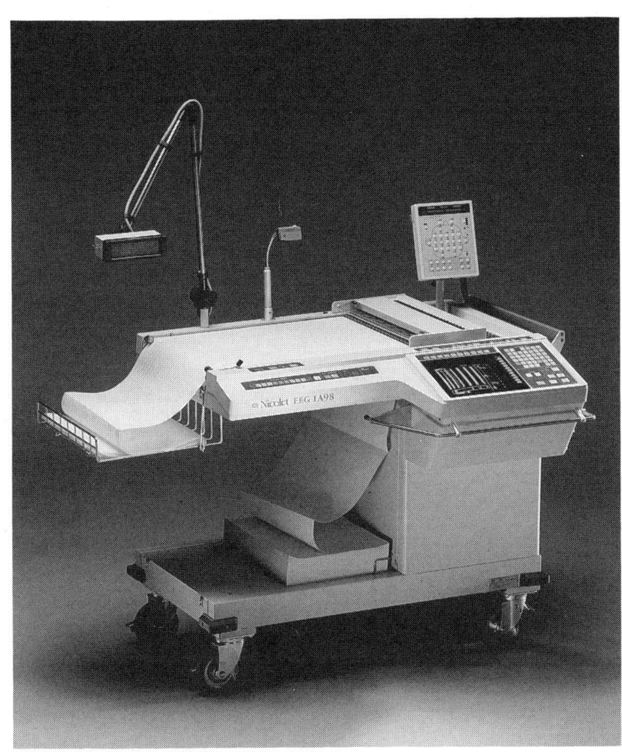

Figure 4-81. EEG (electroencephalograph) machine. (*Courtesy Nicolet Biomedical Instruments, Madison, WI.*)

messy and the patient must have access to a sink or a bathroom to wipe it out of his or her hair afterwards. A thoughtful designer would provide a vanity counter in the bathroom with a paper towel dispenser, a soap dispenser, and a place to hang a coat or handbag. While one does not wish to encourage the patient to shampoo hair in the office, it is necessary to remove the paste at least partially.

The second method of performing EEGs eliminates the paste and instead involves the insertion of small needles. This method, however, cannot be used with children. The third method is generally considered the simplest for both the tech and the patient. It involves the use of an electrode cap that resembles an old-fashioned swimming cap. With this method, there is very little paste to wipe off the hair. The EEG procedure takes about 40 minutes to perform.

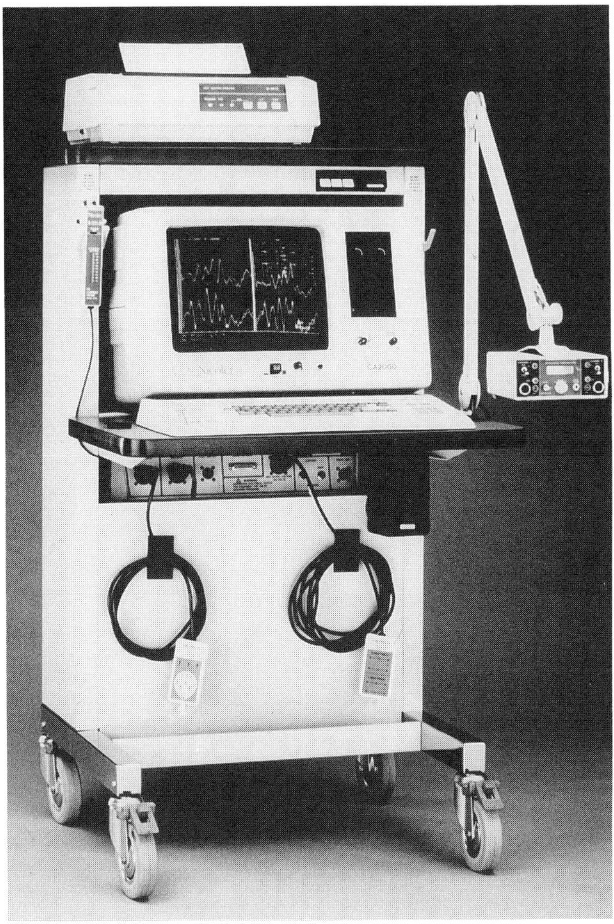

Figure 4-82. Evoked potential and EMG machine. (*Courtesy Nicolet Biomedical Instruments, Madison, WI.*)

Table 4-8. Analysis of Program. Neurology

No. of Physicians:	1	2
Consultation Rooms	12 × 14 = 168	2 @ 12 × 14 = 336
Exam Rooms	2 @ 8 × 10 = 160	4 @ 8 × 10 = 320
Business Office	12 × 14 = 168	14 × 16 = 224
Waiting Room	10 × 12 = 120	12 × 14 = 168
Toilets	5 × 6 = 30	2 @ 5 × 6 = 60
EEG/Control	8 × 12 = 96	8 × 12 = 96
Nurse Station/Lab	6 × 8 = 48	6 × 8 = 48
Storage	4 × 6 = 24	4 × 6 = 24
Subtotal	814 ft^2	1276 ft^2
15% Circulation	122	191
Total	936 ft^2	1467 ft^2

Another commonly performed test is *evoked potential,* which tests the different pathways to the brain (auditory, visual, and somatosensory). Both EEG and evoked potential testing are done by a technician, and both units may be located in the same room (Figure 4-82). A room 10 × 12 feet would be adequate. With the EEG unit, the tech sits at the computerized console during the procedure. If the neurologist prefers that the technician be in an adjoining control room, there must be a large window so that the patient can be observed at all times.

In the test room or the control area, locked storage is needed for drugs used to sedate patients, and somewhere there should be shelves for storage of EEG records that fit into containers resembling small books. The size depends on the particular machine and how many channels it has; however, the boxes are approximately 9 × 10 inches × 3 inches thick. They do not have to be stored in the test room itself. EEG printouts are pre-folded when released from the machine; therefore, there is no need for a mounting area. Lighting in the test room should be able to be dimmed.

Frequently a neurologist will perform EEGs for other physicians but have no personal consultation with the patient. The EEG technician would perform the test, and the printout would be read or interpreted by the neurologist, with a report mailed to the patient's physician. However, the neurologist would not consult with the patient unless the physician, after receiving the report, felt the referral was necessary for treatment of the patient's condition. Therefore a good location for the EEG room is near the front of the suite so that these patients do not have to pass the consultation room or exam rooms in order to reach the test room.

A neurologist may also perform a *spinal tap* (to drain off fluid) in the office. For this procedure, the neurologist would use an exam room with the patient lying on an exam table, which is usually placed against a wall.

Another office procedure is *electromyography,* which shows if a muscle is deteriorating or can be rehabilitated. It measures the strength of a muscle and indicates if the nerve has been affected. This test is performed by the physician, in a dedicated room, with a table placed against the wall. The procedure takes about half an hour, and the reason for putting it in a dedicated room is that it saves time in moving the equipment around and in setting up each patient. The room need only be 8 × 10 feet or 10 × 10 feet. The equipment is on a mobile cart so that the physician can move it around the patient (Figure 4-83).

Other examination rooms will have a physical therapy–type table and a small sink cabinet. In addition, these rooms may have an eye chart and perhaps an X-ray view box. Some neurologists like a scale in each exam room. The patient's evaluation of his or her weight helps the physician gauge a patient's touch with reality.

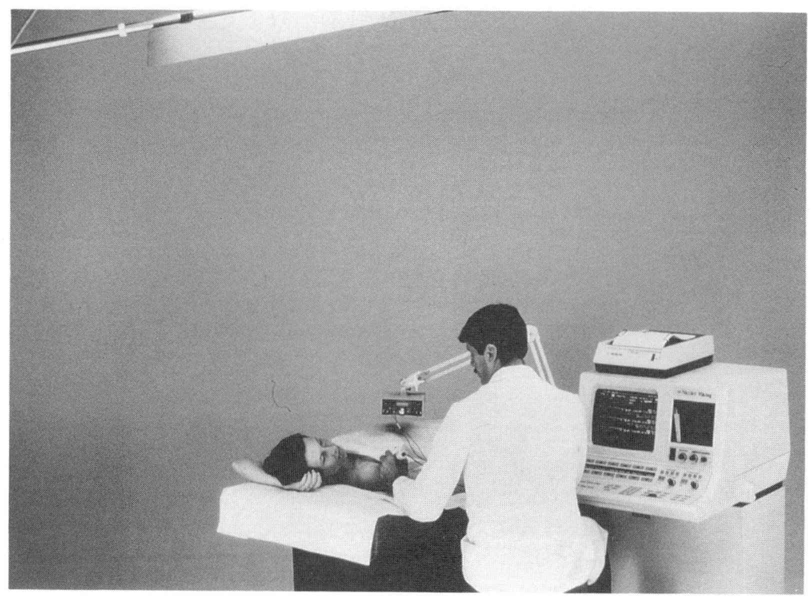

Figure 4-83. EMG (electromyography) machine. (*Courtesy Nicolet Biomedical Instruments, Madison, WI.*)

Interior Design

The consultation room should be large and comfortably furnished, since most patients will be interviewed here. Furnishings in this room, and the remainder of the office, should be tasteful but understated. All colors and patterns should be selected for their restful quality — anything bold is to be avoided. One must be particularly aware of patterns that have a figure-ground reversal or pick up a visual rhythm. Such patterns may cause seizures in people with certain types of neurological disorders.

All rooms in this suite may be carpeted. Carpet should have an anti-static wire woven into it to avoid interference from static electricity that might affect electronic equipment. Lighting should be rheostatically controlled so that it can be dimmed when patients are relaxing and being tested.

PAIN TREATMENT CENTER

These are hybrid-type suites that are becoming increasingly common. They involve a multidisciplinary approach to the treatment of pain. Frequently one will find neurologists, nutritionists, deep tissue massage therapists, chiropractors, psychologists, and biofeedback technicians working together in a holistic manner to change the patient's behavior or symptoms. Some neurologists may have one or more biofeedback rooms and physical therapy massage rooms incorporated into their offices.

People who suffer from chronic pain need a relaxing, comforting environment in which to receive medical treatment. Lighting is especially important. All attempts should be made to do away with 2×4 feet fluorescent lighting in favor of indirect lighting around the perimeter of the room, or from wall sconces, or other semi-concealed sources.

Temperature control is very important, especially in a biofeedback room, physical therapy room, or massage room. When patients are relaxing and/or undressed, if they are too warm or uncomfortably cold, their discomfort will defeat the treatment. With respect to the mechanical system, it is important to zone this suite very carefully and locate thermostatic controls in appropriate rooms.

Rooms used for massage should have built-in shelves and storage specifically designed for massage therapy. A number of salves and creams are used, and there is a need for storage of small pillows used to support limbs. Additionally, a considerable amount of linen is used, which has to be stored. There needs to be a place to hang the patient's handbag and clothing. Most of all, room lighting should be able to be dimmed. Many therapists prepare their own music tapes, and therefore a shelf or storage compartment may accommodate a small tape deck.

Biofeedback rooms should be located in a quiet part of the suite. Patients generally sit in a recliner chair and wear headphones. These rooms need indirect lighting, able to be dimmed, and very soothing colors. Even a piece of artwork may be too distracting.

A pain treatment center would, of course, have the same type of ancillary rooms as any medical suite, including private offices, administrative areas, restrooms, locker/dressing rooms, waiting room, and business office.

NEUROSURGERY

A neurosurgeon's office is often smaller than a neurologist's office and does not include diagnostic testing equipment. All of the tests would be performed in the neurologist's office, and the neurosurgeon would mainly see patients for pre-operative and post-operative consultations. Therefore a small number of examination rooms is necessary, in addition to a business office, bookkeeping area, and a consultation room for each physician (Figure 4-84). One exam room per physician is usually adequate since the surgery schedule rarely permits all physicians to be there at the same time. Each physician may have a private secretary to schedule surgeries and handle correspondence.

GENERAL SURGERY

This is a low-volume practice in large part dependent upon referrals from primary care physicians. The suite can be small, because most of a surgeon's work is done in a hospital. Patients are examined and interviewed pre-operatively and post-operatively in the office, and sutures may be removed or dressings changed.

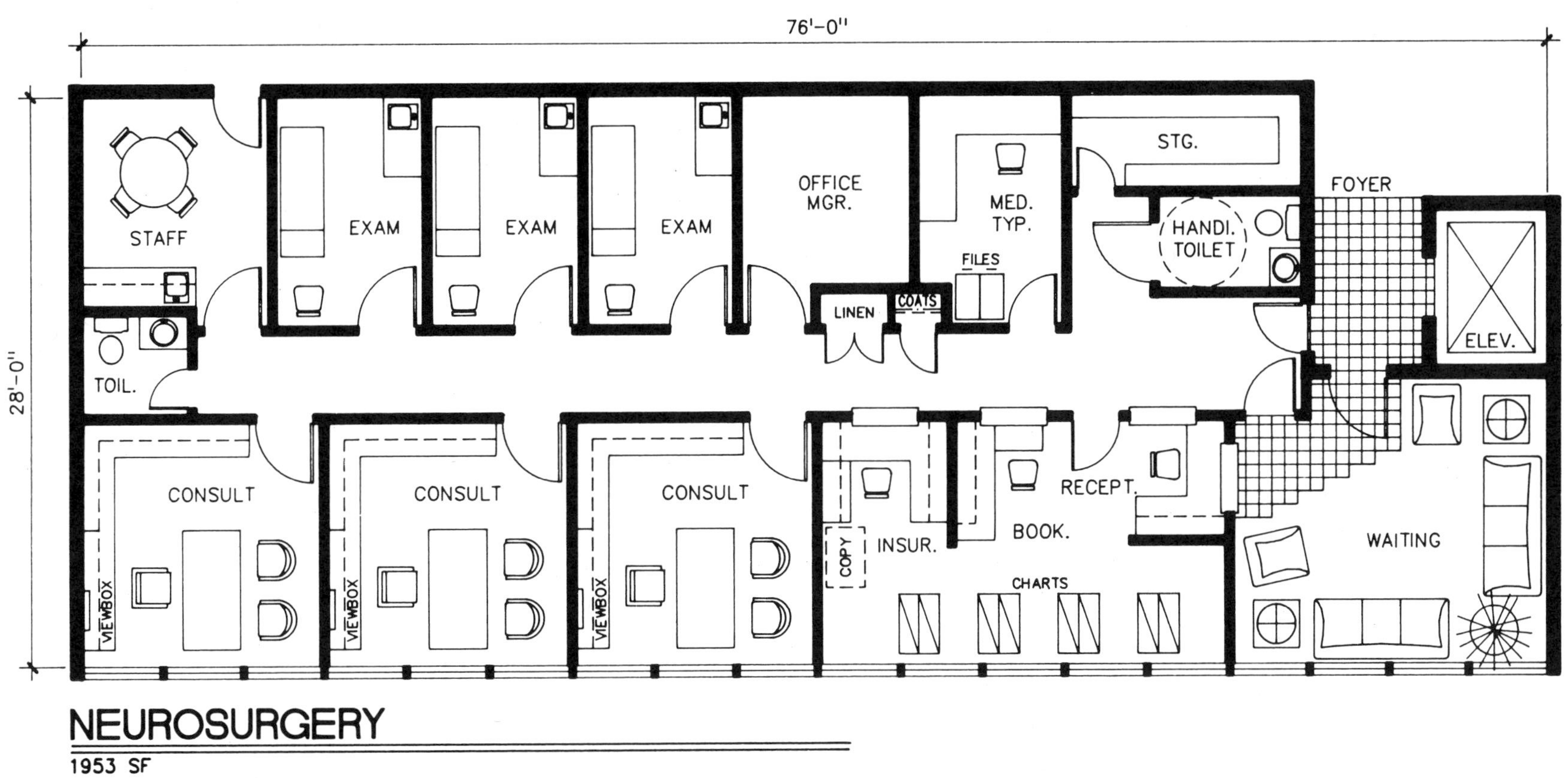

Figure 4-84. Suite plan for neurosurgery, 1953 square feet.

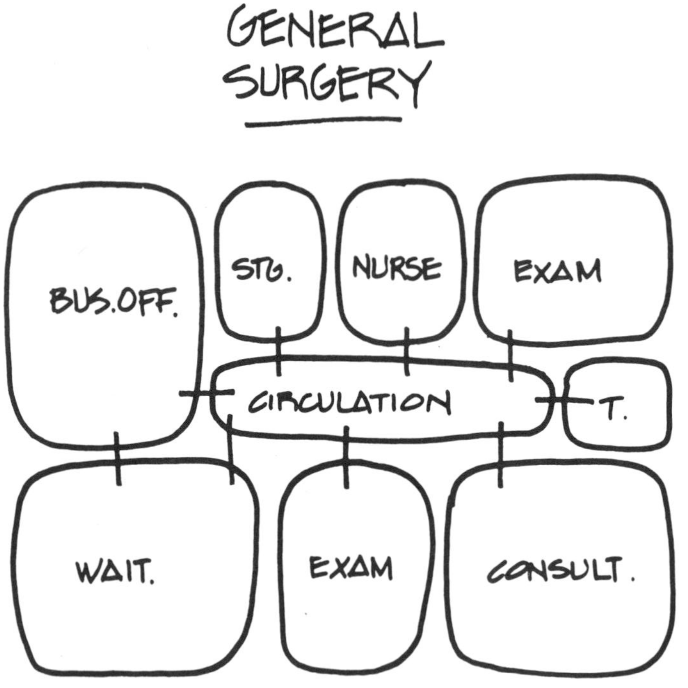

Figure 4-85. Schematic diagram of a general surgery suite.

A surgeon's office will usually contain two standard-sized exam rooms, a large consultation room (12 × 12 or 12 × 14 feet), small business office, a waiting room, and a restroom. (If one exam room is larger — 10 × 12 feet — it can be used for minor surgery.) A small nurse station, a niche in the corridor, will suffice for the sterilization of instruments and storage of dressings and supplies (Figure 4-86). An under-counter refrigerator should be built into the cabinet.

The waiting room need not accommodate more than six chairs, since patients are well scheduled and usually do not have to wait a long time. Surgeons usually perform surgery in the morning and see patients in the office during the afternoon. The consultation room is larger than for many medical specialties because it is used for consulting with patients. A double-panel X-ray view box should be located near the desk.

In a one-physician practice, one employee can usually run the business office — answering the phone, booking appointments, handling insurance, and billing patients. A three- or four-physician practice will have an expanded business office with two or more staff per-

Table 4-9. Analysis of Program. General Surgery

No. of Physicians:	1	2	3
Exam Rooms	2 @ 8 × 12 = 96	3 @ 8 × 12 = 288	5 @ 8 × 12 = 480
Waiting Room	12 × 12 = 144	14 × 14 = 196	14 × 18 = 252
Business Office	12 × 12 = 144	12 × 14 = 168	14 × 18 = 252
Nurse Station	4 × 6 = 24	4 × 6 = 24	6 × 8 = 48
Consultation Rooms	12 × 12 = 144	2 @ 12 × 12 = 288	3 @ 12 × 12 = 432
Toilets	5 × 6 = 30	2 @ 5 × 6 = 60	2 @ 5 × 6 = 60
Storage	4 × 6 = 24	4 × 6 = 24	6 × 8 = 48
Staff Lounge	—	—	10 × 10 = 100
Subtotal	702 ft²	1048 ft²	1672 ft²
15% Circulation	105	157	251
Total	807 ft²	1205 ft²	1923 ft²

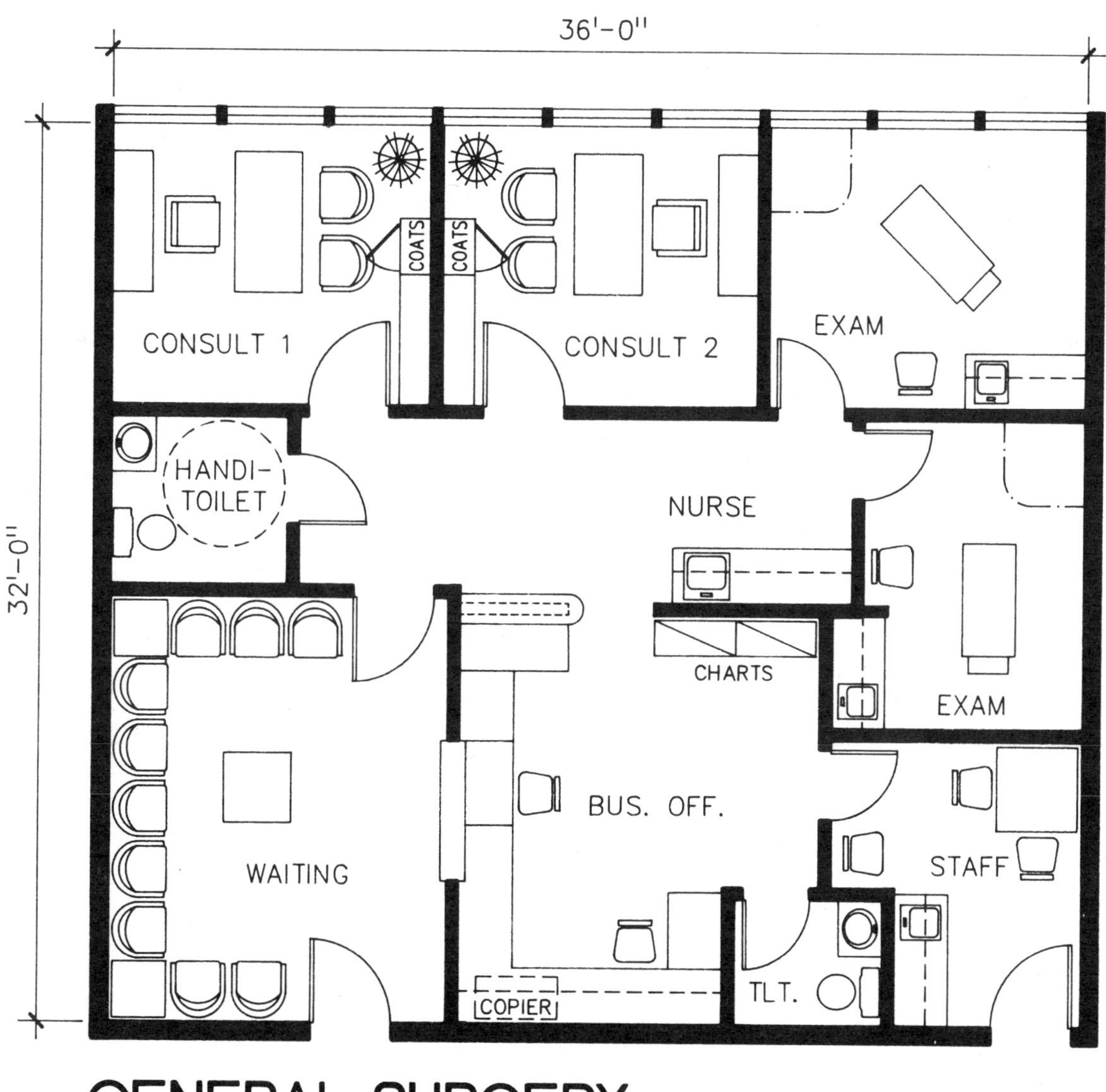

Figure 4-86. Suite plan for general surgery, 1152 square feet.

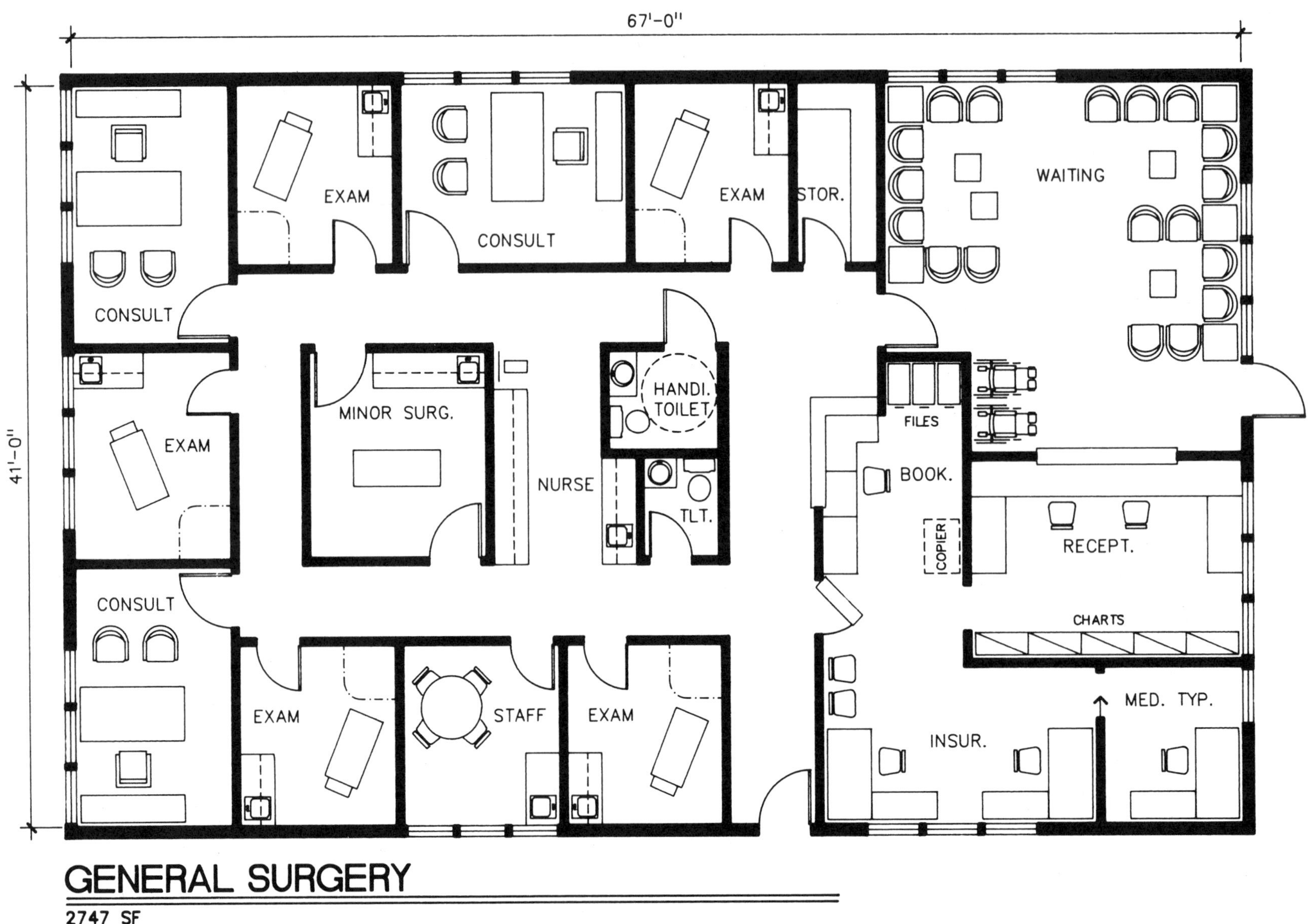

Figure 4-87. Suite plan for general surgery, 2747 square feet.

forming the tasks of reception, bookkeeping, and insurance (Figure 4-87).

All rooms of this suite may be carpeted. The decor should be cheerful with warm colors but, above all, it must convey a solid, conservative image due to the nature of the specialty. A patient wants to think of a surgeon as a serious person not subject to frivolities and trendy decor.

UROLOGY

A urologist treats diseases of the genitourinary tract. Thus each patient must submit a urine specimen before being examined. The toilet room should be located close to the laboratory and have a specimen pass-through to the laboratory. Sometimes a toilet room is located between two exam rooms. Urologists perform most of their own lab work in the suite, and a minimum of 12 lineal feet of countertop should be provided in the laboratory. In addition, a solo practitioner would need two examination rooms, a cystoscopy (cysto) room, a business office, a waiting room, and a consultation room.

Patient flow is from the waiting room to the bathroom to the exam room, and then to the cysto room if necessary. The components of this suite are standard, with the exception of the cysto room. A patient with a inflammation of the urinary bladder would be diagnosed by a cystoscopic procedure to determine the presence of an obstruction or an infection in the urinary tract. The cysto room is often designed as an X-ray room with darkroom, control area, and lead-shielded walls (Figure 4-90). (If the urologist does retrograde cystoscopic examinations, he or she will need a room equipped for radiography.) The reader is referred to Chapter 3, General Practice, for design of an X-ray room.

The cysto room may have a ceramic tile floor pitched to a floor drain. If the budget does not permit a ceramic tile floor, a good-quality sheet vinyl flooring with a self-coved base is recommended, pitched to a floor drain. A cysto room not equipped with X-ray may be as small as 11 × 12 or 12 × 12 feet. With X-ray, it will be about 12 × 18 feet including the darkroom, and the room should have a 9-foot ceiling height. Open-shelf filing of X-ray films should be located in the corridor adjacent to the cysto rooms. Cysto rooms often have a 5-foot-high ceramic tile wainscot on all walls and may have a wall-mounted urinal. Furthermore, the room should have an exhaust fan. The examination table used in this room is pictured in Figure 4-91.

It should be noted that some urologists, in deference to their budgets, use a bucket for waste disposal instead of a floor drain and vinyl asbestos tile instead of ceramic tile or sheet vinyl on the floor. Many do not provide a private dressing or recovery area in the cysto room.

Interior Design

There are no special requirements in this specialty in terms of interior design. However, there are some urologists who have built a large practice in a subspecialty, male sexual dysfunction. If this is the case, one may want to design the suite in a more masculine style, perhaps using artwork with a western theme, or a sports or hunting theme.

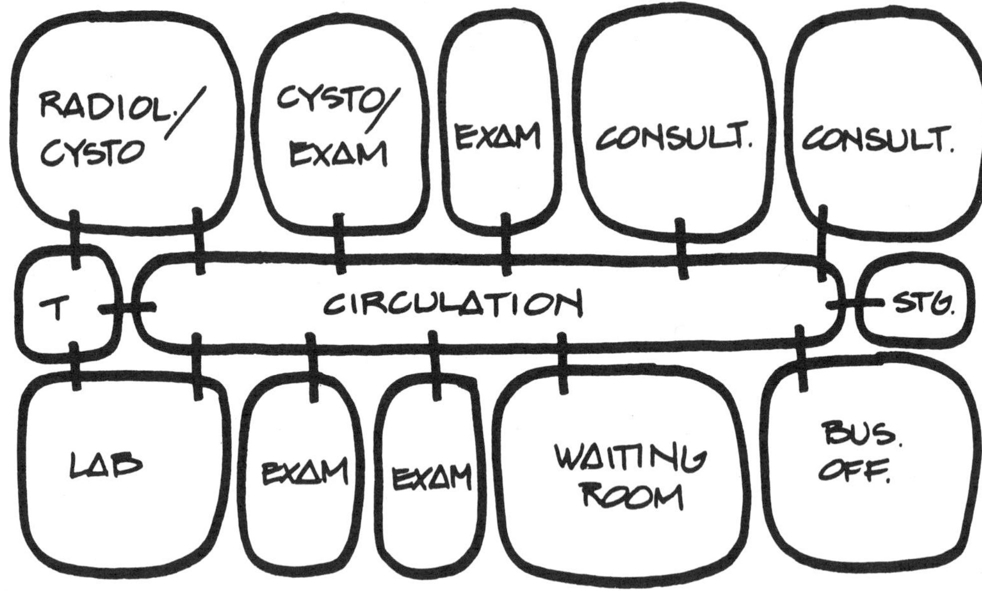

Figure 4-88. Schematic diagram of a urology suite.

Table 4-10. Analysis of Program. Urology

No. of Physicians:	1		2		3	
Business Office	12 × 14 =	168	16 × 18 =	288	16 × 20 =	320
Waiting Room	12 × 16 =	192	12 × 18 =	216	14 × 20 =	280
Toilets	2 @ 5 × 6 =	60	3 @ 5 × 6 =	90	3 @ 5 × 6 =	90
Storage	6 × 8 =	48	6 × 8 =	48	8 × 8 =	64
Consultation Room	12 × 12 =	144	2 @ 12 × 12 =	288	3 @ 12 × 12 =	432
Exam Rooms	2 @ 8 × 12 =	192	4 @ 8 × 12 =	384	6 @ 8 × 12 =	576
Cysto/Exam (no X-ray)	—		12 × 11 =	132	2 @ 12 × 11 =	264
Cysto (with X-ray)[a]	12 × 18 =	216	12 × 18 =	216	12 × 18 =	216
Laboratory	10 × 10 =	100	10 × 10 =	100	10 × 16 =	160
Subtotal		1120 ft²		1762 ft²		2402 ft²
15% Circulation		168		264		360
Total		1288 ft²		2026 ft²		2762 ft²

[a]Includes darkroom, control, film filing and dressing cubicle.

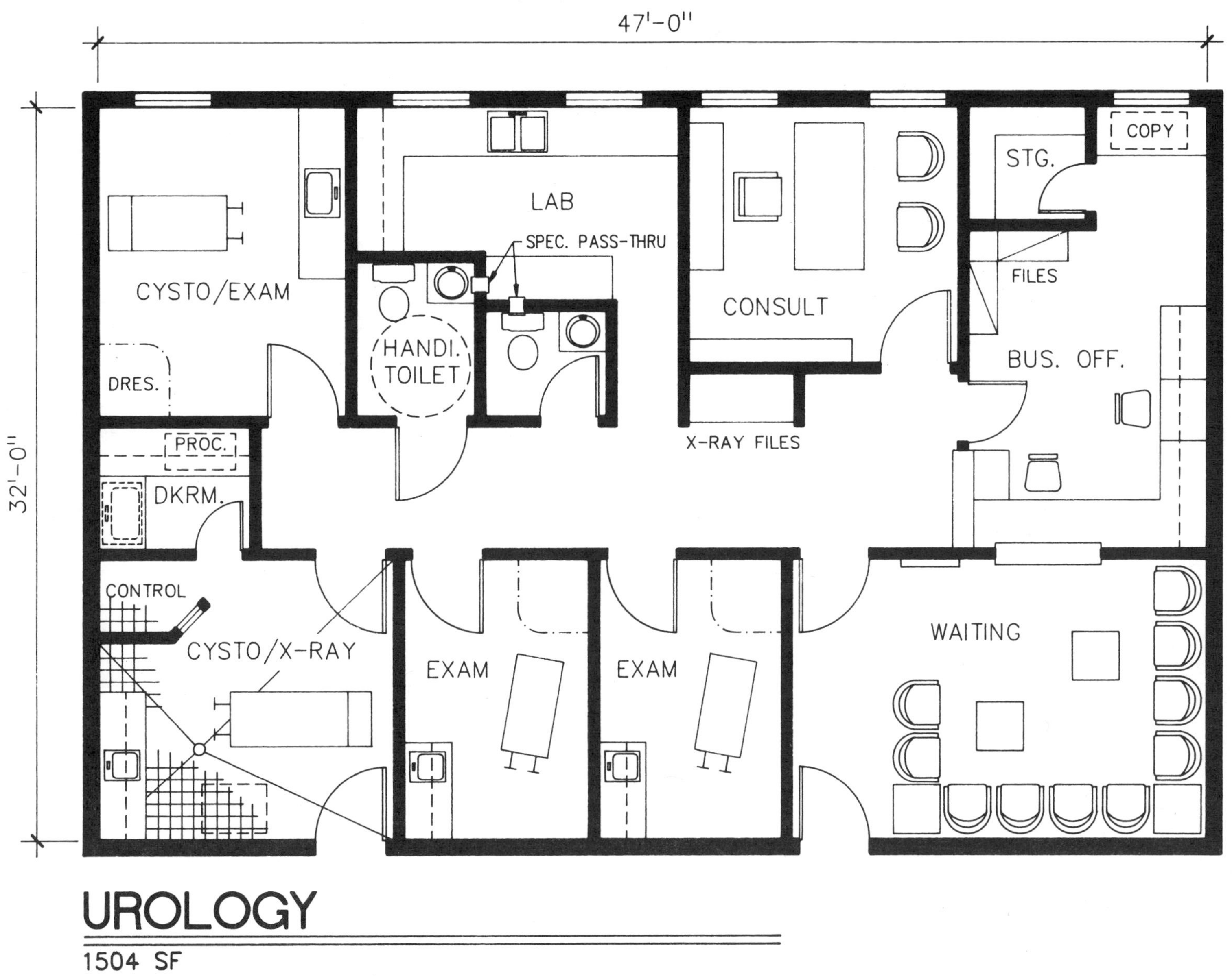

Figure 4-89. Suite plan for urology, 1504 square feet.

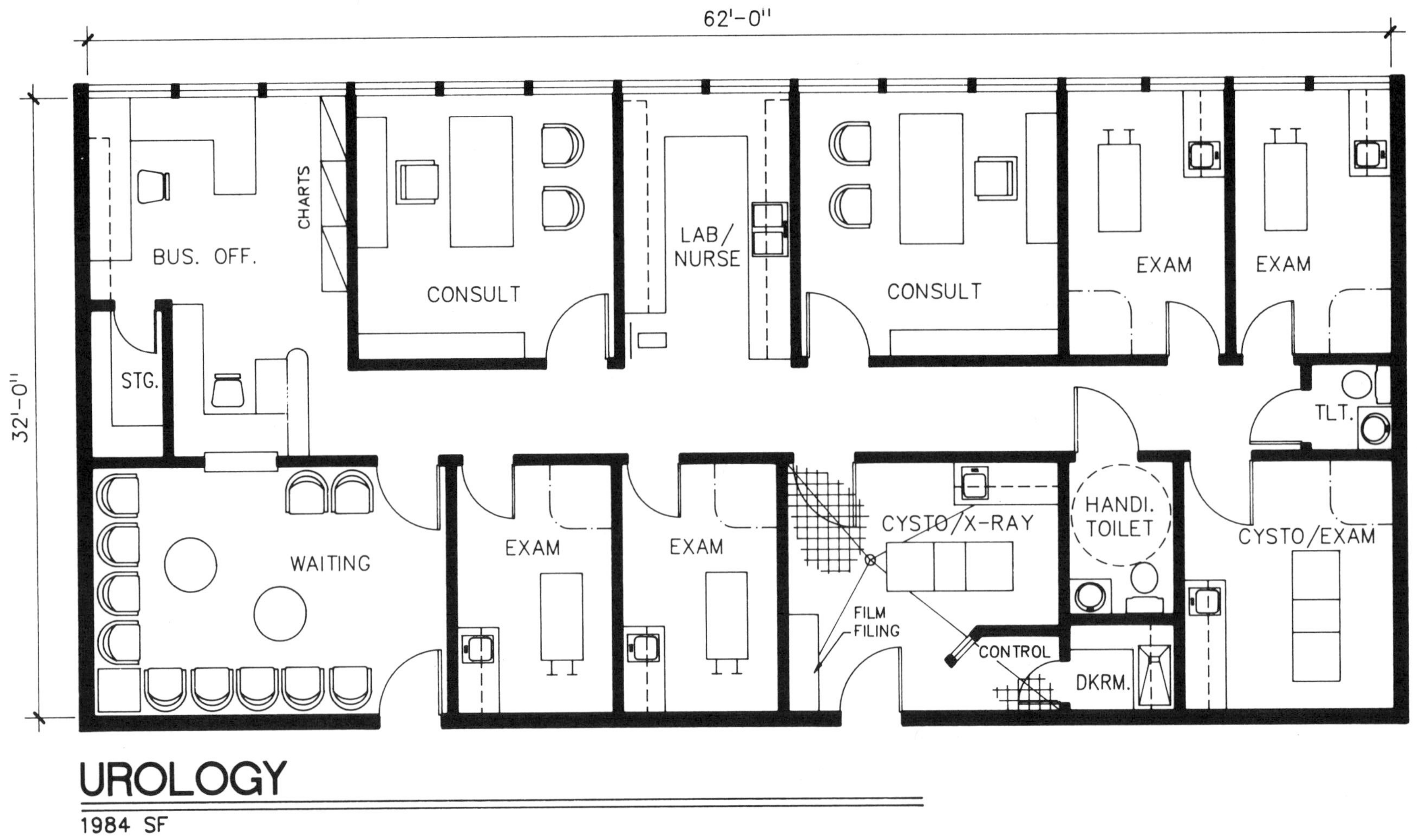

Figure 4-90. Suite plan for urology, 1984 square feet.

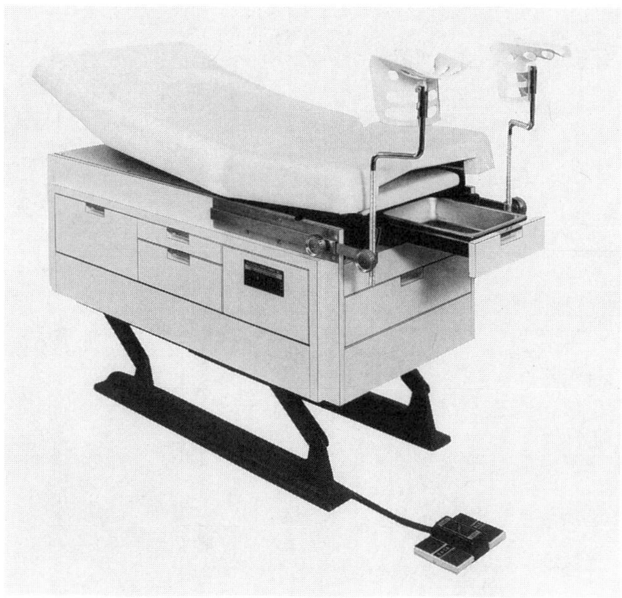

Figure 4-91. Cystoscopy table. (*Courtesy Hamilton Industries, Two Rivers, WI.*)

ORTHOPEDIC SURGERY

An orthopedic surgeon deals with diseases, fractures, or malformations of the bones, as well as arthritis, birth defects, industrial accidents, and sports injuries that affect the bones and joints. Some orthopedic surgeons specialize in hand surgery. With a tendency to group in large practices, it is not uncommon to find six or seven physicians working in the same office (Figure 4-93). Schedules may be arranged so that each doctor performs surgery two days a week, is off one day, and in the office the balance. Therefore all the surgeons are seldom in the office at once.

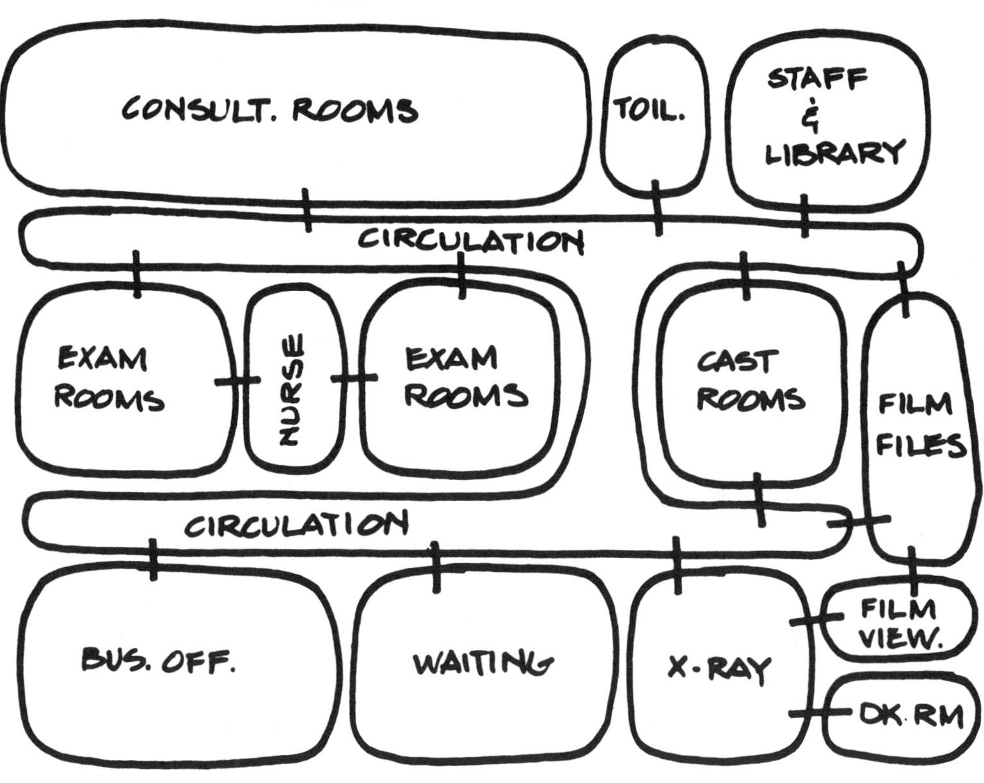

Figure 4-92. Schematic diagram of an orthopedic surgery suite.

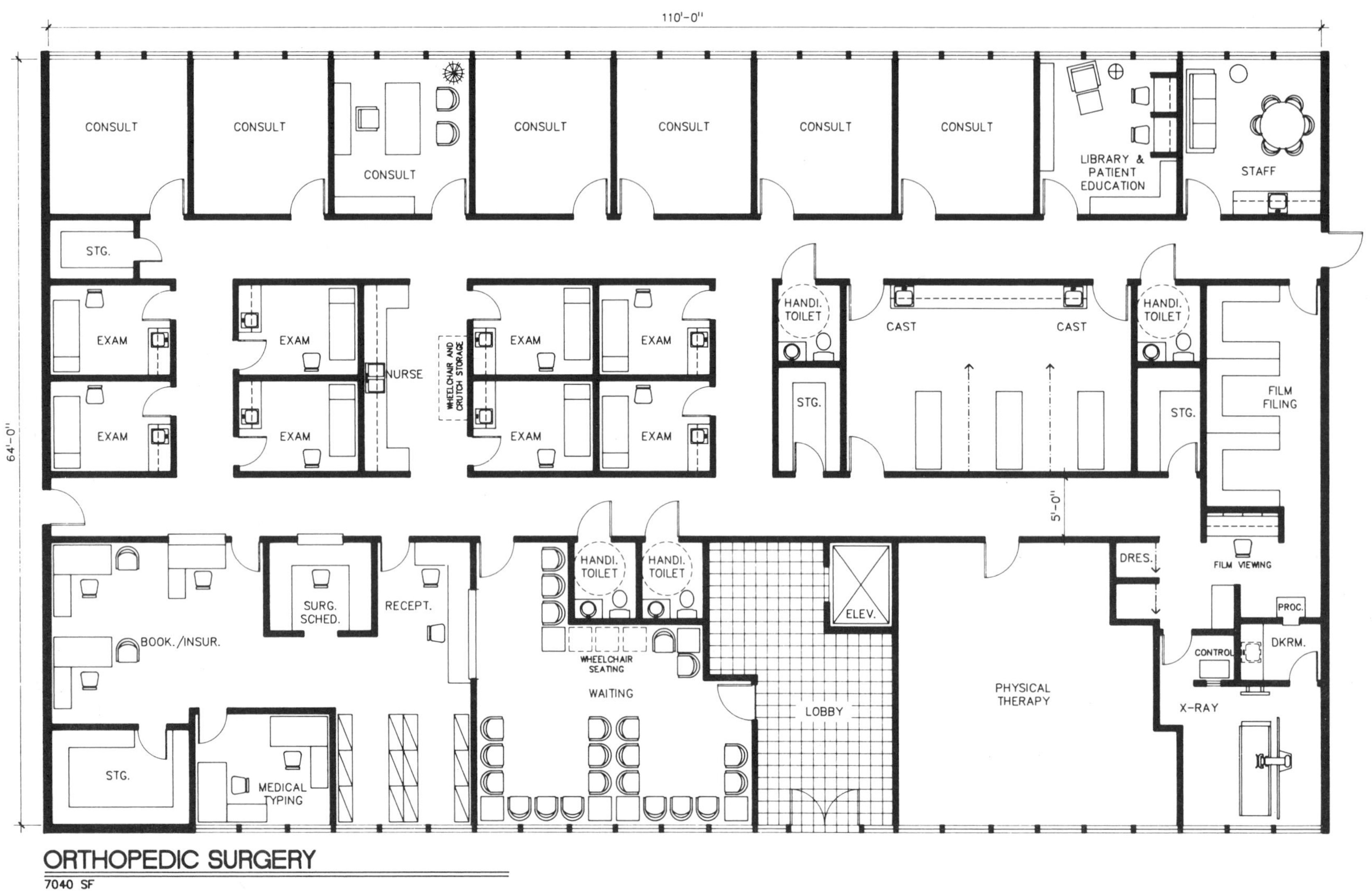

Figure 4-93. Suite plan for orthopedic surgery, 7040 square feet.

Required Rooms

A two-physician practice would typically have four exam rooms, one cast room, a small nurse station, two consultation rooms, a large business office, large waiting room, radiology room and darkroom, toilet room, and large storage and film filing room (Figure 4-94). A larger practice might also have a physical therapy room and a staff lounge, additional cast rooms and exam rooms, and a sit-down film viewing area adjacent to the radiology room (Figure 4-93).

Examination Rooms

Exam rooms may be as small as 8 × 10 feet (if a dressing area is not desired) since an orthopedist uses a 24- to 27-inch-wide by 78-inch-long table (usually custom built), which is frequently placed against the wall, and he or she usually examines the patient from one side only (Figure 4-96). Some orthopedists prefer to place the head of the table perpendicular to the wall so that they can walk around three sides of it (Figure 4-97), in which case the room needs to be 9-feet wide.

The table will frequently have pull-out leaves for examination of limbs, and the lower portion of the table may be closed in for bulk storage. Sometimes a row of drawers is provided alongside the bulk storage portion of the cabinet.

Table 4-11. Analysis of Program. Orthopedic Surgery

No. of Physicians:	2	4	6
Consultation Rooms	2 @ 12 × 12 = 288	4 @ 12 × 12 = 576	6 @ 12 × 12 = 864
Exam Rooms	4 @ 8 × 12 = 384	8 @ 8 × 12 = 768	8 @ 8 × 12 = 768[a]
Cast Rooms	12 × 12 = 144	2 @ 12 × 12 = 288	2 @ 12 × 12 = 288
Business Office	14 × 16 = 224	20 × 20 = 400	20 × 26 = 520
Office Manager	—	10 × 10 = 100	10 × 10 = 100
Toilets[b]	2 @ 5 × 6 = 60	2 @ 5 × 6 = 60	3 @ 5 × 6 = 90
Staff Lounge	8 × 10 = 80	10 × 12 = 120	14 × 16 = 224
Waiting Room	16 × 20 = 320	24 × 30 = 720	24 × 30 = 720
Physical Therapy	—	16 × 20 = 320	20 × 25 = 500
Nurse Station	(Located in corridor circulation area)		
Radiology	10 × 12 = 120	10 × 12 = 120	10 × 12 = 120
Darkroom	4 × 6 = 24	4 × 6 = 24	4 × 6 = 24
Storage and Film Filing	10 × 12 = 120	10 × 12 = 120	12 × 16 = 192
Film Viewing	4 × 6 = 24	4 × 6 = 24	4 × 6 = 24
Subtotal	1788 ft^2	3640 ft^2	4434 ft^2
20% Circulation	358	728	886
Total	2146 ft^2	4368 ft^2	5320 ft^2

[a]In a six-person practice, it is unlikely that more than three or four surgeons would be in the office at the same time.

[b]One toilet room should be equipped for the handicapped.

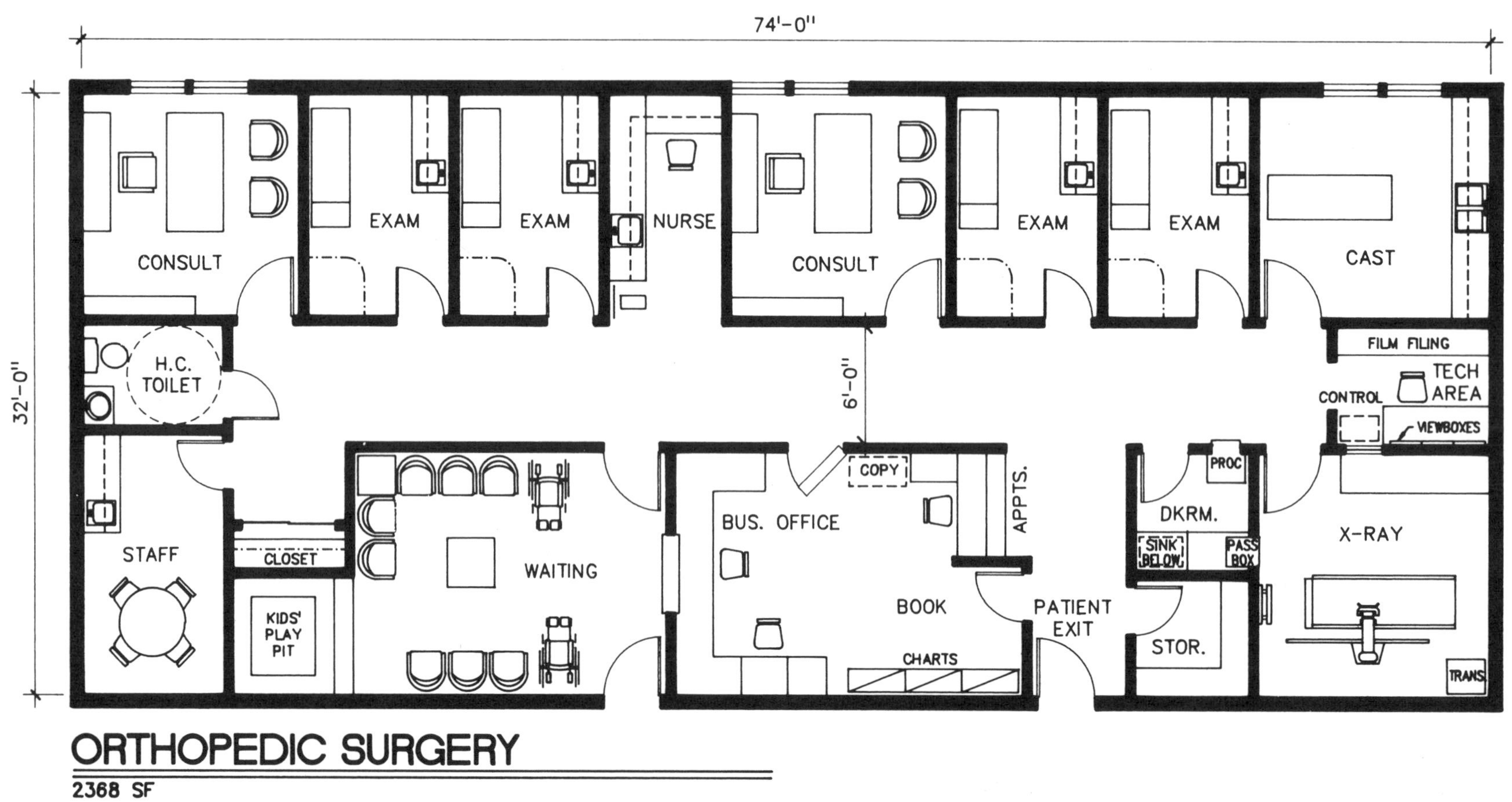

Figure 4-94. Suite plan for orthopedic surgery, 2368 square feet.

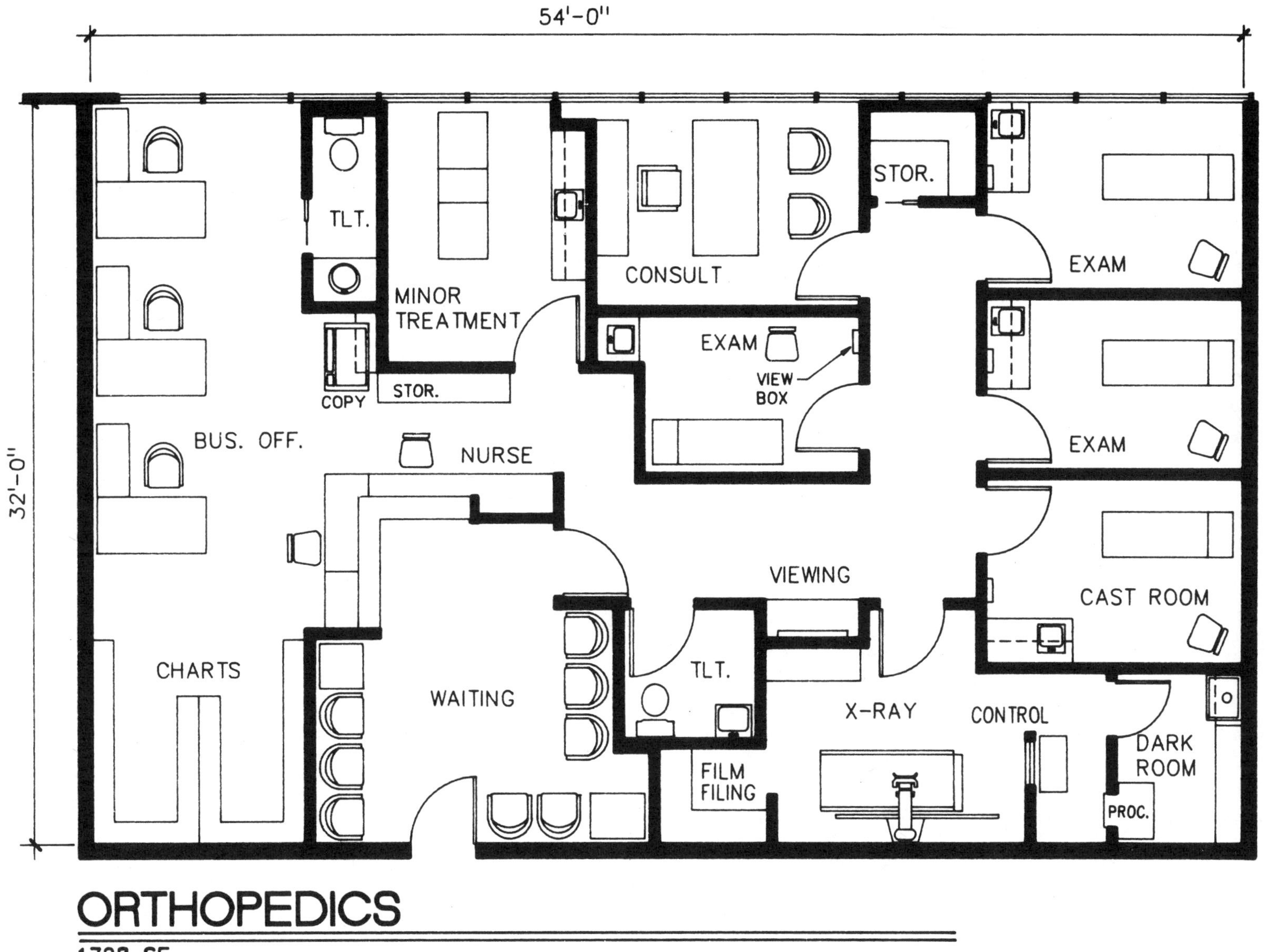

Figure 4-95. Suite plan for orthopedic surgery, 1728 square feet.

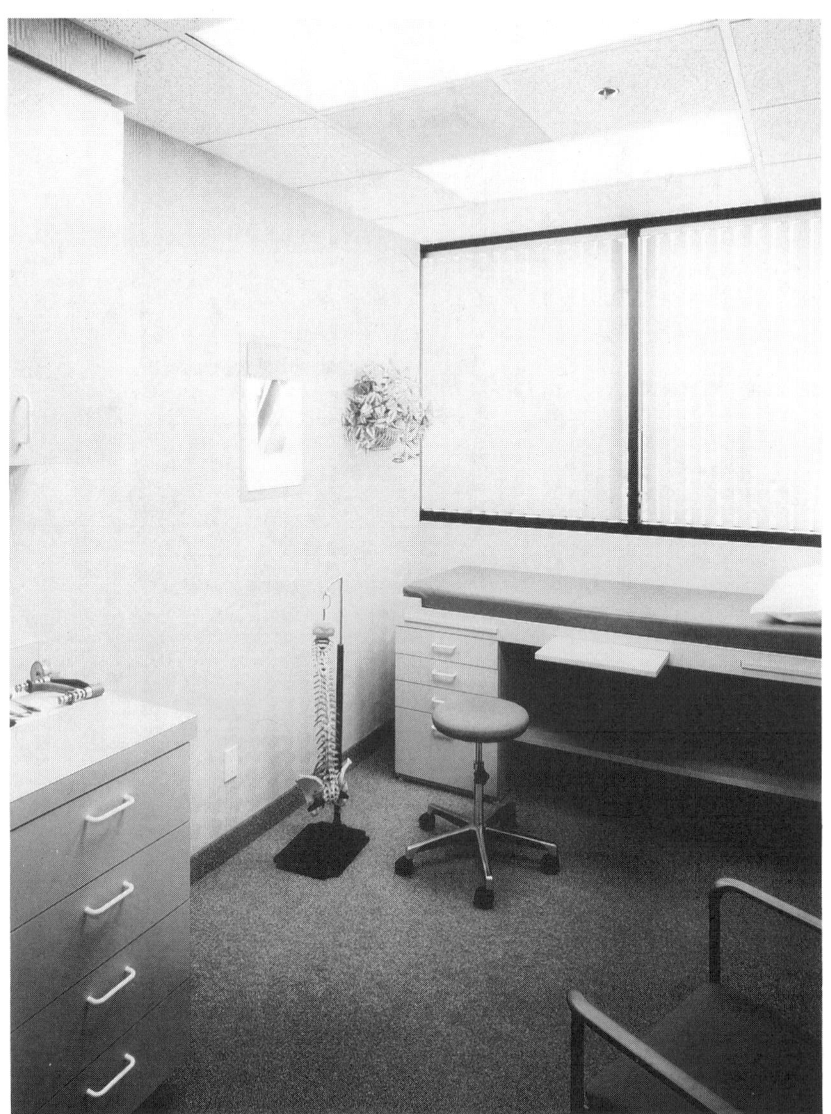

Figure 4-96. Examination room, orthopedic surgery. (*Design: Jain Malkin Inc.; Photographer: John Christian.*)

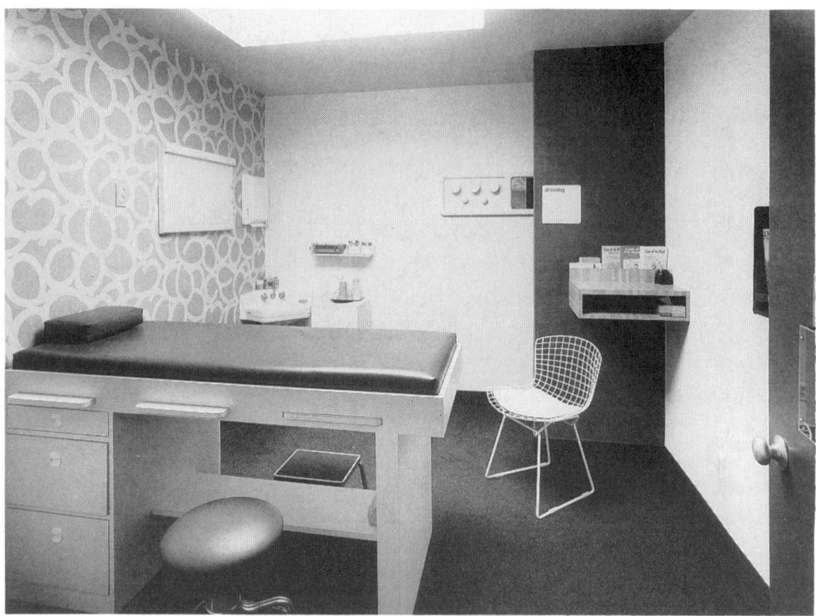

Figure 4-97. Examination room, orthopedic surgery. (*Design: Jain Malkin Inc.; Photographer: Michael Denny.*)

Hand Surgeon

A hand surgeon works at a T-shaped desk (Figures 4-98a and 4-98b). The patient is seated on one side of the stem of the "T" and the surgeon on the other. Drawers and a flip-top countertop hold instruments and tools. This room may be as small as 8 × 8 feet.

A hand surgeon would also require a treatment room or cast room (Figure 4-99) for dressing wounds, removing stitches, and building casts. Each exam room and cast room must have a double-panel X-ray film illuminator (Figure 4-100) recessed in the wall or surface mounted, at a stand-up height (see Appendix).

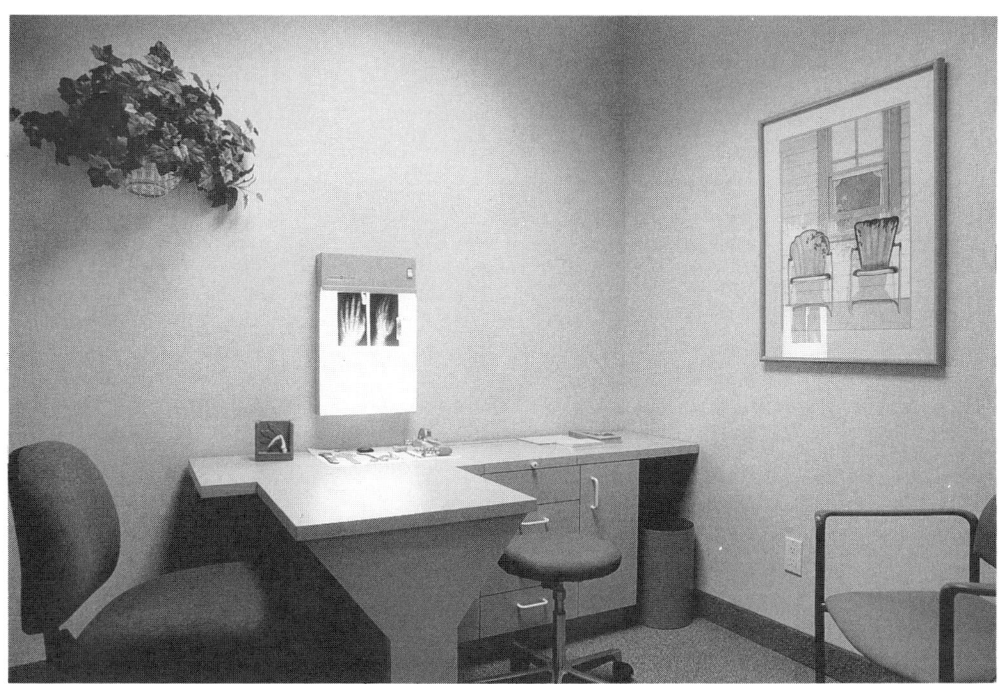

Figure 4-98a. Hand room, orthopedic surgery. (*Design: Jain Malkin Inc.; Photographer: John Christian.*)

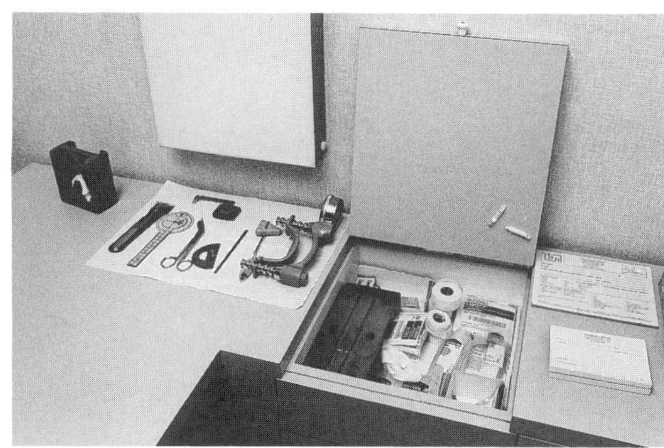

Figure 4-98b. Hand room, detail of cabinet.

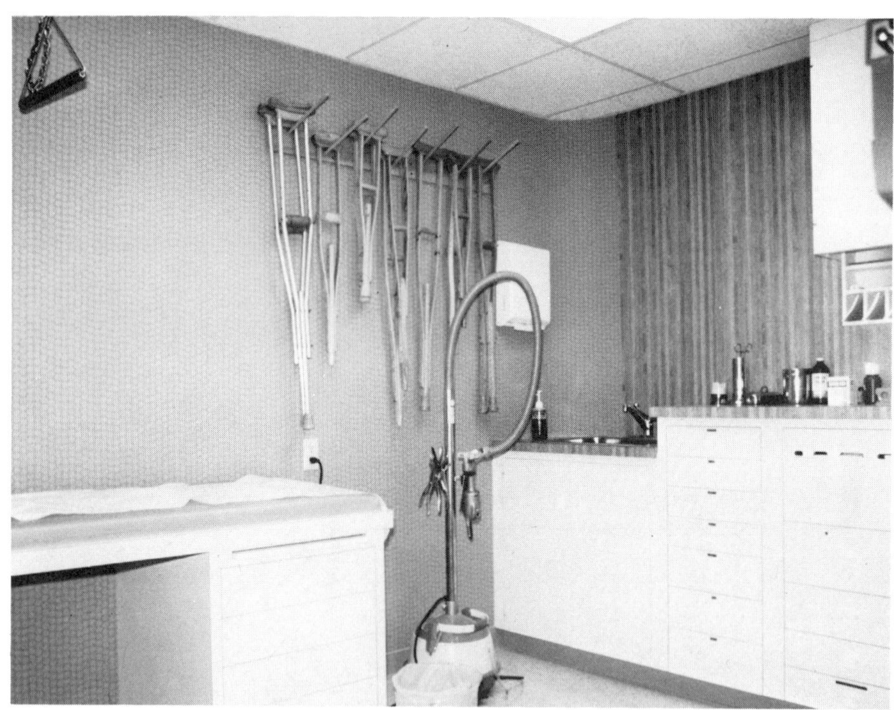

Figure 4-99. Cast room. (*Design: Jain Malkin Inc.*)

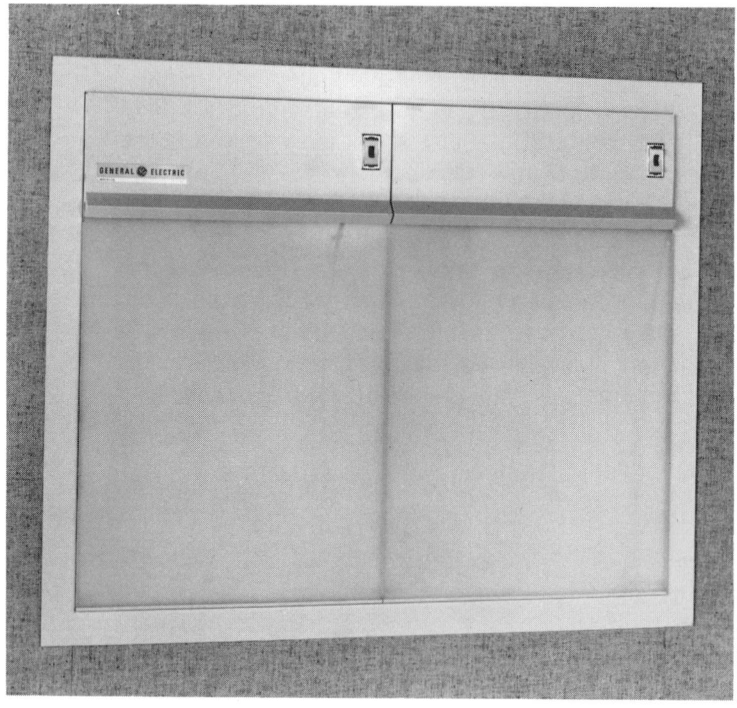

Figure 4-100. Double-panel view box. (*Courtesy GE Medical Systems, Milwaukee, WI.*)

Cast Room

The cast room will have one full wall of cabinets designed precisely to accommodate the numerous splints, bandages, plaster, and required tools (Figure 4-101). The design of a cast cabinet is extremely important to the efficiency of the room. Plaster comes in rolls in widths of 2, 3, 4, and 6 inches. Slots in the face of the cabinet allow the rolls to feed through easily, when pulled. Stockinette may be fed through other slots. Drawers hold padding; open bins hold elastic bandages; and a drawer contains cast tools. Each orthopedist seems to have a preferred arrangement of drawers, slots, and bins on the cast room cabinet, but all cast cabinets are composed, in one arrangement or another, of the above components.

A large hinged trash bin should be built into the cabinet, if space permits. If possible, this bin ought to be vented to the outside, since cast cutoffs have a foul odor. If this is not possible, the room should have an exhaust fan. The sink in the cast cabinet should have a single lever faucet, a gooseneck spout (so a bucket can be put under it), and a plaster trap.

One must bear in mind that surfaces of the cast room must be washable since the room is exposed to plaster dust when casts are sawed off, and wet drippings when new casts are built. A sheet vinyl floor and vinyl wallcovering are recommended.

Orthopedists sometimes use Fiberglas casts. This requires no special accommodation in the cast room as the Fiberglas comes in rolls, like the plaster. The rolls come sealed in foil packets in varying widths. The same type of padding is used for both plaster or Fiberglas casts.

Minor Surgery

Some orthopedists use a minor surgery room for procedures such as removing foreign bodies, installing pins, repairing tendons, removing cysts, or removing toenails, for example.

Consultation Room

The consultation room will usually be used as the doctor's private office and as a place to return phone calls and to review X-ray films. For this purpose, a four-panel illuminated film viewer should be located to the side of or behind the physician at a sit-down height, usually mounted over the credenza (Figure 4-102).

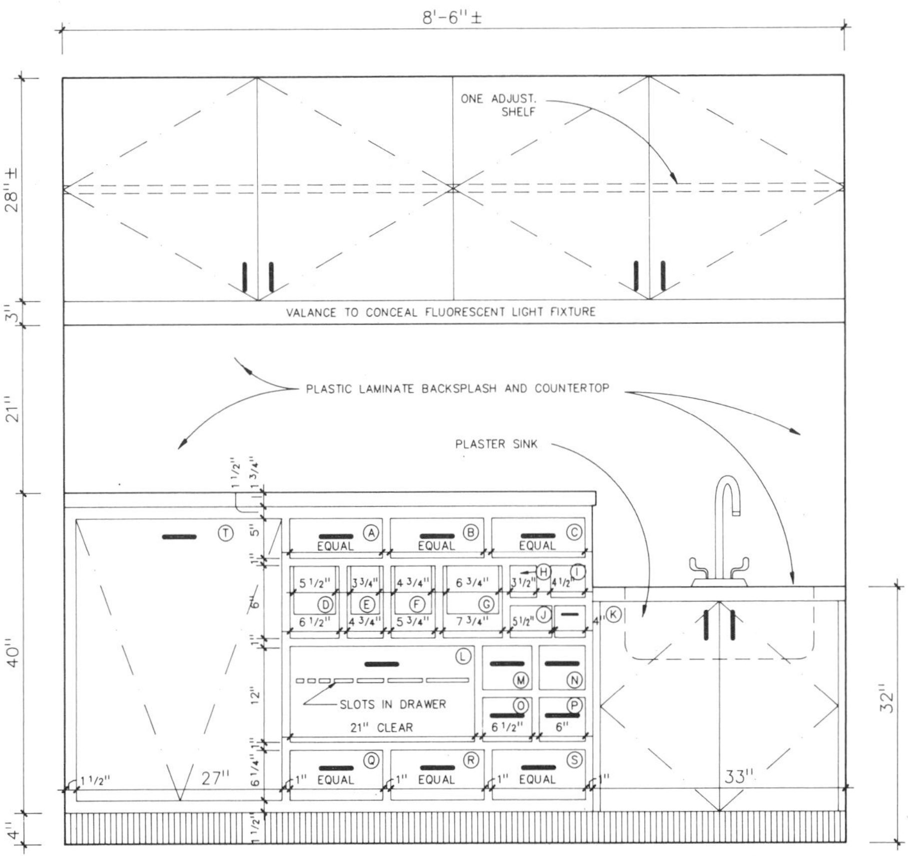

DOOR AND DRAWER SCHEDULE

Ⓐ Ⓑ Ⓒ Ⓠ Ⓡ Ⓢ	DRAWERS WITH SIDE ROLLERS, A, B & C MUST HAVE CLEAR DEPTH OF 4" INSIDE.
Ⓓ Ⓔ Ⓕ Ⓖ	NO SIDE ROLLERS. BOTTOM DRAWER GLIDE ONLY. THESE DRAWERS ARE RARELY OPENED.
Ⓗ Ⓘ Ⓙ	OPEN SHELVES FOR SPINTS (CUBBY HOLES).
Ⓚ	DRAWER FOR 4" BIAS. DRAWER GLIDE ON BOTTOM.
Ⓛ	STOCKINETTE DRAWER. SLOT OPENINGS MUST BE SANDED VERY SMOOTHLY. (NO SNAGS).
Ⓜ Ⓝ Ⓞ Ⓟ	DRAWERS FOR PADDING.
Ⓣ	TILT-OUT TRASH BIN. (HOLDS LARGE PLASTIC TRASH CAN).

CAST CABINET

Figure 4-101. Cast cabinet.

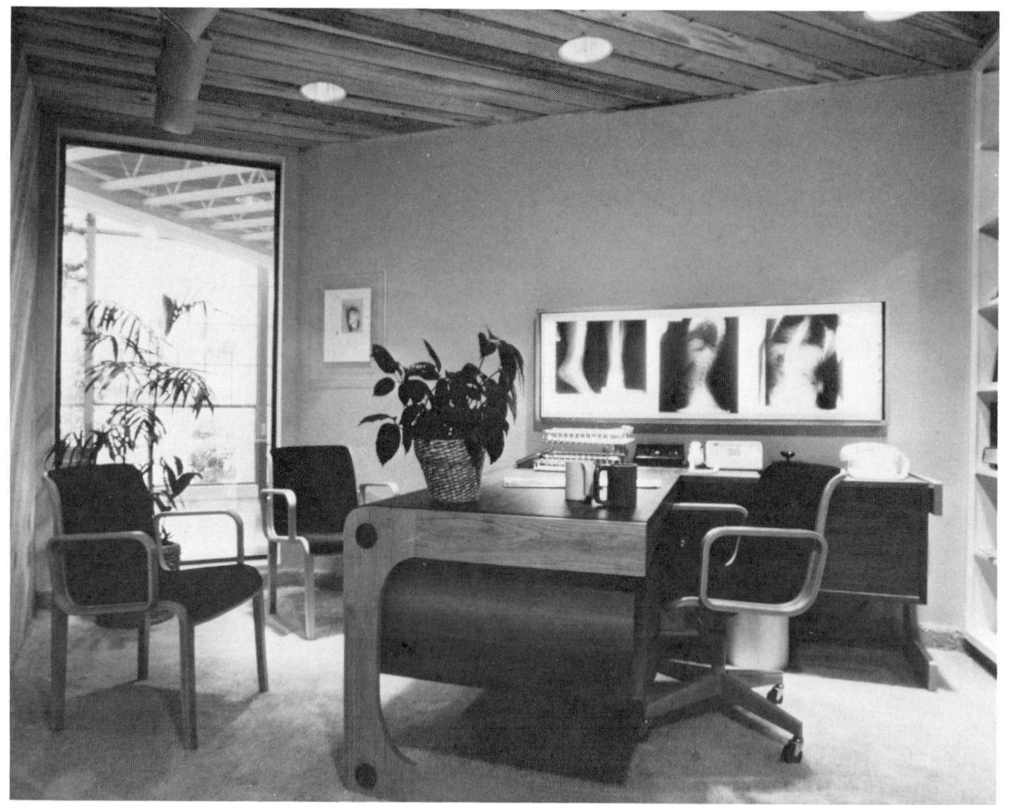

Figure 4-102. Consultation room, orthopedic surgery. (*Design: Jain Malkin Inc.; Photographer: Michael Denny.*)

Adjacency of Rooms

Cast room(s), radiology, and the film viewing area should be located in proximity to each other (Figure 4-103). There should be a tech work area near the cast room and radiology room (Figure 4-104 and see Figure 5-8). It would have a 6-foot-long countertop, and X-ray view boxes and be close to the darkroom and film processor. Sometimes the X-ray tech assists the physician in the cast room.

Radiology Area

The reader is directed to Chapter 3, General Practice, for design of an X-ray room, control area, and darkroom. Open shelves (or lateral file cabinets) must be provided for film filing. Shelves should have vertical dividers every 18 inches, since films are heavy and unwieldy and tend to slump over if not packed tightly between divider supports. X-ray jackets (the paper storage envelope) are 14½ × 17½ inches, and shelves should be shallow enough so that about 2 inches of the film jacket hang over the edge of the shelf for ease of access.

One must be sure that the door to the X-ray room is large enough to move in the equipment. The ceiling height of this room must be at least 9-feet high.

Other Considerations

Corridors of the suite should be 5- to 6-feet wide for easy passage of patients on crutches and in wheelchairs. The corridor is also used as a gait lane. Sometimes a patient education room is included (Figure 4-105). Surgeons find it time-saving to purchase videotapes explaining certain frequently performed

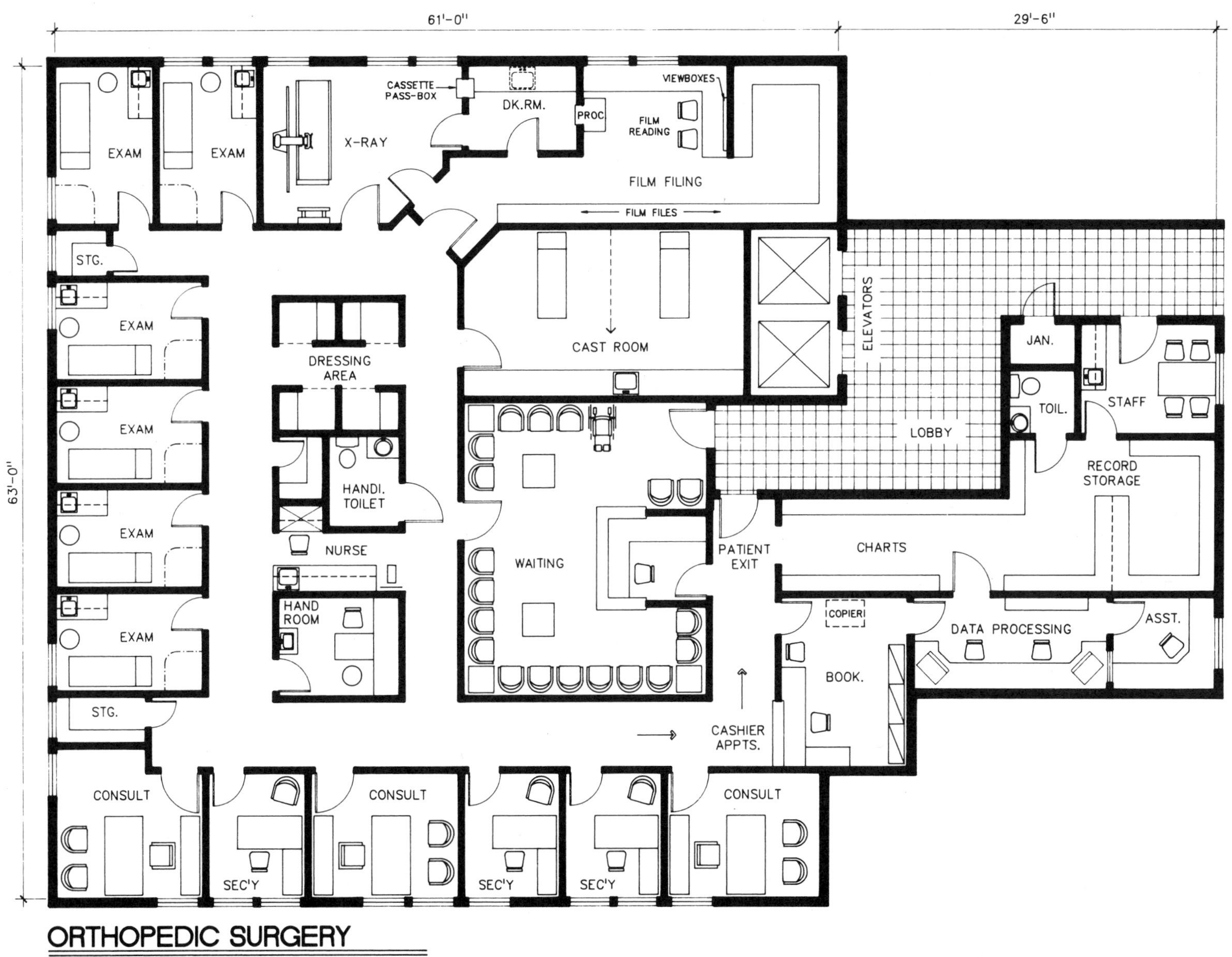

Figure 4-103. Suite plan for orthopedic surgery, 4464 square feet.

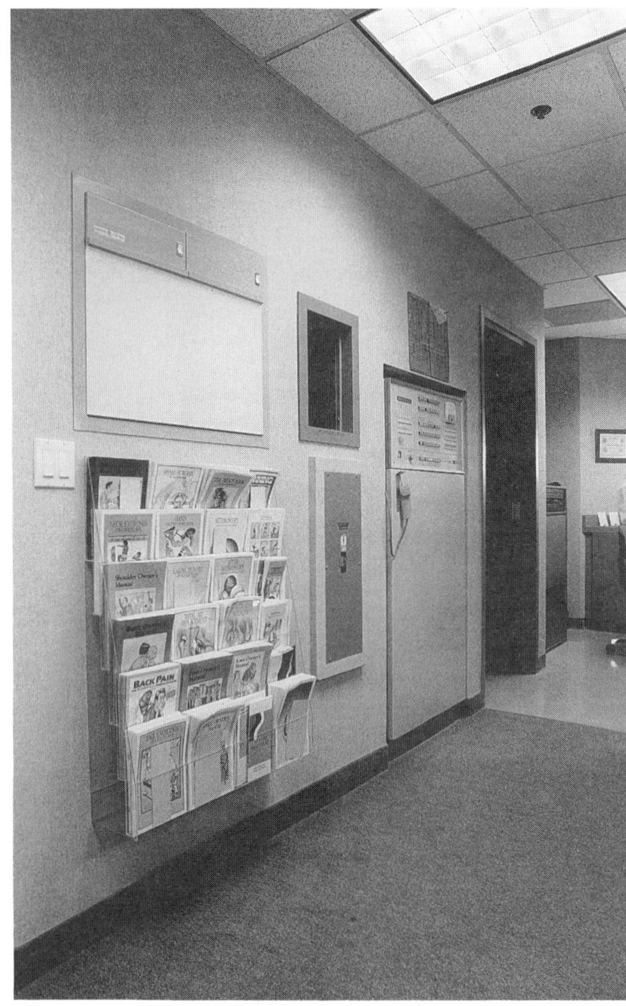

Figure 4-104. Tech work area. Control (generator) for X-ray unit is outside room. Leaded glass window provides view into X-ray room. Emergency electrical shut-off panel located here. Automatic processor and tech viewing area can be seen in rear. (*Design: Jain Malkin Inc.; Photographer: John Christian.*)

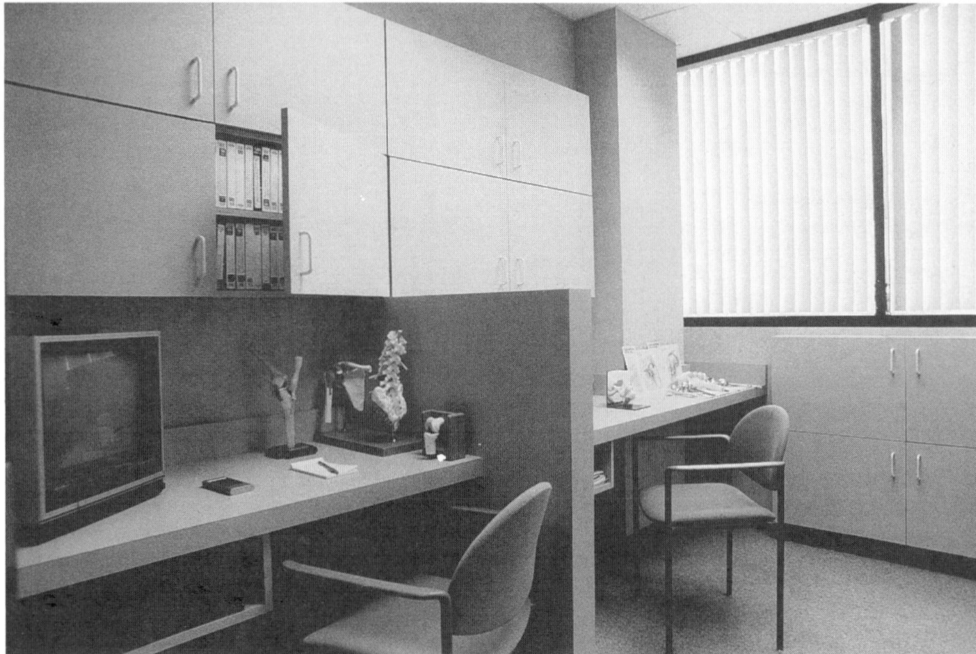

Figure 4-105. Patient education room, orthopedic surgery. (*Design: Jain Malkin Inc.; Photographer: John Christian.*)

procedures to patients (inserting a pin in the hip, arthroscopy, etc.).

Toilet rooms in this suite must accommodate the handicapped (see Appendix) and doors must be 3-feet wide on all rooms.

Interior Design

The interior design of the suite must please patients of all ages. Artwork might include sports photos or perhaps educational exhibits dealing with prevention of sports injuries or other orthopedic topics. All floors except cast rooms and the X-ray room can be carpeted with a level loop commercial carpet glued to the slab without pad. Any other type of installation will be unsuitable for wheelchairs and people on crutches. A firm feeling underfoot is desirable here.

The waiting room needs to be large enough to accommodate people in wheelchairs without ambulatory patients tripping over them. Chairs should be firm, with high seats, and have arms to help arthritic patients, for example, raise themselves out of the chair. Chairs should be well balanced, to avoid tipping when patients lean on them for support (see Color Plate 14, Figure 4-106). It is practical, in an orthopedic waiting room, to offer several types of seating to provide comfort for the widest number of people (Figure 4-107).

If the budget allows, walls (at least corridor walls) should be covered with commercial vinyl wallcovering, since wheelchairs and crutches can damage them.

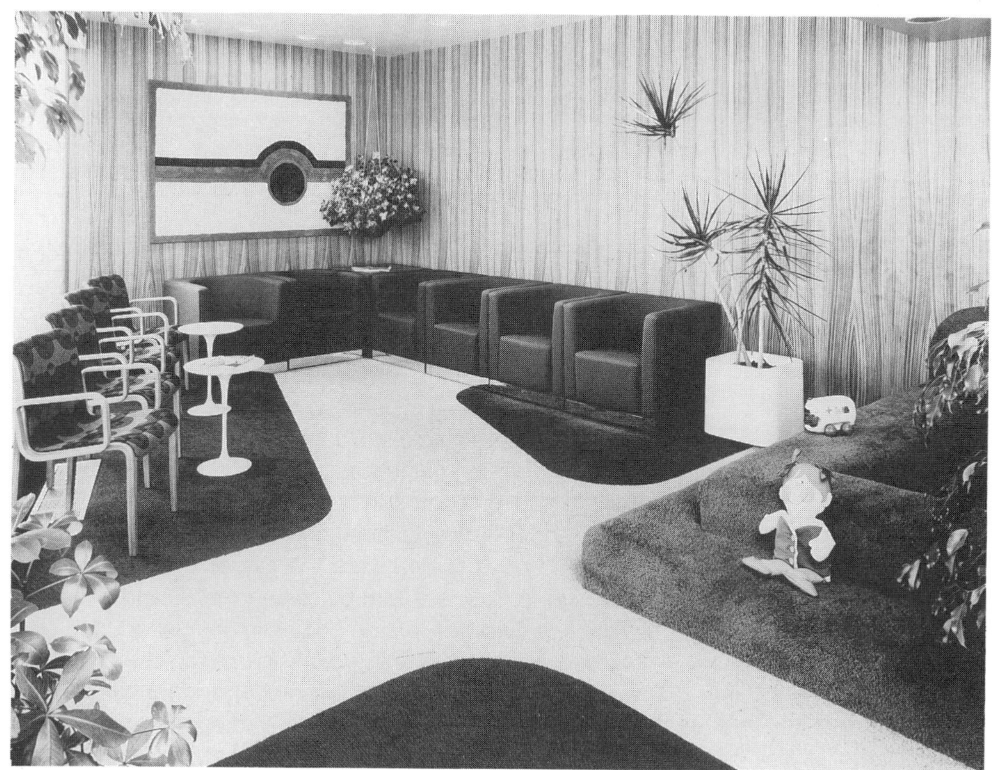

Figure 4-107. Waiting room, orthopedic surgery. (*Design: Jain Malkin Inc.; Photographer: Michael Denny.*)

CHAPTER 5

Diagnostic Medicine

RADIOLOGY

General principles of radiology are commonly understood. A limb is exposed to X-rays, which penetrate body tissues, exposing film mounted on a cassette (film holder) positioned on the other side of the limb. Since body tissues absorb different amounts of radiation, bones, fat, gas, and so on, make different exposures compared with surrounding tissues, which allows the observation of internal body parts without pain and with small exposures to radiation.

In addition to examination of limbs, diagnostic imaging is used to diagnose the presence of gallstones and kidney stones, tuberculosis, arthritis, and bone tumors; to discover foreign bodies in soft tissue, and enlarged or malfunctioning glands; to scan the brain, to reduce tumors (radiation oncology); to monitor a child in the womb (ultrasound); and to diagnose dozens of other diseases. Some forms of diagnostic imaging, such as ultrasound, do not involve radiation.

Making an X-ray film of a leg or the chest requires no special preparation, but filming organs such as the gallbladder or the gastrointestinal tract requires that the patient fast before the procedure and then drink a special liquid or receive an injection that makes the organs visible to the radiologist. Since the designer must understand these procedures in order to plan an efficient suite, a brief outline of diagnostic radiology modalities follows.

Diagnostic Imaging Modalities

Fluoroscopy. Fluoroscopy enables the radiologist to watch internal body structures at work. The patient swallows or receives an injection of a contrast medium — air, barium sulfate, or organic iodine compounds — which causes the soft tissue systems of the body to be outlined. X-rays passed through the body strike the input phosphor of an image intensifier tube, and that image is intensified electronically and can be viewed on a TV monitor. (TV monitors may be ceiling or wall-mounted, or portable, on the floor.) Hard copies (X-ray films) can be made at this time. With a video camera, screen images can be converted into real time studies for future reference.

Contrast media injected into a blood vessel (angiography) travels with the blood supply to a specific organ and allows the radiologist to examine that organ. For a study of the large intestine, a patient is given a barium enema. The radiologist makes sequential spot film radiographs while the barium travels through the large intestine. To study the digestive system, a patient drinks barium and the radiologist films it traveling down the esophagus into the stomach, following it through the small intestines.

Ultrasound. Ultrasound does not involve radiation. A high-frequency sound, much like sonar, bounces off internal body structures. Ultrasound is particularly useful in examining soft pelvic tissue masses, gallbladders, or a fetus in the womb — procedures where even low doses of radiation might be dangerous.

Nuclear Medicine. Nuclear medicine deals with the diagnosis and treatment of disease with radioactive isotopes — chemicals that are unstable and break down, giving off radioactivity. The isotope may be given to the patient orally or by injection. The substance is specific to a particular gland or organ (for example, iodine travels to the thyroid gland). The amount of the isotope absorbed by the gland permits the radiologist to determine the function of the organ and to trace its outline. Nuclear scans are useful for diagnosing brain tumors and malfunctioning of the kidneys, pancreas, and thyroid.

Computed Tomography. Computed Tomography (CT) allows physicians to see cross sections of internal body structures, enabling the radiologist to discover tumors embedded in soft tissue or organs that formerly could not be seen by radiographic procedures. Thus CAT (Computed Axial Tomography) scans have eliminated much exploratory surgery and offer the patient greater safety by reducing the need for more dangerous, often painful, tests.

The patient lies on a table that slides through a rotating doughnut-like enclosure called the gantry. X-rays scan narrow cross sections of the body in a painless, noninvasive procedure. For example, 180 scans just one degree apart may be taken of an area. The numerous images are collected by a detector and reconstructed by a computer into a composite scan of the organ or tissue. CAT scanners represented a major breakthrough in diagnostic imaging technology when they were introduced in 1977.

Mammography. Low-dose mammography, an X-ray of the breast, is considered to be the most accurate and safe means of detecting breast cancer at an early, usually curable stage. The American Cancer Society claims that one out of 11 women in the United States will get breast cancer at some point in her life. Therefore, screening mammographies are recommended on a regular basis for women over the age of 40 and perhaps even earlier for those who have a family history of breast cancer.

Radiation Oncology. Through use of a linear accelerator, tumors are bombarded by very narrowly focused, high doses of radiation in an attempt to kill cancer cells. The course of treatment is carefully plotted and monitored by a radiation physicist and the radiology team. The normal course of treatment runs six weeks, during which time the patient reports three times per week.

Magnetic Resonance Imaging. Magnetic resonance imaging (MRI) has been heralded as a major innovation in diagnostic imaging. It provides exceptional soft-tissue contrast and is especially good for imaging the central nervous system and, in particular, the brain. It permits early and accurate diagnosis of a wide variety of conditions, including brain tumors, strokes, hemorrhage, and multiple sclerosis. Spinal cord compression is more effectively shown by MRI than by other imaging techniques. A pinched nerve or the effects of arthritis can be graphically demonstrated and may prevent the need for a myelogram or CT study. MRI is also effective for diagnosing knee injuries and cancers of the musculoskeletal system.

MRI does not use X-rays, but rather depends on the interaction of radio waves and small particles within the body, called protons, in the presence of a strong magnetic field generated by the MRI equipment. A simplified explanation of a very complex process follows.

Inside the body, protons absorb energy from incoming radio waves of various frequencies and, in turn, give off energy in the form of radio waves. These outgoing signals are recorded by a highly sophisticated computer and reconstructed into an image similar to that produced by CT, but generally with higher resolution, showing more detail and an enhanced view of diseased tissues.

Advantages to the patient are that no special preparations are required before the procedure; no injections of contrast media are generally required; it does not use radiation; and results are available the same day the examination takes place. Although currently MRI examinations are expensive and take longer than a similar CT procedure, that may change as the technology advances. In 1989, statistics indicated MRI was the fastest growing radiology modality, in terms of sale volume. Future applications of MRI include *in vivo spectroscopy* and study of living tissues, providing information on processes occurring inside the cell. A single example of the derived benefit of this would be diagnosing a tumor without resorting to biopsy, based upon the fact that tumors are known to affect cell metabolism.

Planning Considerations

The purpose of this chapter is to introduce the reader to the most common diagnostic imaging modalities and to explain the general parameters of designing rooms to accommodate this equipment. Clearly, one could write an entire chapter on each of these modalities if one wanted to cover thoroughly all aspects of design and construction. The focus of this discussion is the *outpatient radiology facility* that would commonly be found in a medical office building, as opposed to one within a hospital.

Before a space planner can begin to lay out the suite, the radiologist has to provide a program detailing the number and type of diagnostic imaging rooms that will comprise the suite. There is no way a space planner can second guess this, as it depends on a number of considerations. First, if the radiology group has CT at another office not too far from this one, it may not want to duplicate this equipment. Second, the number of physician tenants in the building and their respective specialties will influence the type of equipment the radiologist buys. Third, the medical building's proximity to a hospital and the type of imaging modalities available at the hospital may influence the selection of equipment for the facility, especially if the same radiology group staffs the department at the hospital.

These are the four basic planning considerations:

1. Equipment
2. Patient Flow
3. Staff Flow
4. Function

Equipment. A number of manufacturers offer equipment for each imaging modality. Room size and critical dimensions vary considerably, as do utility requirements. There are numerous accessory or ancillary items that may be added to each major piece of equipment, thereby increasing the size of the room. The space planner, therefore, may be faced with a number of possible combinations of equipment for an individual room. The radiologist will make these selections, but the space planner must obtain from each manufacturer a planning guide and specifications for each unit. Clearly, equipment dictates the size of each room, with function and future requirements being the two important considerations.

When equipment is placed in the room, function is achieved when proper clearances are preserved for items that swivel, extend, or tilt, and for travel of the tabletop. Other aspects of function are patient access and staff ability to move around the room. For example, if a patient needs to be transferred from a stretcher or gurney, there must be ample space to move the gurney alongside the X-ray tabletop. Finally, each procedure room must have an area within it, or outside of it, for controls. Within the room, the control area is a lead-lined partition with a window in it. The tech stands behind it to operate the generator that controls the equipment.

It is optimal, when designing major radiography or radiography/fluoroscopy rooms (abbreviated R&F or R/F) to size them generously in order to accomplish future purchases of equipment. Radiographic rooms are very expensive to remodel due to lead shielding and other construction features.

Patient Flow. The overall layout of the radiology suite is driven by a desire to separate patient circulation from the staff work area (Figure 5-1). In Figure 5-2, patient dressing rooms are toward the front of the suite. Patients circulate around one side of the procedure rooms, while the staff work corridor is on the other side of those rooms. The staff work area includes film processing, film reading, tech sorting and viewing area, staff lounge, staff restrooms, and radiologists' private offices. In this plan, the control area for each procedure room is outside the room in the control corridor. This suite plan keeps patients out of staff work areas and, additionally, prevents them from overhearing staff conversations and from casually seeing X-ray films on view boxes in the tech area. It is desirable to protect the patient from overhearing or seeing anything that might cause anxiety or discomfort.

The suite in Figure 5-2 separates traffic to the women's center, which is typically a high-volume unit. The sub-waiting area is dedicated to the women's center. This unit functions independently from the rest of the suite and has its own daylight film processor located in the tech work area.

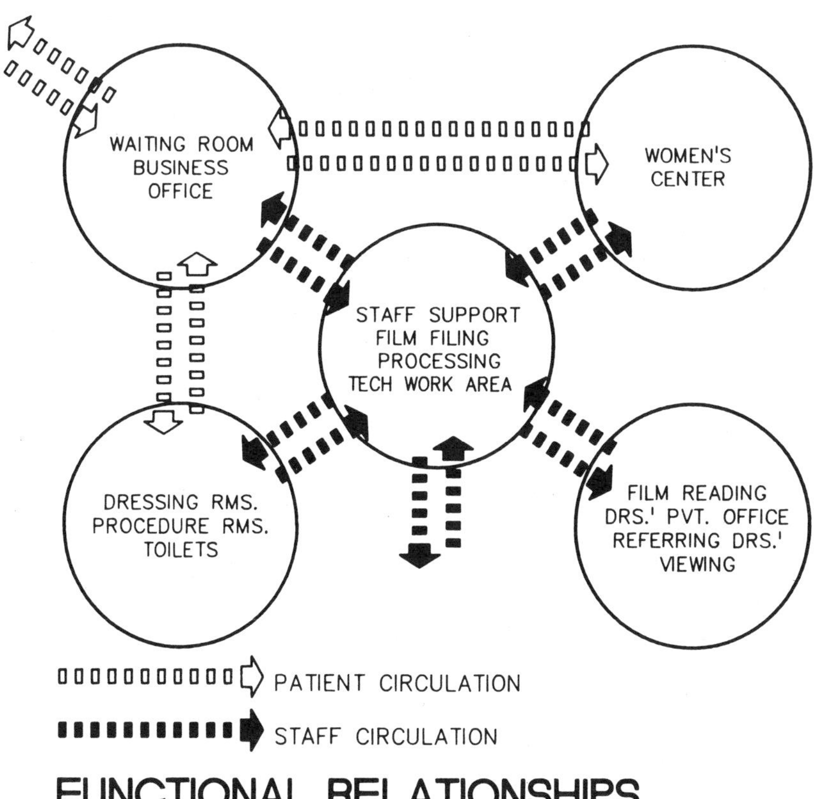

Figure 5-1. Functional relationships, radiology.

Table 5-1. Analysis of Program. Radiology

No. of Physicians:	1		2	
Waiting Room	14 × 16 =	224	16 × 18 =	288
Women's Center, sub-waiting[a]	10 × 12 =	120	10 × 12 =	120
Business Office	14 × 16 =	224	16 × 20 =	320
Dressing Cubicles	6 @ 4 × 4 =	96	10 @ 4 × 4 =	160
General Radiography	14 × 16 =	224	14 × 16 =	224
Radiography/Fluoroscopy	16 × 18 =	288	2 @ 16 × 18 =	576
Barium Prep Area	5 × 8 =	40	5 × 8 =	40
Ultrasound	10 × 12 =	120	10 × 12 =	120
Mammography	10 × 12 =	120	10 × 12 =	120
Nuclear Medicine	—		14 × 16 =	224
Hot Lab	—		6 × 8 =	48
CT Scanner Suite[b]	—		16 × 34 =	544
Toilets	3 @ 6 × 7 =	126	5 @ 6 × 7 =	210
Darkroom/Processing	10 × 10 =	100	10 × 12 =	120
Tech Work Area	6 × 8 =	48	6 × 8 =	48
Film Filing	10 × 14 =	140	14 × 16 =	224
Private Office	12 × 12 =	144	2 @ 12 × 12 =	288
Physicians' Viewing Area	8 × 8 =	64	8 × 8 =	64
Storage	6 × 8 =	48	8 × 10 =	80
Staff Lounge	10 × 12 =	120	12 × 12 =	144
Subtotal		2246 ft^2		3962 ft^2
20% Circulation		450		792
Total		2696 ft^2		4754 ft^2

[a]Optional

[b]Includes procedure, equipment, control, and diagnostic viewing room. Note: The above sizes are an approximation, since radiography rooms must also have control areas, which may be inside or outside the room. Some radiologists may have both a private office and a film reading area; others, only a private office, which then serves as the film reading area.

In Figure 5-3, patient flow is split off into several directions. Those going to the women's center move in one direction; those going to nuclear medicine may undress, be examined, and leave, without ever going through the R/F portion of the suite; those arriving for radiation therapy may enter through the lobby and proceed to the secondary waiting area, or if they are arriving on a gurney, would enter through the rear of the suite and proceed directly to the therapy holding area. Patients going to ultrasound need not mix with the R/F patients. Finally, patients going to radiography or R/F move from the lobby straight down the corridor to the dressing rooms.

Staff Flow. Staff flow must be planned carefully with the X-ray technologists who will work in the clinic. Certain imaging modalities such as CT, ultrasound, and nuclear medicine have dedicated technologists. There must be ample space for all of these technologists to pass one another in corridors and process their films without bumping into one another, and a place to sort and view films.

Figure 5-4 presents a schematic layout for a radiology suite in a square configuration, with the staff work area in the center core. The procedure rooms are arranged around the perimeter of the suite. Figure 5-5 shows a small radiology suite with the tech work area behind the darkroom and around the sides of it. In this plan, the only patients who walk through the tech viewing area are those going to the one R/F room in the lower left corner of the suite.

It is desirable to provide a separate staff bathroom because patient bathrooms are often in use, and those serving the R/F rooms can get messy.

Front office staff function as they would in any medical practice, although the high volume of patients in a radiology suite may necessitate a larger waiting room and a wider reception window.

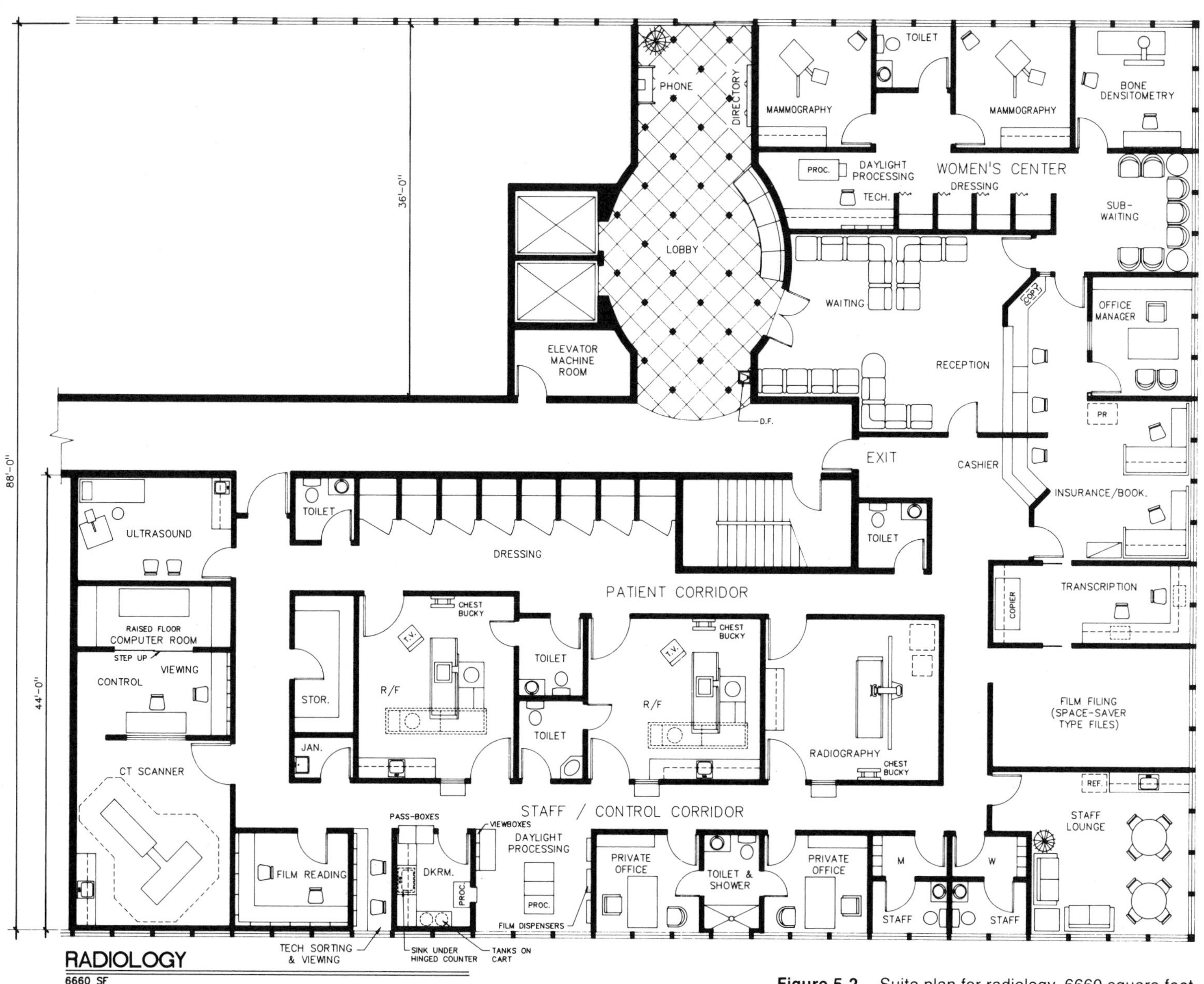

Figure 5-2. Suite plan for radiology, 6660 square feet.

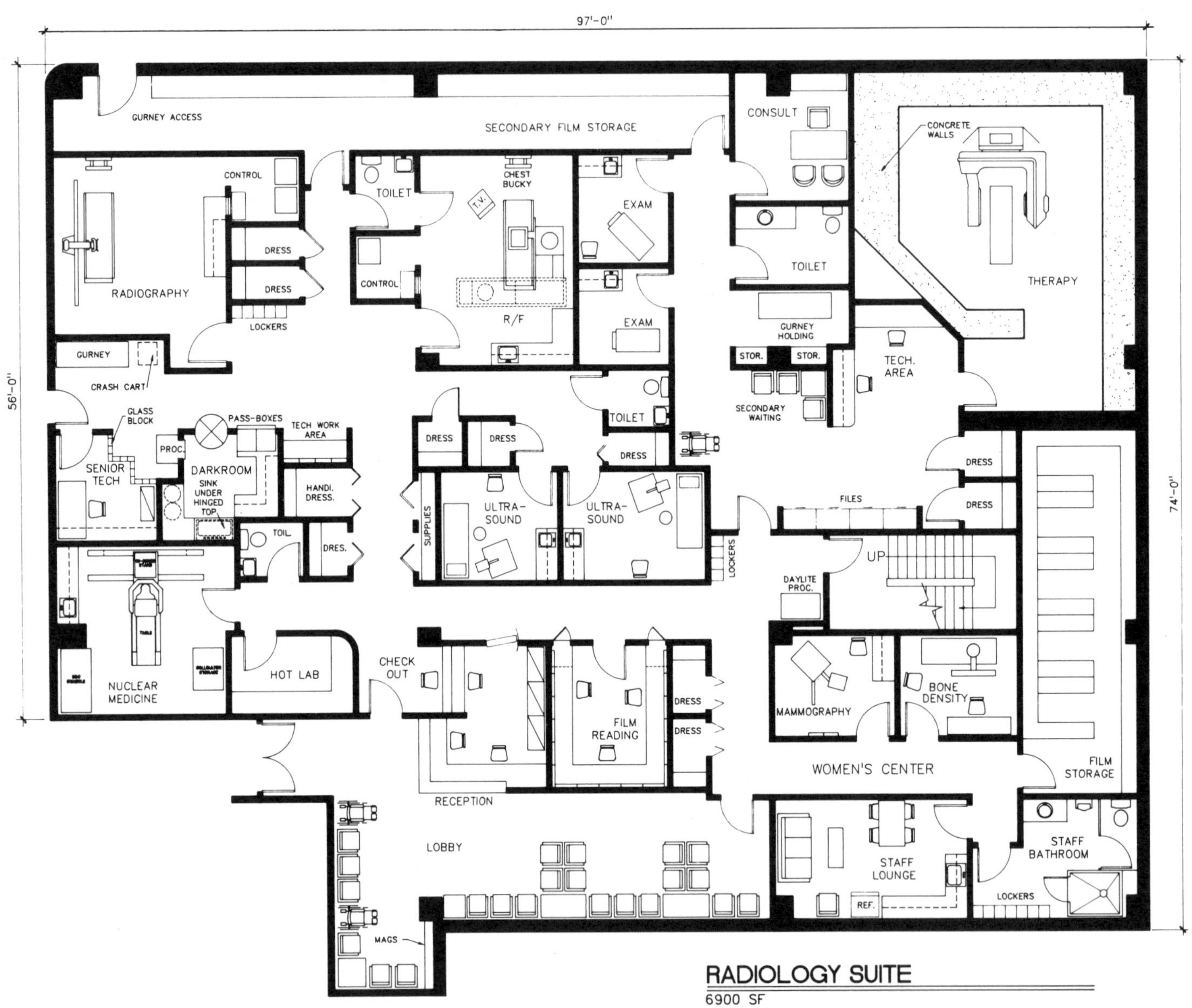

Figure 5-3. Suite plan for radiology, 6900 square feet.

Function. A functional layout would be one that separates patient and staff flow, as discussed above, and one that has a logical placement of rooms based upon patient volume and other considerations. For example, the patient dressing area should be near the front of the suite, as should the referring physicians' viewing area. If possible, locate the film filing room close to the referring physicians' viewing area; thus, physicians can pull films they wish to view and refile them without the assistance of a tech.

If there is a dedicated radiology room for chest films, it would best be located near the front of the suite. These are short examinations, but can be high volume, necessitating a number of dressing rooms nearby. The radiologist's private office, on the other hand, should be located in the most remote and quiet part of the suite.

Components of a Radiology Suite

These are the basic components of a radiology suite, and each will be discussed in detail:

1. Waiting Room
2. Business Office
3. Patient Dressing
4. Tech Work Area
5. Film Reading and Consultation
6. Film Filing
7. Film Processing
8. Darkroom

The various types of radiography and imaging rooms will be described separately.

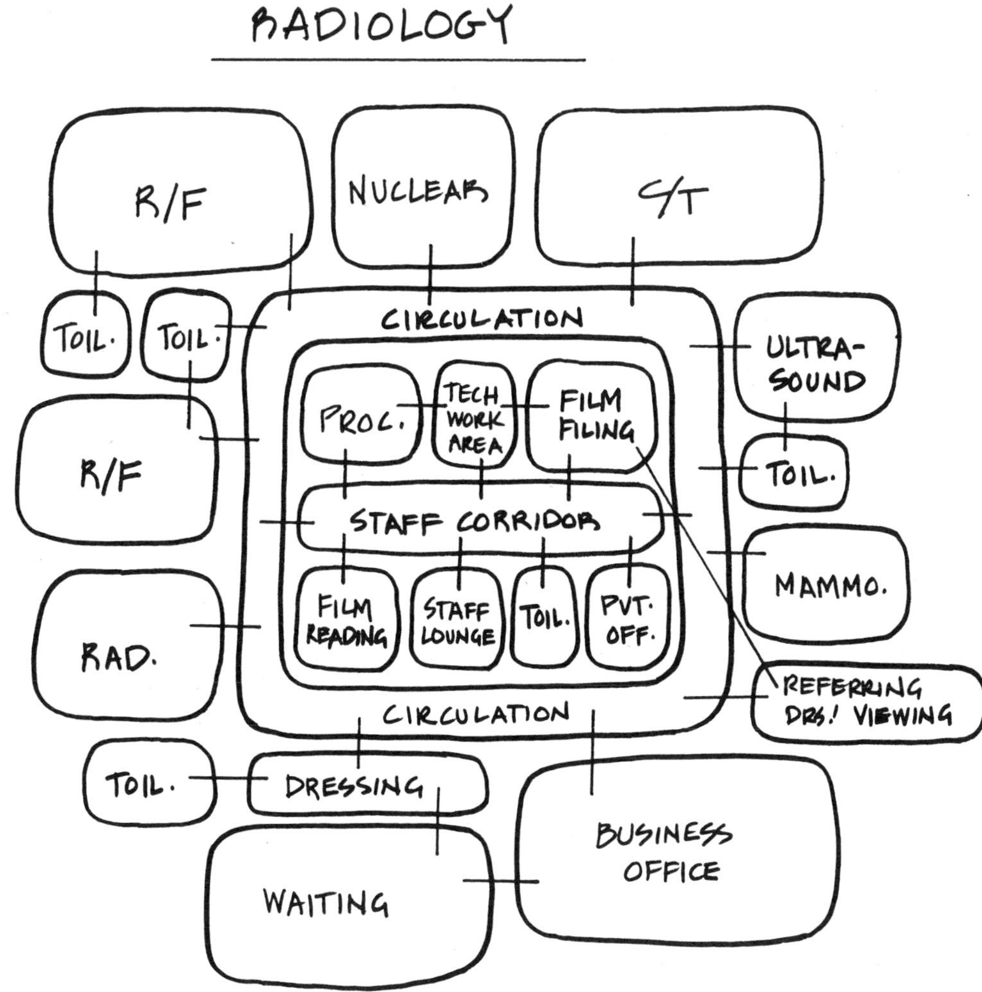

Figure 5-4. Schematic diagram of a radiology suite.

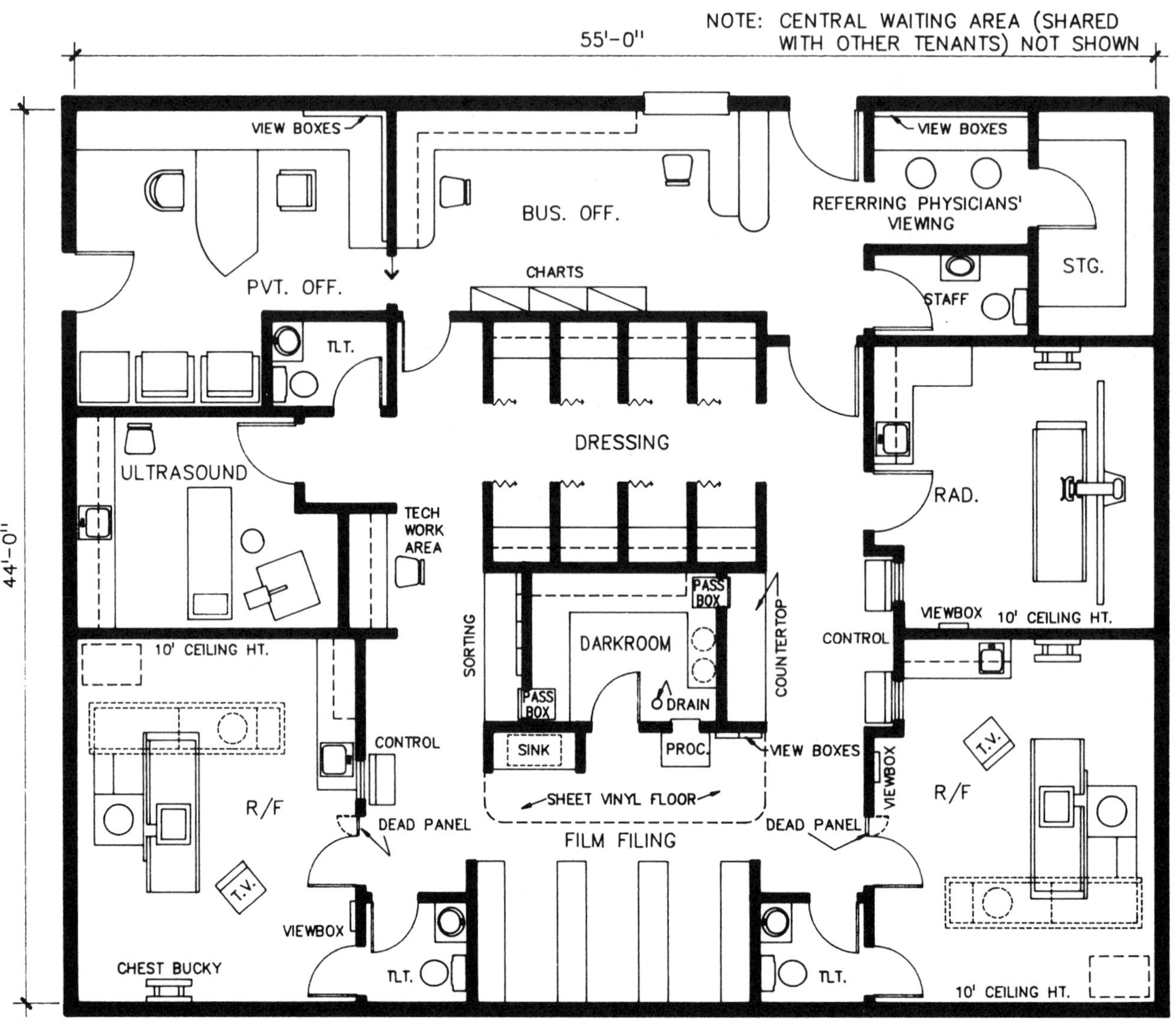

Figure 5-5. Suite plan for radiology, 2420 square feet.

Waiting Room. Allow 2.5 waiting room seats per procedure room and provide a suitable space out of the traffic lane for a patient in a wheelchair. At times a patient may be brought in on a stretcher or gurney. This should be taken into account when laying out the space. A 2- × 6-foot stretcher must be able to be wheeled from the waiting room (or a private staff entrance) through the corridor and into a procedure room, without causing damage to walls or needlessly jostling the patient.

Business Office. The business office is generally not large in a radiology suite, because this is a referral practice, and the patient's medical record remains with the referring physician. The radiologist stores only the X-ray films and a brief report on each patient. Billing and bookkeeping may be done within the suite or at another location.

It is common for radiology groups to sign contracts with hospitals to staff their radiology departments. It is not unusual for one large radiology group to staff three hospitals in a city, in addition to staffing and owning a number of outpatient radiology clinics in various medical buildings throughout the city. If such is the case, bookkeeping and billing might be done off-site, at a centralized location, for all of the clinics.

Patient Dressing. Allow two dressing rooms for each procedure room. Rooms may be as small as 3-feet wide × 4-feet deep, but they should have a chair or built-in bench, mirror, shelf for disposable gowns, and one or two hooks for clothing (Figure 5-6). Sometimes dressing rooms have an emergency buzzer for summoning staff. In a clinic with a sufficient number of dressing rooms, patients may leave their personal effects in the dressing rooms. Each room may have a small lockable compartment for handbags, briefcases, or jewelry.

In other clinics, patients are asked to store their clothing in lockers outside the dressing room, so that others may use the room. The dressing area should be carpeted, since patients may be walking barefoot. Sometimes one dressing cubicle is made double-width so that the built-in bench may serve as a recovery cot in case a patient feels ill. This oversized dressing room also accommodates a patient in a wheelchair.

Tech Work Area. A discussion of the technologists' work space must begin with a clarification of terms. Although often used interchangeably, there is a difference between *technician* and *technologist* initiated by the change in name of the American Registry of X-ray

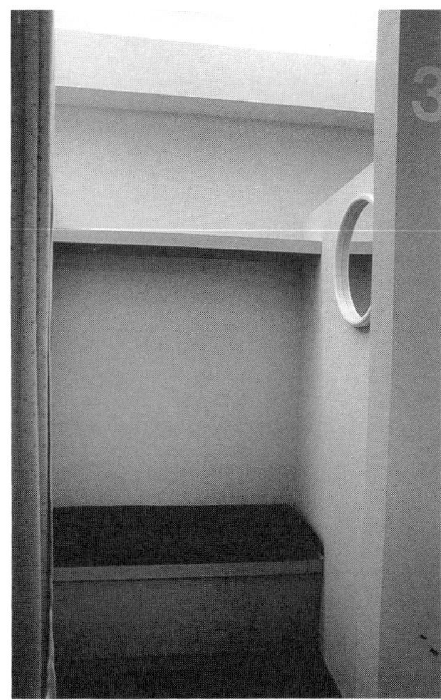

Figure 5-6. Patient dressing room. (*Design: Jain Malkin Inc.; Photographer: John Christian.*)

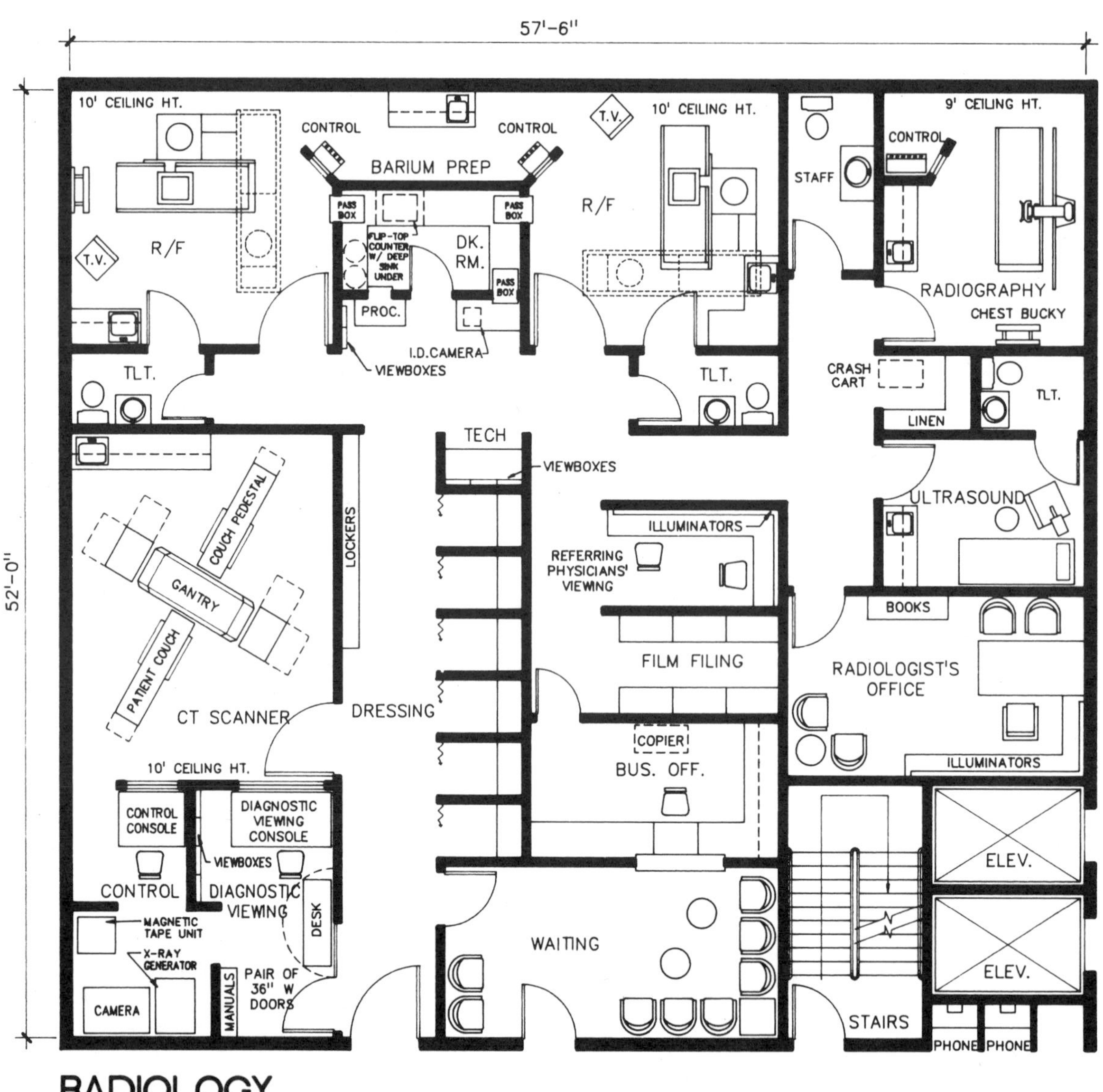

Figure 5-7. Suite plan for radiology, 2990 square feet.

Technicians to the American Registry of Radiologic Technologists. The term "technologist" recognizes the evolution of education and skills — the X-ray technician has become a radiologic technologist.

Many diagnostic procedures are performed entirely by the X-ray technologist, without the radiologist being present. The tech greets the patient, gives instructions for the examination, sets up the equipment, positions the patient, makes the exposure, processes the film, and places the finished films in the radiologist's viewing room for reading.

The darkroom should be located close to the procedure rooms to save steps for the tech who walks back and forth, picking up unexposed film cassettes from pass boxes located in the darkroom wall and, later, returns to the pass box the exposed film to be fed into the processor.

A suite with three or more procedure rooms will generally have a dedicated darkroom technician who continually replenishes the pass boxes with film cassettes and feeds the exposed film into the processor. The processed film drops out of the processor on the daylight side, where the tech picks it up, checks it on the view box, sorts a series of films, puts it in X-ray film jackets, and later delivers it to the film viewing room for the radiologist to interpret. Note that techs need access to film filing, as they often have to pull older films for the radiologist to compare with new ones.

Before the film is fed into the processor, it must have patient identification placed on it. The patient identification camera could be on the countertop outside the darkroom or may be inside the darkroom.

Each tech requires a stand-up height countertop work surface for sorting and viewing films. Mounted over the countertop would be a four- to six-panel view box illuminator, and below, a rack with a number of vertical dividers for sorting films (Figures 5-8 and 5-9). In addition, a double-panel view box must be provided immediately adjacent to the processor on the daylight side, for checking films as they exit the processor. (See Appendix for mounting heights of view box illuminators.)

The control area, discussed in detail below, is also the tech's work area. It may be located in the corridor outside the room or inside the room, behind a lead-lined partition.

Control Area. Note when laying out radiographic rooms, that *tables tilt so that the right side goes down, and the left up, when one is standing on the working side* (see Figure 5-27). The control area, therefore, should be on the right end so that the technologist can see the patient at all times. Some tables do not tilt, making this issue less critical, but it is still optimal for the technologist to have the patient in view.

Figure 5-7 shows a frequently used layout with a control and barium prep area that runs between two radiography rooms. The problem with this, although it is convenient with respect to the darkroom, pass boxes, and barium prep area, is that a right-handed and a left-handed room have been created. The R/F room on the right, puts the control area behind the patient's head, whereas the R/F room on the left keeps the patient in full view of the tech, especially when the table is tilted. In the room on the right, when the table is tilted, the patient would be totally out of view of the tech. (As a point of information, all R/F tables tilt.) Note that in Figure 5-3, the control area for the R/F room is located so that the tech has a good view of the patient when the table is tilted.

The control area may be outside the radiography room as in Figures 5-2 and 5-5 (the operator or technologist looks through a lead-shielded window at the patient as in Figure 5-10), or it may be in the radiography room (see Figures 5-3 and 5-7), provided the control partition and window are lead-shielded. Prefabricated, lead-lined control partitions and lead-shielded windows may be purchased from X-ray supply dealers.

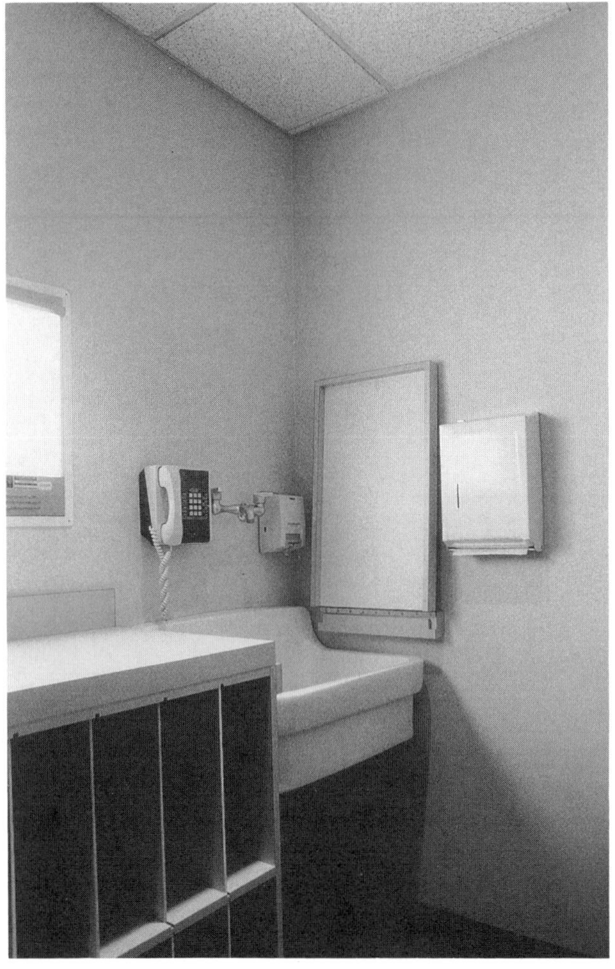

Figure 5-8. Tech work area, sorting and viewing counter. Note sink under hinged countertop. (*Design: Jain Malkin Inc.; Photographer: John Christian.*)

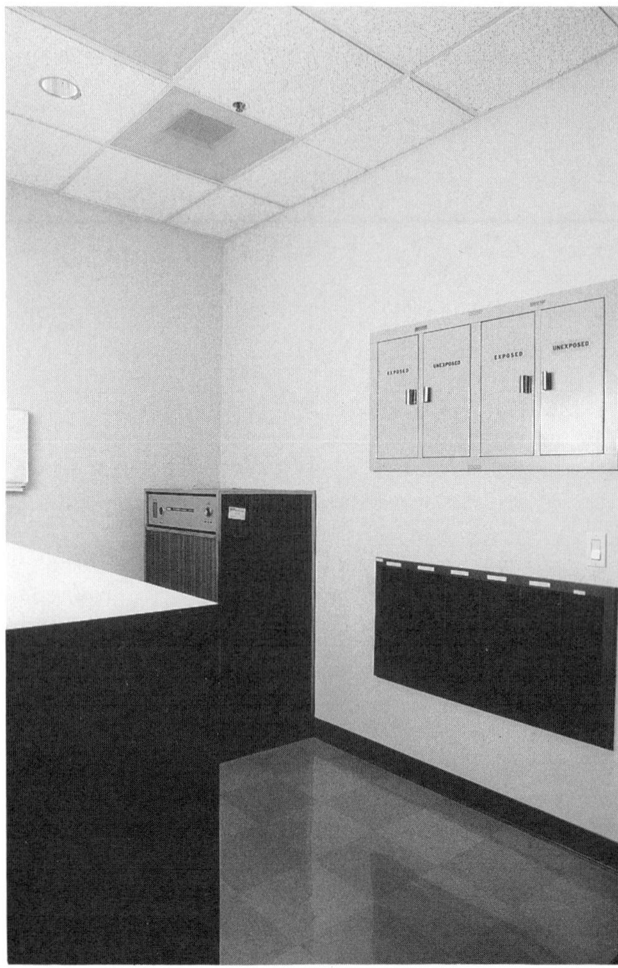

Figure 5-9. Tech work area (opposite side). Note pass boxes to darkroom and automatic processor.

If the control area is outside the room, a lead-lined speaking grille in the wall will enable the technologist to communicate instructions to the patient. As a safety precaution, the control console may be wired to a red signal light outside of each radiographic room to prevent entry when the machine is in use (Figure 5-10a).

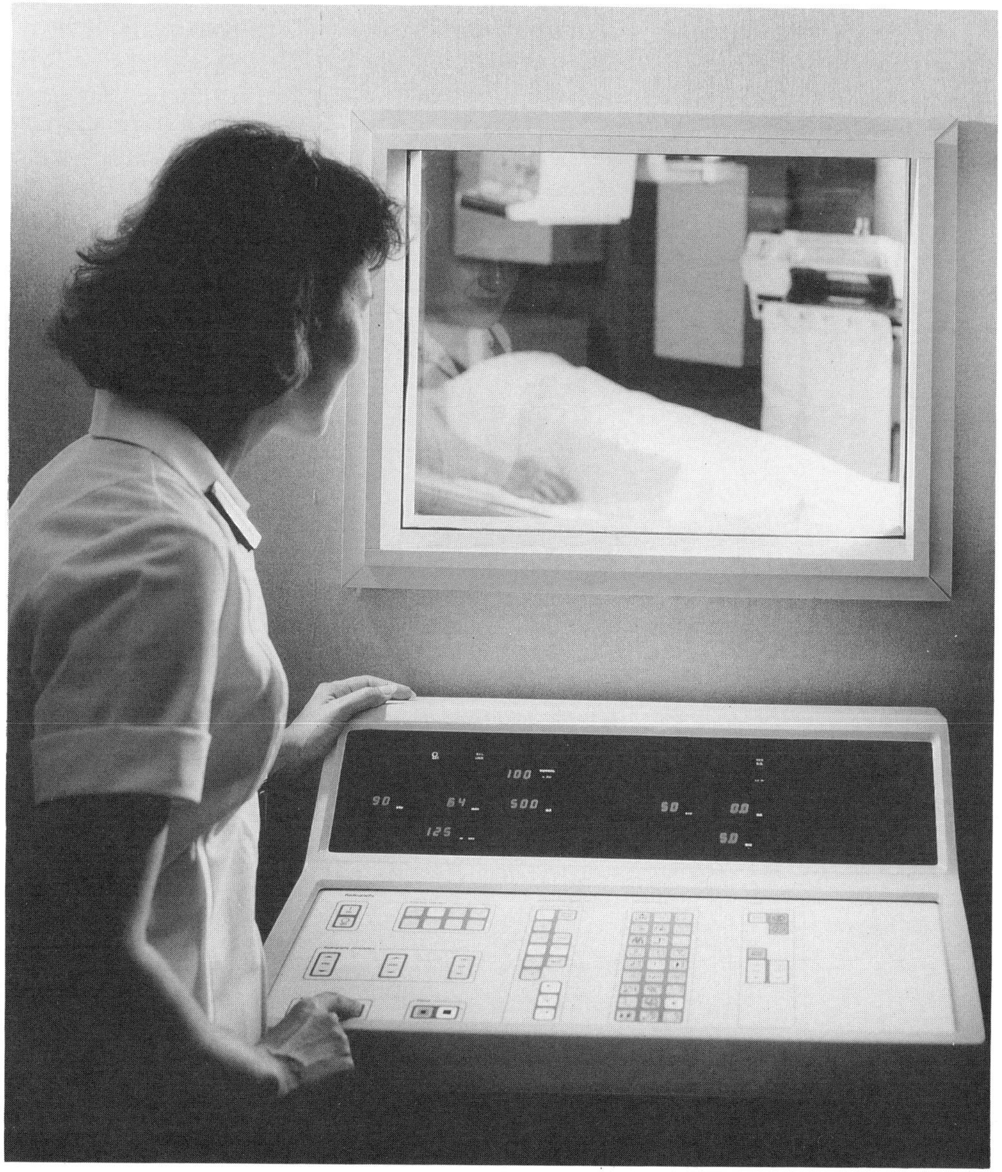

Figure 5-10. Computerized generator, control area. (*Courtesy GE Medical Systems, Milwaukee, WI.*)

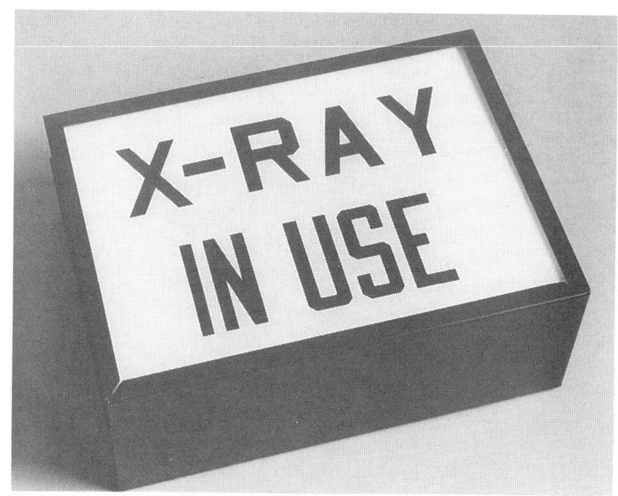

Figure 5-10a. "X-Ray in Use" sign.

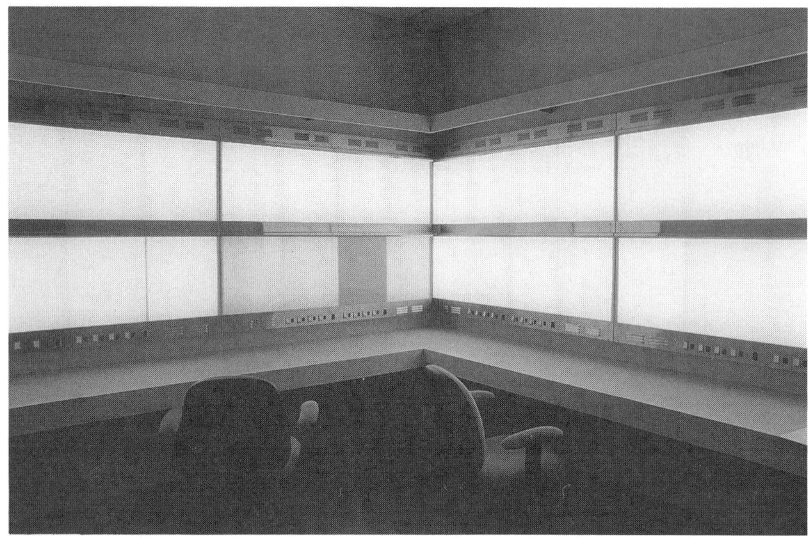

Figure 5-11. Radiologists' reading room. (*Design: Jain Malkin Inc.; Photographer: John Christian.*)

Film Reading. The film reading room is where the radiologist interprets the films. It is approximately 10 × 12 or 10 × 14 feet in size, with a countertop along one or two walls at sit-down height. Above the countertop are two tiers of view box illuminators lining the room, wall to wall (Figure 5-11). The countertop needs to be completely clear underneath so that the radiologist can move freely from side to side. A cantilevered countertop can be accomplished with steel reinforcement inside the wall, extending underneath the countertop.

Ideal room lighting would be a perimeter valance (with dimmer control) running along two or three walls of the room (Figure 5-11). This would provide glare-free indirect illumination.

This room should be located in the staff work area or at the rear of the suite, where it is quiet. It should not be in the front of the suite or in the hectic patient circulation area.

Referring Physicians' Viewing. This is generally an alcove off of the corridor (see Figures 5-5 and 5-7), where referring physicians may come to review their patients' X-rays. A four-panel view box is generally sufficient. This would usually be at sit-down height, but could be a stand-up consultation area (Figure 5-12). Some radiology facilities provide closed-circuit TV in the physician's viewing room to enable referring physicians to observe a fluoroscopy procedure in progress.

This room should be positioned in the suite so that physicians' discussions will not be overheard by patients. If located near the front of the suite, doctors would not have to intrude upon patients in the examination area. Additionally, by locating it near the film filing area physicians may pull their own films for viewing, but this is not an essential requirement.

Radiologist's Office/Consultation. The radiologist usually does not consult with patients, but does consult with referring physicians. This may take place in the private office or in the referring physician's viewing area. (Those who do consult with patients would use the private office.) Most radiologists will have view box illuminators in their private offices (four-over-four or perhaps eight-over-eight panels) mounted on the wall behind and to the side of the desk, with a sorting shelf underneath (Figure 5-14). This room should be located in the quietest part of the suite.

Film Filing. Sufficient storage for X-ray films must be provided in lateral file cabinets. Films are placed in color-coded paper jackets and stored on open shelves for easy retrieval (Figure 5-13). (X-ray film jackets are 14½ × 17½ inches in size.) Many radiology suites use space-saving movable aisle type filing systems, which may be manually operated or motorized. A word of caution: The weight of these file cabinets, loaded, must be carefully calculated in order to design the floor to support it.

Film Processing. Film processing may be done in a darkroom or by a daylight process that does not require a darkroom. However, many suites that use daylight processing also have a small darkroom. The large central darkroom that necessitates long travel routes has been replaced, in large clinics, by a number of processing areas distributed in a *decentralized* fashion throughout the suite, adjacent to procedure rooms.

Advantages of decentralized darkrooms are several. They free the tech from carting cassettes back and forth, which can be tiring. Shorter walking distances allow the tech to spend more time with patients who, in turn, have a shorter wait because films are processed more rapidly. This improves the operational efficiency of each procedure room, thereby generating more revenue.

In an effort to increase efficiency, some X-ray equipment manufacturers have developed certain types of radiography units with integrated (attached) film pro-

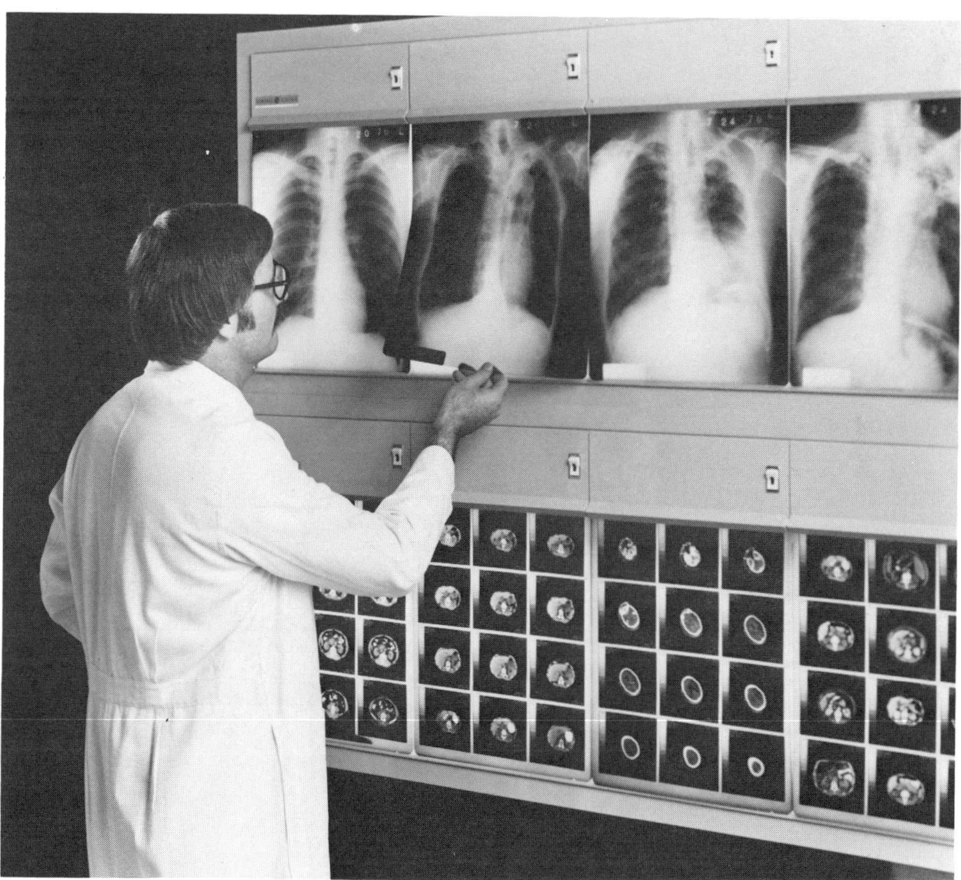

Figure 5-12. Six-over-six view boxes. (*Courtesy GE Medical Systems, Milwaukee, WI.*)

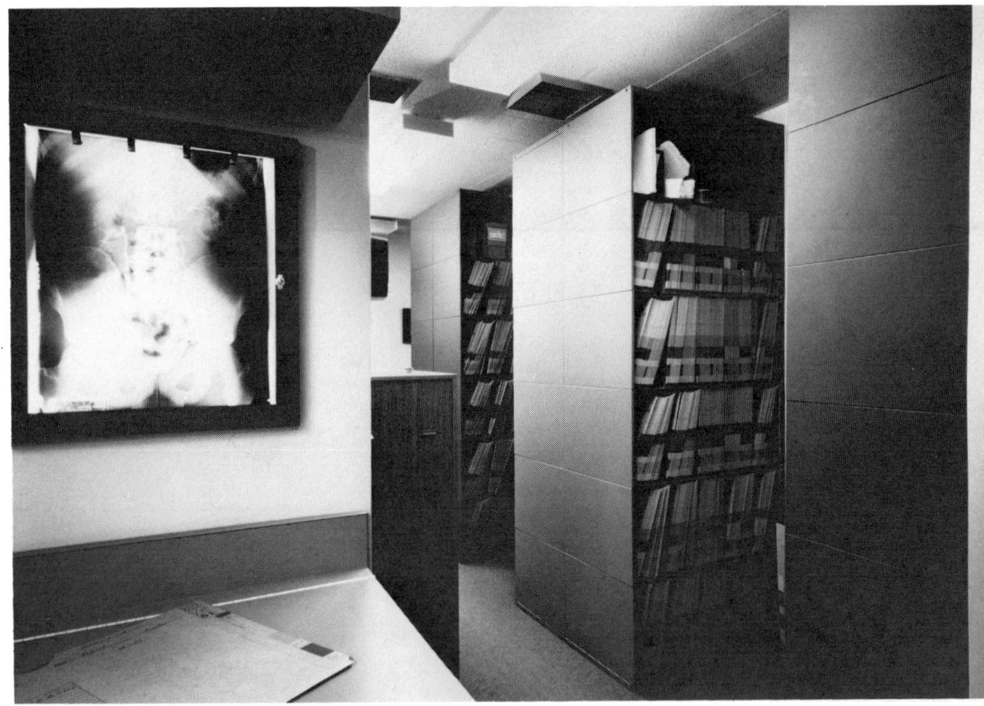

Figure 5-13. X-ray film filing. (*Design: Jain Malkin Inc.*)

cessors. The X-ray unit has its own film supply magazine and a permanently attached film processor, which accomplishes all of the goals stated above.

From the planning point of view, there are four different possibilities for routing exposed film to the processor.

1. Single-film cassette
2. Transportable film magazine
3. Daylight system
4. Integrated (attached) film processor

The *single-film cassette* is used in all conventional fluoroscopic and radiographic procedures. Single cassettes are loaded and stored in lead-lined cassette pass boxes (Figure 5-15).

The *film magazine* accommodates a large quantity of exposed films that are processed sequentially, together, in the processor.

Daylight systems allow the film processor to be located in a lighted room. This system can be used for all types of imaging including CT, MRI, nuclear medicine, general radiography, mammography, ultrasound video imaging, and even 35mm Cine films. Advocates of this system claim that daylight processing saves 20 percent of the total patient examination time, allowing the tech to spend more time in the room with the patient, rather than running back and forth to the darkroom.

There may be some savings in utilization of space as well. A darkroom can be used only for opening and processing film, whereas a daylight area is all usable space. Furthermore, a daylight processor can sometimes be placed in the procedure room itself; thus, the tech would not have to leave the patient in order to develop the film. The compact unit in Figure 5-16 is one such unit.

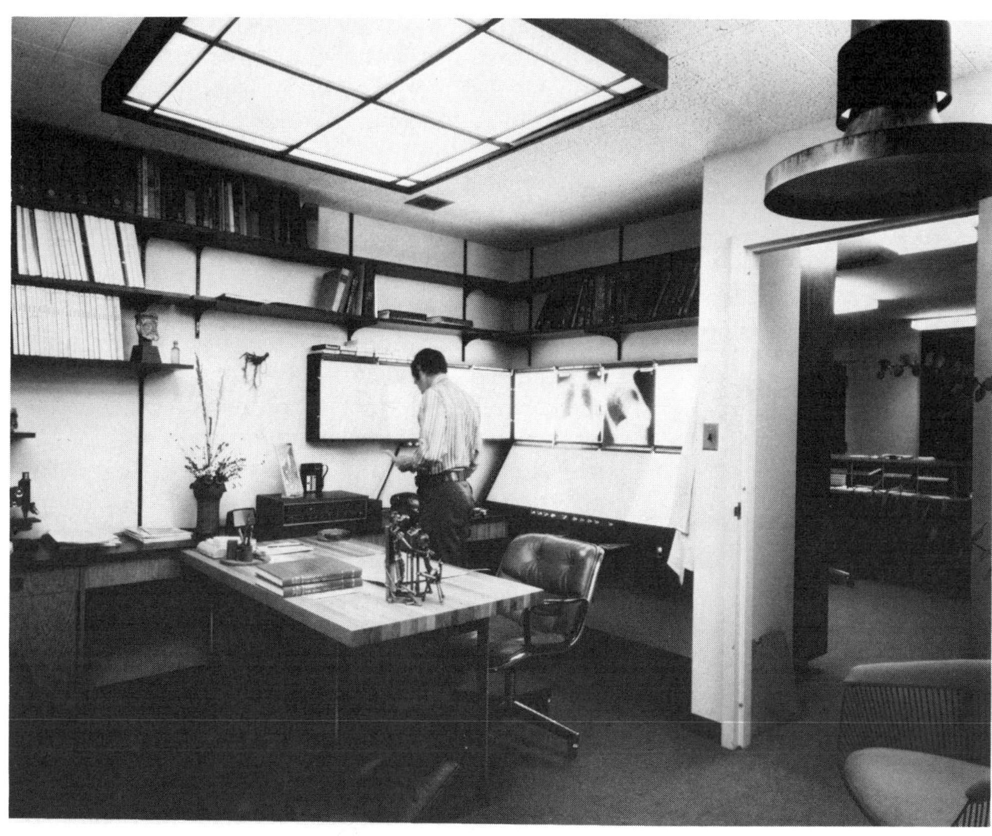

Figure 5-14. Radiologist's private office. (*Design: Jain Malkin Inc.*)

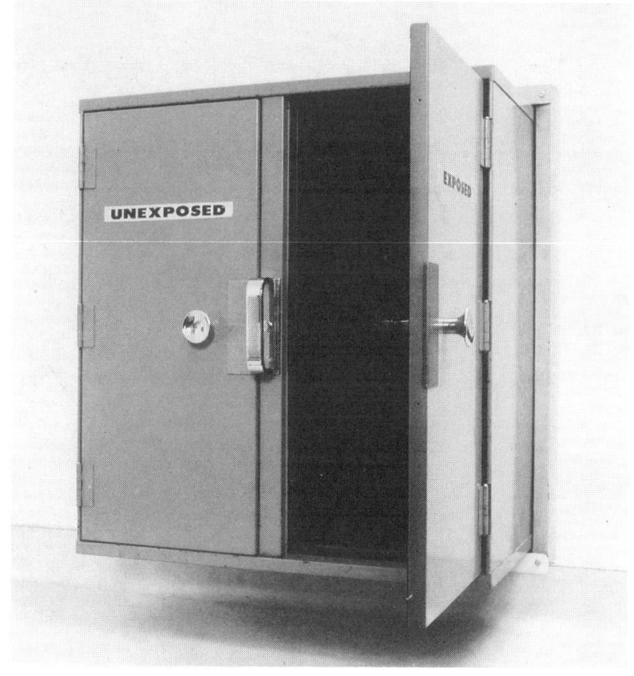

Figure 5-15. Cassette pass box. (*Courtesy GE Medical Systems, Milwaukee, WI.*)

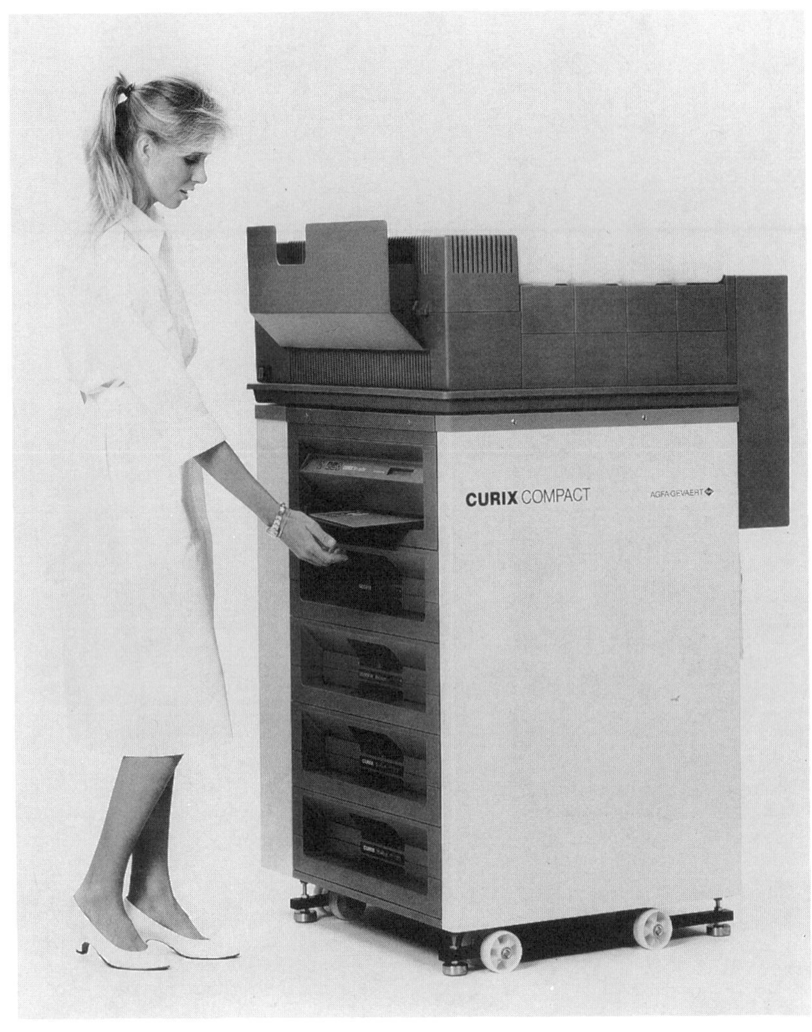

Figure 5-16. Daylight film processor. (*Courtesy Agfa-Gevaert Inc., Ridgefield Park, NJ.*)

Integrated film processing refers to a radiography unit that has its own attached film processor. There is a popular unit that does chest films, which allows a high volume throughput of patients.

Darkroom. All radiology suites contain one or more darkrooms unless they are dedicated to daylight film processing. Even then, they may have a darkroom for storage of film or for loading odd-sized film into magazines. The system by DuPont (Figures 5-17 and 5-18) needs no darkroom due to the wall-mounted daylight film dispensers. However, if it is not possible to extinguish room lights for servicing, then a portable darkroom is needed to remove unprocessed film from the upper storage section of the dispenser. The daylight processing units in Figures 5-16 and 5-19 by Agfa-Gevaert require a small darkroom for loading film into magazines. This system does not require any wall-mounted film dispensers.

The size and design of the darkroom and processing area depends upon the equipment, the number and arrangement of radiographic rooms around it, whether there is one central darkroom or several decentralized ones, and the volume of film to be processed. In any case, there would be a "wet" side and a "dry" side. The wet side is where the automatic processor and the replenisher tanks are located. Either inside the darkroom or in the tech work area outside, there needs to be a large sink (size 18 × 24 × 9 inches deep) for washing the rollers of the processor. This sink should have hot and cold water as well as a sprayer attachment. Since it is not used on a daily basis, it is advisable to put it under a hinged countertop (see Figure 5-8) to preserve more working space.

The dry side of the darkroom is where the film storage bin (which requires an electrical outlet) is located and where cassettes are loaded with film. One or more cassette pass boxes will be built into the wall for the transfer of unexposed and exposed film cassettes. Since these are very heavy lead-lined boxes, the wall in which they are supported will require reinforcement. Pass boxes will be located in the wall of the darkroom closest to, or contiguous with, the radiography rooms (see Figure 5-7). If the darkroom is not contiguous with the radiography rooms (see Figure 5-5), pass boxes would be located on a darkroom wall accessible to the radiography room corridor. Daylight processing systems do not require pass boxes.

The automatic processor (Figure 5-20) may be located inside the darkroom or more commonly, outside the darkroom, feeding through a light-sealed opening in the wall into the darkroom. (The unit would be outside the darkroom with the feed tray extending into the darkroom.) Exposed film would be fed from inside the darkroom into the tray, and the processed film would be delivered on the daylight side of the tech work area.

Older processors require hot and cold water and a temperature mixing valve (Figure 5-21); however, new models require only cold water, as temperature is controlled within the unit. The processor shown in Figure 5-20 is the standard in the industry; therefore, its planning requirements will be noted. It needs 18 inches clear on the right side as that's where it is opened for servicing. It requires little space on the left side but, to repair occasional leakage that may occur, it is wise to allow 12 inches if possible.

The unit requires a floor drain or, preferably, a floor sink inside the darkroom and a vent to the outside for exhaust. Exhaust comes out of the processor from the rear, which can be handled by connecting a flexible duct that runs exposed along the inside darkroom wall, or it can be run concealed inside the wall at the proper location to connect with the vent hole exhaust pipe at the rear of the processor. The unit requires 208 VAC, 30-ampere service with a 30-ampere breaker.

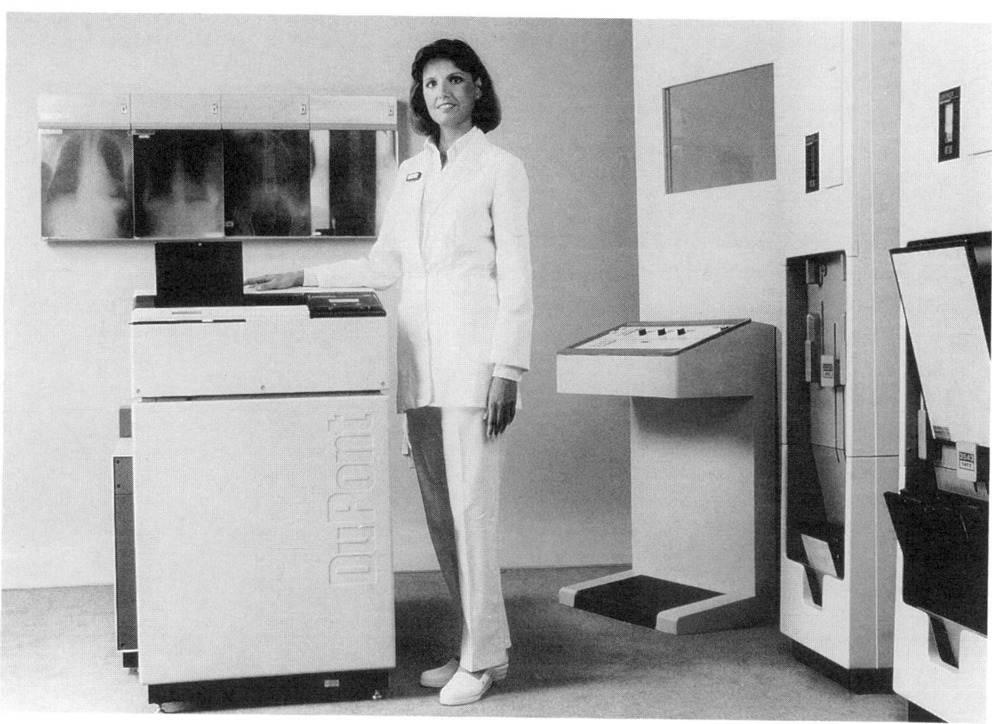

Figure 5-17. Daylight processing system. (*Courtesy Du Pont Co., Wilmington, DE.*)

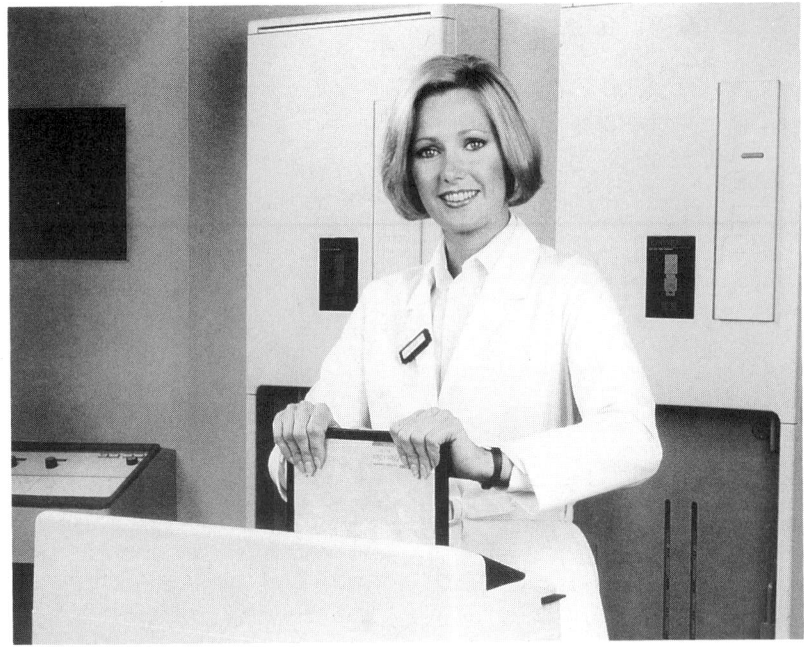

Figure 5-18. Feeding cassette into daylight processor. (*Courtesy Du Pont Co., Wilmington, DE.*)

Two 50-gallon replenisher tanks of developer would be located under the countertop on the wet side of the darkroom, close to the processor. These tanks may also be placed on a rolling cart. The area under the processor, including the path between the processor and the sink used for washing rollers, must have a hard surface flooring, preferably sheet vinyl. Carpet should not be used in the tech work area outside the darkroom.

A darkroom needs two sources of light. A 100-watt incandescent fixture, either recessed or surface-mounted to the ceiling, will serve for general illumination, but a red safelight must be provided for work with exposed film. The safelight can be plugged into an outlet at 60 to 72 inches off the floor, and it can work by a pull chain or be wired to a wall switch (Figure 5-22). If the latter, the switch should be located away from the incandescent light switch, so that the technologist does not accidentally hit the wrong switch while working with exposed film. The safelight shown in Figure 5-23 can sit on a countertop or be bracketed to the wall. Any recessed light fixtures and the exhaust fan must have light-sealed housings. Similarly, the darkroom door must have a light seal. Codes in some cities require a lightproof louver ventilation panel in the darkroom door.

Countertop work surfaces in a darkroom may be at a 36-inch or 42-inch height, depending on personal preference. Open shelves may be provided above the countertop for storage of various items. There is no need for closed storage in a darkroom. As for color of walls, some techs prefer dark walls and others prefer a light color.

An option for a darkroom door is that shown in Figure 5-24. This revolving door provides lightproof entry into the darkroom, allowing one tech to enter while another is working with exposed film. If this type of door is not used, it is important to have a red warning light

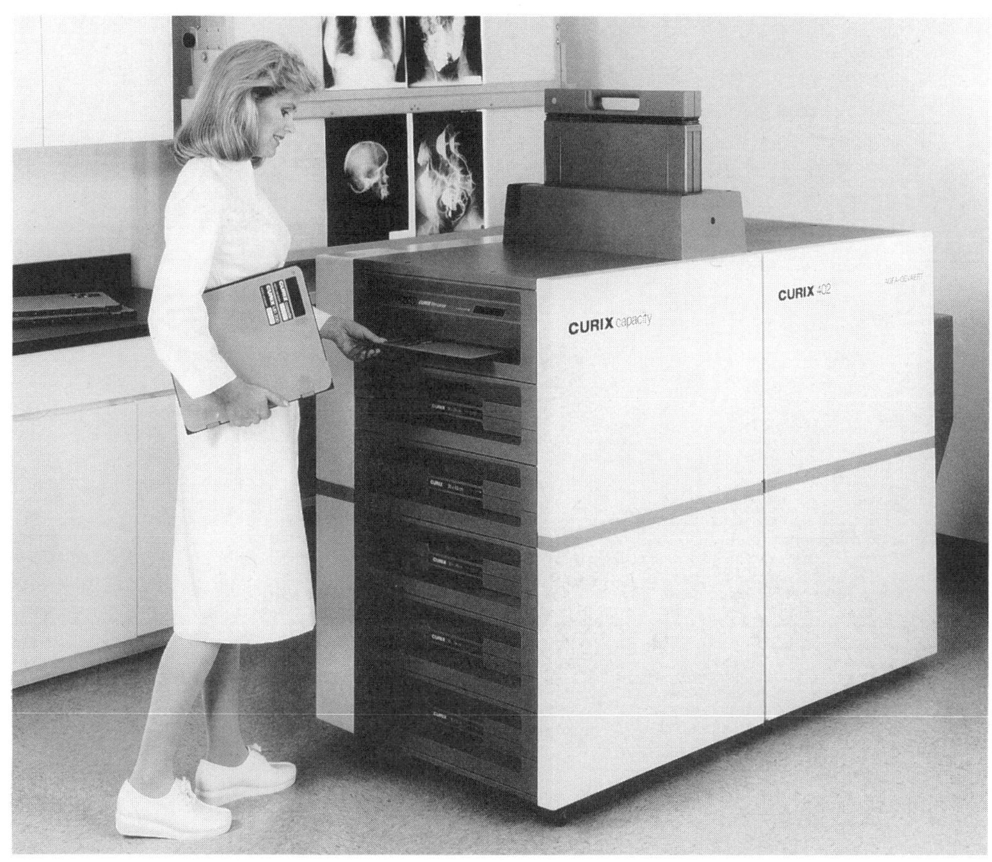

Figure 5-19. Daylight processor. (*Courtesy Agfa-Gevaert Inc., Ridgefield Park, NJ.*)

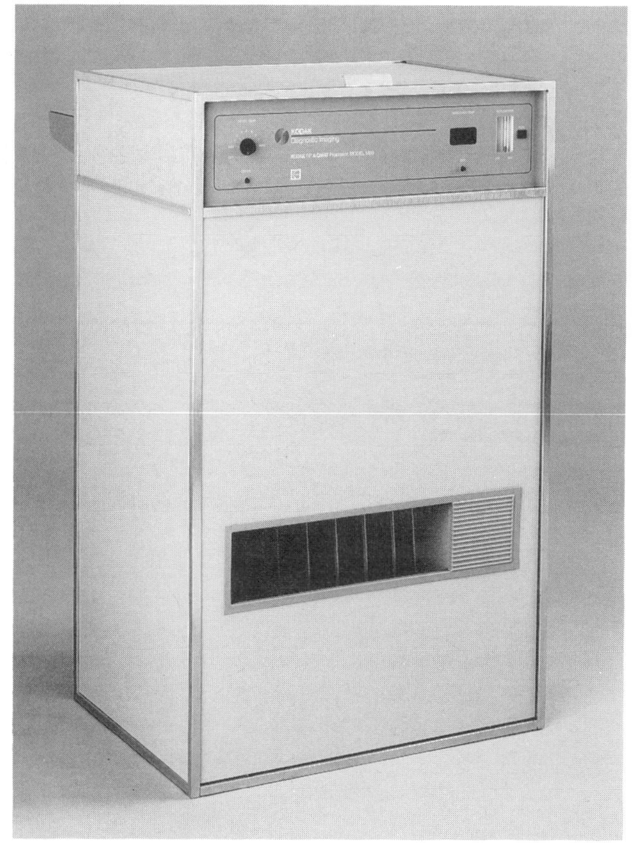

Figure 5-20. *X-OMAT* automatic film processor. (*Courtesy Eastman Kodak Co., Rochester, NY.*)

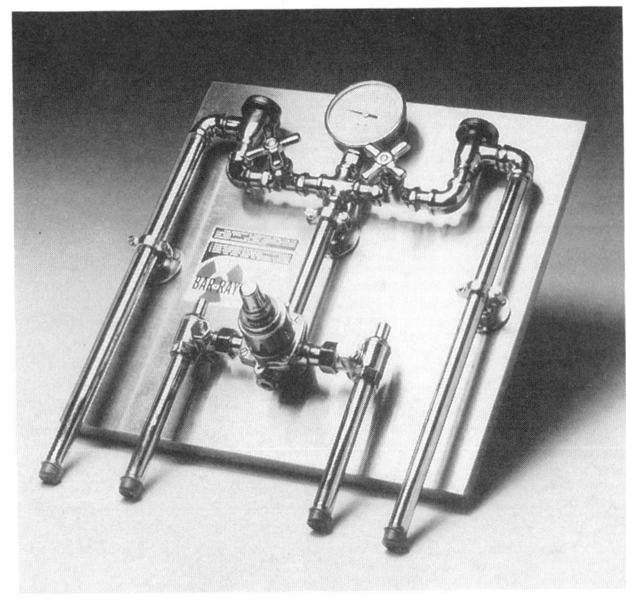

Figure 5-21. Temperature mixing valve, for darkroom. (*Courtesy GE Medical Systems, Milwaukee, WI.*)

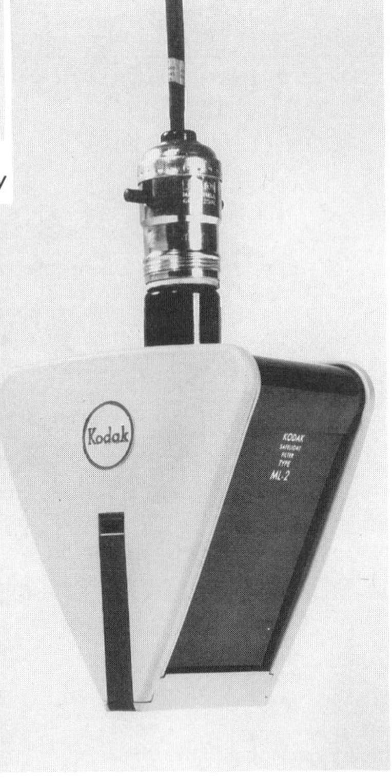

Figure 5-22. Safelight. (*Courtesy Eastman Kodak Co., Rochester, NY.*)

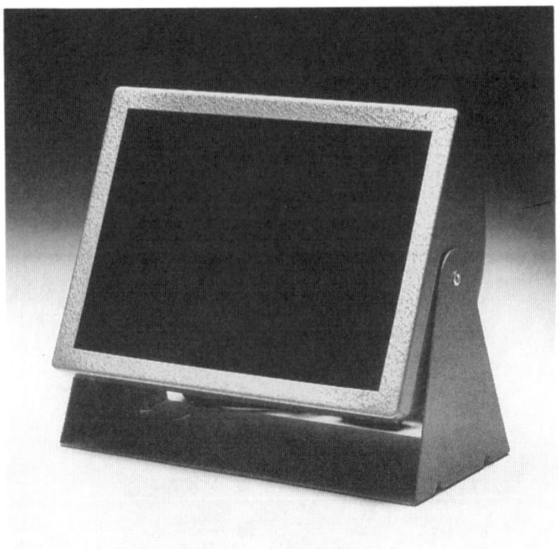

Figure 5-23. Safelight. (*Courtesy GE Medical Systems, Milwaukee, WI.*)

over the door that is automatically activated (tied into the film bin) whenever cassettes are being loaded or unloaded.

The darkroom water supply must be filtered, and the processor may need a silver recovery unit (Figure 5-25), depending upon local codes. When disposing of waste chemicals or water, regulations of local agencies must be followed. If used liquids are allowed to be fed into the sewer system, piping must be of polyethylene up to the main line (vertical disposal pipe). Additionally, waste lines must have vacuum breakers.

Daylight Processing. There are a number of daylight processing systems as well as options within each system. As with any selection of equipment, it depends upon an analysis of needs. The layout of the suite, availability of space, number and type of radiology examinations, anticipated work flow, availability of personnel and, of course, cost must all be factored into the decision. Manufacturer's literature must be consulted for suggested equipment layouts, critical distances between various components, weight, and utility requirements.

The system in Figures 5-17 and 5-18 has four components: 1) *wall-mounted film dispensers,* 2) *daylight cassettes,* 3) *daylight unloader,* and 4) *processor.* The tech loads the cassette from the wall-mounted film dispenser, carries it to the procedure room, makes the exposure, brings it back to the daylight processing area, and puts the cassette into the unloader where it automatically receives patient identification via an integrated I.D. system built into the unloader.

From the unloader, the film proceeds to the processor, and the finished film is delivered in 90 seconds. If the daylight processing area is laid out contiguous with or between two or three procedure rooms, it is possible to place the control area for those rooms within the processing area. Thus the tech can complete the entire radiographic process just a few feet away from the patient. Films can be checked for resolution, immediately, as they drop out of the processor.

The daylight processing system shown in Figures 5-16 and 5-19 requires a darkroom for loading film into magazines. The patient I.D. camera (not integrated into the equipment) sits on a countertop or on top of the cassette storage cart. The unit in Figure 5-16 may be located in a mammography room or in an area just outside the room, so that the tech does not have to leave the patient.

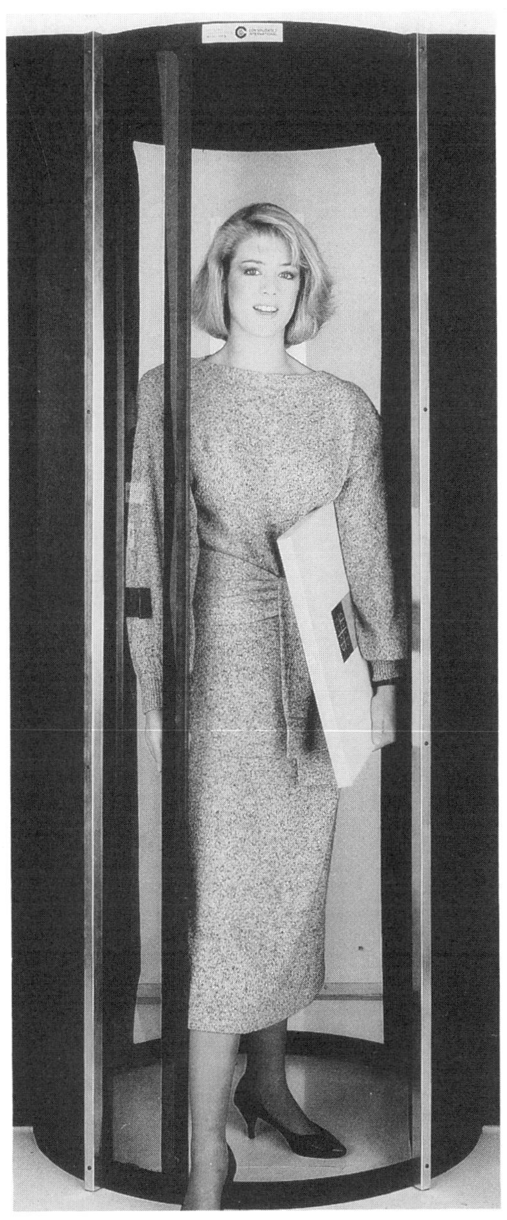

Figure 5-24. Revolving darkroom door. (*Courtesy Consolidated International, Chicago, IL.*)

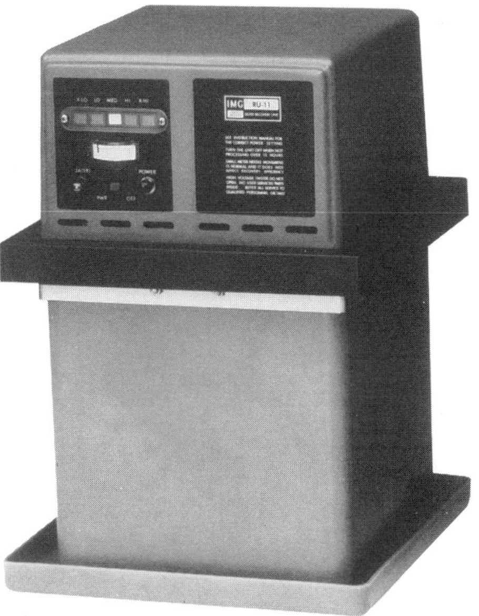

Figure 5-25. Silver recovery unit. (*Courtesy GE Medical Systems, Milwaukee, WI.*)

Today it is popular to create a women's center within a radiology suite. For marketing purposes, this area is generally located near the front of the suite and may even have a private entrance (see Figures 5-2 and 5-3). This means that the tech would have quite a distance to walk to a central darkroom or processing area; therefore, a compact daylight processor is the ideal solution.

Certain issues need to be considered with daylight processing systems. All machine functions are monitored and controlled by microprocessors; therefore, manufacturers' recommendations for relative humidity and ambient temperature must be heeded. There are two methods of discharging waste, water, and chemicals (fixer and developer): central discharge into the sewer system, or collection of waste into storage tanks. If local codes allow for chemicals to be discharged into the public sewer system, waste liquids would be run straight to the drain through a hose. Polyethylene piping will be needed for the drain as far as the main riser (vertical downpipe). An alternative to this is a waste disposal trolley with containers to collect the chemicals.

Additional accessory items that may be internally integrated into the processing system or may be accessory attachments are a water filter, replenisher tanks, a silver recovery unit, or a chemical mixer. As with any automatic processor, a deep, large sink (with sprayer hose attachment) is necessary for washing rollers. Most daylight processors require a cold water supply, dedicated circuit, good ventilation in the processing area, controlled water pressure, and a 3- to 4-inch diameter exhaust connect from the processor, vented to the plenum or to the outdoors, as local codes dictate.

GENERAL RADIOGRAPHY ROOMS AND RADIOGRAPHY AND FLUOROSCOPY ROOMS

Not all radiography rooms are equipped for fluoroscopy. A diagnostic imaging facility may have two general radiography rooms plus one radiography and fluoroscopy (R/F) combination room or perhaps one general radiography room and two R/F rooms. The R/F room should be a minimum of 14 × 16 feet in size and may even be 16 × 18 feet.

The size of the radiography room will vary in accordance with the size of the X-ray unit and the ancillary equipment. As the room is equipped for taking radiographs of all parts of the body in standing, sitting, or angled positions, the room will have freestanding, wall-mounted, and ceiling-suspended equipment. Because there are a certain number of variables from one manufacturer to another, the space planner must obtain suggested room layouts that note critical distances between various components, along with specifications of required utility connections from each manufacturer.

To begin with, electrical cables connect the control unit (generator) to the X-ray tube stand and the transformer. The most unobtrusive way of handling this is to trench the floor and bury them under the coverplate. Conduit or cabling can also be run, exposed, at the base of the wall. (The transformer is generally located in one corner of the radiography room.)

An R/F room must have a toilet attached to it. The toilet often has one door to the R/F room and another to the corridor as shown in Figures 5-3 and 5-7. The patient needs to discharge immediately the barium enema after the lower G.I. (gastrointestinal) procedure.

The patient exits the bathroom via the corridor door, adjacent to the dressing area. If he needs to use the bathroom again, he may enter from the corridor side, as the next patient would not be using it immediately. (A certain amount of clean up time and prep is required before examining the next patient.)

In addition to a toilet room, an R/F room must have a barium prep area, which is a countertop with sink and plaster trap for preparation of barium or contrast media and an under-counter refrigerator. This may be done within the procedure room as in Figure 5-5, or it may be an area outside the room, as shown in Figure 5-7.

The fluoroscopy room is the workroom for the radiologist. He or she will watch the TV monitor as the patient is turned in different positions, and the contrast medium moves through the organs.

The size of the fluoroscopy room is largely determined by the amount of ceiling equipment. The ceiling tube-mount (Figure 5-26) moves on ceiling-mounted tracks, supported by a Unistrut system above the finished ceiling. When a room has a table that tilts (Figure 5-27) and a ceiling-mounted tube-stand, a 10-foot ceiling height may be required.

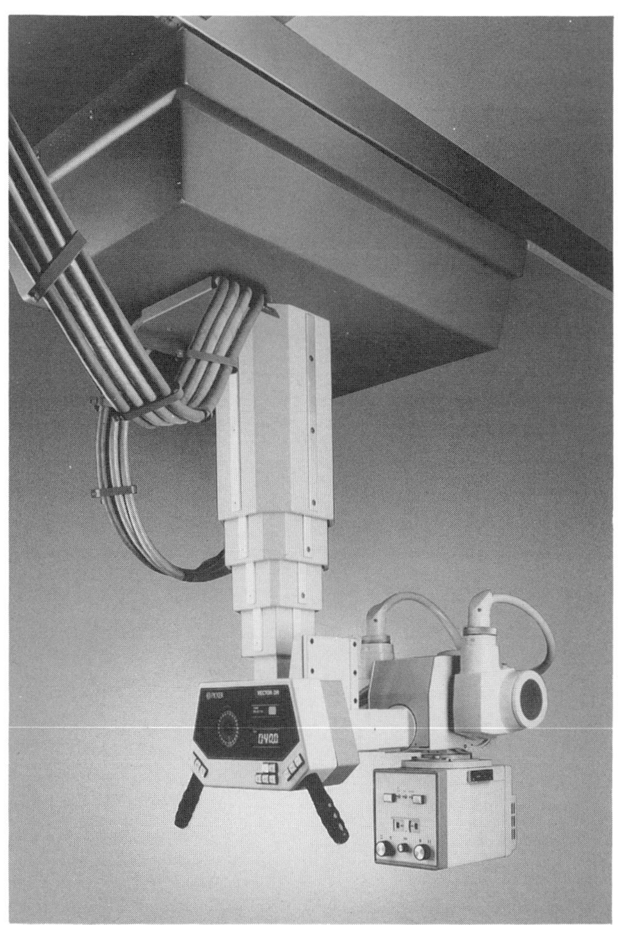

Figure 5-26. Ceiling tube-mount. (*Courtesy Picker International, Highland Heights, OH.*)

Radiography Room without Fluoroscopy

A radiography room without fluoroscopy may be as small as 12 × 16 feet or 14 × 16 feet. The X-ray table shown in Figure 5-28 is a compact one designed for rooms where space is tight. No wall or ceiling mounting is required because support tracks and the X-ray tube-column are mounted directly to the table. If a radiography room is used by a technologist only (as is often the case), the room may be smaller than if it is used by

Figure 5-27. Radiography/Fluoroscopy system. (*Courtesy Siemens Medical Systems, Inc., Iselin, NJ.*)

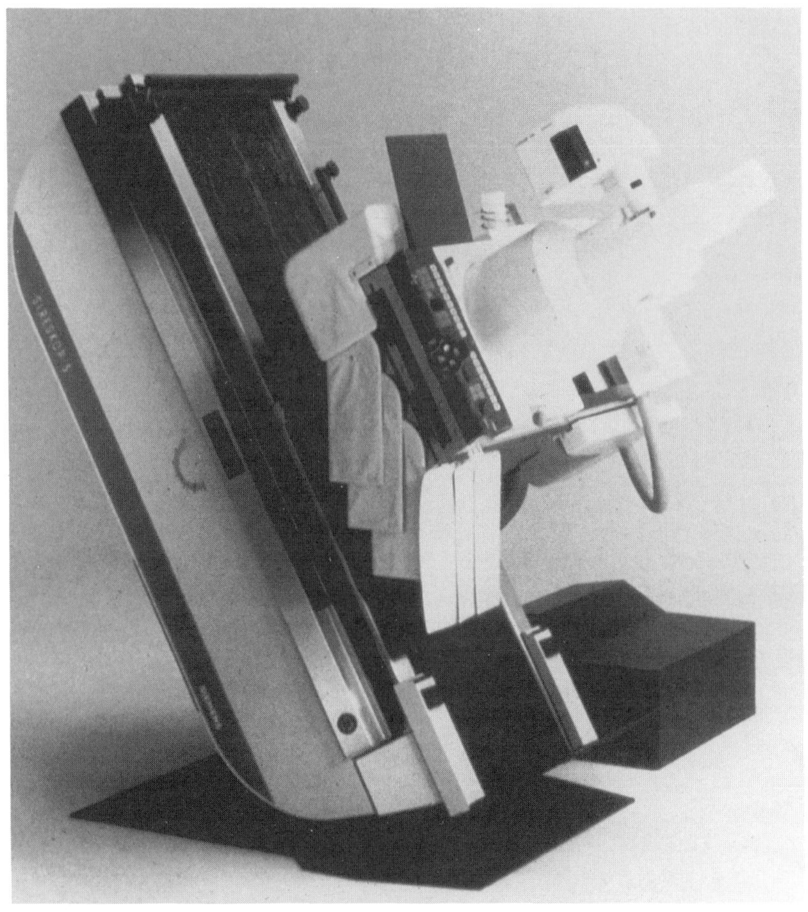

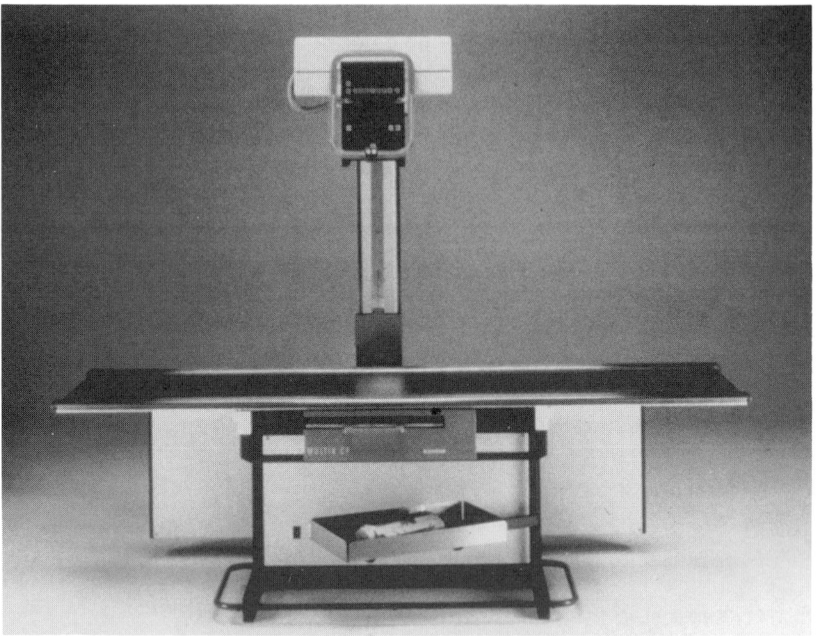

Figure 5-28. Radiography unit, compact model. (*Courtesy Siemens Medical Systems, Inc., Iselin, NJ.*)

the radiologist, who may do special procedures requiring more than one person to be in the room and perhaps use additional portable equipment.

Chest films would typically be done in this room. A wall-mounted film holder, called a *bucky,* would be located at the "head" end of the X-ray table. Another common procedure, an IVP (*intravenous pyelogram*), used to study the kidneys, uterus, and bladder, is performed in a general radiographic room that has tomographic capabilities. For these studies, a bathroom must be nearby, but need not be attached to the room.

Radiography rooms without fluoroscopy need not have sinks, but do require a cabinet and shelves for storage of patient positioning devices such as sandbags and foam wedges, and for disposable items needed for procedures.

The door to a radiography room must be large enough to move equipment in and out. It should be noted that a lead-lined door is very heavy and will require a heavy-duty closer. Figure 5-5 shows a 3-foot-wide door with a 4-foot-wide frame and a 1-foot dead panel (lead-lined) that can be removed when equipment has to be brought into, or removed from, the room. Figure 5-7 shows 42-inch-wide doors, without the dead panel.

As with any radiographic equipment, the space planner must consider the weight in order to design the floor to support it. As an example, the R/F table shown in Figure 5-29 weighs close to 3000 pounds.

Lead Shielding. Once a radiology suite is designed, a radiation physicist must be consulted to prepare a study of lead shielding requirements. In order to do this, the physicist will need to know full specifications on the equipment for each room, the anticipated volume of films, the location of a particular X-ray room with respect to adjacent rooms in the suite, and the location of the suite itself within the medical office building.

For example, if a radiology room is on the third floor of a building and has two exterior walls, the lead shielding requirements would be considerably different than if the room were contiguous with an office where someone sits at a desk all day. If the suite is located on the ground floor of a building and the radiography room is on an exterior wall, with passersby walking to a parking lot, the physicist evaluates the volume of foot traffic and the amount of exposure in order to "protect the genes of future populations." Of course, placement of equipment in the room will determine the direction of radiation scatter.

Figure 5-29. Radiography/Fluoroscopy system. (*Courtesy Picker International, Highland Heights, OH.*)

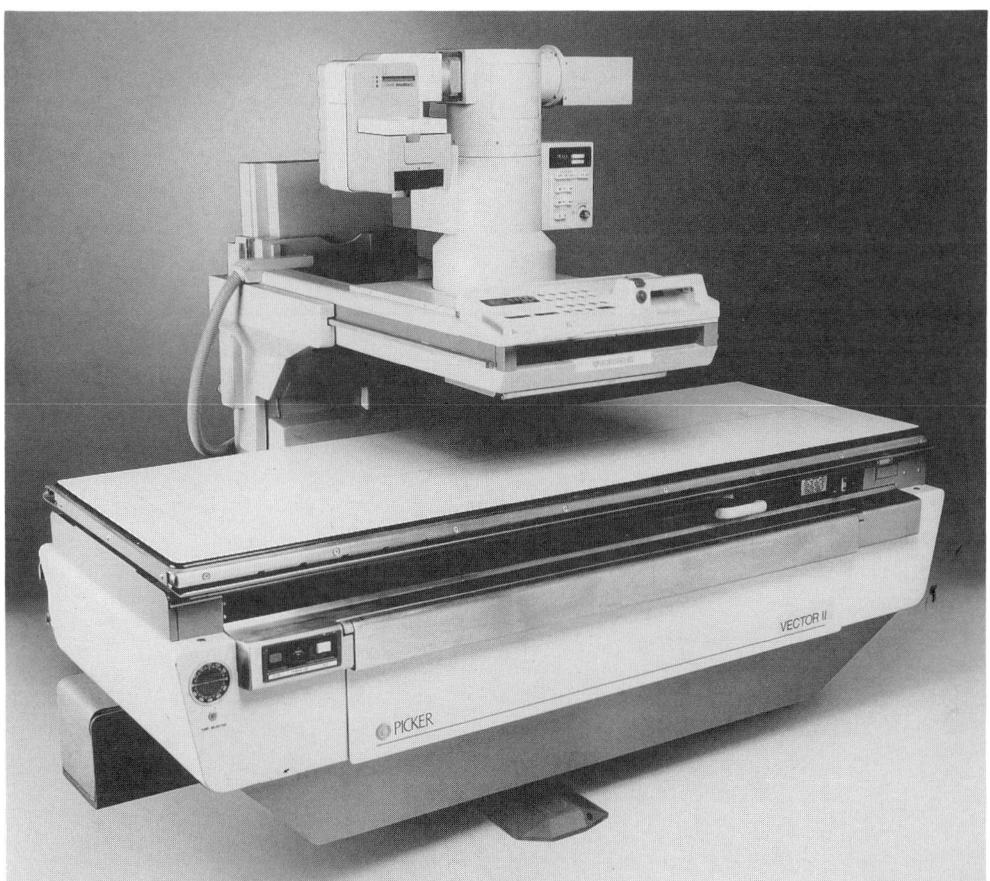

Odor Control. To prevent the spread of odors from the R/F rooms and darkroom, the ventilation system should be designed so that a negative air pressure, relative to adjoining corridors, is maintained. This can be accomplished by exhausting more air from these rooms than is supplied to them, and by reversing this procedure in the corridors. *Air from fluoroscopic radiography rooms should not be recirculated when these rooms are in use, unless adequate odor removal equipment is incorporated in the ventilation system.*

Emergency Precautions. When laying out a radiology suite, thought must be given to the possible evacuation of a patient on a stretcher. Since most radiology suites are located on the ground floor, this may be accomplished by a secondary exit that leads directly to the parking lot, enabling an ambulance to pick up a patient without the patient having to be carried through the waiting room or the building lobby. Additionally, resuscitation equipment on a crash cart should be readily available to the procedure rooms. Radiologists sometimes request emergency call buzzers for procedure rooms, patient dressing rooms, and toilet rooms. The annunciator panel would be located at the reception desk.

Lighting. There should be two types of lighting in an R/F room: overhead fluorescents and indirect perimeter lighting, switched separately. Perimeter lighting should be able to be dimmed, as fluoroscopy procedures are done in a dark or dimly lit room.

ULTRASOUND

Since ultrasound does not use radiation, there is no need for lead shielding. The room may be as small as 10 × 12 feet or 10 × 14 feet in size. The patient lies on a physical therapy type table, and the technologist works to the right side of the patient. The equipment is portable (Figure 5-30), approximately 24 × 34 × 54 inches high, and consists of microprocessor, videotape recorder, video printer, multiformat camera, and TV monitor. The equipment has no special electrical requirements, except for a dedicated circuit. However, the room is darkened for the procedure, and an ideal type of lighting would be indirect perimeter lighting that can be dimmed.

An ultrasound room must have a toilet immediately adjacent, to accommodate voiding studies of the bladder. A cabinet with sink should be provided in the ultrasound room.

NUCLEAR MEDICINE

Nuclear imaging equipment is not commonly found in the outpatient setting. Hospitals generally have a multiple-room nuclear medicine department such as that shown in Figure 5-31. Statistics indicate that 75 percent of nuclear medicine imaging is hospital-based. This discussion, then, will familiarize the reader with the type of nuclear imaging equipment that will occasionally be found in an outpatient radiology facility.

While there are numerous variables in equipment, these are the basic components:

1. Computer console
2. Workstation
3. Gamma camera
4. Columnator and stands
5. Patient bed (may be part of detector stand)

A nuclear imaging room does not require lead shielding, as the gamma camera emits no radiation; it picks

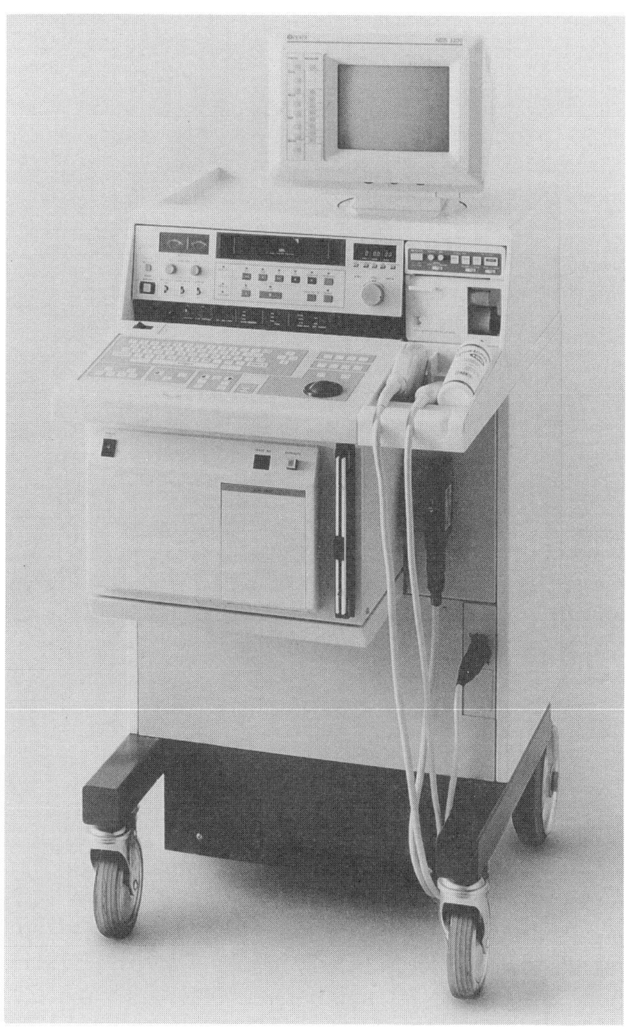

Figure 5-30. Ultrasound imaging system. (*Courtesy Picker International, Highland Heights, OH.*)

up the small amount of radioactivity released by the organ being imaged. (The patient ingests or is injected with a small amount of a radiopharmaceutical that travels through the bloodstream to the specific organ being studied.)

There are many types of nuclear medicine scans, including bone scans, liver scans, thyroid scans, lung scans, and gallbladder scans, to name a few. The time between administering the radioactive compound and taking the scan may vary, depending on the compound used and how long it takes to accumulate in the part of the body being studied. Some scans are performed a few hours after the injection, while others may be performed immediately. The scan itself may take any-

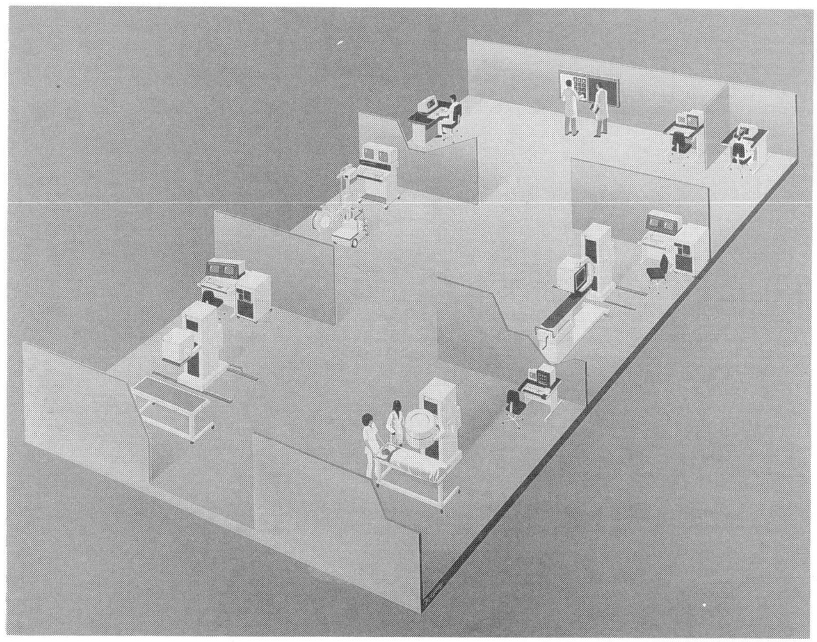

Figure 5-31. Hospital nuclear medicine department. (*Courtesy Picker International, Highland Heights, OH.*)

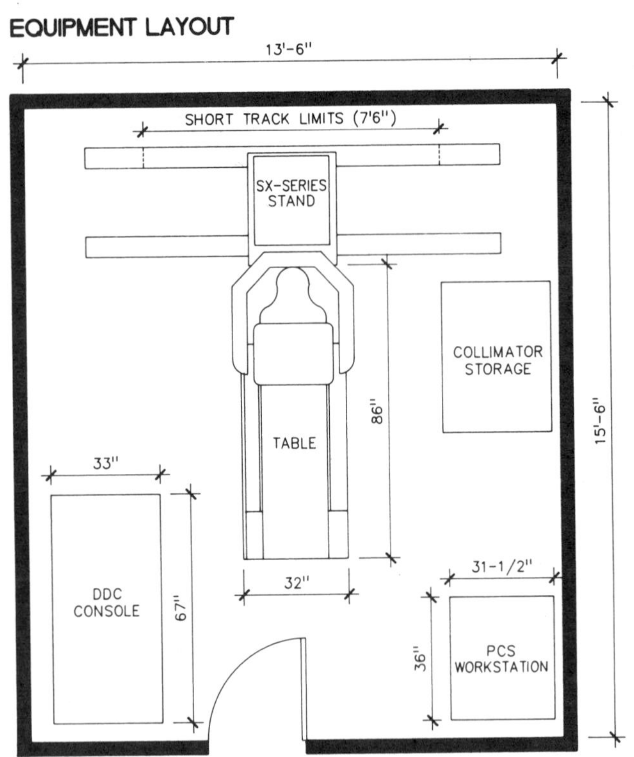

Figure 5-32. Layout, nuclear imaging room. (*Courtesy Picker International, Highland Heights, OH.*)

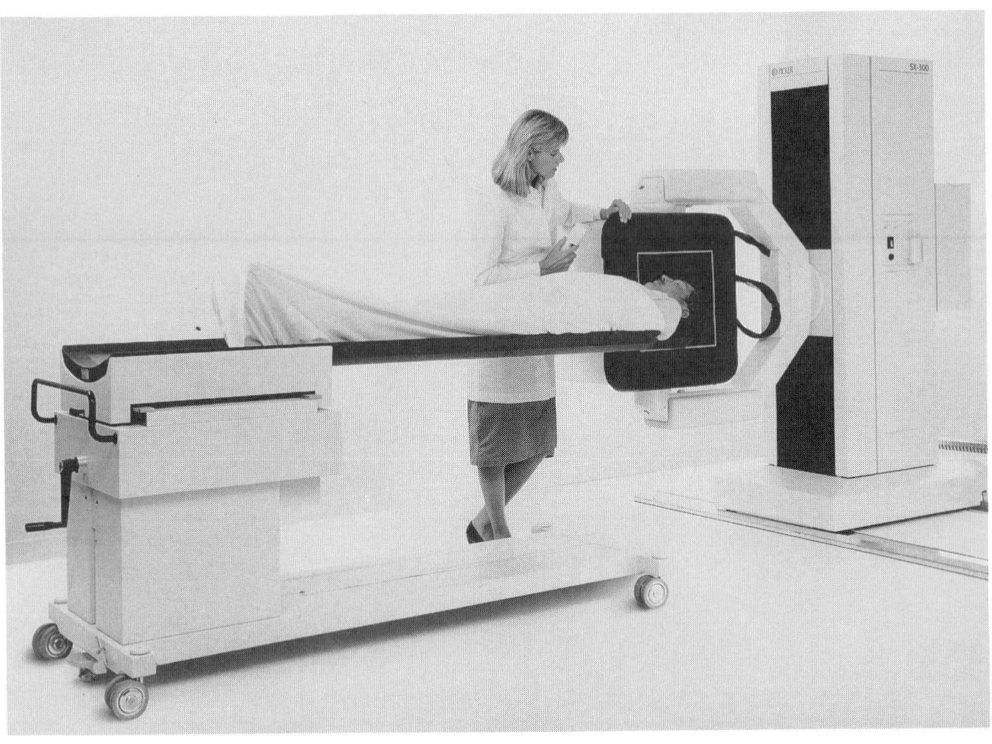

Figure 5-33. Nuclear imaging system. (*Courtesy Picker International, Highland Heights, OH.*)

where from 30 minutes to two hours, again depending upon the part of the body being studied. Figure 5-32 shows the manufacturer's suggested layout for equipment shown in Figure 5-33, whereas Figures 5-34 and 5-35 are layouts for another manufacturer's nuclear imaging equipment. Note that nuclear imaging consoles vary considerably in size (Figure 5-36).

The space planner may encounter the terminology *SPECT* in regard to nuclear imaging procedures. It refers to *single photon emission computed tomography* capability.

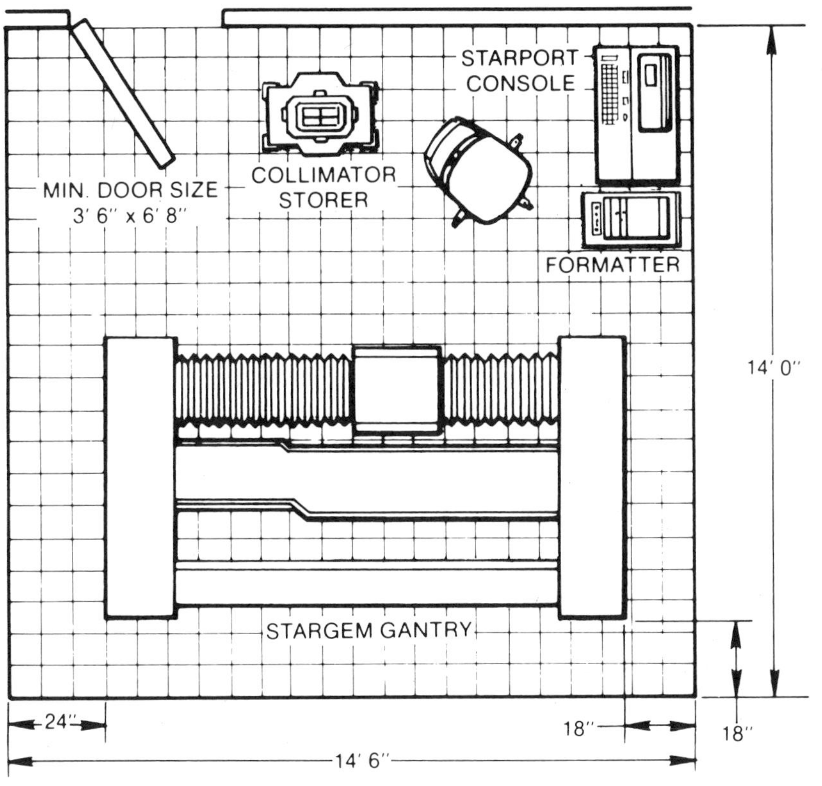

Figure 5-34. Layout, nuclear imaging room. (*Courtesy GE Medical Systems, Milwaukee, WI.*)

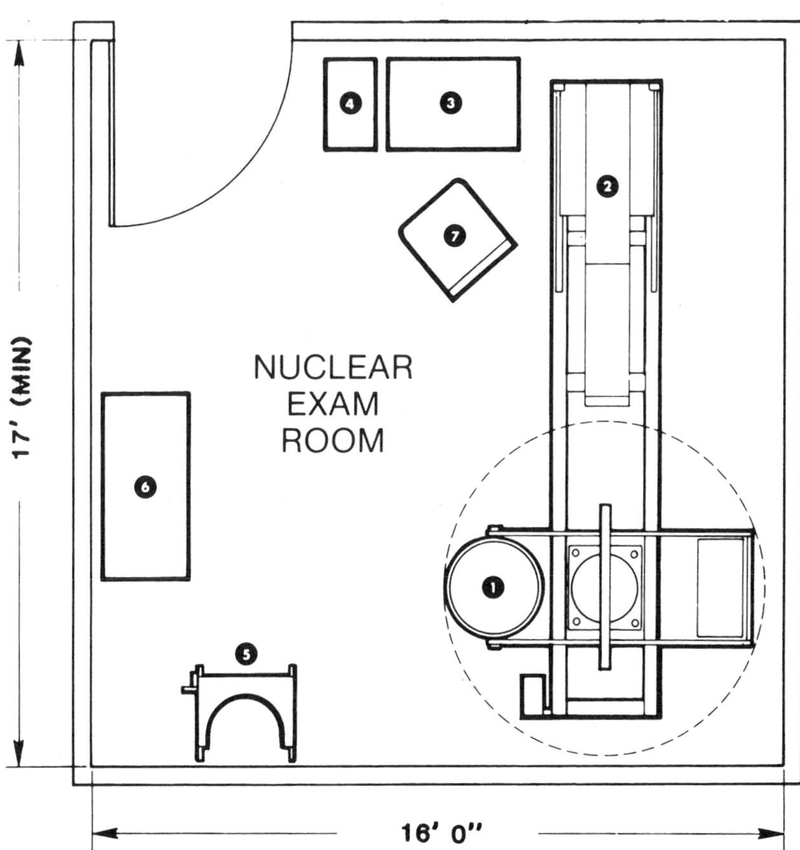

1. Imaging Detector and Counterbalance Assembly
2. ECT, PBC or WB Imaging Table
3. Electronics Console
4. Video Formatter
5. Collimator Crane
6. Collimator Shelf
7. Chair

Figure 5-35. Layout, nuclear imaging room. (*Courtesy GE Medical Systems, Milwaukee, WI.*)

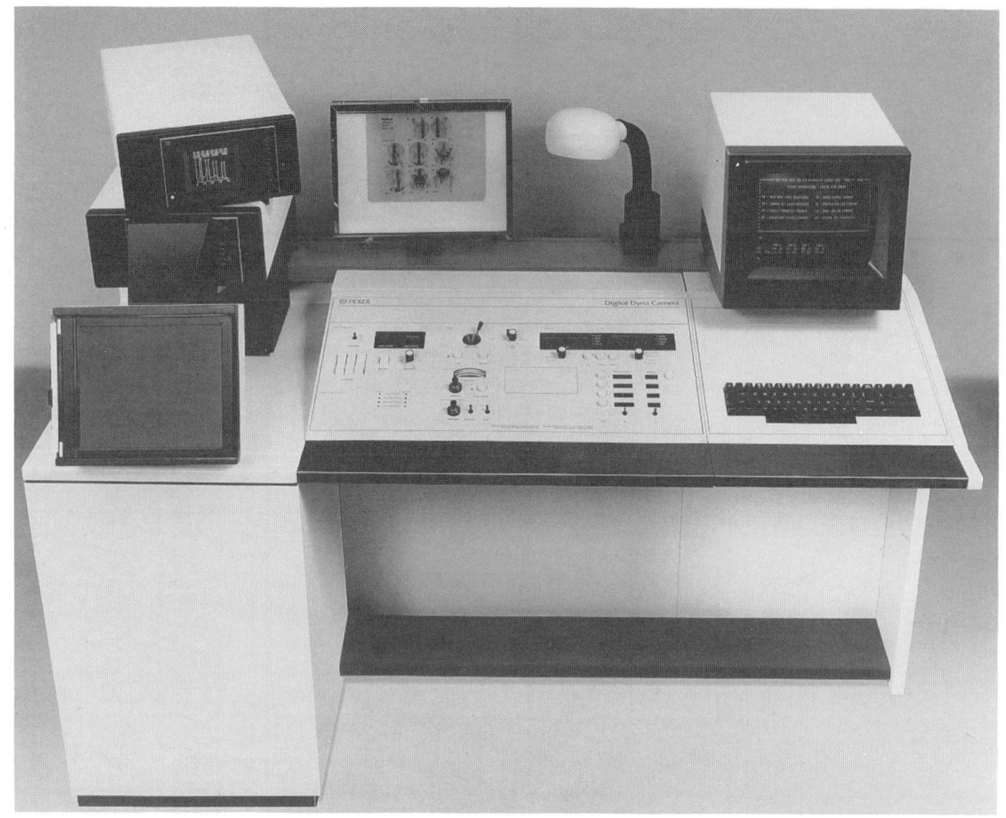

Figure 5-36. Operator's console, nuclear imaging. (*Courtesy Picker International, Highland Heights, OH.*)

Nuclear Stress Test

This is used in conjunction with a dynamic EKG. The room would have a nuclear cardiology unit such as that shown in Figure 5-37, a computer console for the tech (Figure 5-38), and a treadmill or exercise bicycle. A room 12 × 12 feet would be appropriate.

Ventilation Studies

The ventilation lung scan is performed by breathing in, through a mouthpiece, a tasteless, odorless radioactive gas called Xenon. The study shows the location of any obstructions or other types of breathing abnormalities. This can be done in a room as small as 8 × 8 feet. The tech stands at the Xenon delivery system (Figure 5-39), while the patient sits on the other side breathing into a mouthpiece at the end of a hose, attached to the machine. This particular unit features an integral gas trap to assure that room air does not become contaminated.

Tech Shielding

Sometimes tech shielding is required. The nuclear medicine mobile barrier in Figure 5-40 features lead-impregnated acrylic. The oversized window permits unobstructed viewing of the patient. This barrier may be positioned close to the patient table, and it shields the tech from patient-emitted radiation.

Hot Lab

This is a room perhaps no larger than 6 × 8 feet, where radiopharmaceuticals are prepared. This is best located in a part of the suite where there is not a lot of traffic. The room would have 36-inch high countertops

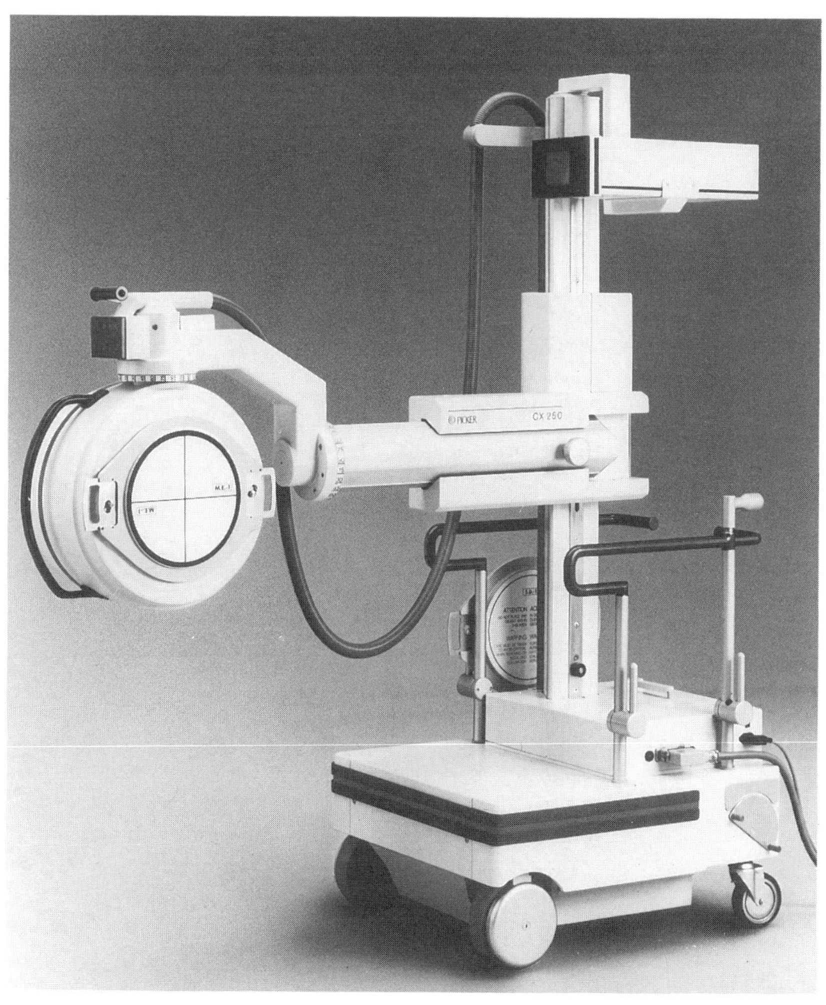

Figure 5-37. Nuclear cardiology imaging unit. (*Courtesy Picker International, Highland Heights, OH.*)

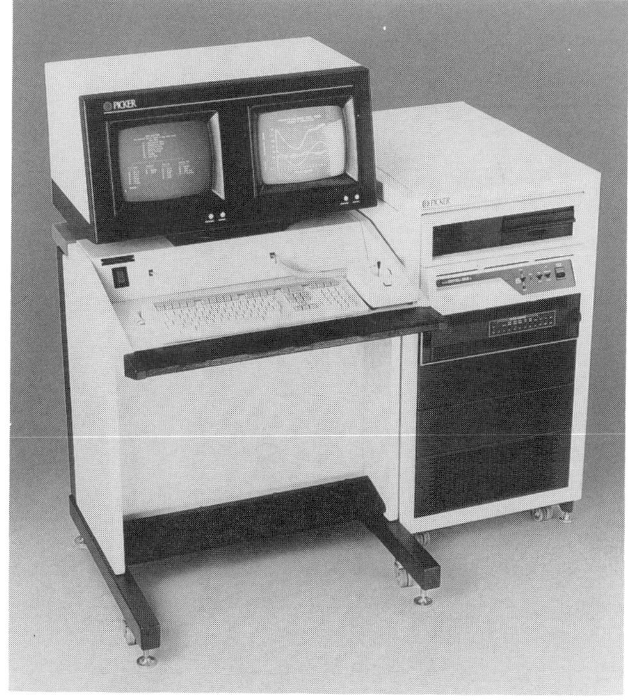

Figure 5-38. Operator's console, nuclear cardiology imaging. (*Courtesy Picker International, Highland Heights, OH.*)

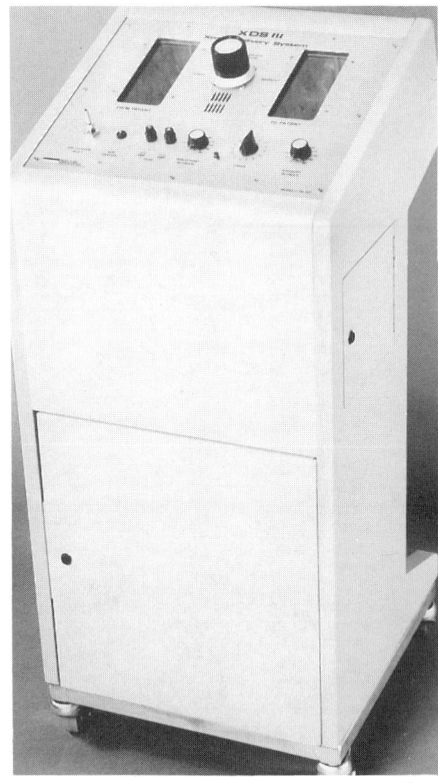

Figure 5-39. Xenon delivery/trap system, used for nuclear ventilation studies. (*Courtesy Nuclear Associates, Carle Place, NY.*)

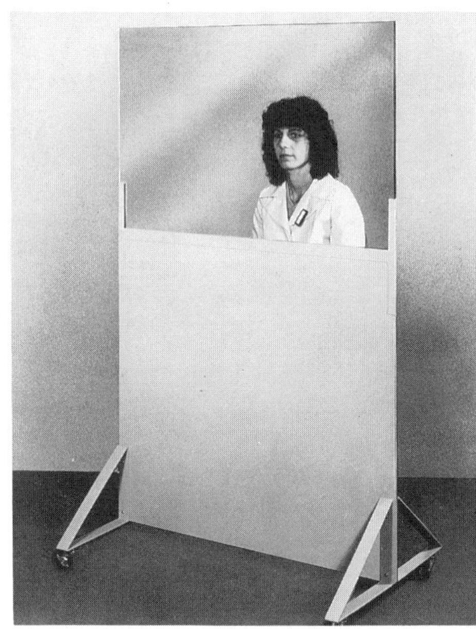

Figure 5-40. *Clear-Pb* nuclear medicine mobile barrier. (*Courtesy Nuclear Associates, Carle Place, NY.*)

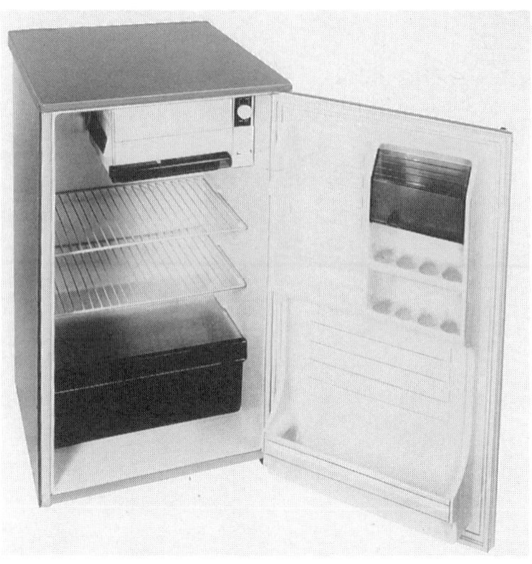

Figure 5-41. Lead-lined refrigerator, for hot lab. (*Courtesy Nuclear Associates, Carle Place, NY.*)

with a single compartment sink, lead-lined under-counter refrigerator (Figure 5-41), with some open shelves and hinged door storage under the countertop. Note that the countertop must be steel reinforced in order to support the interlocking lead bricks (Figure 5-42) that will be placed on it. These may total as much as 500 pounds. It may be more practical to buy a pre-fabricated work bench designed specifically for handling, storing, and disposing of radioactive materials (Figures 5-43 and 5-44). The modules of these work benches are lead-lined and encased in steel. Stainless steel countertops allow for easy cleaning and decontamination.

Radioisotopes are stored in *vial shields* (Figure 5-45) from which the contents are dispensed. Vial shields of radiopharmaceuticals are stored in a small *safe* made up of interlocking lead bricks or in a lead container such as that shown in Figures 5-46 and 5-47.

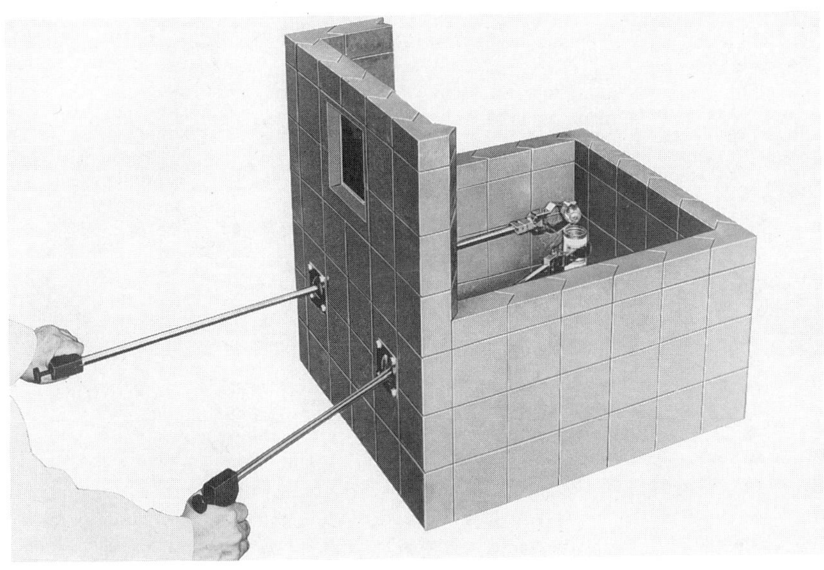

Figure 5-42. Interlocking lead bricks. (*Courtesy Nuclear Associates, Carle Place, NY.*)

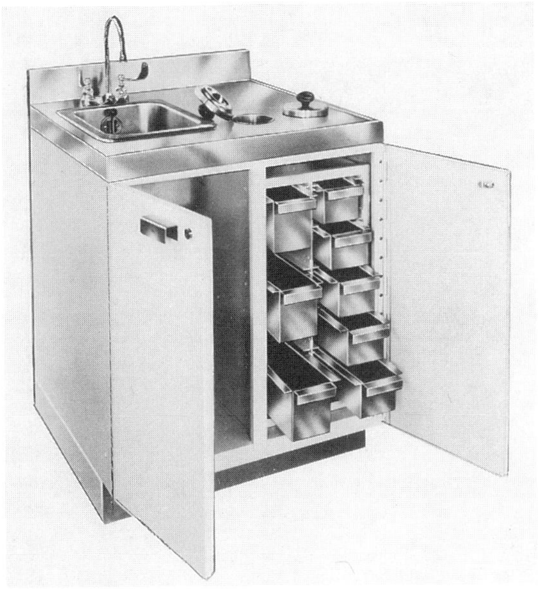

Figure 5-43. Work bench for handling radioactive materials. (*Courtesy Nuclear Associates, Carle Place, NY.*)

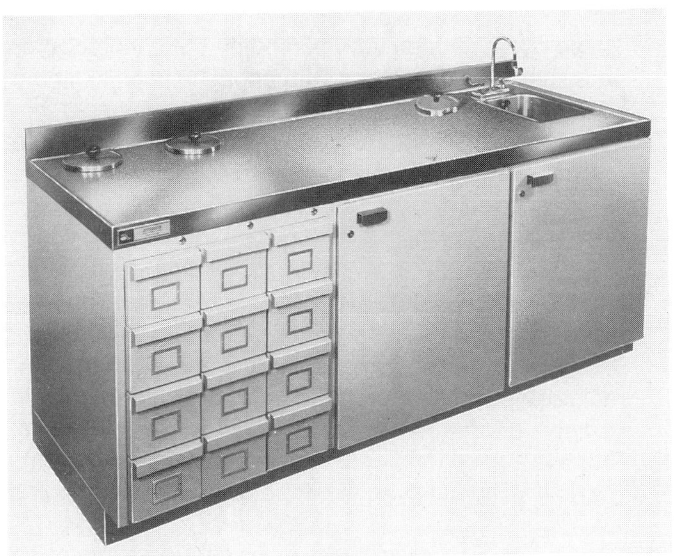

Figure 5-44. Work bench for handling, storing, and disposing of radioactive materials (stainless steel countertop). (*Courtesy Nuclear Associates, Carle Place, NY.*)

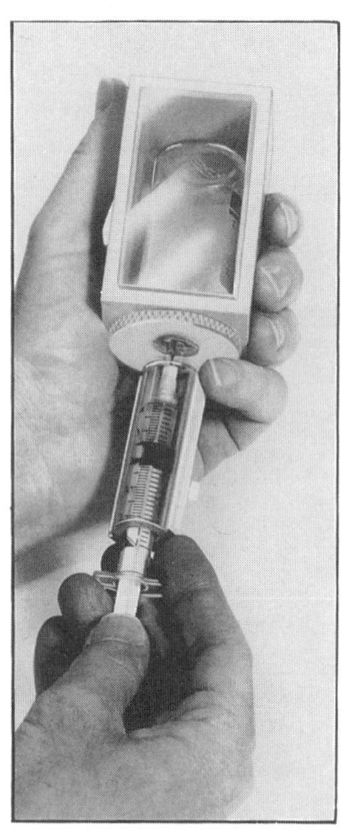

Figure 5-45. Vial shield for viewing, handling, and dispensing radioactive liquids. (*Courtesy Nuclear Associates, Carle Place, NY.*)

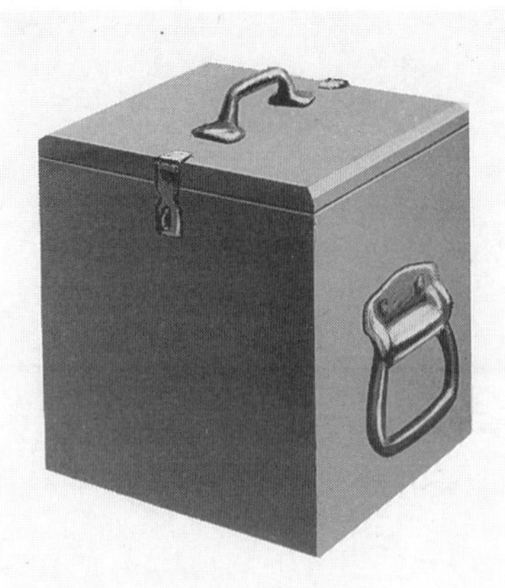

Figure 5-46. Square lead container for storing radioactive materials. (*Courtesy Nuclear Associates, Carle Place, NY.*)

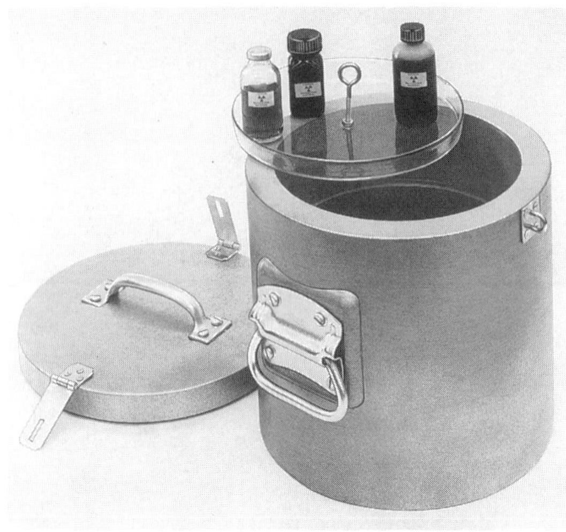

Figure 5-47. Lead storage container (safe) for storing radioactive materials. (*Courtesy Nuclear Associates, Carle Place, NY.*)

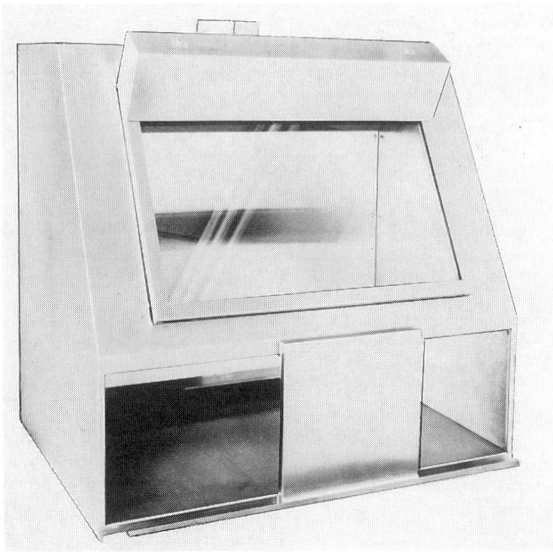

Figure 5-48. Preparation and fume hood enclosure, for hot lab. (*Courtesy Nuclear Associates, Carle Place, NY.*)

These containers may be placed on the countertop or on a shelf under it — one with enough space to lift the lid and access the contents of the safe. Remember that safes range from 125 to 200 pounds in weight. Figure 5-48 shows a preparation and fume hood enclosure which is lead-lined and used for working with gaseous radiopharmaceuticals.

Figures 5-49a and 5-49b show clear *bench-top shields* that provide a protective lead barrier from radiation exposure when working with radionuclides.

Electrical outlets are required over the countertop for radioisotope calibrators (Figure 5-50), the wipe test counter (Figure 5-51), and other accessory items. There is a need for storage of items used to mix agents such as vials and syringes, for gloves, and for gripping tools.

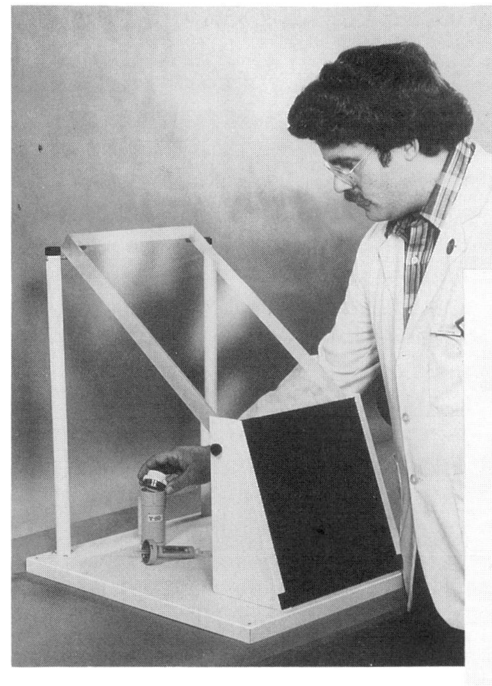

Figure 5-49a. Protective lead barriers for benchtops, hot lab. (*Courtesy Nuclear Associates, Carle Place, NY.*)

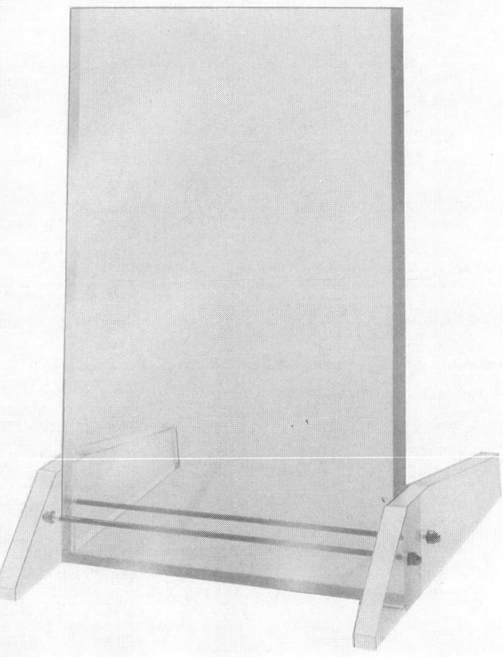

Figure 5-49b. Protective lead barriers for benchtops, hot lab. (*Courtesy Nuclear Associates, Carle Place, NY.*)

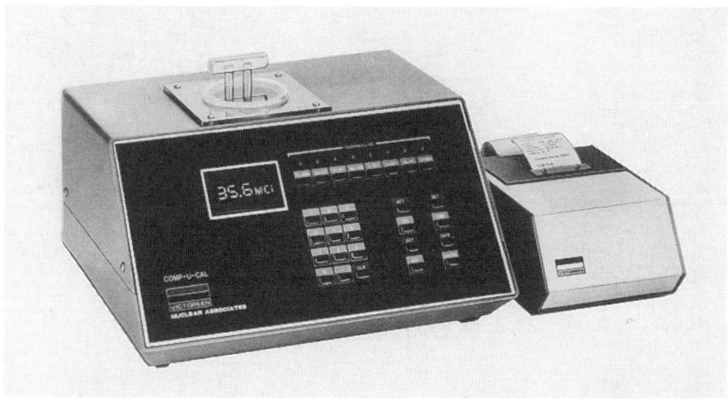

Figure 5-50. Computerized radioisotope calibrator. (*Courtesy Nuclear Associates, Carle Place, NY.*)

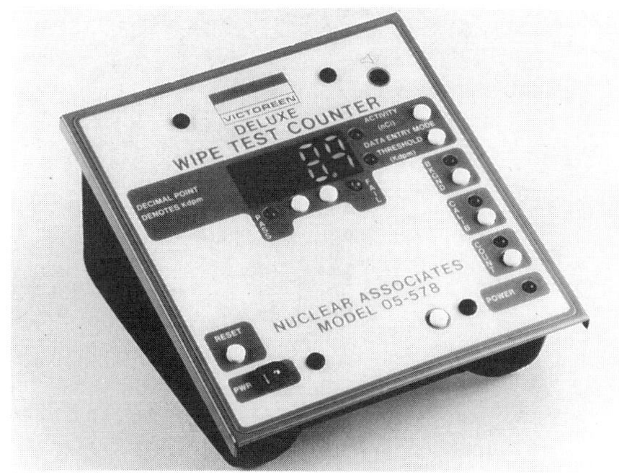

Figure 5-51. Wipe test counter. (*Courtesy Nuclear Associates, Carle Place, NY.*)

Structural Support

Nuclear imaging equipment is very heavy. One manufacturer's specifications state 66 pounds per square inch floor loading for the imaging detector gantry assembly.

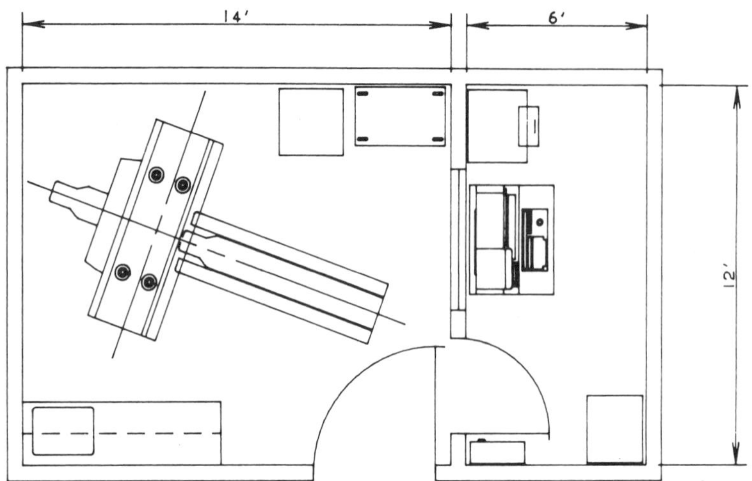

Figure 5-52. *Tomoscan CX™, CT scanner, microprocessor-based system. (Courtesy Philips Medical Systems Inc., Shelton, CT.)*

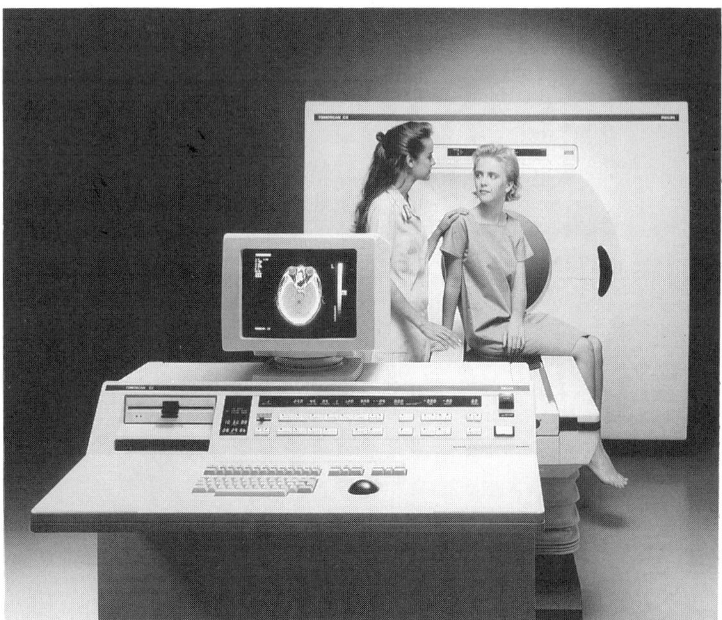

COMPUTED TOMOGRAPHY

The CT suite consists of a scanner or procedure room, an equipment room, a control room, and a diagnostic room. Manufacturers will supply engineering data sheets with alternative suggested layouts, critical dimensions, floor loading, and utility requirements.

There is a difference, in terms of space planning requirements, between CT systems based on large mainframe computers, and those that are microprocessor-based. Those with a large computer require a separate equipment room with a raised floor for access to cables and special climate control.

However, there is a trend toward microprocessor-based systems, which makes possible a reduction in the size of all components. Additionally, the microprocessor (computer) may be incorporated in the operator's console. A raised computer floor is no longer necessary, nor is special climate control. The equipment in Figures 5-52 and 5-53 is of this type. Another advantage to microprocessor-based systems is that they can be retrofitted into an existing radiography room (provided the size is correct) without major expense in terms of construction modification.

There are options with respect to how and where the radiologist views the CT scans. The finished films may, of course, be viewed on standard view box illuminators, but if the radiologist wants to manipulate the image (by changing contrast or by enlarging or reducing it in order to study a portion of the diseased organ more closely), he or she will have to work at the operator's control console or at a separate diagnostic viewing console, as shown in suite plan Figure 5-7.

While a CT suite used to occupy approximately 900 square feet of space, manufacturers have continually worked to reduce the amount of space required, without sacrificing image quality or restricting the range of procedures. The average space requirement currently is 600 to 650 square feet, while the unit shown in Figure 5-52 can be installed in as little as 240 square feet and that in Figure 5-53 requires only 340 square feet.

The space planner should note that these are minimum space requirements, and larger spaces may be desirable. Remember that, for patient safety, sufficient access around the scanning unit must be maintained in case a patient becomes ill to allow the resuscitation team unobstructed access.

The *procedure room* is where the scanner gantry is located. The patient is positioned on a table that slides back and forth under a rotating doughnut-like enclosure. The size of the procedure room will vary with different brands of equipment, but 15 × 20 or 18 × 20 feet is an average. In addition to the gantry, the room needs a built-in cabinet with sink, and storage for clean linen, patient positioning devices, contrast media, and IV materials. A cart for soiled linen is also required. An 8-foot-long base cabinet with a wall cabinet above would be adequate. A couple of drawers might be partitioned for storage of alcohol preps, disposable syringes, injectables, contrast media, tubes, tape, and vomit pan.

The ceiling of the room is normally 9-feet 6-inches high and the door should be at least 48-inches wide, with heavy-duty closer. The walls and door will have to be lead-shielded according to recommendations of the radiation physicist.

Room lighting must be controlled by a dimmer. Indirect lighting around the perimeter of the room will keep glare out of the patient's eyes. The massive size of this equipment can be frightening to patients, even though it does not have exposed cables or clutter. A room with cheerful colors and a mural or artwork on the walls would be comforting.

The *equipment room* is where the computer would be located, if the equipment is not microprocessor-based. This room must be air-conditioned and humidity controlled. Normally located adjacent to the control room, it often has sliding glass doors so that one can see into it (see Figure 5-2). The room should be well illuminated since this is where a technician has to work when the unit needs repair.

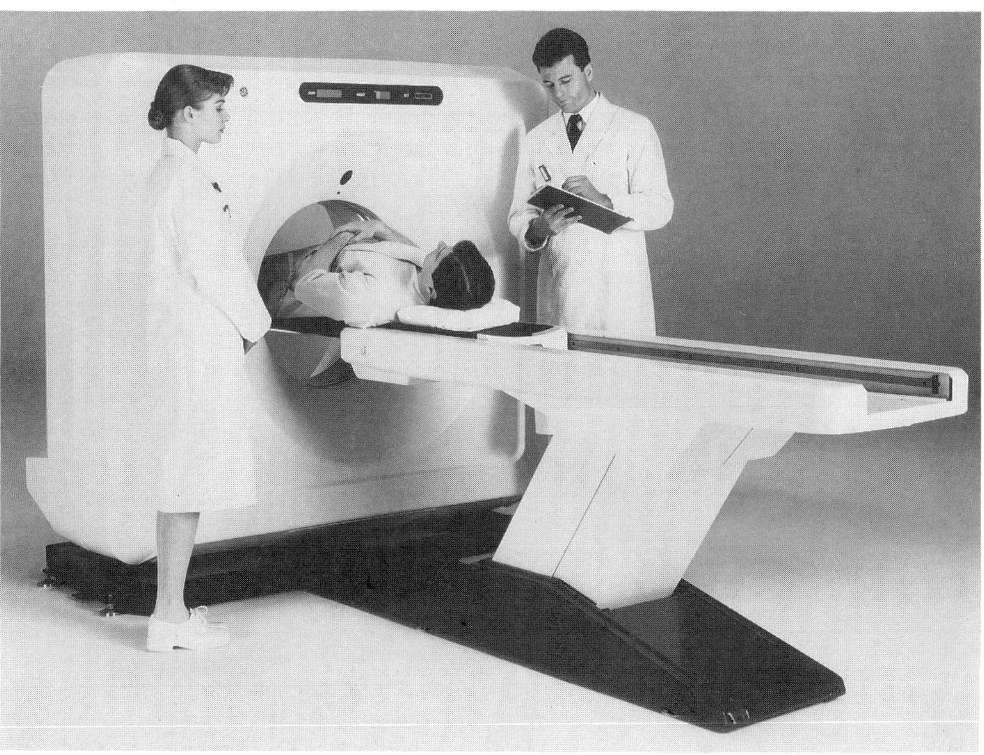

Figure 5-53. *CT Pace*™ scanner system, microprocessor-based. (*Courtesy GE Medical Systems, Milwaukee, WI.*)

The *control room* is where the technologist sits during the procedure. It must have a lead-shielded window facing the procedure room so that the patient is always in view. The operator's console is located here (Figure 5-52). The dimmer control for room lighting should be accessible from the control room. Although the size of this room depends upon the brand of equipment and the number of accessory items to be accommodated, 8 × 10 or 8 × 12 feet is usually adequate.

It should be noted that the pass boxes within the general diagnostic radiology area of the facility can be used for CT; it is not necessary to provide a dedicated pass box.

The *diagnostic viewing room* is where the radiologist works. This may be part of the CT suite as shown in Figure 5-7, or it may be located remotely in another part of the clinic. As explained above, scans may be read at the radiologist's viewing room, or the radiologist may work at a CT viewing console.

After the scanner has scanned the patient's tissue, multiple images are reconstructed by the computer and appear on the diagnostic viewing console (VDT screen). It is here that the radiologist makes the diagnosis. It is interesting to note that the entire examination is held in the computer's memory, and hard copies (X-ray films) are made with a multiformat camera after the patient has been released.

Alongside the viewing console, or at right angles to it, should be a built-in countertop work surface with multiple film illuminators mounted above and film sorting compartments below it. Room lighting should be indirect (eliminates glare on VDT screens) and able to be dimmed.

Storage of magnetic tapes should be provided either in the equipment room or the control room. A small bookcase for technical manuals may be located in the control room or the viewing room.

MAMMOGRAPHY

A room of 10 × 12 or 12 × 12 feet is adequate for a mammography room. Most manufacturers' equipment is approximately the same size, except the unit made by Xerox (the technique is called *Xerography*) has its own processor which sits in the same room (Figure 5-54). There will generally be a built-in cabinet in the room, but there is no need specifically for a sink, provided that there is a sink somewhere nearby for technologists to wash their hands. Mammography examinations are often performed in a women's center, as shown in Figure 5-2.

An independent daylight processing unit is ideal here so that the tech does not need to leave the patient and travel to the darkroom to process the film. Mammography equipment incorporates an attached leaded-glass protective screen behind which the operator stands. There are no unusual utility requirements for this equipment, and sometimes the walls may not need to be lead-shielded. As with any radiography equipment, however, a radiation physicist must be consulted.

A radiology suite having two or more mammography rooms often has equipment by more than one manufacturer, as some units are reputedly better for examining the chest wall, and others are preferred for exposing tumors in soft tissue.

Film processors, located within the room, produce considerable heat and may require two air exhausts. Specifications for each manufacturer's equipment must be studied carefully.

Indirect lighting (Figure 5-54), is optimal for this type of room, and decorative wallpaper, carpeting, and attractive artwork make the patient's experience more pleasant (Figure 5-55).

RADIATION ONCOLOGY

Also known as radiation therapy, radiation oncology is designed to bombard tumors with high doses of radiation. This tends to be a hospital-based modality and

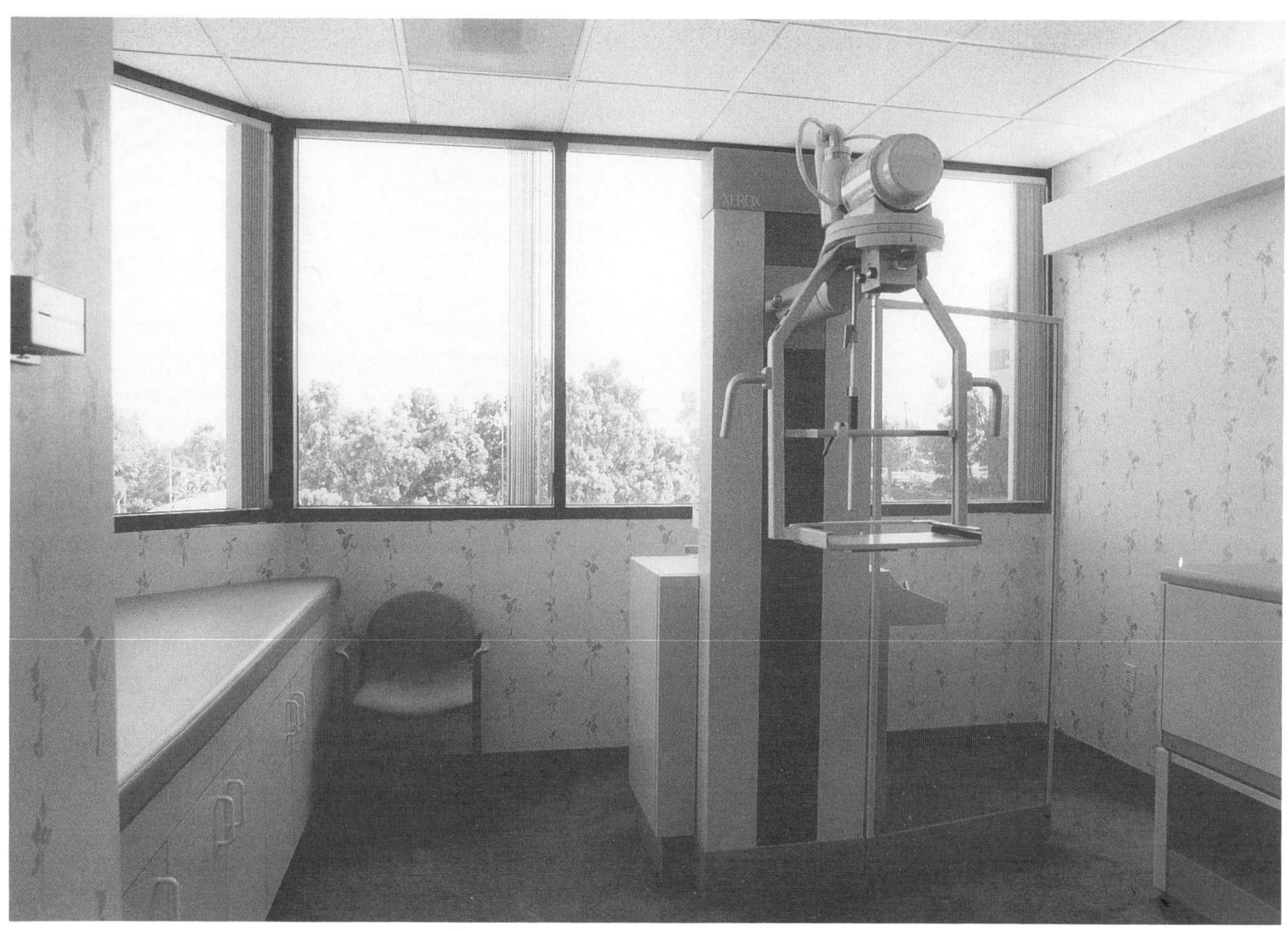

Figure 5-54. Mammography room with Xerox system. (*Design: Jain Malkin Inc.; Photographer: John Christian.*)

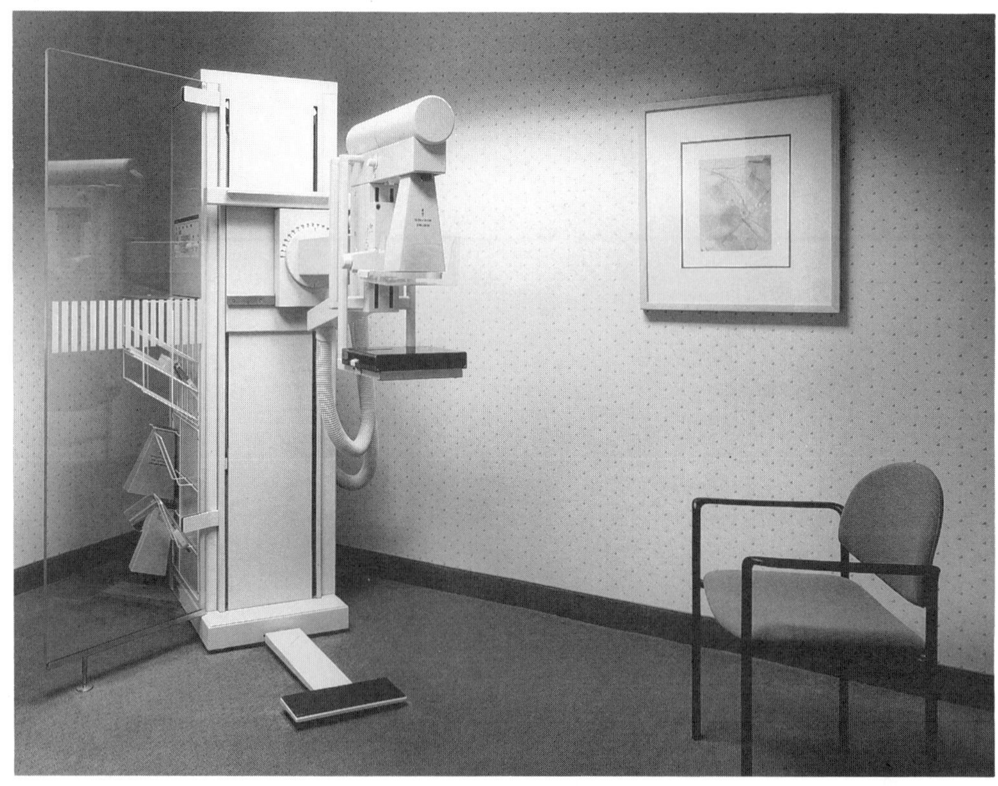

Figure 5-55. Mammography room with Philips system. (*Design: Jain Malkin Inc.; Photographer: Kim Brun.*)

is not commonly found in a medical office building. However, there is no reason why it cannot be located in a medical office building except that it is mandatory that this tenant be identified while the building shell is being planned.

The room containing the linear accelerator (Figures 5-56 and 5-57), will have concrete walls of varying thickness of anywhere from 24 to 36 inches. Sometimes this room can be situated on the site where the ground slopes, to enable the room to be either partially or totally underground, reducing somewhat the radiation shielding requirements.

The radiation therapy suite in Figure 5-3 illustrates the required ancillary rooms. Patients arriving for therapy may be ambulatory or may arrive on a gurney; therefore, both types of traffic must be accommodated. It is desirable to have a dedicated sub–waiting area for radiation therapy so that those patients need not wait with diagnostic radiology patients. Radiation treatment often results in hair loss and skin irritation, sometimes making people self-conscious about their appearance.

Dressing rooms need to be provided, as do examination rooms, radiation physicist's office, and tech work area. The tech work area has TV monitors that allow techs to view patients in the therapy room. Some suites may have a conference room in which the physicist, radiation technologists, and other members of the treatment team can meet to plan treatment for each patient. All rooms of this suite may be carpeted. The treatment room is greatly enhanced by special design features, such as the *trompe l'oeil* (fool the eye) mural shown in Figure 5-57, which is so realistic, it provides a psychological escape for the patient.

MAGNETIC RESONANCE IMAGING

Magnetic resonance imaging (MRI) is considered by many to be the most revolutionary imaging technology of the century. Manufacturers of radiology equipment have committed large sums of money to engineering, research, and product development to continually expand the capabilities of MRI. For example, advances in magnet technology have continually reduced the area of magnetic field influence (the *Gauss field*) surrounding the equipment.

This discussion is aimed at acquainting readers with the basic principles of MRI facility planning and design. As each brand of equipment varies in terms of magnet size, space requirements, extent of magnetic field protection required, radio frequency (RF) shielding requirements, system dimensions and weight, and environmental conditions, the manufacturer's MRI planning division must be consulted for specific guidelines.

Planning Considerations

Imaging magnets are of three types: *resistive, permanent,* and *superconducting.* As the trend seems to be toward the larger superconductive magnets (Figures 5-58 and 5-59), planning considerations for other types of magnets will not be discussed.

A number of issues must be evaluated before defining the site for an MRI facility.

1. Magnet's effect on the surrounding environment
2. Environment's effect on the magnet
3. Corridor/door sizes for transport of magnet during installation

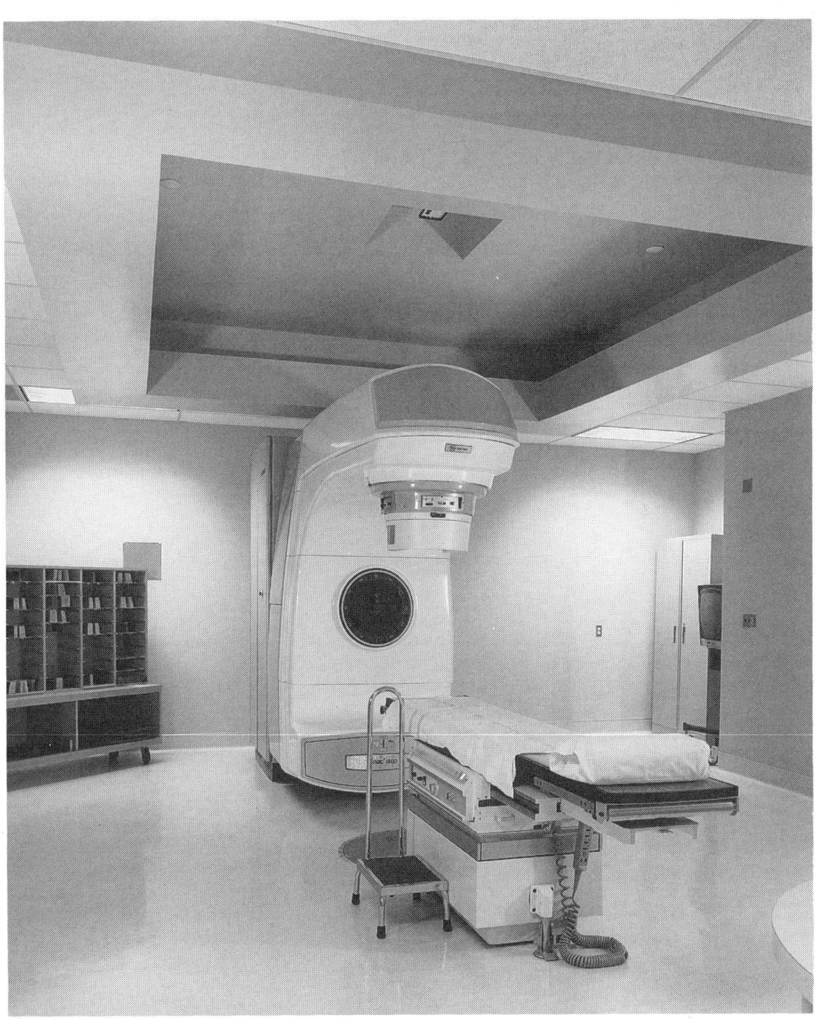

Figure 5-56. Linear accelerator, radiation therapy room. (*Interior Design: Jain Malkin Inc.; Architecture: Brown Leary Associates; Photographer: John Christian.*)

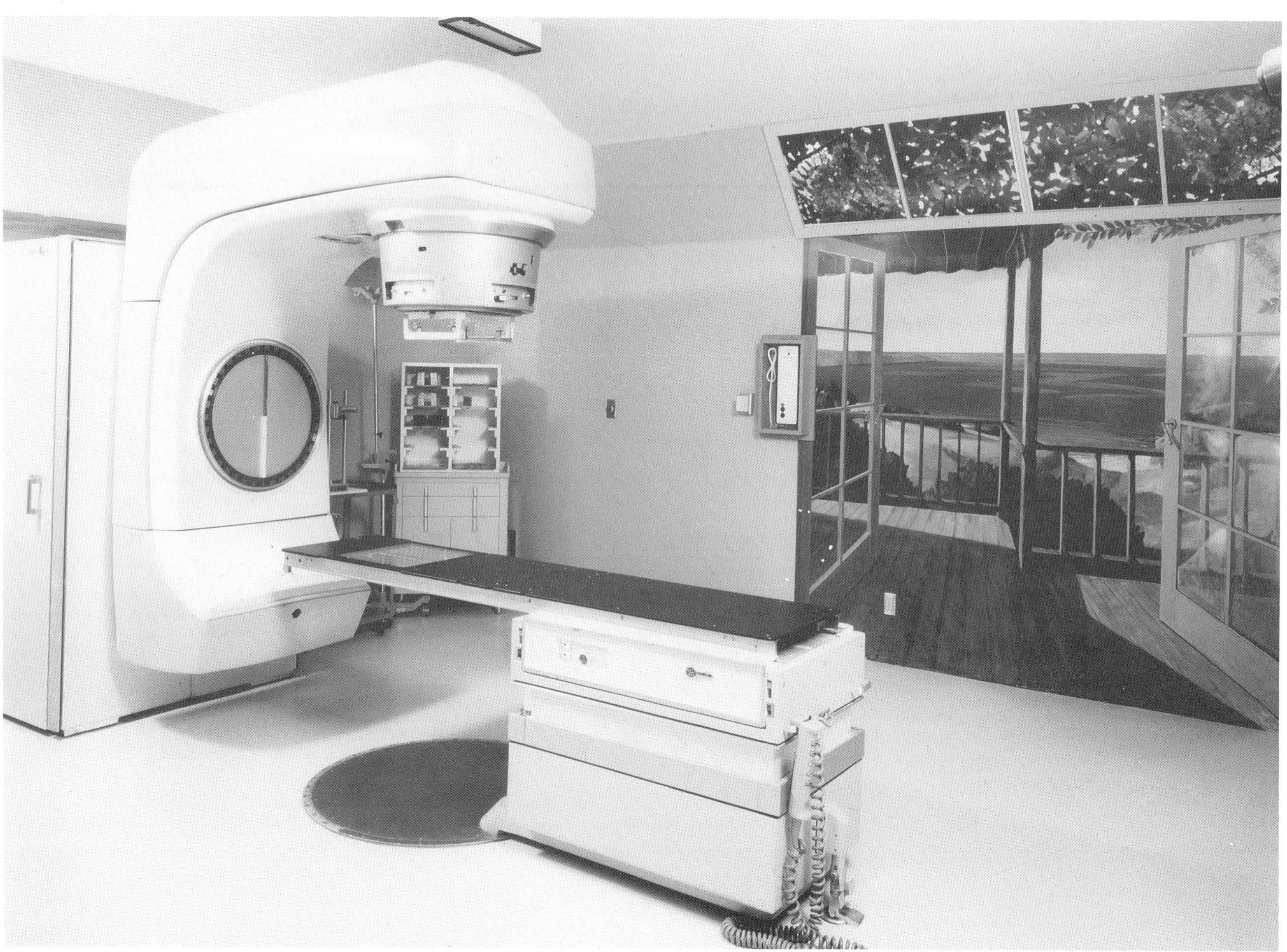

Figure 5-57. (*facing page*) Linear accelerator, radiation therapy room. Note *trompe l'oeil* mural, providing a psychological escape. (*Design: Jain Malkin Inc.; Photographer: John Christian; Cibachrome films in lenses of light fixtures: Joey Fischer.*)

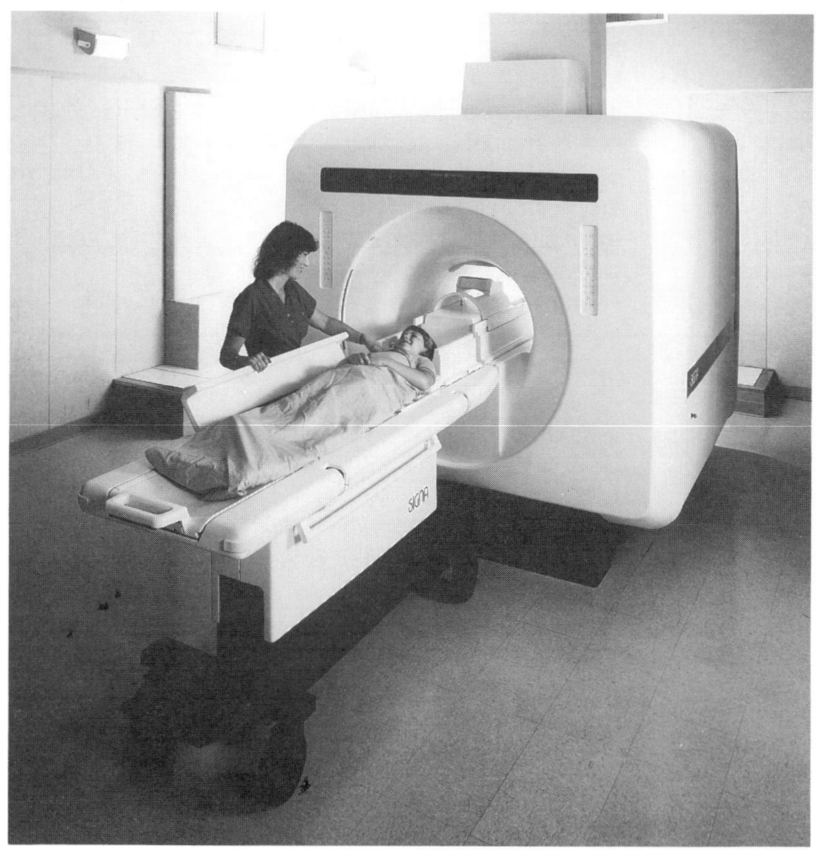

Figure 5-58. Magnetic resonance imaging system. (*Courtesy GE Medical Systems, Milwaukee, WI.*)

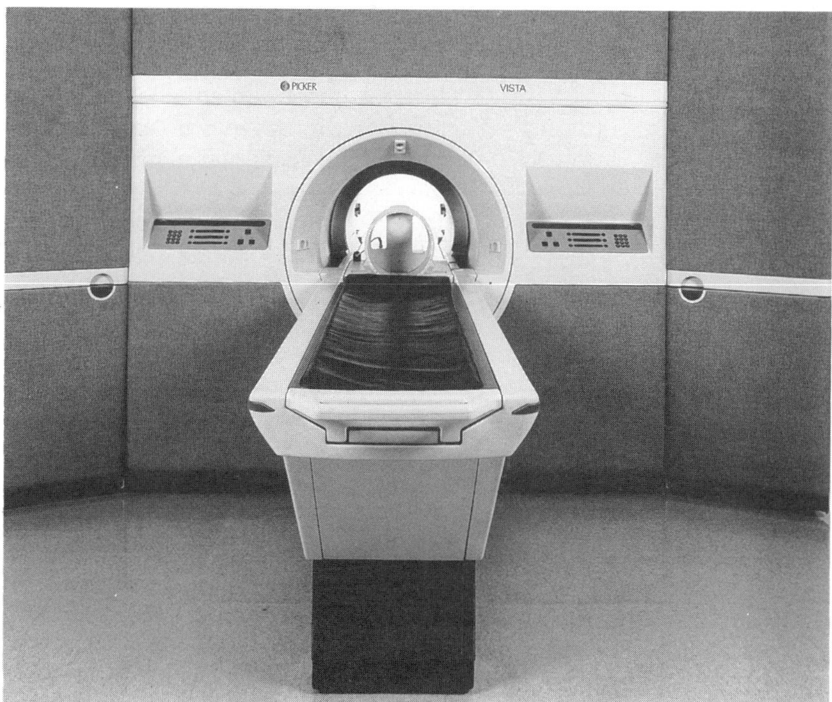

Figure 5-59. Magnetic resonance imaging system. (*Courtesy Picker International, Highland Heights, OH.*)

4. Convenient access for filling of dewars, for magnet cryogen replenishment, and for servicing the equipment
5. Area of magnetic field influence
6. RFI shielding
7. HVAC
8. Power requirements
9. Floor loading
10. Interior design

Magnet's Effect on Environment. The influence of a strong magnetic field upon the surrounding environment is illustrated in Figure 5-60. It is important to protect the immediate environment from the effect of the magnetic field. People with heart pacemakers are especially vulnerable, as are any sort of electronic or electromagnetic systems. Information on credit cards or magnetic tapes may be erased.

Magnetic fields are three-dimensional, extending outward on all sides, above and below, measured from the exact center of the magnet. Related to the magnet's maximum operating field strength, the *fringe magnetic field* (the measurable stray field around the magnet) decreases in strength the farther one is from the center of the magnet.

Persons with cardiac pacemakers must be kept outside the 5-Gauss line (Figure 5-60). (*Gauss and Tesla are units of measurement of magnetic field strength. 1 Tesla = 10 kilogauss.*)

One often sees MRI facilities surrounded by chain link fences or other barriers to keep people outside the 5-Gauss line. Even more sensitive are cathode ray tubes, image intensifiers, or other types of electronic equipment commonly found in radiology systems. These must be kept out of the 1-Gauss line.

An assessment of all adjacent areas within the influence of the magnet is required to identify carefully the presence of equipment, people, or materials that may be sensitive to the magnetic field. It is possible to reduce the area of magnetic influence with shielding. The entire room may be shielded; part of the room may be shielded; or the equipment itself may be shielded. The thickness and permeability of the shielding material have a direct effect on the extent of reduction of the magnetic field of influence.

Environment's Effect on Magnet. The presence of ferrous material within the vicinity of the magnet can adversely affect the equipment's performance. Ferromagnetic material may be either stationary or moving. Moving objects include an elevator in the vicinity of the magnet, a passing automobile, or a piece of garden maintenance equipment. Structural steel beams and reinforced concrete in floors, ceilings, or walls are examples of stationary materials that may interfere with a distortion-free image.

The negative effects of stationary material can sometimes be minimized by positioning the magnet symmetrically between and/or parallel to the ferromagnetic objects. *Shims* (energized coils that provide a magnetic field opposite to the one causing the disturbance) are another method of compensating for stationary ferrous objects.

It is critically important to estimate, by taking physical measurements of the site, the influence of moving ferrous objects that may produce an image artifact. Each manufacturer supplies an overlay grid that indicates, in concentric circles, the Gauss field and indicates the distance in feet, moving away from the center of the magnet.

There are a number of other issues that should be considered. Light fixtures within the 5-Gauss field must be of nonmagnetic material. Fluorescent lighting must not be used within the RF shielded room containing the magnet. Rheostatic-type light dimmers may be used within the magnet room, but SCR-type dimmers may

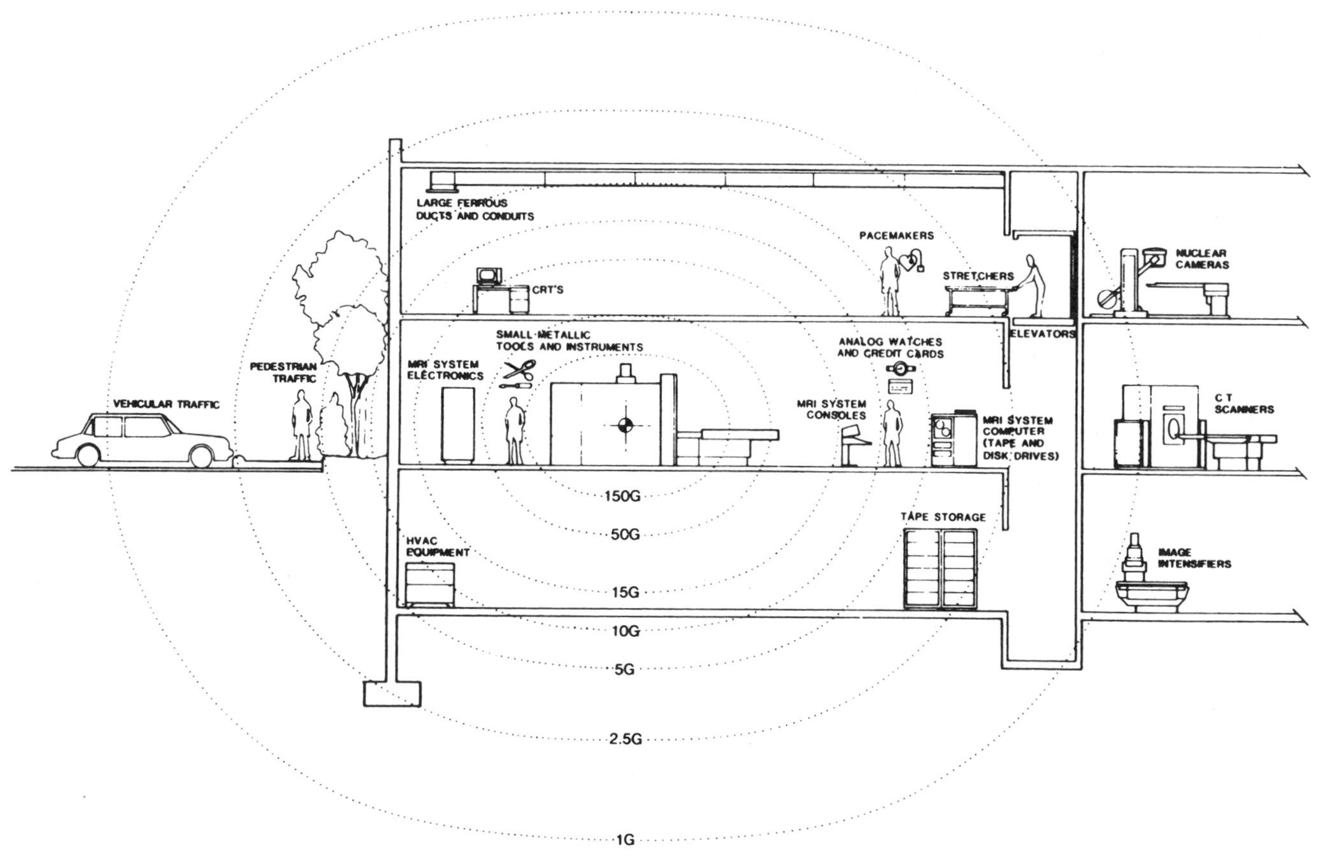

Figure 5-60. This diagram represents recommended minimum distances from an MR system and self-selected magnetically influential objects and occurrences. These distances are based on non-magnetically shielded system. (*Courtesy Picker International, Highland Heights, OH.*)

not be used. Commonly used medical accessory items such as oxygen cylinders, IV poles, and gurneys may not be used within the 5-Gauss line. Framework for suspended ceilings must be of aluminum.

Magnet Transport Access. Consideration must be given to the transport of a magnet during installation. Corridor and door sizes, as well as floor strength, must be adequate to handle a 16,000-pound superconductive magnet. This piece of equipment cannot be broken down into smaller components.

Cryogenic Replenishment. Superconductive magnets carry electrical current resistance-free only at cryogenic temperatures, necessitating cooling by liquid helium and nitrogen. Storage cylinders containing liquid helium and liquid nitrogen are called *dewars.* The dewars are on casters and must be located so that they can be moved to the magnet to replenish it from time to time. In addition, the dewars have to be replenished.

Magnetic Field Influence. As discussed previously, the extent of the magnetic field of influence would be determined by the size of the magnet. A 2.0T (Tesla) size superconductive magnet has a larger field of influence than a less powerful one. Minimum safety distances for objects in the magnetic fringe field must be carefully assessed. Inside the facility, a strict protocol regarding patient screening, the use of metal detectors, and architectural barriers can be utilized to protect visitors, as well as protect the magnet. A ferrous object in a person's pocket can become a lethal projectile.

The freestanding magnetic dome, shown in Figure 5-61, is designed to be a cost-effective method of magnetic shielding. It protects the homogeneity of the magnetic field, thereby preserving optimum image quality, and it contains the fringe magnetic field to within desired limits, preventing interference with magnetically sensitive equipment located nearby.

RFI Shielding. There are two types of shielding in an MRI facility. One is shielding to contain the magnetic field, and the other is shielding from radio frequency interference (RFI). Noise generated by stray radio frequencies distorts the image. Any penetrations in the room, such as doors, windows, light fixtures, or mechanical ductwork must be filtered to prevent radio frequency interference. Some brands of equipment are internally shielded from RFI, thereby eliminating the cost of shielding the room.

HVAC. A careful analysis of the heat output of the equipment must be made, and each area must be individually environmentally controlled so that the heat load in one room does not adversely affect the temperature and humidity of other rooms. An audible thermal alarm may be required in the computer room to alert the operator if the ambient temperature exceeds operating limits. An air filtration system may be required in the computer equipment room. Some units need chilled water for cooling the power supply, while others are air-cooled, eliminating the need for water.

A vent system must be provided to exhaust helium and nitrogen to the outside of the building. Precautions must be taken to ensure that the exit end of the exhaust duct does not allow gases to be vented into a closed area or allow access to passersby within 10 feet of the duct, in order to protect people from cold burns.

Power Requirements. A power conditioner unit is a component of most MRI systems to assure a clean, continuous power source with minimum fluctuation. A power management system or power conditioner controls electrical surges and spikes that are the principal causes of computer malfunction.

Floor Loading. MRI magnets average 16,000 pounds, concentrated in a relatively small area. The floor space immediately under the magnet is of critical concern with respect to allowable amounts of ferrous material

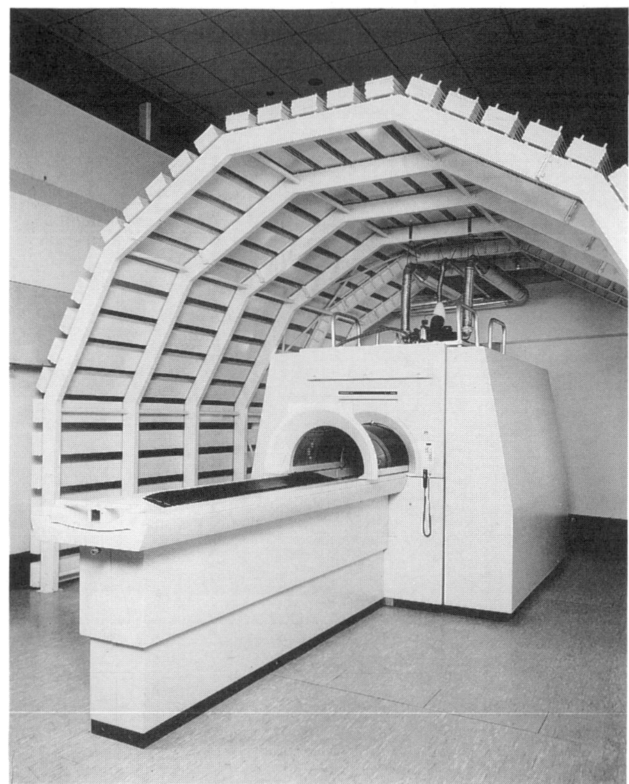

Figure 5-61. Freestanding magnet shielding dome. (*Courtesy Philips Medical Systems, Shelton, CT.*)

used in construction of the slab. Manufacturers' recommendations must be carefully followed in this regard.

Interior Design. When MRI was first introduced, it was thought that any ferrous substance would negatively affect image quality. Very expensive construction techniques using totally nonferrous materials were standard procedure. Wood beams, glued connections, stainless steel nails, Fiberglas, copper, and aluminum were considered appropriate construction materials. Now, however, manufacturers generally agree that shimming of the magnet is able to compensate for *static* ferrous building materials. The use of conventional construction techniques and materials greatly reduces the expense of constructing an MRI facility.

Carpeting may be used in the examination (magnet) room as well as in the control room (Figure 5-62). Manufacturer's specifications must be checked to verify that the carpet has the proper amount of static control. The computer room, and a portion of the exam room, will generally have computer-access type flooring, making this an optimum condition for installation of carpet tile (Figures 5-63 and 5-64).

The ceiling height of the magnet room will generally be 12 feet for a superconducting magnet. Ancillary areas will usually be 9 feet in height.

Diagnostic imaging equipment is often frightening to patients. This is especially true with equipment as large as MRI. A creative interior designer would attempt to make the unit appear built-in by surrounding the housing of the magnet with acoustic panels, wrapped with fabric. This texture softens the room, and the acoustic panels absorb noise generated by the equipment.

A view of the outdoors can be simulated with a *trompe l'oeil* mural painted on the wall or by using an acrylic material that looks like glass block installed either as a full wall or as an upper window. Behind this might be artificial plant material and a computer-operated system of colored lights that simulate sunrise, daylight, and sunset. Care must be taken in the selection of both interior finish materials and construction techniques, so as not to interfere with RF shielding or disturb the magnetic field.

Case Study

The freestanding MRI facility in Figures 5-65*a* and 5-65*b* illustrates many of the design principles previously discussed. Designed by architects Harvard, Jolly, Marcet and Associates of St. Petersburg, Florida, the

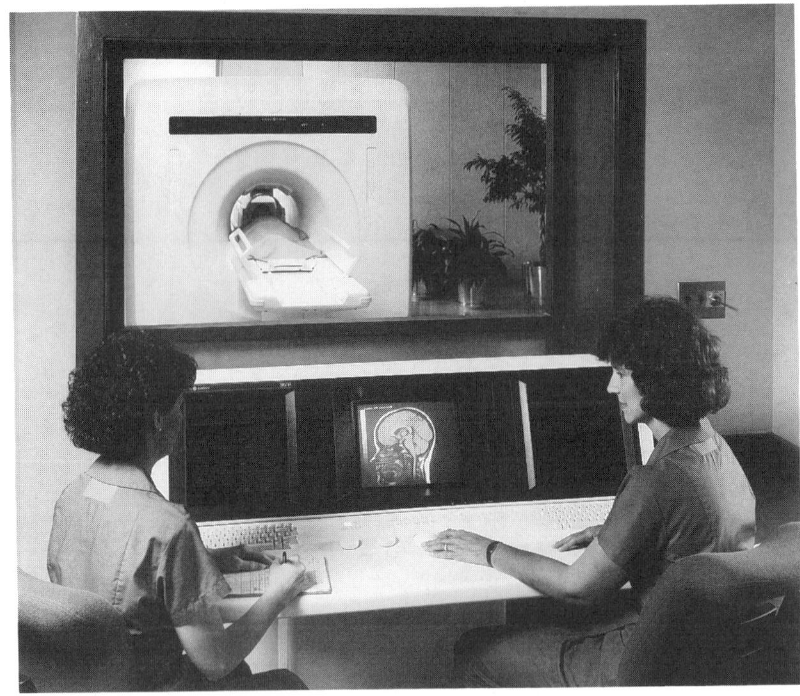

Figure 5-62. Control room, magnetic resonance imaging suite. (*Courtesy GE Medical Systems, Milwaukee, WI.*)

AUX. EQUIP.
CRYOGEN STORAGE
SYSTEM ELECTRONICS
EXAM AREA
FOYER
CONTROL
5G
15G
0 2 4 6 8 10

PLANNING CODE

		WIDTH	DEPTH	HEIGHT	WEIGHT (LBS)	HEAT (BTU/HR)
1	Operator Console	28″	33″	46″	210	500
2	Viewing Console	28″	33″	46″	210	500
3	Superconductive Magnet	82″	94½″	90 3/16″	11,000	5000 (During Scan)
4	Patient Handling System	21½″	117″	38″	420	—
5	RF Transmitter Cabinet	22″	32½″	67¾″	420	3000
6	Gradient Cabinet	22″	32½″	67¾″	380	6800
7	Gradient Cabinet	22″	32½″	67¾″	380	6800
8	Gradient Cabinet	22″	32½″	67¾″	380	6800
9	Sequence Interlock Cabinet	22″	32½″	67¾″	420	1800
10	Central Power Distribution Cabinet	22″	32½″	67¾″	660	1800
11	Shim Power Supply	22″	32½″	67¾″	440	0 *
12	Magnet Power Supply	22″	32½″	67¾″	595	0 *
13	Computer System	48″	36″	59″	1000	25,000
14	Multi-Format Camera	22½″	27″	52″	190	2000
15	Dewars (2)	25″ dia.	—	60″	645	—
16	Power Conditioner	62″	36″	78″	3500	10,900

*-Chilled water supply required for cooling.

Figure 5-63. Layout, magnetic resonance imaging suite. (*Illustration courtesy Picker International, Highland Heights, OH.*)

3700-square-foot facility, located on a hospital campus, was designed for future upgrading of a 0.6-Tesla magnet to a 1.5-Tesla magnet.

The radial shape of the floor plan is derived from flux lines emanating from the scanning device. Interior planning takes into account magnetic areas of influence, keeping unscreened visitors, the computer, and mechanical equipment outside the critical zone lines.

The interior space works well because patients and staff have separate, well-defined circulation patterns. The staff entry doubles as the service and cryogen delivery entrance and allows the radiologist to come and go without walking through patient areas. The landscaped entry court provides an attractive, nonclinical introduction to the facility. Inside, vistas of gardens and a soft color palette combine to relax patients.

As the patient passes into the most restricted zones to be prepared for scanning, the on-deck waiting area is a final staging point prior to proceeding through the control area into the magnet room.

Outside the building, features such as the reflecting pool and the landscape buffer zone are an aesthetically pleasing way to keep people and vehicles out of critical magnetic zones.

MRI facilities present new and unique challenges to architects and designers. In coming years, there will no doubt be a proliferation of these facilities, and planning for them will become more standardized. MRI installations seem to offer interesting investment opportunities for entrepreneurial physicians who often form a joint venture with a hospital for these projects. The fact that these are often freestanding facilities adjacent to a hospital or medical office building facilitates this type of investor arrangement. For these and other reasons, projected growth in MRI technology makes it imperative that architects and designers understand how to design these facilities.

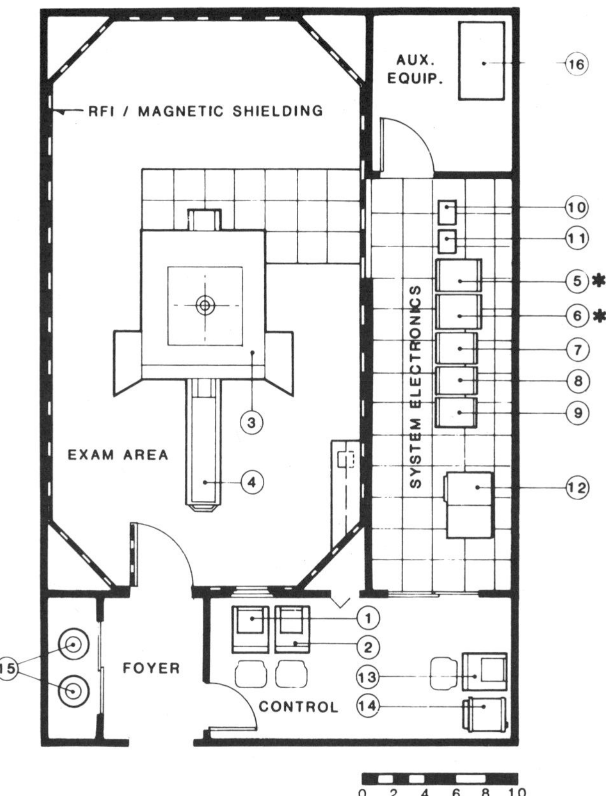

PLANNING CODE

#	EQUIPMENT	WIDTH	DEPTH	HEIGHT	WEIGHT (LBS)	HEAT (BTU/HR)
1	Operator Console	28″	33″	46″	210	500
2	Viewing Console	28″	33″	46″	210	500
3	Superconductive Magnet	96″	113½″	89⅝″	16000	5000 (During Scan)
4	Patient Handing System	26″	99¼″	37¼″	420	—
5	Shim Power Supply	23½″	35″	72″	440	0 *
6	Magnet Power Supply	23½″	35″	72″	440	0 *
7	RF Amplifier Cabinet	22″	32½″	84″	660	3400
8	Gradient Cabinet	22″	32½″	84″	660	10,200
9	Central Power Distribution Cabinet	22″	32½″	84″	660	850
10	Blower Cabinet	20″	10″	16″	50	—
11	Blower Cabinet	20″	10″	16″	50	—
12	Computer System	51″	34½″	69″	1000	25,000
13	Remote Viewing Console (Optional Purchase)	28″	33″	46″	210	500
14	Multi-Format Camera	26″	28″	72¾″	1848	680
15	Dewars (2)	25″ dia.	—	60″	645	—
16	Power Conditioner	62″	36″	78″	3500	10,900

*-Chilled water supply required for cooling.

Figure 5-64. Layout, magnetic resonance imaging suite. (*Illustration courtesy Picker International, Highland Heights, OH.*)

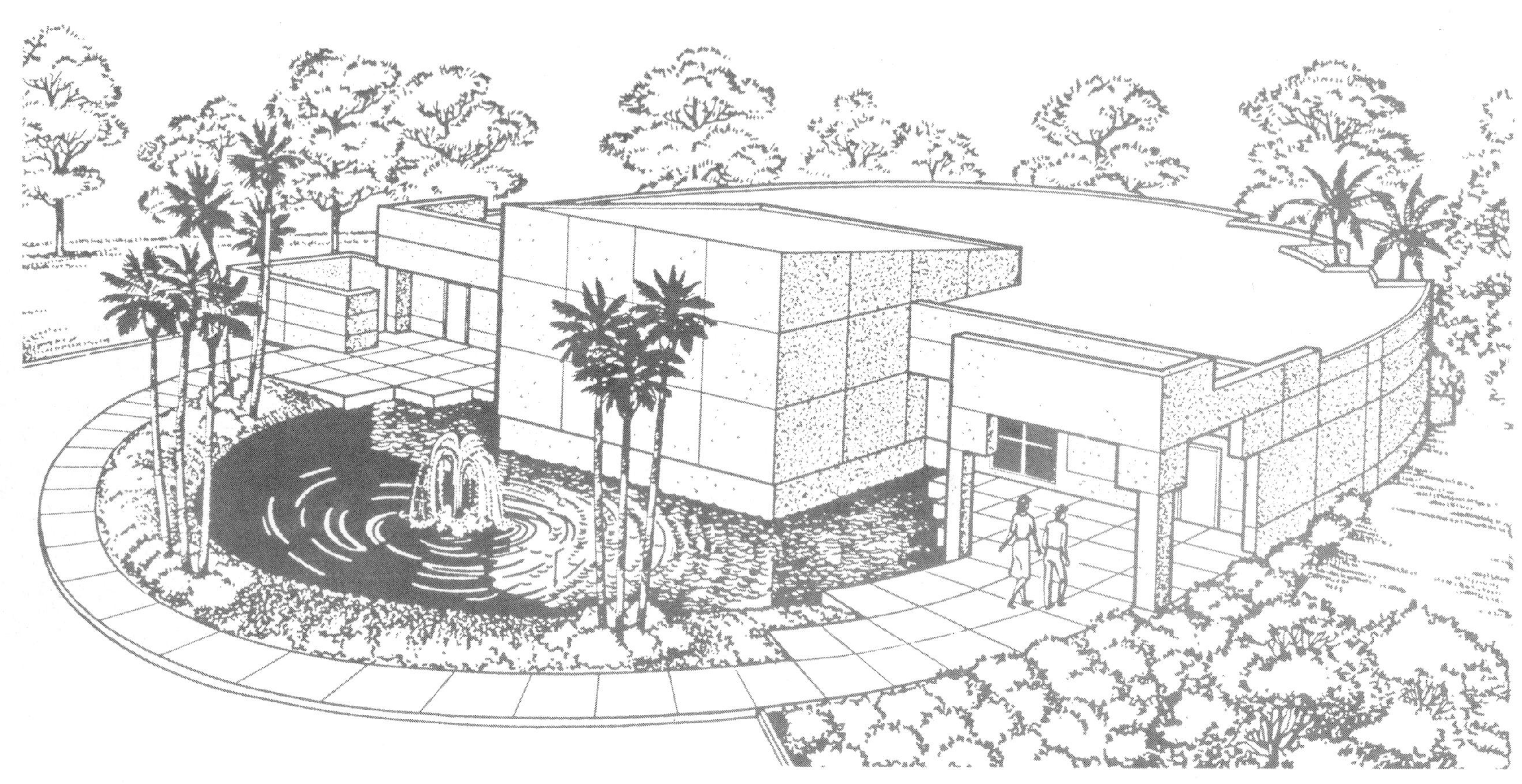

Figure 5-65a. MRI clinic, exterior view. (*Courtesy Harvard, Jolly, Marcet & Associates, P.A., AIA, Tampa and St. Petersburg, FL; Photographer: George Cott, Chroma, Inc., Tampa, FL.*)

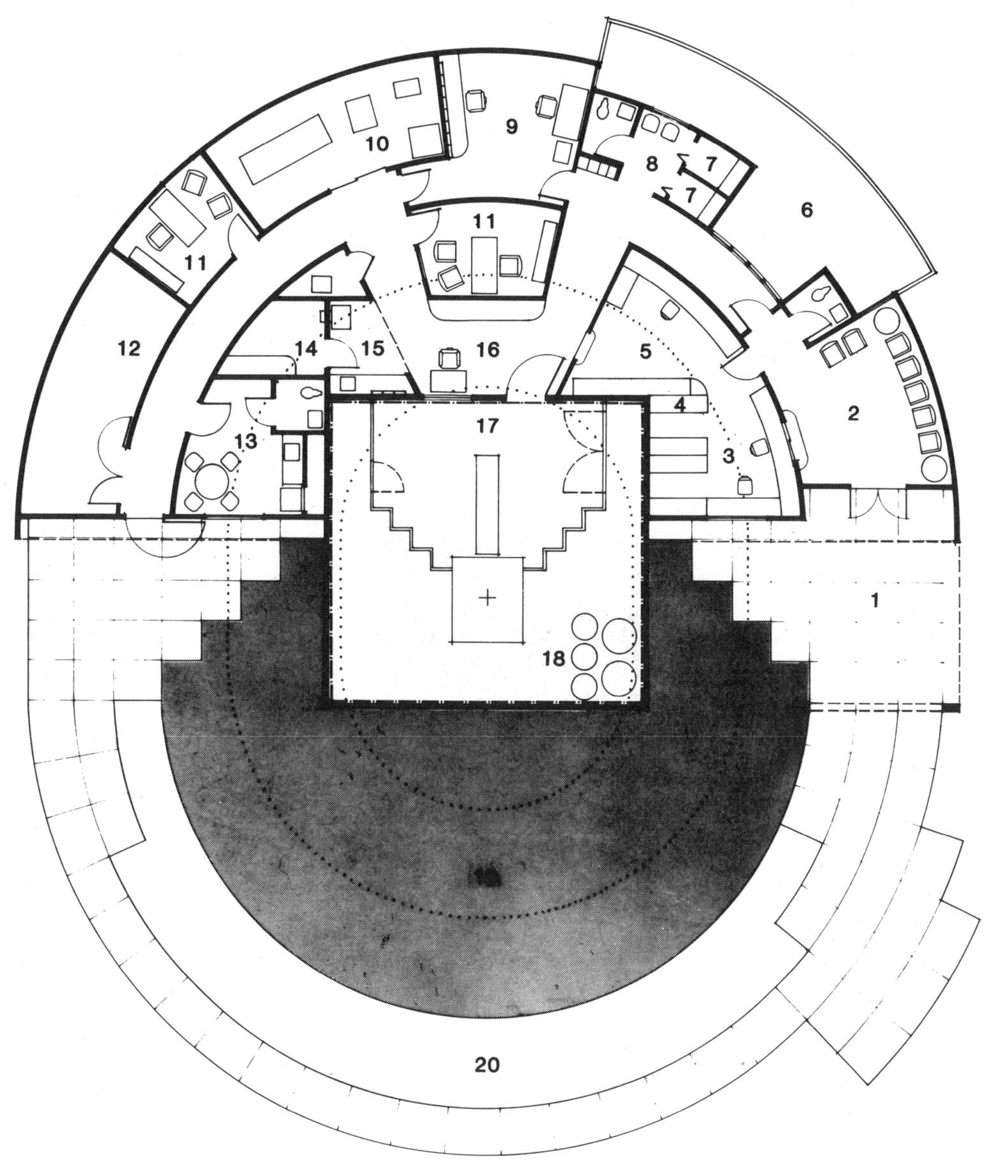

1. Entry Court
2. Waiting
3. Reception
4. Film Files
5. Business
6. Planter
7. Dressing
8. On-Deck Waiting
9. Viewing
10. Computer
11. Office
12. Mechanical
13. Lounge
14. Dark Room
15. Sorting
16. Control
17. Scan Room
18. Cryogens
19. Pool
20. Landscape Buffer

Figure 5-65b. MRI clinic, floor plan. (*Courtesy Harvard, Jolly, Marcet & Associates, P.A., AIA, Tampa and St. Petersburg, FL.*)

CLINICAL LABORATORY

Laboratory tests are a vital tool in diagnosing disease. A basic part of a thorough examination, these studies may be performed in a small room within the physician's office or in a sophisticated clinical laboratory located within a medical office building, or the lab may be located in an adjacent hospital. A physician may take a blood or urine specimen from a patient, but send it out for processing. Others will do simple tests in the office, but send out the more complicated ones.

The designer of a medical office building will most often encounter small clinical labs. Large labs, employing a pathologist, will usually be designed by a lab specialist experienced in the planning of such facilities. It is unlikely that a large clinical lab will be included in a medical office building if that building is adjacent to a hospital. This discussion, then, is limited to introducing the reader to basic laboratory processes and space requirements — some of which will occur in a small laboratory facility.

Development of the Program

As with all medical suites, the success of a well-designed laboratory is dependent upon a thorough understanding of the program — a written description of all requirements that must be incorporated into the design.

The following checklist will serve as a guide.

1. List the procedures that are to be performed. They will vary with the medical specialties of the building's tenants.
2. Analyze the space in terms of projected equipment and personnel in three areas:
   a. Administrative
   b. Technical
   c. Support (includes washing, sterilizing, storage, and locker facilities)
3. Review sizes and specifications of major pieces of equipment. Tabulate the lineal feet of countertop space required for each item or area, and note required adjacencies.
4. Determine which procedures may be combined in the same work area and which require separate areas.
5. Divide technical areas by functional units: hematology, chemistry, parasitology, microbiology, histology, urinalysis, serology.
6. Projected volume of tests in each functional unit will indicate the number of tech work stations required.
7. Review desirable functional adjacencies. For example, hematology can be combined with urinalysis or with chemistry. In addition, hematology would be adjacent to the blood draw station located near the waiting room. Small laboratories have a limited staff; therefore, technical modules need to be clustered together so that staff working in each unit can support each other. The glass-washing/sterilization room should be principally closest to microbiology, and secondarily close to chemistry (Figure 5-66).
8. If any units are expected to expand in terms of physical space, they would best be located at the end of the suite where expansion may occur.
9. Carefully review utility requirements for all equipment. Separate electrical circuits are required for many instruments in order to avoid fluctuating voltage which adversely affects the accuracy of the instruments.
10. Note any equipment (refrigerators, centrifuges, fume hoods, freezers, and incubators) that may be shared by technicians from different work stations.
11. Each technical module needs storage space for supplies used on a daily basis. A storage room would be used for bulk purchase of supplies.
12. Consider environmental factors such as ventilation, color reflectance, light, and isolation of equipment that may be noisy or produce heat when used.

Technical Modules

The following descriptions of technical modules will familiarize readers with standard methods of processing samples. Electronic, automated clinical analyzers are widely used even by small labs. Instrument manufacturers in recent years have designed automated equipment specifically for this market, the price of which has been brought in line with what small laboratories can afford.

Hematology. This is the study of the cellular components of blood. Procedures performed in this area are those most frequently ordered by a physician; thus it should be located close to the *phlebotomy* (blood drawing) station for most efficient workflow (Figure 5-67).

One half of the module should be set aside for procedures such as sedimentation rates (a level, stable work surface is needed), the hematology analyzer, and slide staining. Another portion of the work surface (at 30-inch height) should have kneespaces for sit-down work at the microscope. The microhematocrit centrifuge, due to its noise and vibration when in use, should be placed in an area where it will not disturb anyone or interfere with the microscopic examination of slides. Generally, a hematology module will have both a large centrifuge and a small, microhematocrit one. A refrigerator, desk, and computer terminal (if applicable) should be centrally located for use by hematology, urinalysis, and chemistry. If, because of the physician mix or the presence of an ambulatory surgical center, coagulation tests, such as prothrombin time, are to be done, they would be performed in this unit.

Chemistry. A variety of chemical procedures are performed here. Most work is done at a 36-inch-high countertop, but a lowered kneespace area should be provided for seated procedures. One countertop will have

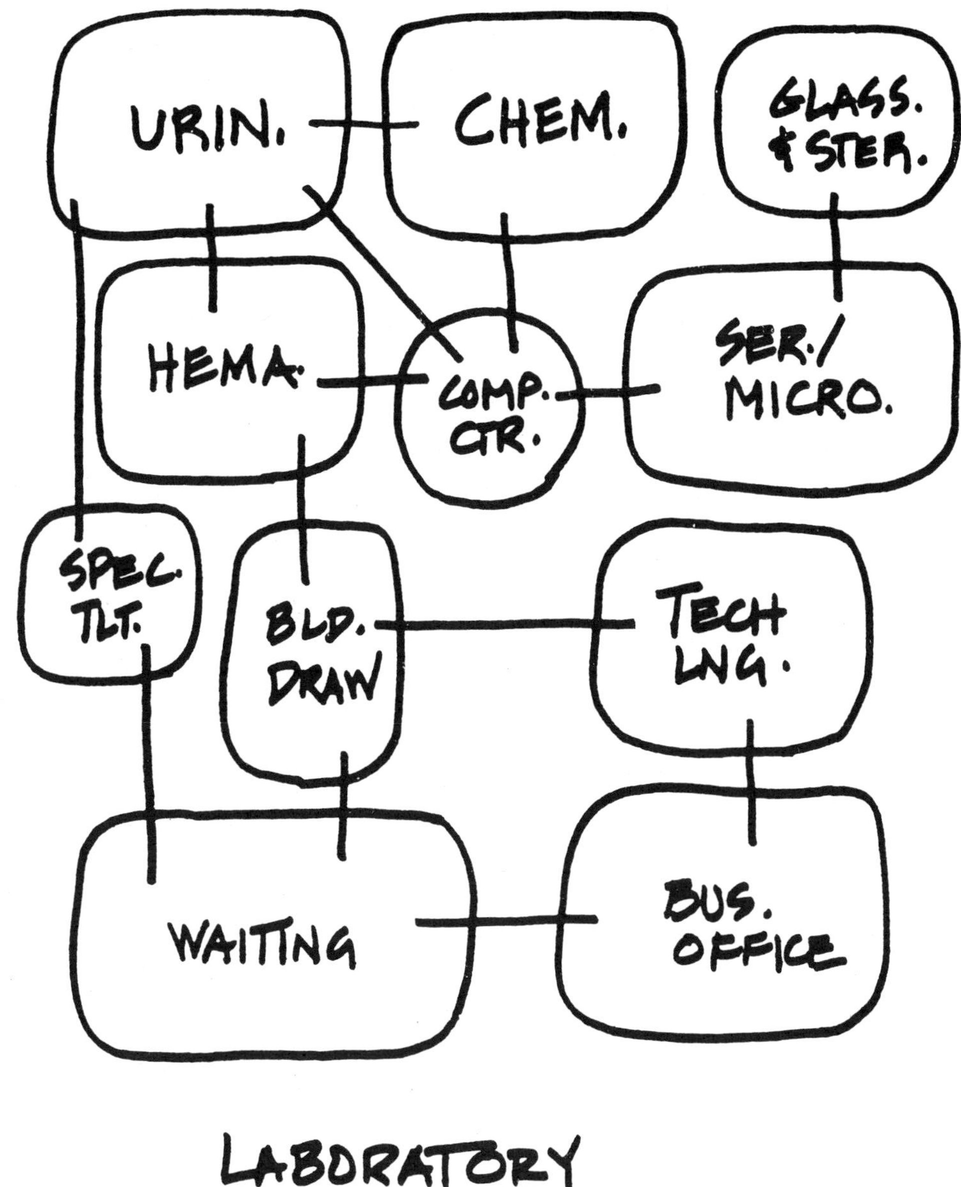

Figure 5-66. Schematic diagram of a clinical laboratory.

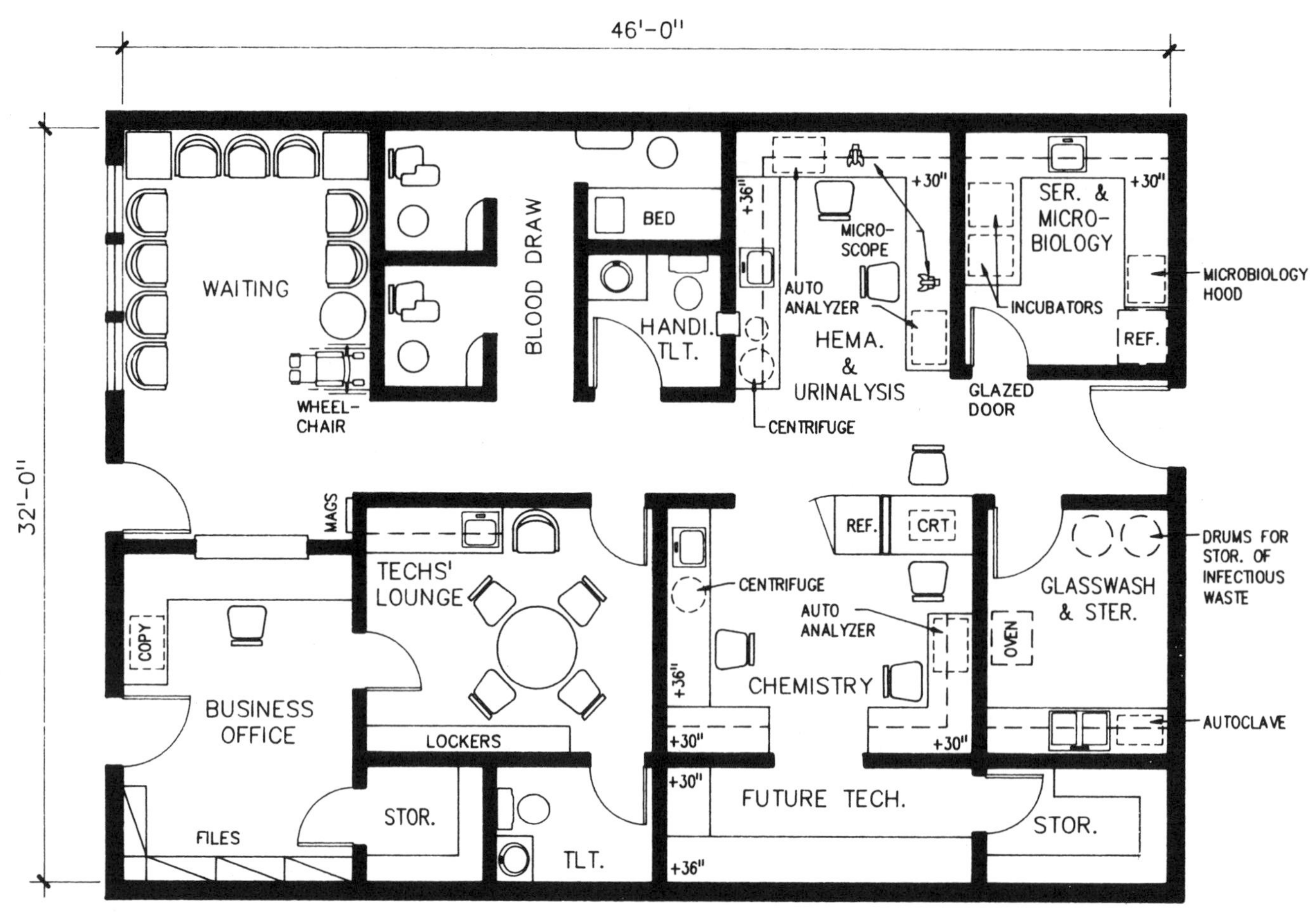

CLINICAL LABORATORY

1472 SF

Figure 5-67. Suite plan for clinical lab, 1472 square feet.

open shelves above for chemicals used during procedures. However these shelves should have a protective barrier such as a 3-inch-high Plexiglas band at the edge to prevent the fall of items in case of an earthquake or accident. A sink is required in each chemistry work area and built-in cabinetry would consist of drawers and hinged door storage below the countertop.

An instrument table (36 inches high) or countertop area should be located away from the prep and test area for the spectrophotometer, electrolyte analyzer, and chemistry analyzer. The area will require countertop space for a centrifuge. Depending upon the volume of work performed in the laboratory, this centrifuge could be shared with urinalysis and coagulation (hematology). In this case, chemistry should be adjacent to the hematology/urinalysis module.

Urinalysis. This unit may be located in the hematology or the chemistry module. One half of the urinalysis work counter is used for microscopic examinations and the other half for chemical procedures. The work surface should be 30 inches high and should have a sink. Urinalysis could share a centrifuge with another department.

Serology-Microbiology. Serology is the study of serum and the body's immunological response to infection. Microbiology is the study of infectious organisms. These units are usually combined. Parasitology, the study of parasites (normally performed on feces), is often included in the microbiology module. Since most work is done in a seated position, the countertop should be 30 inches high with a kneespace for the technologist, space for a centrifuge, and open shelves above, for reagents. A refrigerator is needed for the storage of purchased media and reagents. Floor or countertop space must be allocated for both a 37°C and a CO_2 incubator. A sink is needed for staining slides and for hand washing. As with other technical modules, drawers and undercounter cabinets are necessary.

A microbiological hood is required to prevent the spread of infection during preparation of specimens for tuberculosis, fungus, viruses, bacteria, or parasite isolation and identification. This hood must be either vented to the outdoors or run through a HEPA filter. If at all possible, separate the microbiology module from other modules by full-height partitions and a glazed door to reduce contamination of air and the chance of infection being transmitted to other lab personnel.

Histology. This is the study of tissues. Thin slices of diseased specimens are examined by microscope. During surgery (or autopsy), for example, sections of tumors would be sent to the lab for a pathologist's report on possible malignancy or other cellular deformities. Small labs in a medical office building would not have a histology unit or a pathologist. Normally this work would be performed in a hospital lab. Thus the requirements in equipment and work space will not be discussed here.

Automated Analyzers

Many laboratories now have microprocessor-based hematology and chemistry analyzers, which considerably reduce the number of technologists required and eliminate much of the equipment necessary for manual analysis. Automated analyzers vary considerably in their size and capabilities. All of them are aimed at speed and total automation, freeing the technologist to walk away while samples are being processed.

One may place a blood or urine specimen into the machine, and in less than one minute, the analyzer will complete 12 tests simultaneously and produce a printout with the results. Large analyzers (Fig. 5-68) process upwards of 180 samples per hour and do a

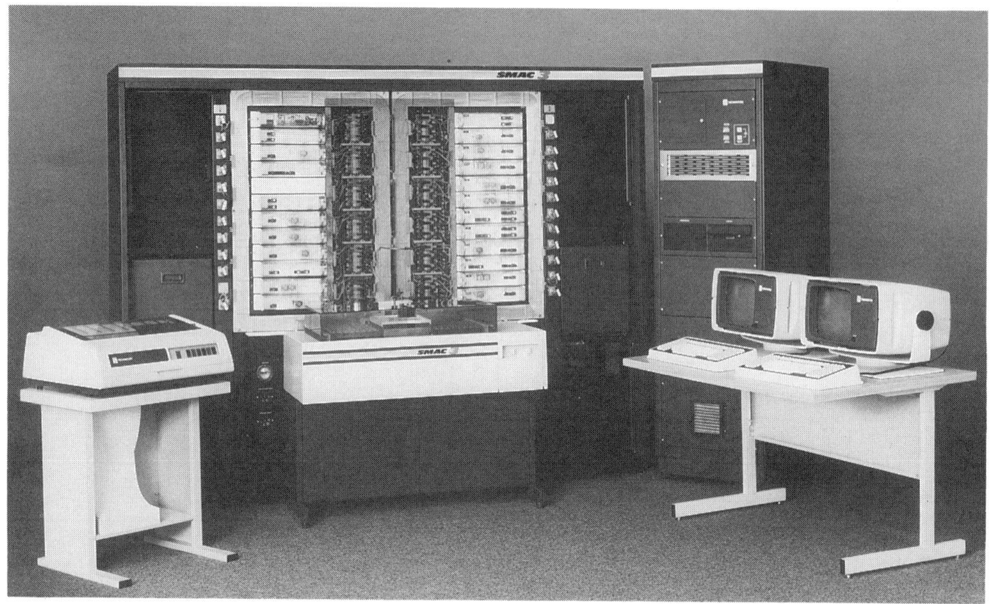

Figure 5-68. Chemistry analyzer, SMAC® 3 system. (*Courtesy Technicon Instruments Corp., Tarrytown, NY.*)

thorough analysis—error free — of each, thus fractionalizing the time required by lab techs to perform these tests individually and manually. Some analyzers fit on a countertop (Figures 5-69 and 5-70) while others require floor space (Figure 5-71).

Administrative Area

The administrative area consists of waiting room, business office/reception room, staff lounge and locker room, and sometimes a private office for the pathologist or director of the lab. These areas should be separated from clinical areas so that non-lab personnel need not enter the clinical work space.

Dressing Area for Employees. A lab will often include lockers and a dressing area where technicians may change clothes. A staff toilet room at this location is convenient. The dressing area may be combined with the staff lounge. Since food cannot be stored or eaten in the lab, it is important to provide a room to be used for breaks and lunch.

Specimen Toilet

The toilet room for collection of urine specimens should have a small pass-through in the wall (see Appendix) that opens into the clinical area so that urine samples can be picked up by the technician without the patient having to carry the cup out of the bathroom. This toilet room, as in any medical or dental suite, should be designed to accommodate the handicapped.

Blood Drawing

Blood drawing (phlebotomy) can be performed either in a small booth or cubicle (equipped with a straight chair and a 24- × 36-inch table) or in a prefabricated special blood drawing chair with tablet arm (Fig. 5-72), located in an open room without any enclosure or behind a screen. The screen protects those waiting from the view of blood being drawn. Often, persons watching become faint. If space allows, it is a good idea to have a private cubicle large enough to accommodate a built-in bed or bench for drawing blood of patients who may feel faint and for babies or small children.

Central Communication Center

The modern laboratory is directly linked by computer to physicians' offices and to reference laboratories. Communication into and out of the laboratory is of critical importance. A personal computer may be used for laboratory record keeping. If the lab sends out a substantial amount of work to a reference laboratory, a CRT and printer allow quick access to results from the reference laboratory specimens. This is best located at a desk convenient to all of the technical modules (see Figure 5-67).

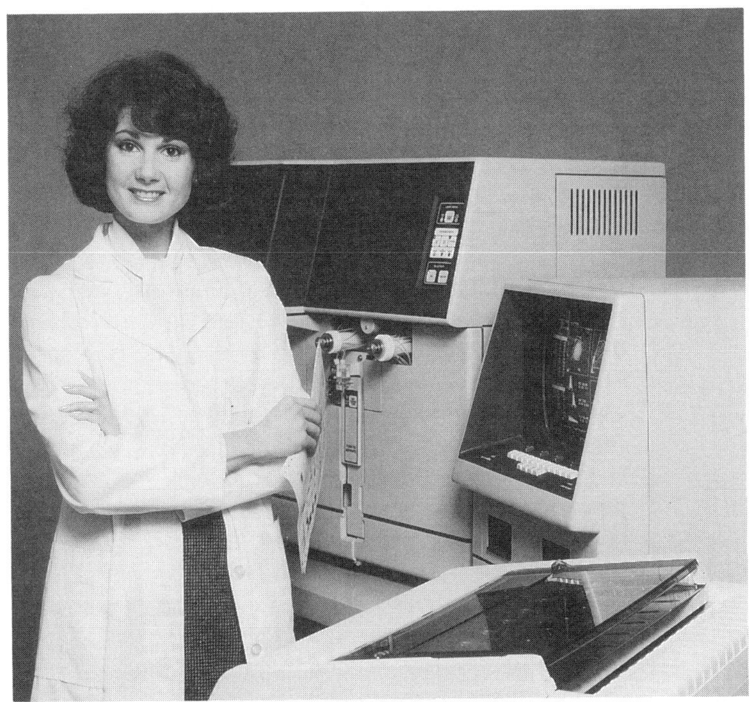

Figure 5-69. Hematology analyzer, H-I® system. (*Courtesy Technicon Instruments Corp., Tarrytown, NY.*)

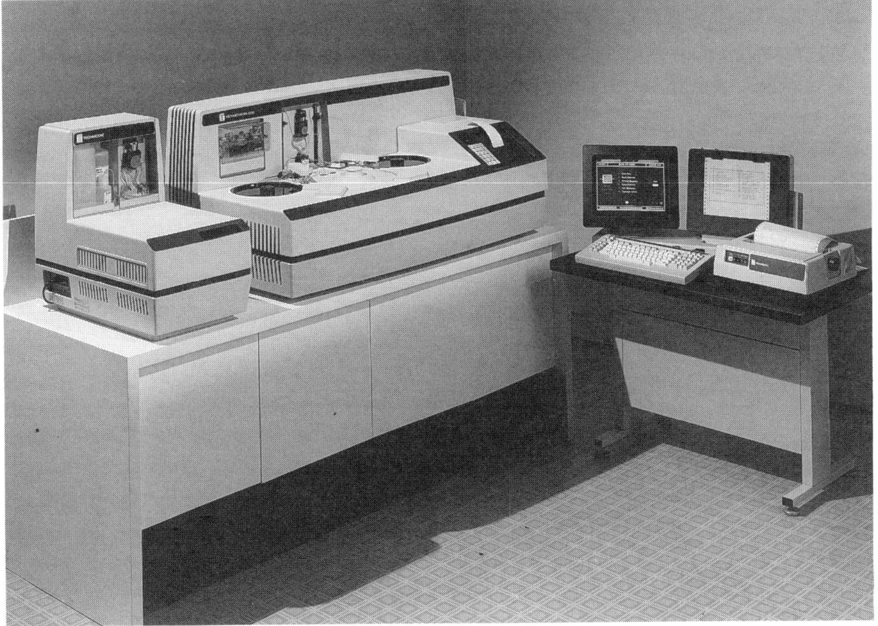

Figure 5-70. RA-1000® chemical analyzer with data manager system. (*Courtesy Technicon Instruments Corp., Tarrytown, NY.*)

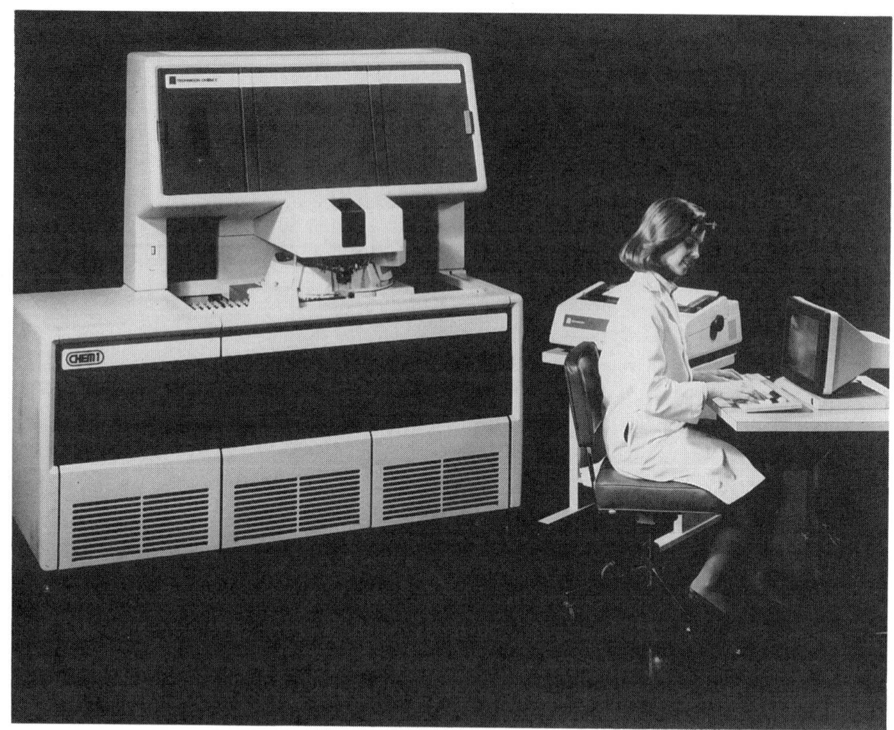

Figure 5-71. Chemistry analyzer, CHEM I® system. (*Courtesy Technicon Instruments Corp., Tarrytown, NY.*)

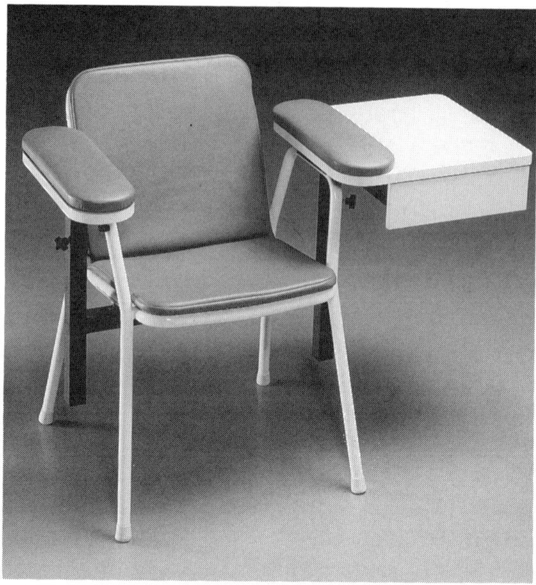

Figure 5-72. Blood draw chair. (*Courtesy Midmark Corp., Versailles, OH.*)

Accessioning of Specimens. The lab should have an area designated for accessioning (recording) of specimens and tests performed. Recording may be done manually or by computer. If done manually, there should be an area in each module for performing paperwork. If the laboratory uses a computer for keeping track of patient specimens and results, it is efficient to have a telephone nearby for answering inquiries about results.

Auxiliary Services

Disposal of Infectious Waste. Regulations for the disposal of infectious waste dictate that an area be allocated for the storage of laboratory specimens, disposable supplies, needles, syringes, and other items which may have come into contact with patient specimens until these contaminated items are collected by licensed disposal companies. Presently OSHA standards require storage in special red bags placed in closed containers in a labeled, secured area. This waste cannot be stored for more than four days.

The laboratory has the option, however, of autoclaving its infectious waste prior to its being picked up by the standard refuse collection agency. If the laboratory chooses this option, an additional space large enough to accommodate this equipment will be required in the sterilization room. Currently, government agencies are establishing new regulations for physician-operated laboratories. Criteria for the handling of hazardous materials (i.e., potentially carcinogenic or infectious waste) must be reviewed before designing a laboratory that must meet certification and licensure requirements.

Glass-washing and Sterilization. Today with the use of disposables and premade reagents, the need for a glass-washing and sterilization area has been reduced. This area used to be larger when lab procedures were done manually. This module should be located close to the serology-microbiology and chemistry units, since they use these services more frequently than do other modules. This unit may contain deionized water equipment, sterilizer, drying oven, and pipette washer, depending upon the laboratory's test volume and mix of procedures. Storage of glassware, chemicals, reagents, and paper supplies should be provided in cabinets. A ventilation hood over the sterilizers would exhaust heat and moisture generated by the equipment.

Future Technology

As with any medical space, there should be some flexibility in the layout to allow for future space requirements as technology evolves. Note the expansion area provided in Figure 5-67.

Utilities

A clinical lab may require gas, suction, and compressed air. Because of the need for continuity of service, piping of utilities should be easily accessible (but not exposed) and should have an ample number of valves, traps, and cleanouts to facilitate repairs. Each individual piping system may be color coded and must be of an acid-resistant material, including the plumbing drains and the "U" joint. Waste from pipes may be discharged to a dilution pit or may be carried to a point in the system where the discharge material will be diluted by waste from other areas. It is important to know local codes regarding requirements for waste disposal. Laboratory sinks should be of a noncorrosive material and countertop work surfaces may be chemical-resistant plastic laminate or special ceramic lab tops.

Air Conditioning and Ventilation

The need for a well-planned, functional air-conditioning and ventilation system is critical in a laboratory. Chemical fumes, vapors, gases, heat from equipment, plus the impracticality of open windows, create a health hazard to those in adjacent medical suites as well as to the laboratory staff who suffer repeated exposure. It is not adequate simply to exhaust these vapors out of the roof of the building without considering the dispersion to nearby persons and buildings.

Ventilation requirements for each work unit must be studied so that airflow patterns can be regulated by proper location of supply and exhaust grilles. A competent mechanical engineer should be consulted to prepare this study. Exhaust air from fume hoods should be conducted through noncorrosive ducts to the roof of the building and not be recirculated. The microbiology module should have a higher air pressure than the surrounding rooms to reduce the possibility of infiltration of aerosols that might contaminate specimens being processed. A slightly negative air pressure between the lab and the medical building should be maintained in order to prevent odors and contaminants from spreading.

Power Requirements

A laboratory demands maximum flexibility; thus each work surface countertop should have a continuous plug-mold strip and a separate circuit every 8 to 10 feet. Because certain pieces of equipment may draw as much as 15 amperes when warming up, a careful inventory must be made of the power requirements of each major piece of equipment. Automated analyzers are sensitive to voltage fluctuations and may require a constant voltage regulator as well as a separate circuit. It should be noted that a centrifuge or shaking equipment cannot be put on the same circuit as a computer because it will create severe electrical interference.

Work areas need shadow-free light, requiring that a fluorescent "shelf" light be mounted below the upper cabinets. Otherwise, light may be supplied totally by ceiling-mounted fluorescent luminaires in sufficient quantity to assure a level of at least 100 footcandles for close work and 50 footcandles for general illumination.

Consideration must be given, when designing and specifying lighting, to the elimination of glare from data management display monitors associated with clinical analyzers. This may necessitate indirect lighting that bounces off the ceiling for general illumination. The issue would be the same as that encountered in any office where video display terminals are in use.

Interior Design

For years, laboratories have been designed in a neutral color palette because the reflection of colors made it difficult to match samples to a standard or to analyze colors. Today, with automated equipment, matching of specimens to a standard is no longer done visually. Walls may be any pleasant color the technologist prefers, and subtle patterns may be considered for plastic laminate countertops. The floor might have an attractive design created with several colors of vinyl composition tile or it may be sheet vinyl with a confetti pattern.

In patient areas, a thoughtful designer will provide a place where patients can hang their coats, handbags, and stow their packages or briefcases. This should be located principally in the blood drawing area. The waiting room needs a secure place for hanging overcoats and umbrellas and for stowing boots.

The Small Laboratory

The small laboratory which may be part of a group practice suite would perform the more common and simple laboratory tests. (This is also known as a STAT lab, because the tests are generally urgently required.) Specimens requiring complex bacteriological or chemical procedures would probably be sent to an outside laboratory. Diseased tissue specimens would be sent to a pathologist at a nearby hospital. Thus the small lab (650 to 750 square feet) would have separate areas for hematology, chemistry, urinalysis, and microbiology, allowing approximately 8 lineal feet of countertop for each, plus two blood draw cubicles, specimen toilet, small reception/waiting area, storage room, and glass-washing/sterilization area.

CHAPTER 6
Group Practice

The point of origin for all group practices is the Mayo Clinic. Founded in 1897, it became the prototype for others that followed, including the prominent Menninger Clinic in Topeka. The Mayo Clinic is reputed to be the world's largest medical clinic. While few aspire to this level of achievement, many of the principles upon which the Mayo Clinic was founded apply to smaller group practices as well. These are: the sharing or pooling of knowledge, a division of labor that allows physicians to concentrate on their specialty, and a desire to stay on the cutting-edge of new technology. It is a teamwork approach to the delivery of medicine.

There is an ever-increasing trend toward group practice. Economics and the threat of for-profit chains dominating the market have encouraged many solo practitioners to band together in groups to enhance their strength and presence. Although some physicians do not feel psychologically geared to practice in a large organization, and some fear a loss of individual authority in medical matters, group practice does increase a physician's productivity and may lower the cost of health care.

In theory, each physician can be made more productive by eliminating the waste and inefficiencies inherent in a solo practice. A solo practitioner may work a 60-hour or 70-hour week, but about a quarter of his or her time is spent on office management — bookkeeping, scheduling, ordering supplies, etc. A group practice provides a division of labor with sufficient personnel to perform these nonmedical tasks, thereby enabling physicians to concentrate solely on medical matters.

Another advantage of group practice is the convenience of having a fully staffed radiology department and clinical lab right in the physician's own office. Equipment that might be too costly or underutilized in the small medical office can easily be justified in a large group practice. Other benefits of a group practice are greater freedom with regard to leisure time. Partners can cover for one another with no lack of continuity in care for the patient. And physicians in a multispecialty group provide one another with immediate access to specialists in other fields. This pooling of resources provides patients more efficient and complete professional services than each physician could provide individually.

Of course, economics plays a prime role in motivating physicians to practice together. Eight physicians in private practice would require eight business offices, eight waiting rooms, six to eight X-ray rooms, six to eight minor surgery rooms — a great duplication of space and personnel. Together, as a group, the eight could do with two minor surgeries, two X-ray rooms, one large waiting room, and one centralized business office. More efficient use of space and personnel means more take-home profit for physicians and perhaps lower costs for patients. In addition, certain lab tests or X-rays that might otherwise be sent out could be done within a properly equipped suite, netting extra fees for the group practice to reduce office overhead.

In fact, as physicians' fees for services are reduced in coming years, predictions are that there will be much more reliance on billing of ancillary services to make up the difference. This will attract many to a group practice where the vertical integration of services enhances physicians' income.

TYPES OF GROUP PRACTICES

There are four types of group practices. The *single-specialty group* consists of physicians (rarely more than eight) who are all of the same medical specialty. This type of group permits a physician a great deal of freedom since patients usually will accept treatment from any member of the group. This allows for better utilization of all the doctors' time.

The *multispecialty group* might typically be a large clinic offering internal medicine, OB-GYN, urology, pediatrics, family practice, ENT, or any combination of medical specialties. A group such as this could offer many of the outpatient services provided by a hospital: clinical lab studies, diagnostic radiology, physical therapy, respiratory therapy, renal dialysis, and multiphasic medical screening. A multispecialty group might consist of 20 physicians to several hundred physicians as in a health maintenance organization (HMO).

The *internal medicine group* might be a group of general internists plus those with various subspecialties: pulmonary medicine, cardiovascular disease, hematology, oncology, gastroenterology, or endocrinology. A large enough group could support its own clinical lab, radiology department, cardiovascular rehabilitation lab, and pulmonary function lab.

The *general practice group* enables general physicians to expand beyond their individual resources in purchasing equipment and staffing an office. Large general practice groups are often found in small towns, and sometimes they have one or more specialists on staff in an effort to offer the community a wider range of services.

Health Maintenance Organizations

Any of these groups may be organized as a health maintenance organization, although HMOs tend to be multispecialty groups offering services to a group of members on a prepaid fee basis, or they may charge a fee at the time the service is rendered, as do the majority of physicians. It should be remembered that HMOs stress health maintenance (it is less costly to keep people healthy than to treat them when they are sick), so any clinic set up as an HMO should be designed to accommodate many more patients than would a multispecialty group of the same number of physicians. Many more paramedic aides will be employed in an HMO to provide health screening and other procedures aimed at preventive medicine. An HMO will usually have a large physical therapy department, inhalation therapy unit, cardiopulmonary lab, and allergy department — all of which may process a large volume of patients daily who do not have to see a doctor.

The bookkeeping system is somewhat simplified in an HMO, since members prepay a monthly fee that entitles them to office visits for a routine flat fee of $2 to $3 plus a minimal charge for lab tests and X-rays. Members are issued an embossed identification card that is presented to the receptionist upon checking in and checking out of the clinic. This saves time in heading up a form for each patient visit, and the identification plate has the patient's billing code and other pertinent information on it. Thus, although an HMO may have more subscribers than a similar-sized multispecialty group that charges a fee for service, the billing procedures are often less complicated (there are no insurance claims to file) and are assisted by data processing and computer systems.

The two main types of HMOs are the *Independent Practice Association* (IPA) and the *Group Practice* model. The latter usually employs its own physicians or engages them on a contract basis, and care is delivered through a number of clinics owned and operated by the HMO. IPA-type HMOs are usually developed by groups of physicians to service employers. The big difference between these and group practice models is that IPAs allow physicians to remain in private practice and to treat subscribers from their own offices. The reader is referred to the Introduction for a more detailed discussion.

Health maintenance organizations are regulated by the state and are subject to close scrutiny by various health planning regulatory agencies. This accounts for the low number of HMOs and also for the fact that they are usually very large multispecialty groups that have met strict requirements with regard to their medical services, utilization of personnel, and schedule of fees.

Single-Specialty Group

This suite would be composed of the same elements as a standard medical office for a solo practitioner except on a larger scale. (The reader is referred to Chapter 3 under General Practice). The functions of administration, patient care, and support services remain the same. It is the *relationship* of rooms that becomes critical as the suite becomes larger. It is no longer possible for all rooms to be close to each other as they are in a small suite. Administrative and support services may be *centralized* or *decentralized* — that is the major decision to be made at the outset. With a centralized plan (also known as an "island" plan), the business office, nurse station, lab, and supply room would be grouped together, forming the core of the suite, with patient areas (exam and treatment rooms, consultation and waiting rooms) grouped around the perimeter of the core (Figure 6-3).

With a decentralized plan, administrative and support services would be divided into units each serving a certain number of exam and treatment rooms. Exam and treatment rooms would be grouped into pods (three to six exam rooms to a pod) with an adjacent nurse station/lab and one or two consultation rooms (Figure 6-6). It would be impractical to have more than one business office, medical records area, or insurance office, so these services would have to be located so that a patient exiting from any pod of exam rooms would follow a path leading him or her past the cashier's desk and appointment desk and back into the central waiting room. Sometimes in a large suite, proper circulation must be reinforced by strategically placed, easy-to-read signage plaques or wallgraphics (Figure 6-5).

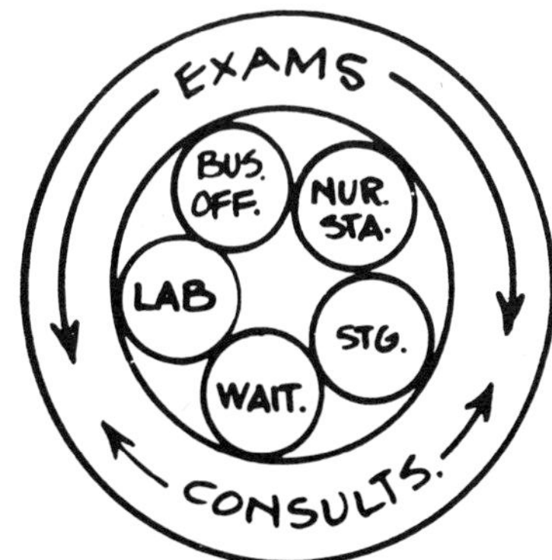

Figure 6-1. Schematic diagram of a centralized plan for a single-specialty group.

Figure 6-2. Schematic diagram of a decentralized plan for a single-specialty group.

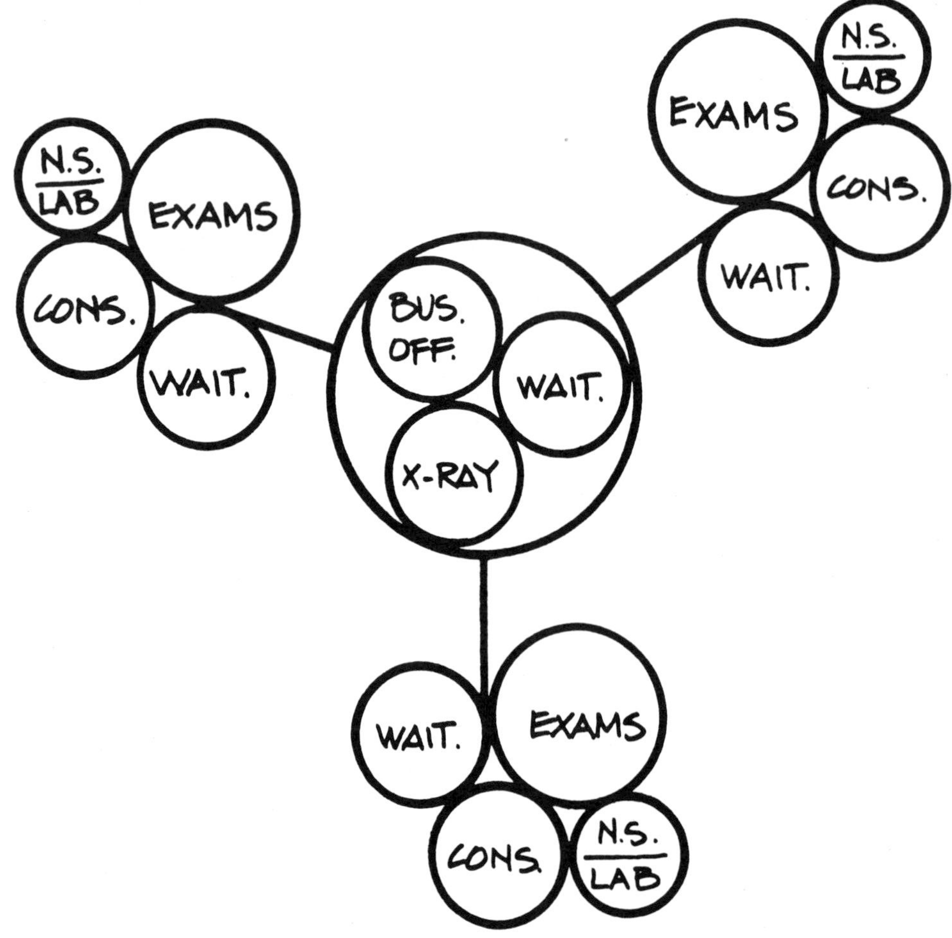

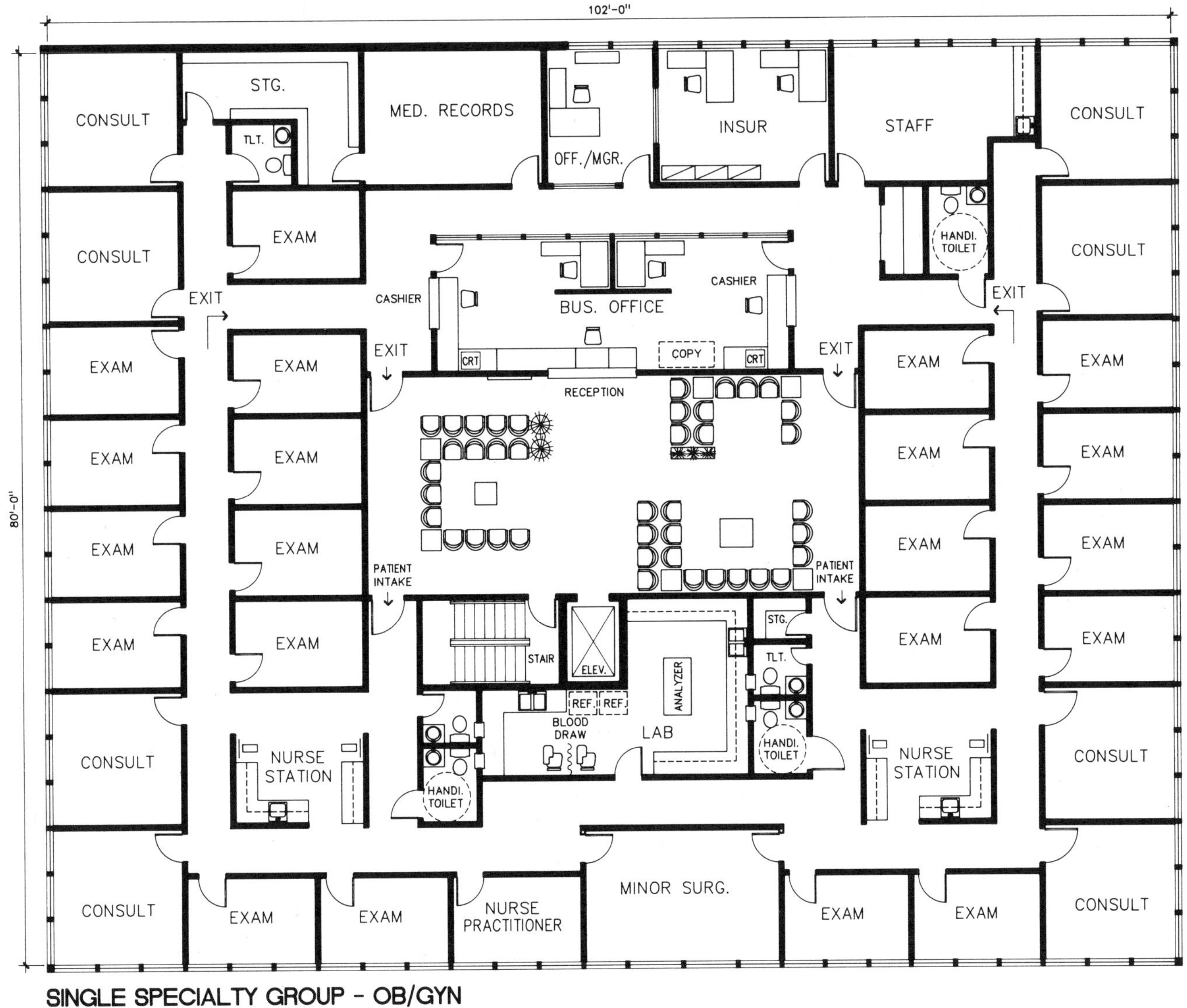

Figure 6-3. Suite plan for single-specialty group, OB-GYN, centralized plan, 8160 square feet.

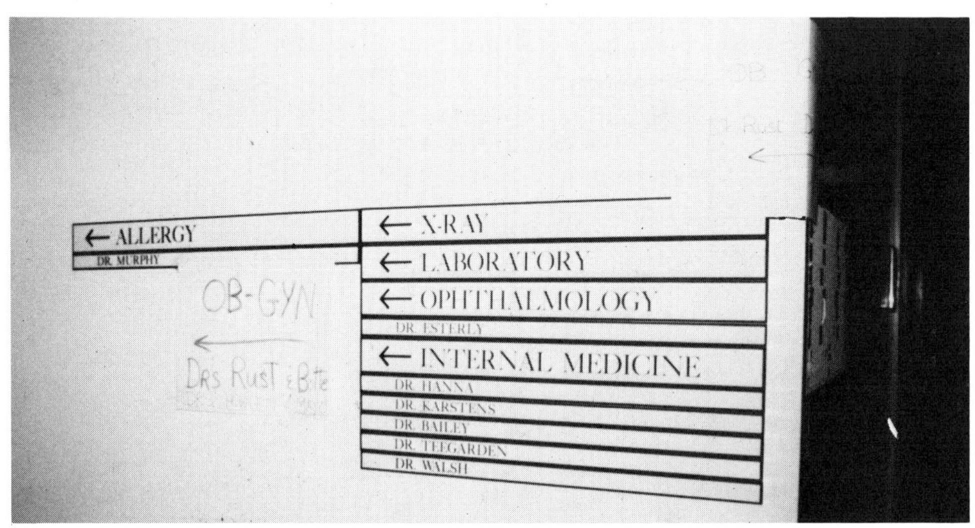

Figure 6-4. Clinic signage system "before."

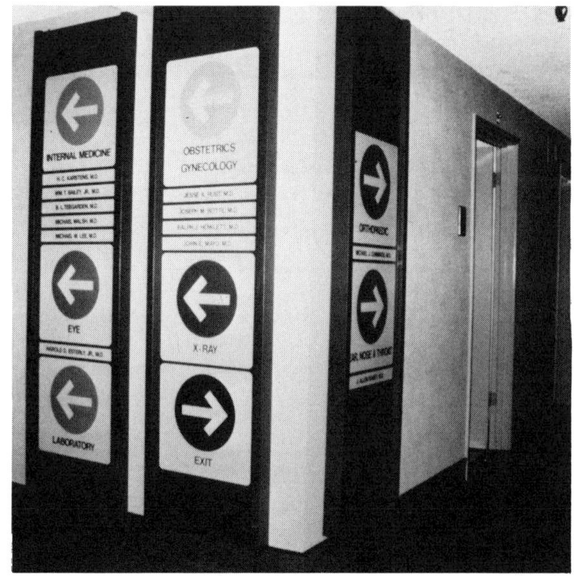

Figure 6-5. Clinic signage system "after": Each medical specialty has a color identification. (*Design: Jain Malkin Inc.; Photographer: Jain Malkin.*)

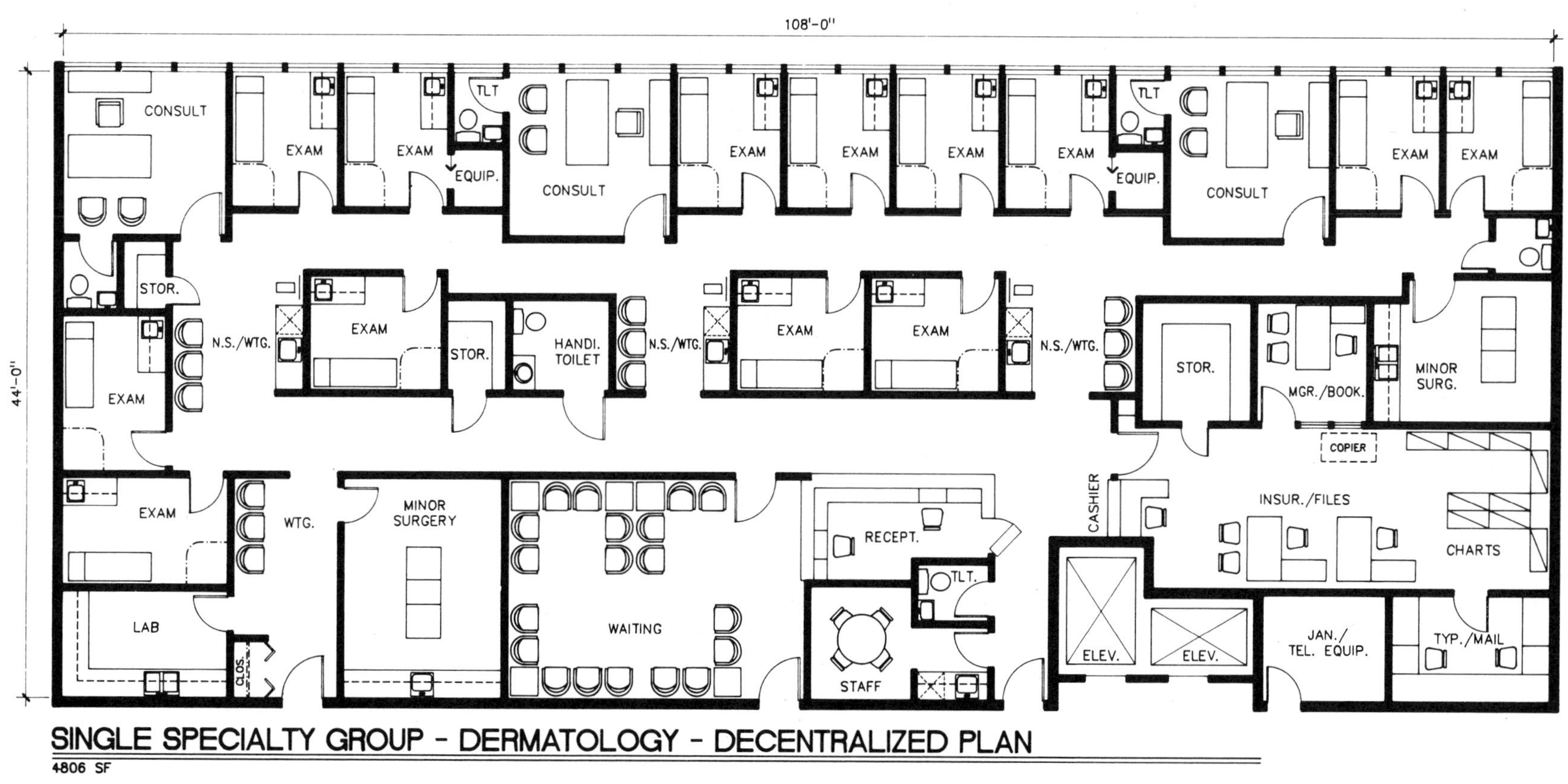

Figure 6-6. Suite plan for single-specialty group, dermatology, decentralized plan, 4806 square feet.

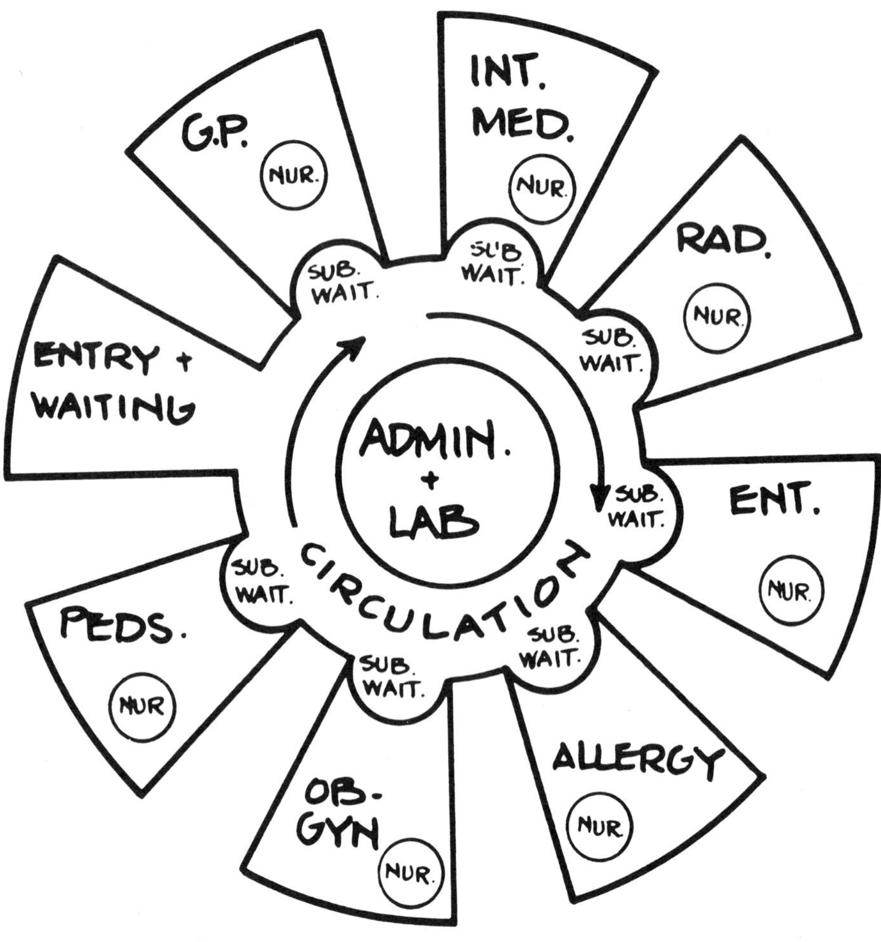

Figure 6-7. Schematic diagram of a satellite plan for a multispecialty group.

Multispecialty Group

This type of clinic offers the greatest challenge to a designer. The space to be planned may be vast, and each specialty must be carefully analyzed for its relationship to other specialties (Figures 6-7 and 6-8). Large multispecialty clinics tend to grow and change a good deal. Physicians leave, and others join the group. Departments are sometimes shuffled around to realign them according to new priorities. The facility should be designed for expansion with anticipation of which departments may outgrow their present limits.

Radiology, for example, tends to expand. New equipment is introduced, and due to the scale of the machinery, a single piece may require its own room. Thus it is a good idea to locate the radiology department on the perimeter of the suite adjacent to the area allocated for expansion. Radiography rooms are very costly to build due to special electrical, plumbing, and lead-shielding requirements; therefore, it would not be economically feasible to abandon existing radiology rooms, tearing them down to remodel for less specialized use such as additional examination rooms or an expanded waiting room. By locating the radiology department contiguous to the area of the proposed future expansion, existing radiology rooms need not be altered, but new rooms could be added.

Medical records is another area that often has to be expanded. However, since this would typically be located in the core of the suite, it is usually difficult to enlarge it. It is better to project a realistic number of charts and growth for a seven-year period (physicians must keep medical records for seven years) and make the room large enough to begin with.

If the building is designed for and owned by the doctors, the architect can take liberties with the design and make the structure of the building really conform to the spatial requirements of the group's practice. A large

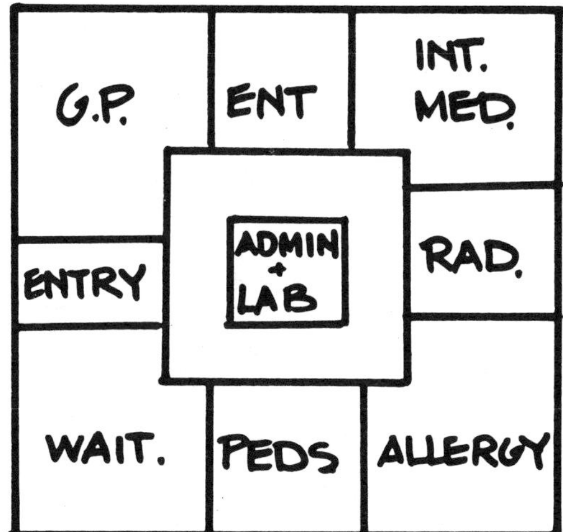

Figure 6-8. Schematic diagram for a multispecialty group, showing the relationship of specialties for optimum function—keeping the highest volume toward the front, pediatrics close to allergy, radiology close to internal medicine, lab and business office central to all.

MULTI-SPECIALTY GROUP

clinic may be laid out with the administrative and support services in the core, with each specialty department radiating out from it like spokes of a wheel. Each "spoke" would have its own nurse station and waiting room, but the clinical lab, medical records, insurance, business office, and so on would be in the core area (Figure 6-9). This is also known as a *satellite* plan.

If the square footage of each specialty department is not great, one large waiting room may be designed near the reception and business office. Patients would be called from there to the various departments. More often, each specialty department would function independently with its own waiting room, reception desk, nurse station, and other support facilities. There may be a central reception desk and waiting room at the entrance of the clinic, where an aide may prepare a

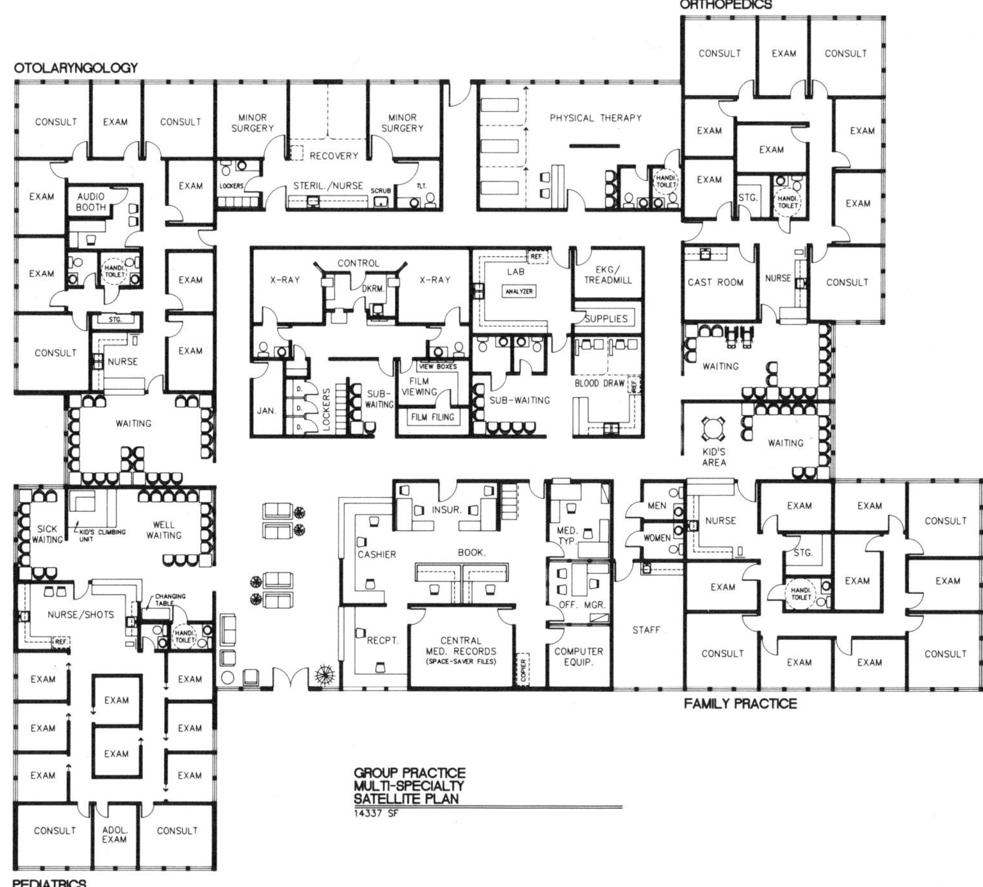

Figure 6-9. Suite plan for mixed-specialty group, satellite plan, 14,337 square feet.

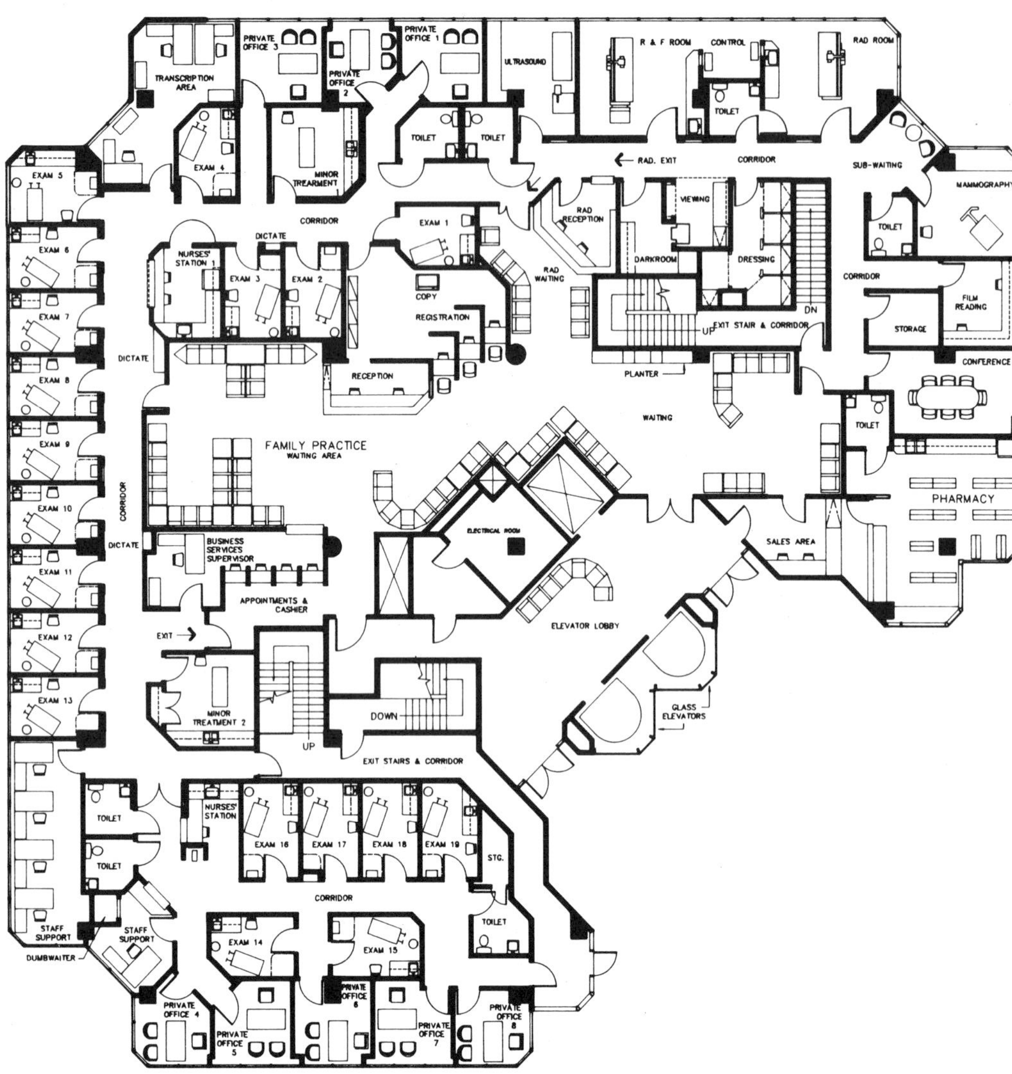

MULTI-SPECIALTY GROUP PRACTICE CLINIC, 30,000 SF MAIN LEVEL FLOOR PLAN

Figure 6-10a, b, and c. Suite plan for multispecialty group, 30,000 square feet.

form that the patient carries to the sub–reception desk located at the specialty department. Upon checking out, the patient may book a future appointment either at the sub–reception desk or at the central reception desk depending upon how the paperwork flow is set up. Payment for services would usually be made at the central reception desk or cashier's counter, if one exists, rather than at the specialty department.

Large medical offices use computer bookkeeping systems. The equipment varies somewhat, depending on the manufacturer and individual requirements, so the designer must carefully review the sizes of computer components, utility requirements, and communication linkage between departments. Computer terminals at each sub–reception desk can give each department access to a patient's ledger or to the appointment schedule without having to phone or walk over to the central business office.

The multispecialty group practice clinic shown in Figure 6-10 is 30,000 square feet in size and located on two-and-one-half floors of a large medical office building. The clinic includes internal medicine, family practice, radiology, pharmacy, vascular lab, cardiopulmonary testing, clinical lab, and a large endoscopy suite. Medical records, conference room/staff lounge, and the clinic administrator's office are on the lower level. Medical charts are brought up from the lower level to the circulation point on each floor via a dumbwaiter.

The clinic functions as a *group practice model* HMO, a PPO, and also accepts fee-for-service patients. On the first visit, the patient registers on the first floor, near the family practice reception desk. There an embossed card is dispensed, paperwork is handled, and a medical chart is prepared. The patient is then referred to the appropriate decentralized reception desk to check in prior to receiving treatment. On subsequent visits, the patient proceeds directly to the re-

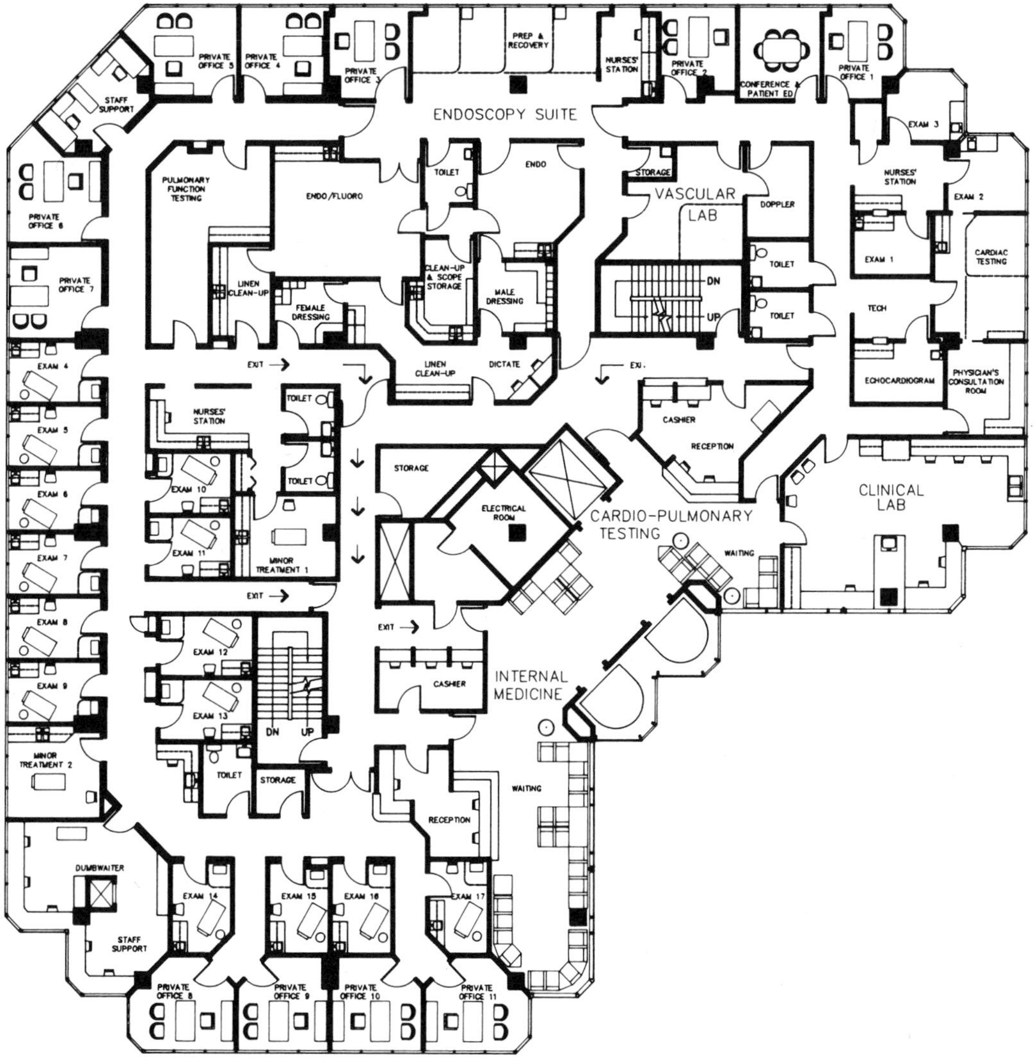

MULTI-SPECIALITY GROUP PRACTICE CLINIC
SECOND LEVEL FLOOR PLAN

Figure 6-10b.

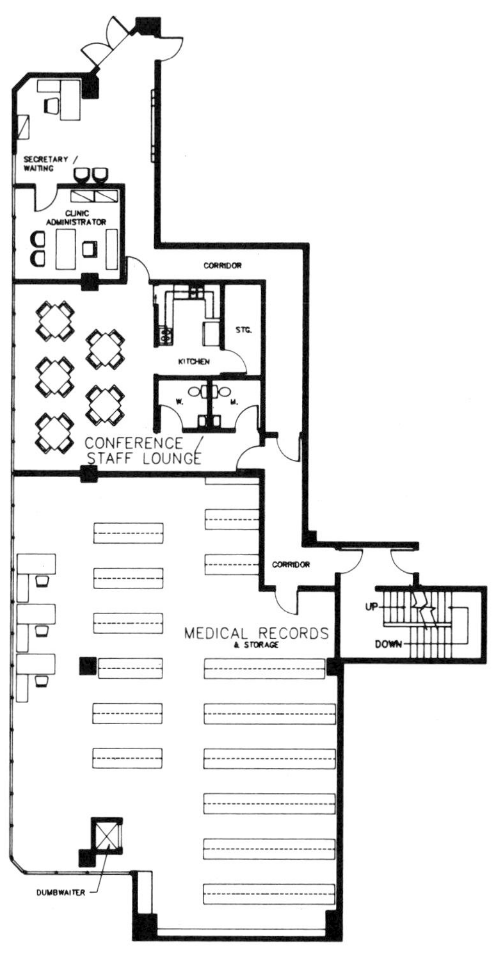

MULTI-SPECIALITY GROUP PRACTICE CLINIC
LOWER LEVEL FLOOR PLAN

Figure 6-10c.

ception desk at the respective department, and does not need to stop at the registration desk.

This is an example of a *decentralized* plan where each specialty department has its own reception and waiting area, with nurse stations, exam rooms, and private offices arranged in pods.

Great attention was paid to circulation patterns to minimize the possibility of patients leaving without passing the cashier desk. On the first floor, inset carpet designs and unique signage properly placed lead patients past the principal cashier station while radiology patients exit through the radiology waiting room. On the second floor, all exiting circulation is directed past two cashier stations. Color Plate 15, Figures 6-14 and 6-15, show an internal corridor and a view of the family practice waiting room. Figures 6-11 and 6-12 show the family practice reception desk and the clinic entrance/ registration area.

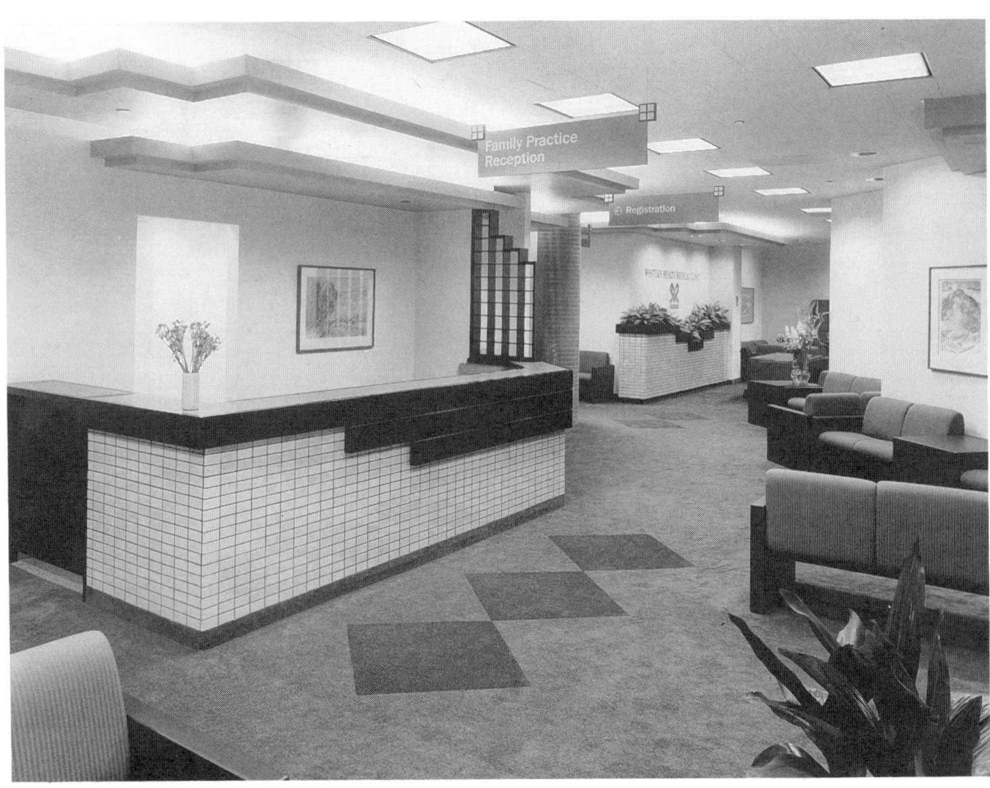

Figure 6-11. Family practice reception desk. (*Design: Jain Malkin Inc.; Photographer: Robinson/Ward.*)

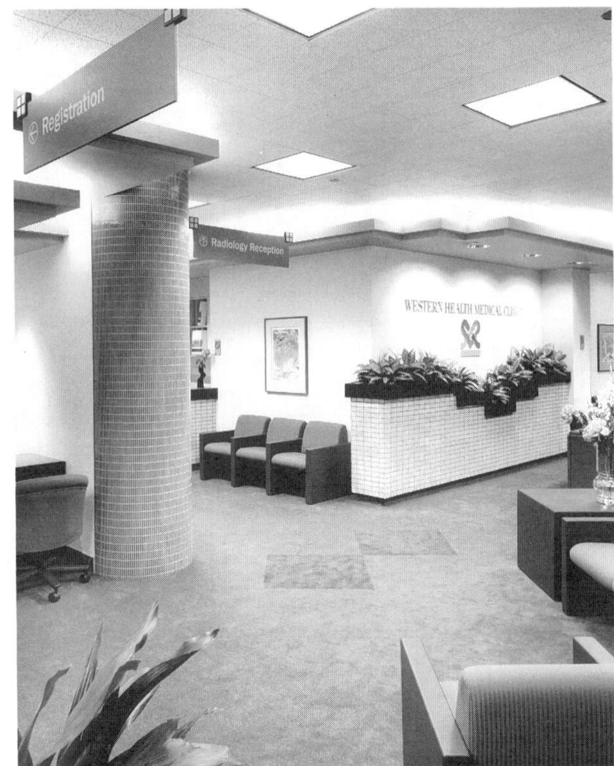

Figure 6-12. Clinic entry and registration area. (*Design: Jain Malkin Inc.; Photographer: Robinson/Ward.*)

Internal Medicine Group

This is a single-specialty group, but due to the many internal medicine subspecialties, more specialized rooms and a larger clinical lab and radiology suite are required than with most single-specialty groups. An internist specializing in cardiology or in pulmonary disease would need an EKG room and a cardiopulmonary lab. One who specializes in gastroenterology would require a proctology room and perhaps an endoscopy suite. If he or she wishes to do the G.I. series of X-rays in the office, a fluoroscopy room with adjoining toilet and barium prep area would be required. Endocrinologists, on the other hand, order many lab studies — some of which require patients to report to the lab in the morning and remain nearby for four to six hours, with blood being drawn every hour. Thus the lab must be of sufficient size to accommodate a high volume of work and should have a comfortable lounge for waiting patients.

The suite for a group practice of internists would typically have five exam rooms for each two doctors (two rooms for each doctor plus a third shared between them), a consultation room for each physician adjacent to his or her pod of exam rooms, a toilet, and a nurse station. The proctology rooms, EKG rooms, cardiopulmonary lab, clinical lab, and radiology suite would be located in the core area central to all exam rooms. The business office, insurance office, cashier's desk, and waiting room would be located at the entrance to the suite so that each patient upon entering and leaving must pass by the reception and cashier's desks (Figure 6-13).

Table 6-1. Analysis of Program. Group Practice—Single Specialty

	Internal Medicine 8 Physicians	General Practice 8 Physicians
Waiting Room(s)	35 × 35 = 1225	35 × 40 = 1400
Exam Rooms	20 @ 8 × 12 = 1920	24 @ 8 × 12 = 2304
Consultation Rooms	8 @ 12 × 14 = 1344	8 @ 12 × 12 = 1152
Nurse Stations	12 × 14 = 168	12 × 14 = 168
Toilets	4 @ 6 × 7 = 168	4 @ 6 × 7 = 168
Storage	12 × 12 = 144	12 × 12 = 144
Staff Lounge	12 × 16 = 192	12 × 16 = 192
Laboratory[a]	24 × 32 = 768	24 × 32 = 768
Minor Surgery	—	2 @ 12 × 12 = 288
Cast Room	—	12 × 14 = 168
EKG Room[b]	2 @ 12 × 10 = 240	12 × 14 = 168
Radiology[c]	12 × 26 = 312	12 × 26 = 312
Procto Room[d]	12 × 15 = 180	—
Business Office[e]	24 × 24 = 576	24 × 24 = 576
Office Manager	12 × 10 = 120	12 × 10 = 120
Pulmonary Function Lab (optional)	16 × 20 = 320	—
Medical Records	12 × 16 = 192	12 × 16 = 192
Insurance	14 × 16 = 224	14 × 16 = 224
Subtotal	8093 ft²	8344 ft²
20% Circulation	1618	1669
Total	9711 ft²	10,013 ft²

[a]Includes lab waiting, blood draw, recovery, toilet.

[b]Includes mounting area.

[c]Includes darkroom, control, film filing, film viewing, dressing area. (Radiography room not equipped for fluoroscopy.)

[d]Includes prep area and toilet.

[e]Includes reception, bookkeeper's office, transcription, computer equipment.

Table 6-2. Analysis of Program. Group Practice—Single Specialty

	OB-GYN 8 Physicians	Orthopedics 8 Physicians
Waiting Room(s)	35 × 40 = 1400	40 × 40 = 1600
Exam Rooms	21 @ 8 × 12 = 2016	12 @ 8 × 12 = 1152
Consultation Rooms	8 @ 12 × 12 = 1152	8 @ 12 × 11 = 1056
Nurse Stations	2 @ 8 × 10 = 160	2 @ 6 × 8 = 96
Toilets	6 @ 6 × 7 = 252	4 @ 6 × 7 = 168
Storage	12 × 12 = 144	12 × 12 = 144
Staff Lounge	12 × 16 = 192	12 × 12 = 144
Lab	12 × 16 = 192	—
Minor Surgery	14 × 16 = 224	14 × 16 = 224
Cast Rooms	—	4 @ 12 × 12 = 576
Radiology	—	12 × 28 = 336
Business Office	16 × 30 = 480	16 × 30 = 480
Office Manager	10 × 12 = 120	10 × 12 = 120
Insurance	14 × 16 = 224	14 × 16 = 224
Medical Records	12 × 16 = 192	12 × 16 = 192
Head Nurse's Office	10 × 10 = 100	—
Physical Therapy	—	25 × 45 = 1125
Subtotal	6848 ft²	7637 ft²
20% Circulation	1370	1527
Total	8218 ft²	9164 ft²

Table 6-3. Analysis of Program. Group Practice—Multispecialty—9 Physicians

This program assumes the following: 2 internists, 3 general practitioners, 3 pediatricians, and 1 otolaryngologist; a central business office and lab will serve all; in addition to the central supply, several small storage rooms would be scattered throughout the facility.

Waiting Rooms	40 × 45 =	1800
Pedo Exam Rooms	2 @ 8 × 12 & 8 @ 8 × 8 =	704
Pedo Nurse Station	10 × 12 =	120
Pedo Consultation Rooms	3 @ 10 × 12 =	360
ENT Exams	2 @ 8 × 12 =	192
Audio Room	10 × 12 =	120
ENT Minor Surgery	12 × 12 =	144
ENT Consultation Room	12 × 12 =	144
ENT Nurse Station	8 × 8 =	64
I.M. Exam Rooms	5 @ 8 × 12 =	480
I.M. Consultation Rooms	2 @ 12 × 12 =	288
I.M. Nurse Station	8 × 10 =	80
Procto Room[a]	12 × 15 =	180
EKG/Cardiopulmonary Lab	16 × 18 =	288
G.P. Exam Rooms	9 @ 8 × 12 =	864
G.P. Consultation Rooms	3 @ 12 × 12 =	432
G.P. Nurse Station	8 × 10 =	80
Cast Room	12 × 12 =	144
Minor Surgery	12 × 12 =	144
Staff Lounge	14 × 16 =	224
Central Supply	12 × 16 =	192
Medical Records	12 × 16 =	192
Office Manager	12 × 10 =	120
Lab[b]	24 × 32 =	768
Radiology[c]	12 × 26 =	312
Toilets	7 @ 6 × 7 =	294
Business Office:		
Reception	10 × 12 =	120
Bookkeeper	14 × 16 =	224
Insurance/Collections	14 × 16 =	224
Transcription	10 × 12 =	120
Computer Equip./Clerical	12 × 12 =	144
Subtotal		9562 ft²
20% Circulation		1912
Total		11,474 ft²

[a]Includes prep area and toilet.

[b]Includes lab, lab waiting, blood draw, recovery, toilet, storage.

[c]Includes darkroom, control, film filing, viewing areas, dressing area.

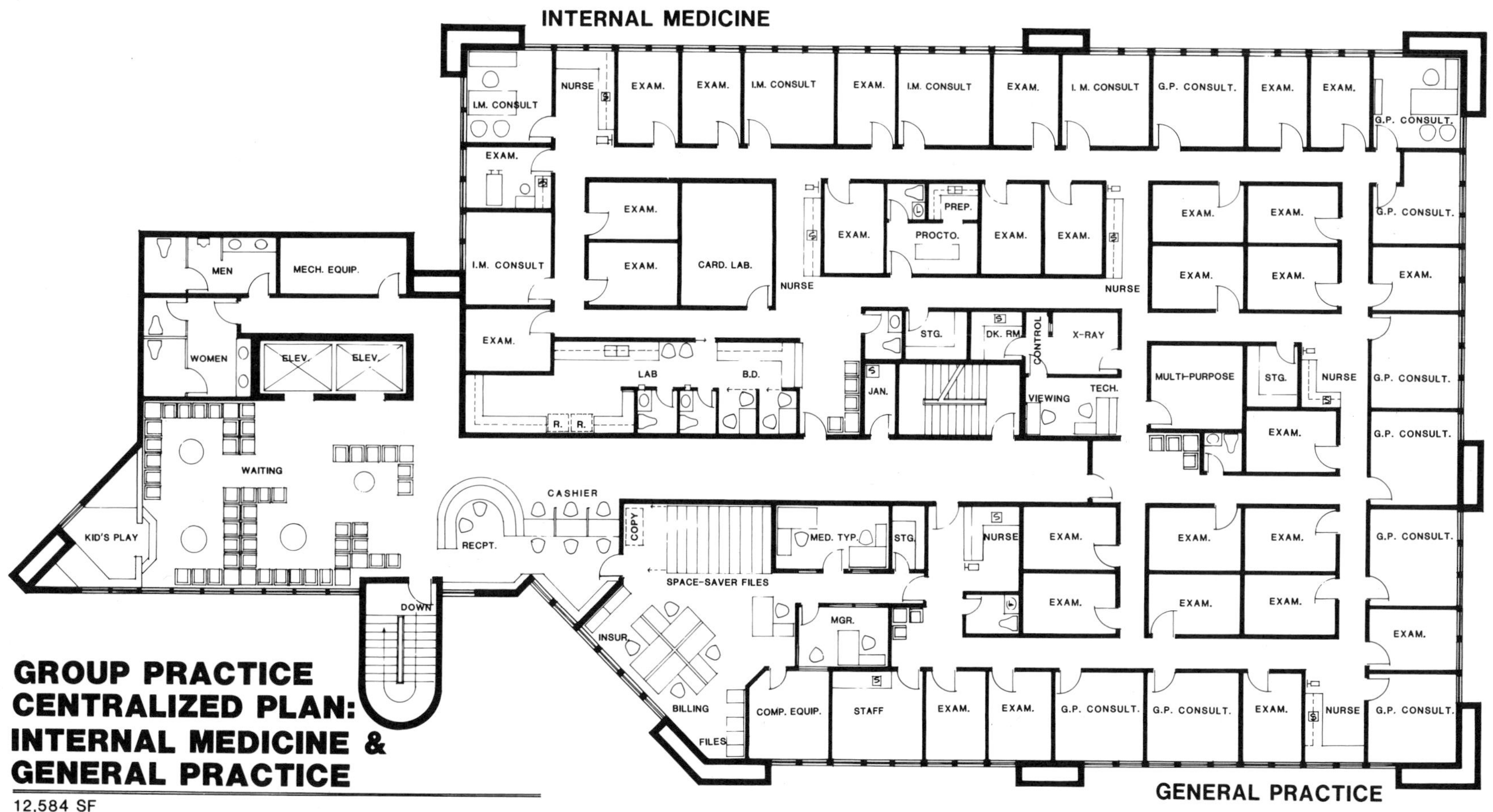

Figure 6-13. Suite plan for group practice, centralized plan, 12,584 square feet.

A large group practice will have a business manager or an administrator who will require a small private office preferably with a window wall (starting at 48 inches off the floor) facing the business office so that he or she can keep an eye on operations at all times.

Patients may at times report to the lab without having to see a physician, so the lab should be located at the front of the suite, enabling a patient to enter and leave without mingling with patients waiting for visits with a physician. In fact, the lab might have an entrance from the street (or public corridor of the medical building) directly into the lab. The reader is referred to Chapter 5 for space planning requirements of a clinical lab.

The waiting room must accommodate one hour's patients per doctor. Thus if each doctor can see an average of four patients per hour and each has 2.5 examining rooms, an eight-physician group would need seating for approximately 44 persons in the waiting room or elsewhere within the suite when all doctors are seeing patients simultaneously. A formula for estimating the required number of seats is:

$$2P \times D - E = S$$

where

P = Average number of patients per hour per doctor
D = Number of doctors
E = Number of exam rooms
S = Seating

The formula assumes that each patient arrives with one other person, a friend or relative.

Allowing that some patients will arrive unaccompanied by a friend or relative and some will be directed to the lab, X-ray, procto room, or EKG room, the 44 required seats might be reduced to 35 at the absolute minimum. Figuring 18 square feet per person, a waiting room that will accommodate 44 persons will have to be approximately 792 square feet in size.

General Practice Group

The suite for a general practice group would be an expansion of a suite for a solo G.P. (refer to Chapter 3). It would also include cast rooms, an X-ray facility, a lab, a private office for a business manager, and maybe a small allergy suite. Often a group of G.P.s will include a general surgeon. The formula discussed above for estimating the number of seats in the waiting room applies here, except that a G.P. can see up to six patients an hour, and each G.P. should have the use of three exam rooms.

CHAPTER 7

Ambulatory Surgical Centers

OVERVIEW

Ambulatory surgery refers to scheduled surgical procedures provided to patients who do not require overnight hospitalization. Ambulatory surgery may be provided in a physician's office — in which case it is called *office-based surgery* — or in a freestanding, independent facility specifically organized to provide scheduled ambulatory surgery.

The practice of ambulatory surgery is not a new concept. The British Medical Association in 1909 reported 7320 operations performed by a Scottish physician on ambulatory patients at the Royal Glasgow Hospital for Children.[1] The results were reported to be as successful as those for inpatient surgery. However, the interest in ambulatory surgery declined somewhat until the early 1960s when the development of new fast-acting anesthetics made ambulatory surgery more practical.

The first successful freestanding ambulatory surgical center (FASC) is generally recognized to be the Phoenix Surgicenter®, which began operations in February 1970. Anesthesiologists Wallace Reed and John Ford established the facility that has become the model for other non-hospital-based ambulatory surgical centers.

The freestanding ambulatory surgical center may be organized according to a variety of operational models that vary according to type of ownership and sponsorship, affiliation with hospitals, and types of services offered. The term *freestanding* may be used to refer to a facility that is physically separate from another, such as a hospital, or it may mean a facility whose program and ownership are independent and legally distinct from any other organization.

Ambulatory surgical centers may be located within a hospital, may be a separate building located on the hospital campus, or may be a satellite facility located off campus. Some ambulatory surgical centers are entrepreneurial enterprises owned and operated by a group of anesthesiologists or surgeons and have no affiliation with a hospital. These facilities are commonly located within a medical office building, or they may be physically freestanding in a single tenant building. It is this last example which is the focus of this chapter — a facility not owned by a hospital and located in a medical office building.

Advantages of Ambulatory Surgery

There are many advantages to ambulatory surgery from both the patients' and the physicians' viewpoints. Some of these advantages follow.

1. Hospitals are geared to traditional inpatient surgery protocols, which are often inappropriate for am-

[1]Thomas O'Donovan, *Ambulatory Surgical Centers,* Germantown, Maryland, Aspen Systems Corp., 1976, p. 4.

bulatory patients, whereas a facility organized for the sole purpose of ambulatory surgery would have a staff trained to meet the specific needs of these patients. Hospitals sometimes find it difficult to merge new protocols with existing systems.

2. Ambulatory surgery patients are not sick; they are candidates for elective procedures. In a hospital, their families may have to share a common surgery waiting room with inpatients' families, which can have a devastating psychological effect. Imagine the stress of sitting next to someone whose husband may be having open heart surgery.

3. Patients often experience psychological stress when entering a hospital. Fear of the unknown is heightened by unexpected sights, such as a view of a patient arriving in an ambulance, or seeing a patient on a gurney with an IV in the arm. Patients are generally less apprehensive when arriving for surgery in a facility located in a medical office building.

4. Physicians and staff often experience greater satisfaction in an FASC because they can tailor operational systems as they wish, with no bureaucratic red tape.

5. There is much greater flexibility in scheduling procedures in an FASC. In a hospital, ambulatory patients will be bumped to open up the schedule for urgent or emergent patients. Both physicians and patients find ease of scheduling an advantage in an FASC.

6. Ambulatory surgery provides for better utilization of hospital beds and generally costs less than doing the same procedure in a hospital. The major saving is due to elimination of a hospital stay, and insurance providers often stipulate they will pay for certain procedures only if done within an ambulatory surgical center.

7. Ambulatory surgical patients receive less medication both pre- and postoperatively, and they often return to work sooner than people who have those same procedures as inpatients. Perhaps this is due to the fact that FASCs promote a wellness philosophy, treating patients as if they are healthy, and allowing them to take responsibility for a large part of their own care.

Economic and Regulatory Issues

Prior to designing an FASC, it is necessary to understand the facility's goals with respect to licensing, certificate-of-need (CON) requirements, accreditation, and reimbursement by Medicare/Medicaid and commercial insurance carriers.

Licensure. A facility owned and operated by a physician group practice generally need not be state licensed, provided that non-owner surgeons are not allowed privileges. A physician's license to practice his or her specialty meets the requirements. Surgical procedures are usually done on a small scale and are performed within the context of the physician's practice. State agencies typically do not regulate office-based surgery. However, when a facility is organized specifically for the purpose of ambulatory surgery, and a surgeon need not be an owner to be awarded privileges, then licensure of the facility becomes an issue.

Only in the last few years have state regulatory agencies become concerned with licensing facilities other than hospitals. Licensing is often a requirement for receiving state reimbursement, and insurance payers may require that a facility be licensed for their participation. Furthermore, licensed facilities may be eligible for rate discounts from liability carriers.

NFPA 101 Life Safety Code and state building codes are the standard for all licensing and certification requirements. The designer must check with the state fire marshal, state facilities' development agencies, and the local building department to ensure that all requirements are identified. The cost of designing a facility initially to meet licensing requirements will be comparatively small compared with retrofitting it later to achieve compliance. Licensing offers a certain amount of economic security in that it assures the facility of receiving the maximum amount of reimbursement offered by payers.

CON/Health Systems Agency Review. Each state is unique in its approach to regulating FASCs. The Health Planning and Resources Development Act of 1974 mandated that state governments establish Certificate-of-Need (CON) programs to regulate health care facilities and services. In some states, a CON may be required for an FASC, whether it be owned by a hospital or another entity. The purposes of the CON are to prevent duplication of highly specialized facilities and equipment, and to keep a lid on rising health care costs. Some states exempt facilities from the CON process if they are non-hospital-owned.

In many states, the CON process starts with review by the local Health Systems Agency (HSA), which must endorse the project and make recommendations to the state. Early in the planning stages of an FASC, it is essential to ascertain whether a CON may be required, and whether HSA endorsement is mandatory. If a local HSA does not exist, there may be another areawide health planning agency that should be consulted. It should be noted that many states have abandoned their CON programs since the federal government ceased funding them. The national trend toward deregulation allows FASCs a much easier path to their goals.

Accreditation. The Joint Commission on Accreditation of Hospitals (JCAH) can accredit freestanding ambulatory surgical centers that are not owned by hospitals; however, accreditation by the Accreditation Association for Ambulatory Health Care (AAAHC), established in 1979, is more common. This is a voluntary accreditation program aimed at quality assurance in all aspects of patient care. The agency publishes a handbook of standards for ambulatory health care as well as a code checklist for ambulatory surgical facilities based on compliance with NFPA 101 Life Safety Code.

It should be noted that there is a national organization for freestanding ambulatory surgical centers called FASA (Federated Ambulatory Surgical Association), with national headquarters located in Alexandria, Virginia.

Certification. Medicare certification is a requirement for receipt of federal reimbursement for patients eligible to receive these benefits. With respect to the physical plant, Medicare does not stipulate sizes of rooms or number of scrub sinks per operating room, but rather relies entirely on compliance with NFPA 101 Life Safety Code. Medicare engages a local state fire marshal to conduct the survey of a new facility to verify compliance. Medicare certification paves the way for approval by other reimbursement agencies and insurance carriers. It constitutes the seal of approval, so to speak. In reality, there is little difference between licensure and certification with respect to design criteria, because both rely upon compliance with the Life Safety Code.

Reimbursement Policies. The total charge for a surgical procedure has two components. One is the anesthesiologist's and surgeon's professional fees, and the other is the facility fee — the charge for the surgical suite, operating room staff, and supplies. Third-party payers vary in their reimbursement policy with respect to these two components.

Physicians are generally reimbursed a reasonable and customary fee for their services regardless of whether the facility is licensed or certified; however, third-party payers will not pay for the use of the facility unless it meets certain criteria. These usually involve a strict adherence to the Life Safety Code. Therefore, Medicare certification and/or state licensure assure that the FASC will be reimbursed for the use of the facility.

Marketing Considerations

Among the most attractive features of surgery in a freestanding facility is the element of choice. A physician may have privileges at several facilities and may offer the patient the opportunity to choose the preferred setting. Along with that choice comes the expectation of care delivered in a small-scale, nonclinical, friendly environment. Patient satisfaction is necessary for a facility's success, and many FASCs are keenly aware of guest relations.

The interior environment is a critical element of patient satisfaction. The entire facility should use color to relax and soothe patients, and texture should be introduced in carpets and wallcoverings, whenever appropriate (in terms of maintenance and infection control). Artwork and accessories should not be overlooked as a means of distracting patients and making the facility less threatening.

However, patients and their families are not the only ones who benefit from a well-designed environment. In order to attract top quality physicians and nursing staff and to keep morale high, staff areas must be properly designed so that they are functional, and they should look as attractive as patient areas.

Survey of Surgical Procedures

It is helpful to understand, prior to designing a facility, the types of procedures that are normally performed in an FASC. A survey of 880 facilities nationwide is represented in Table 7-1, indicating that nearly 60 percent of procedures fall into three specialty categories.

Table 7-1. Specialty Surgical Procedures Performed in Freestanding Surgery Centers in 1987

Type of Procedure	Percentage
Ophthalmology	27.2
Gynecological	20.4
ENT	10.8
Orthopedic	10.2
General	9.1
Plastic	8.9
Urology	3.8
Podiatry	4.9
Dental/Oral	1.8
Other	2.9
	100.0

Source: Freestanding Outpatient Surgery Centers Report and Directory, June 30, 1988. SMG Marketing Group, Chicago, Illinois.

FACILITY DESIGN

An enormous amount of careful planning precedes the establishment of an ambulatory surgical center. Feasibility studies analyze the demographics of the area and determine the demand for such a facility. In terms of codes and regulatory agency review, an FASC is certainly the most complicated of any outpatient facility.

Location

The feasibility study will identify, among other things, the geographical area from which patients will be drawn. Travel time factors heavily into the equation.

FASCs, after all, are designed to be convenient for patients; therefore, driving distance and site accessibility are important. Traffic patterns near the location, parking space, visibility from the street, and building appearance all require consideration.

What makes an FASC so sensitive to these factors is that the best marketing efforts cannot create an increased demand within a given area for surgical services. Business must be generated from within the existing demand of the area served. Marketing studies will reveal whether there is excess demand, whether existing facilities are underutilized, or whether projected growth will support the additional service.

Transfer Agreement

The preference for a facility to be located near a hospital is a matter of individual consideration. The incidence of need for patient transfer to a hospital has been much lower than was originally anticipated. Those transfers which have occurred were nearly always for pain control or for persistent bleeding. Transfer for life-threatening conditions has been almost unheard of according to studies done by the Federated Ambulatory Surgical Association (FASA). This is the result of careful patient screening to determine potential risks and careful selection of types of procedures successfully performed on an outpatient basis.

Codes

The FASC has many characteristics of a hospital inpatient surgery unit, and must comply with many, but not necessarily all, of the same requirements imposed upon hospitals. To receive certification and/or licensure, which may or may not be required depending upon jurisdiction, state administrative codes and NFPA 101 Life Safety Code must be followed. Federal guidelines focus almost entirely on operational procedures of the facility, and they make virtually no demands above state requirements for the built environment.

Explosion/Fire/Electrical Shock. Codes are designed to prevent a variety of hazards in the operating room and recovery areas, and to reduce fire hazards elsewhere. The National Electrical Code (NEC) is widely used across the nation to set standards for the use of electricity. This code, like the others described here, is implemented through adoption by state and local jurisdictions, and exact requirements vary somewhat from region to region. For instance, explosive anesthetic gases, which might be ignited by a stray spark, are virtually never used in an FASC, yet some states require that conductive flooring and isolated electrical power be used. Other states recognize that this is unnecessary.

NFPA 101 concentrates on fire protection and prevention. NFPA 99 is the industry standard for storage and distribution of hazardous gases, vacuum systems, essential electrical systems, and respiratory therapy.

Power Failure. Emergency power for certain medical equipment and for exit lighting is required. The capacity and intended use are described in the NEC, section 517. It gives requirements for ORs and recovery areas, and defines which features are required to enhance life safety.

Infection Control. The most pervasive risk in the surgery setting is that of infection. This involves two issues: contamination of the open wound and staff exposure to HIV or hepatitis virus. Facility design, internal protocols for handling infectious waste, and proper protection during surgery are the three principal ways of reducing this hazard.

Patient and staff circulation patterns bear significantly on the spread of infectious microorganisms. This often poses a challenge for the space planner, since program requirements often exceed available space, sometimes reducing circulation alternatives. State building codes usually establish standards for smooth and washable finishes, and for special air handling requirements within specific areas, but there is little of a definitive nature in the way of regulatory codes to assist the designer in laying out the suite to minimize the spread of infection. Common sense, experience, and guidance of the OR supervisor often dictate proper alternatives.

Today, the risk of AIDS is the major health hazard to be encountered whenever working with blood or body fluids. Extreme care must be taken in the surgery setting to protect both patients and staff. The Centers for Disease Control in Atlanta and the Association of Operating Room Nurses in Denver offer written guidelines on facility design and patient handling to control the risk of infection.

Operational Protocols

FASCs adhere to very strict procedural protocols. In order to assure life safety and quality of care, and to move patients and supplies through the facility with ease and efficiency, it is imperative that each task be performed routinely, in the same manner, by all personnel. The AAAHC guides facilities on protocols for medical record keeping, patient discharge procedures, quality assurance/peer review, patients' rights, and so forth.

Every aspect of patient handling is based on a protocol developed by the individual facility, to assure that nothing is forgotten or overlooked. While many of these protocols do not actually have an impact on the physical design of the facility, it is important for a successful project to include in the planning process representatives of all staff functions including anesthesiologists, surgeons, and nursing and administrative staff. The space planner must avoid making any assumptions about a center's operations that could inadvertently defeat operational effectiveness.

Patient Flow

There are seven stages of patient flow through the facility: *pre-admitting, arrival, patient prep, induction, recovery, post-recovery,* and *discharge.* The patient's first encounter with the facility may be a day or two prior to surgery, to complete pre-admission forms, have laboratory tests, and receive dietary instructions.

This may be the first time the patient has ever had surgery, or perhaps the first time the patient has had ambulatory surgery, and he or she may have no frame of reference upon which to rely to defeat fear and anxiety. Therefore, it is important that the pre-admitting process give the patient confidence about the experience. After all, a patient truly cannot evaluate the quality of the clinical care or the surgeon's competence, but patients do make judgments nevertheless, based on interactions with staff and an assessment of the interior environment.

A patient's confidence can be bolstered by an understanding of exactly what to expect on the day of surgery. Nursing staff, anesthesiologists, and surgeons all play a significant role in educating and reassuring the patient. If the facility is designed well, circulation patterns will be predictable and convenient, allowing easy access for patients, staff, and family. Good design should make it easy for staff to do things right.

The patient arrives on the day of surgery anywhere from one and one-half to three hours prior to the scheduled surgery time, accompanied by an escort.

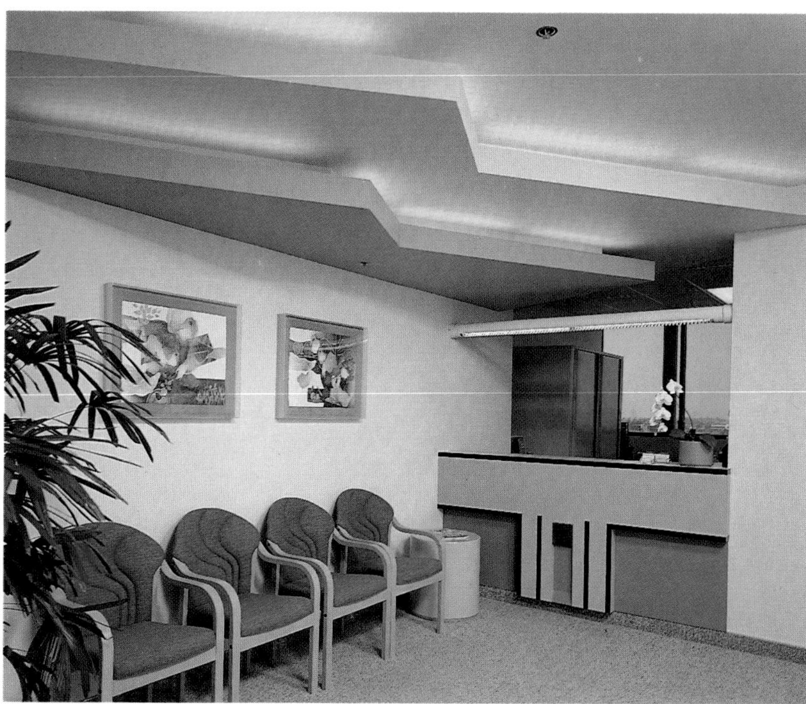

Figure 3-2. Waiting room. (*Design: Jain Malkin Inc.; Photographer: John Christian.*)

Figure 3-3. Pediatric play area. (*Photo courtesy Richard Foster Associates, Architects and Interior Designers, Greenwich, CT; Photographer: Copyright Norman McGrath 1985.*)

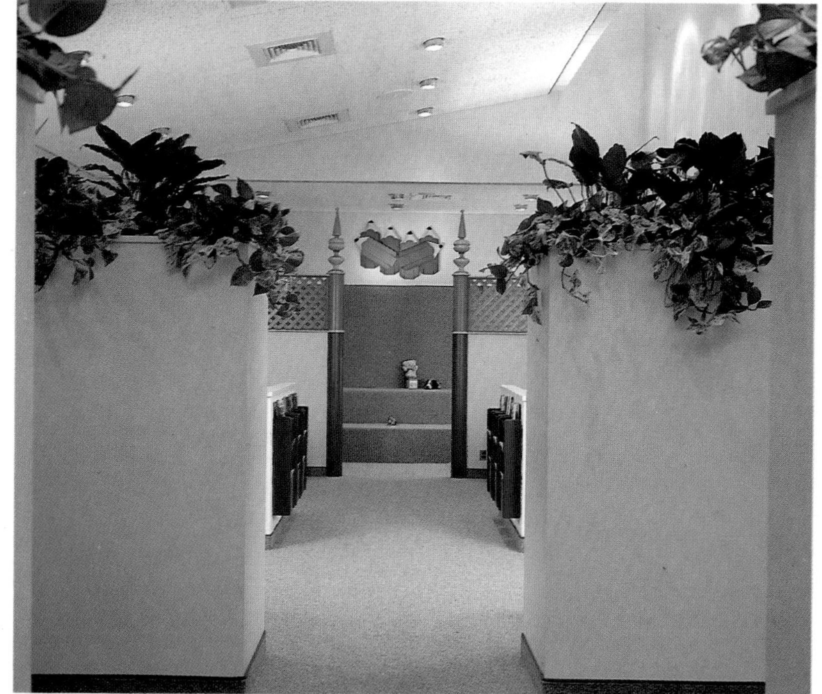

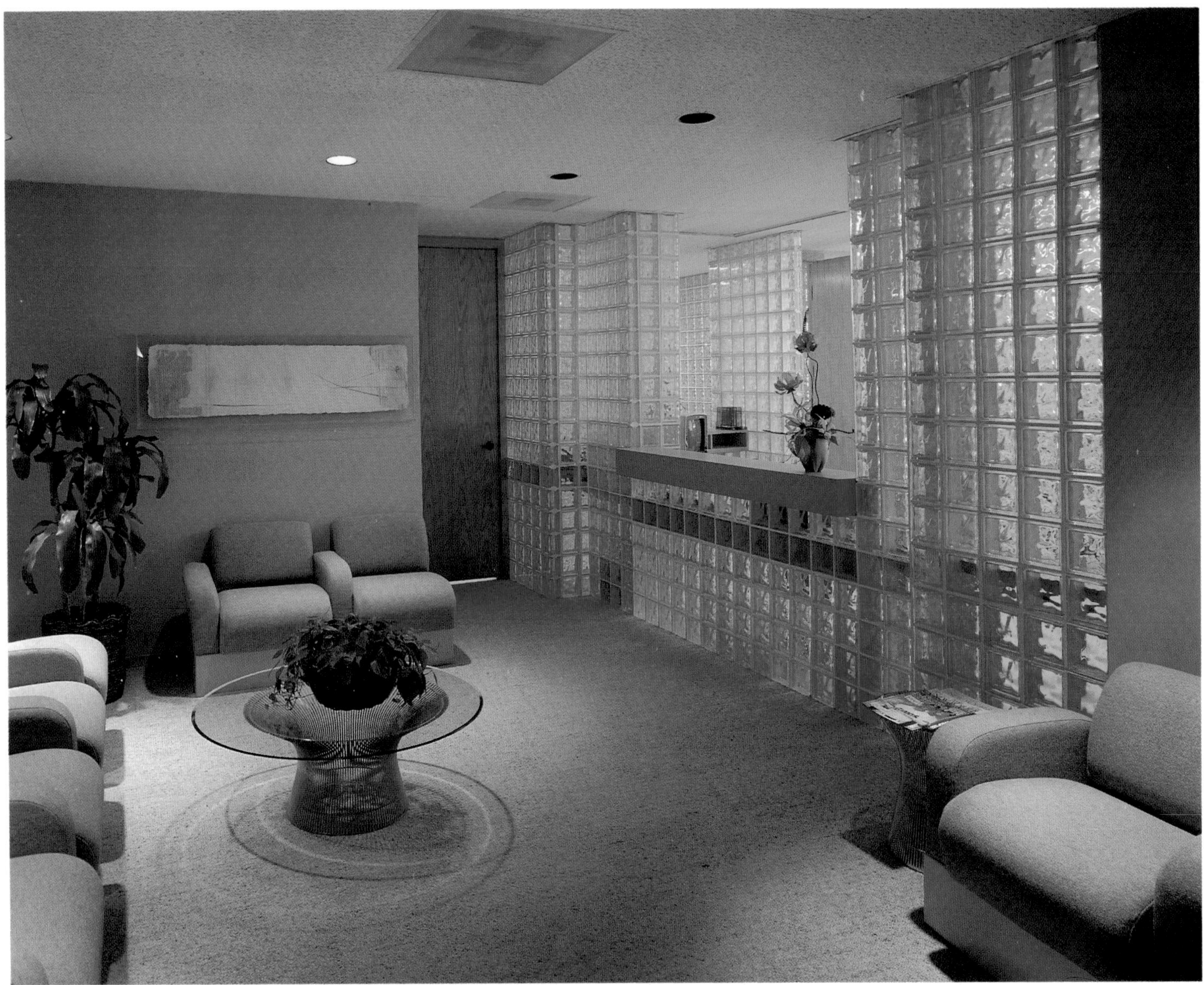

Figure 3-56. Waiting room, cardiac surgery suite. (*Design: Jain Malkin Inc.; Photographer: John Christian.*)

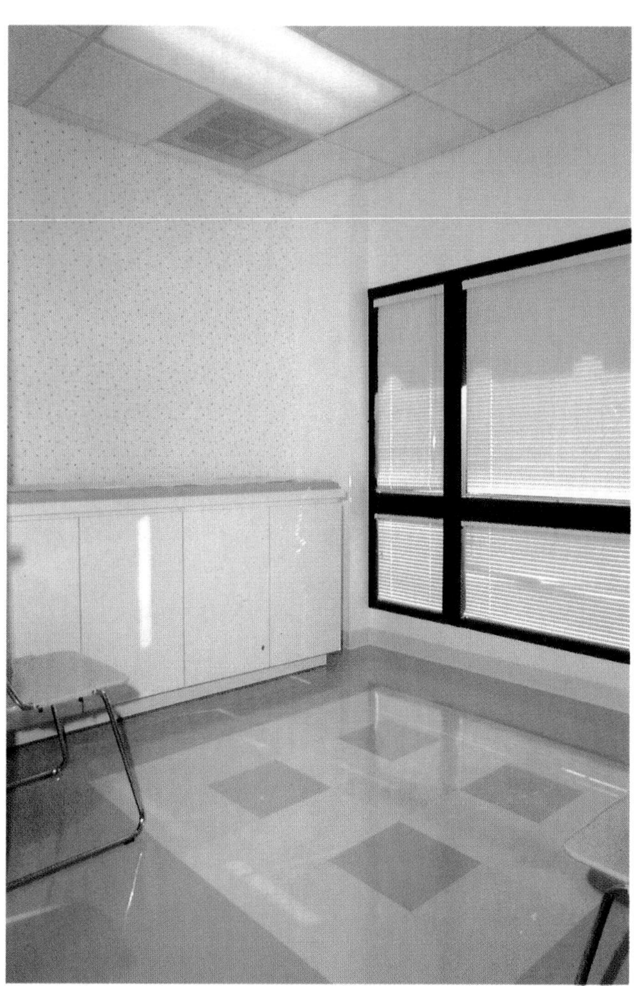

Figure 3-77. Pediatric examination room. (*Design: Jain Malkin Inc.; Photographer: Jain Malkin.*)

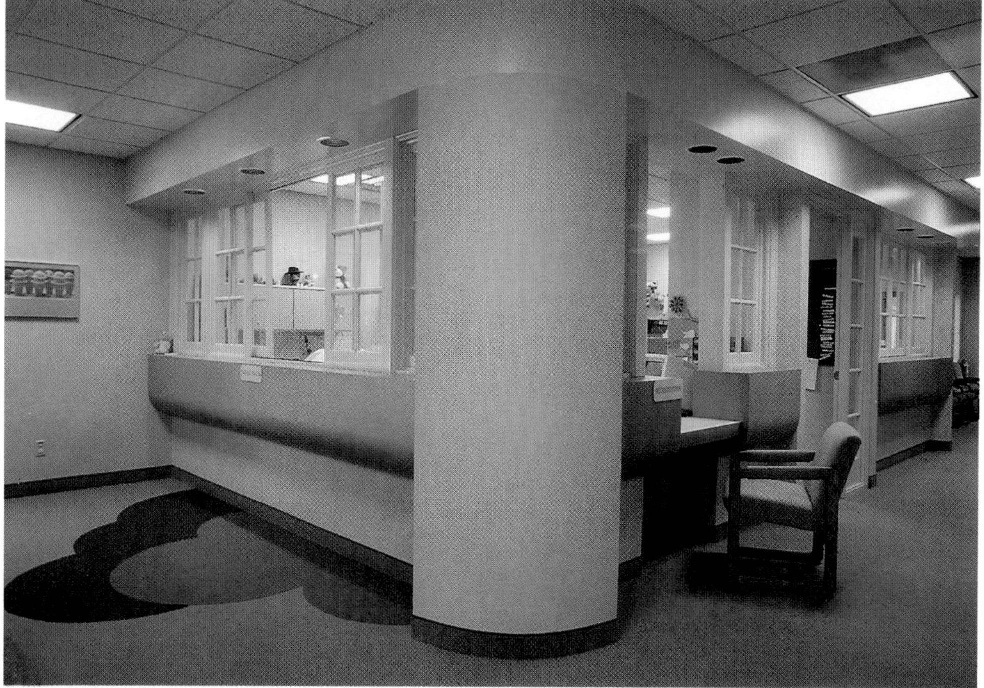

Figure 3-79. Reception window, pediatrics clinic. (*Design: Jain Malkin Inc.; Photographer: John Christian.*)

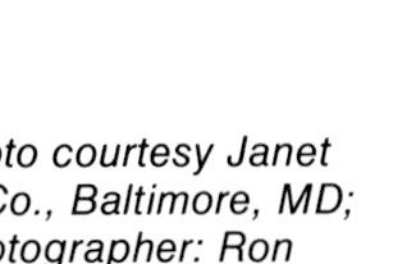

Figure 4-12. Waiting room, OB-GYN suite. (*Photo courtesy Janet K. Richardson, ASID, formerly of the Chambers Co., Baltimore, MD; currently principal, RHA Ltd., Baltimore, MD; Photographer: Ron Solomon*)

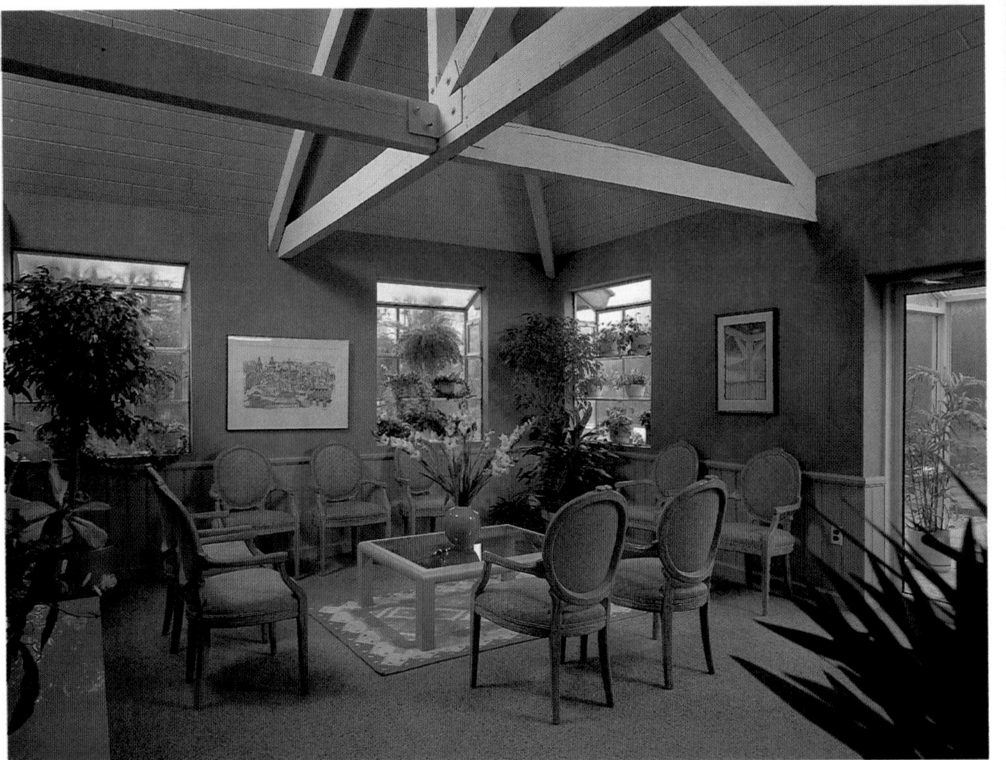

Figure 4-3. Children's area. (*Design: Jain Malkin Inc.; Photographer: Michael Denny.*)

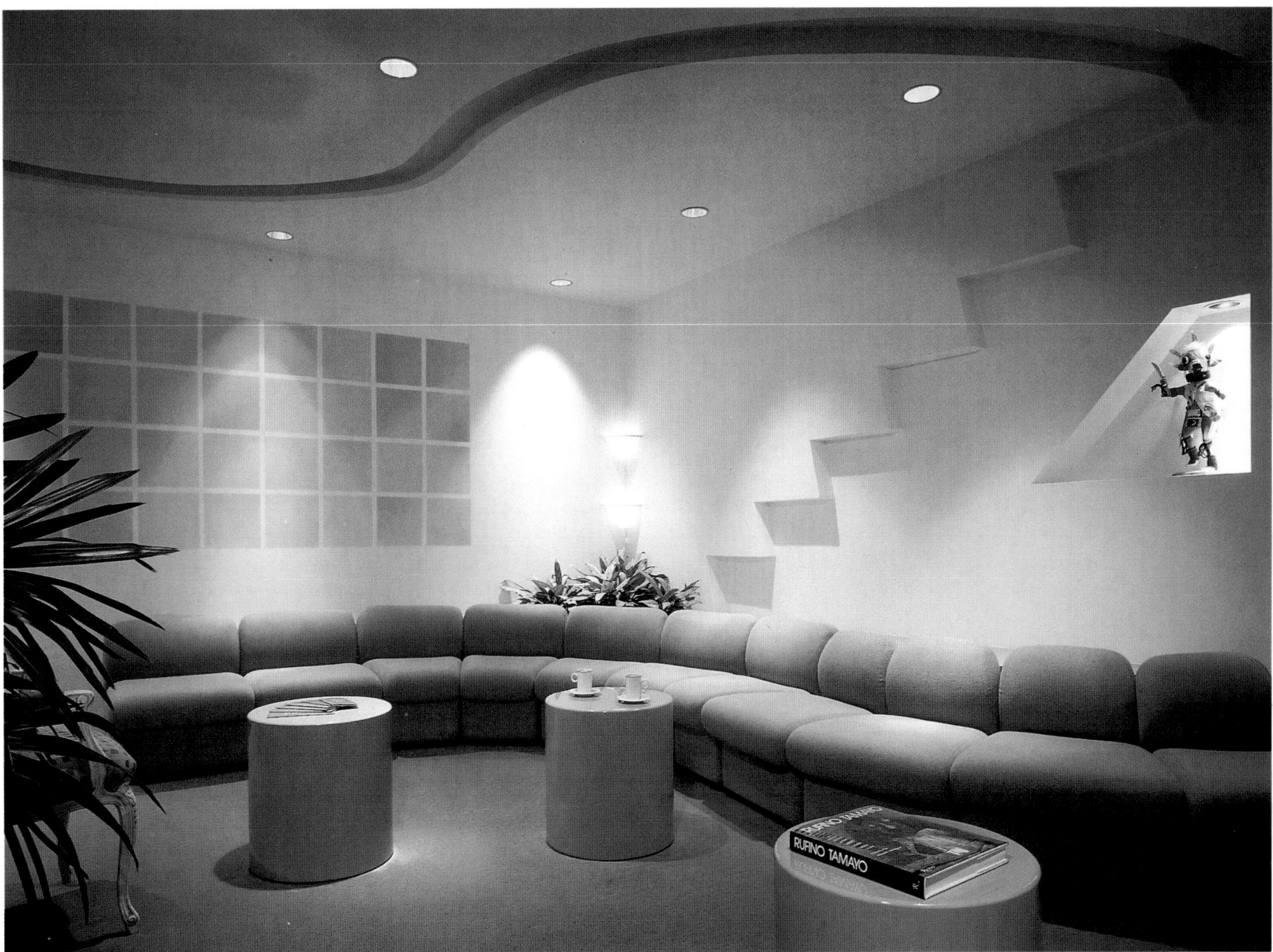

Figure 4-13. Waiting room, women's clinic. (*Design: Jain Malkin Inc.; Photographer: Kim Brun.*)

Plate 6

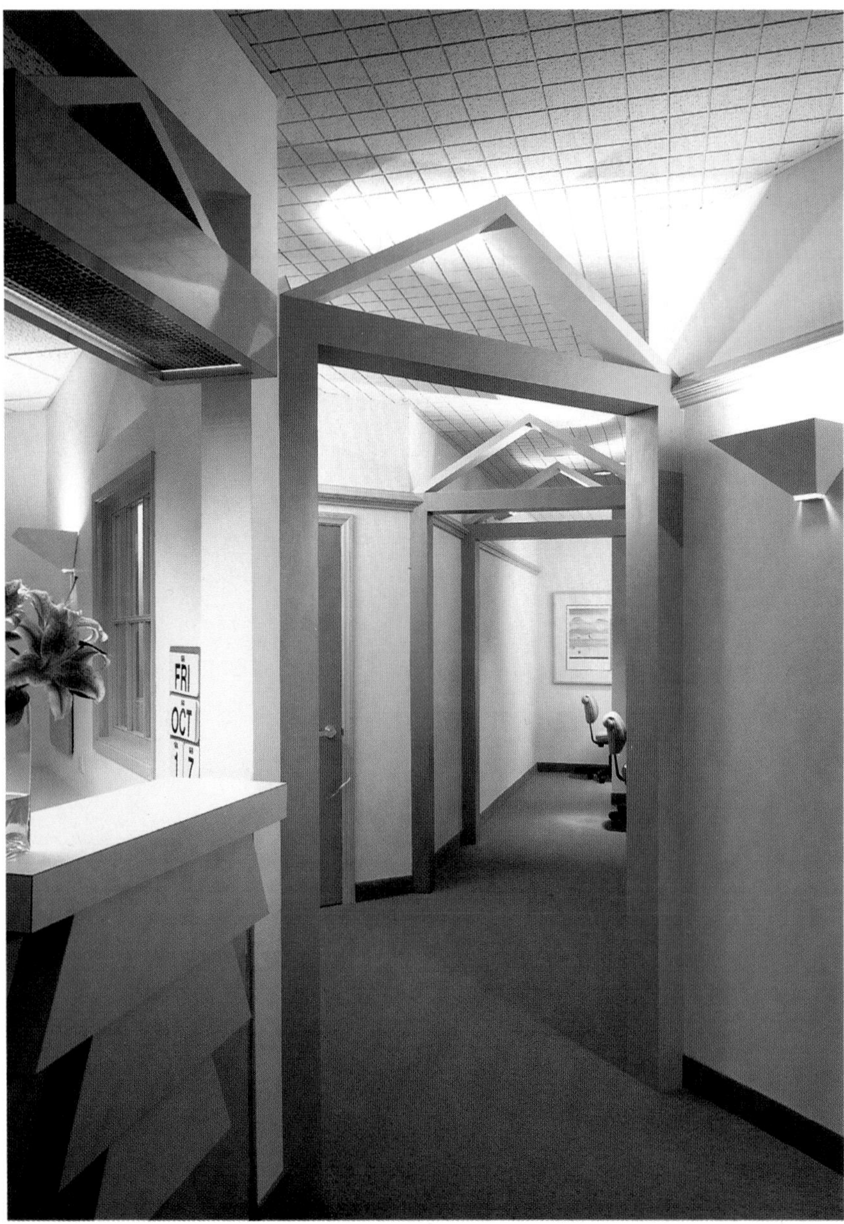

Figure 4-14. Corridor, women's clinic. (*Design: Jain Malkin Inc.; Photographer: Kim Brun.*)

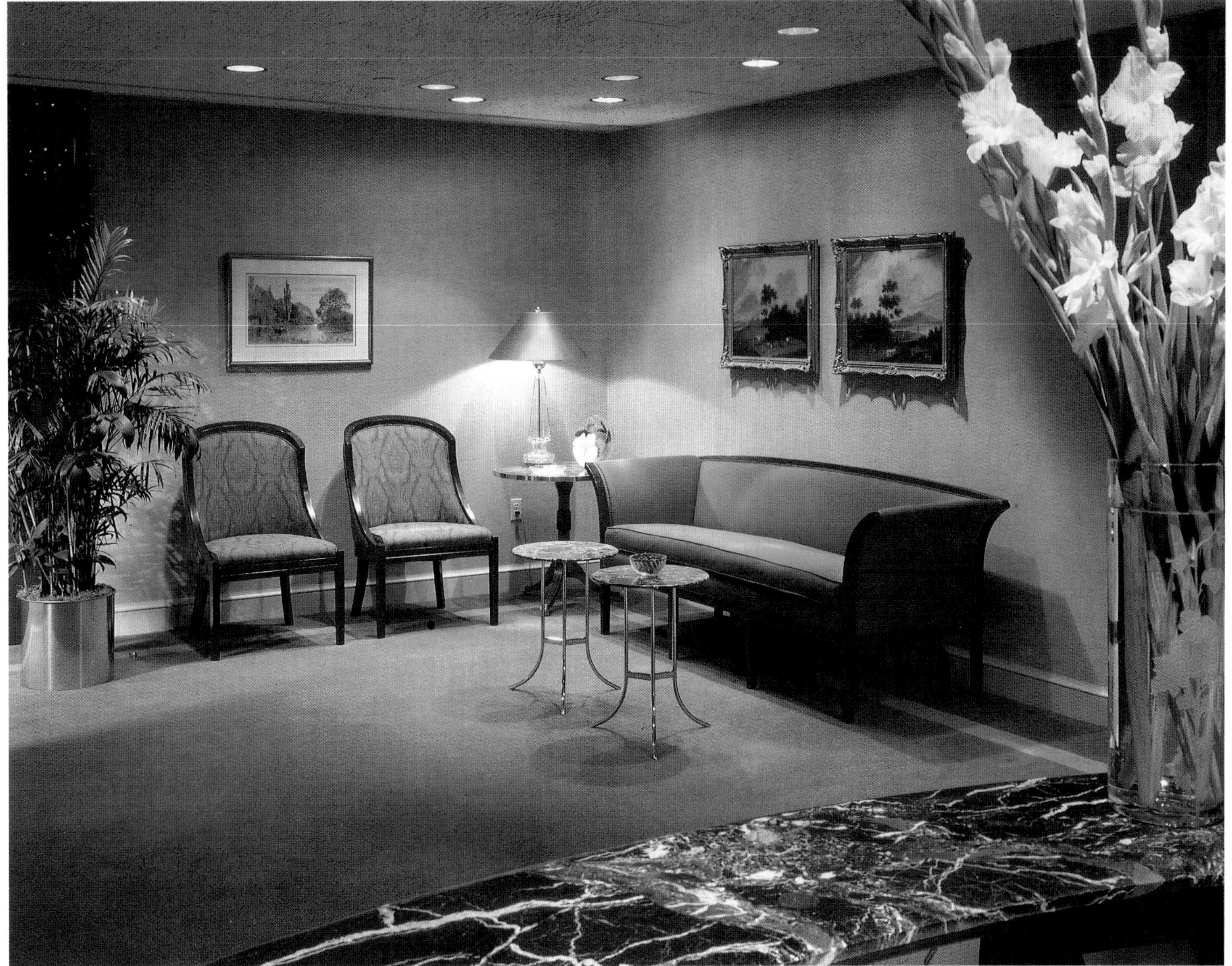

Figure 4-39. Waiting room, ophthalmology. (*Photo courtesy Ann Ascher, Inc., Los Angeles, CA; Photographer: Ron Solomon Photography, Glyndon, MD.*)

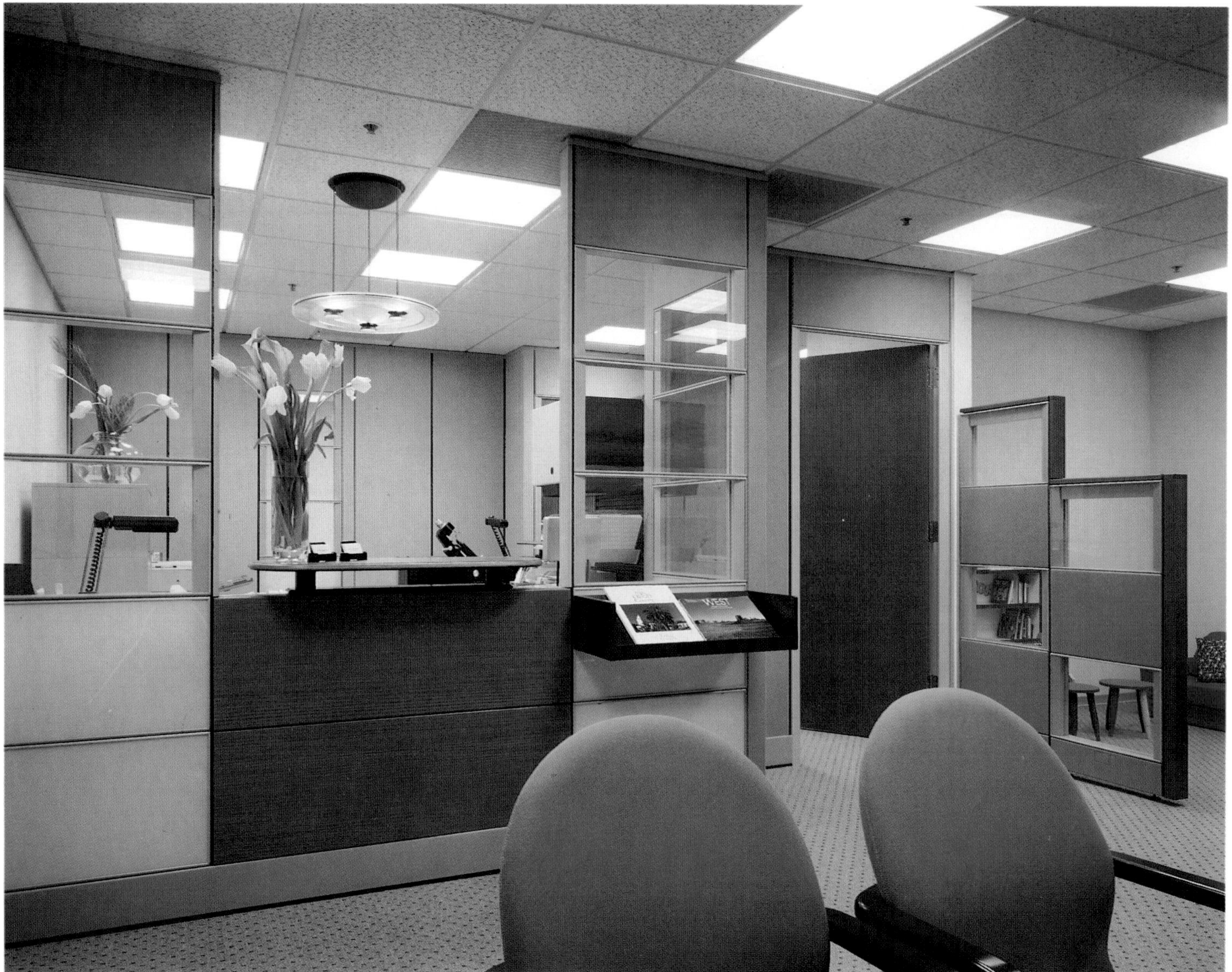

Figure 4-40. Reception window, ophthalmology suite. (*Photo courtesy Carmel Repp, Ltd., Interior Design Associates, San Diego, CA; Design: Phyllis C. Morris, R.N., M.P.H.; Photographer: Kim Brun.*)

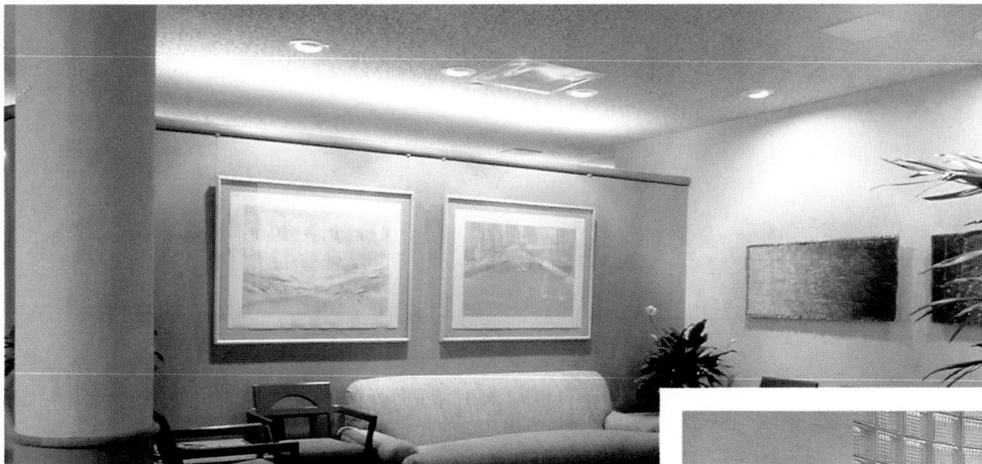

Figure 4-49. Waiting room, dermatology. (*Architecture/Interiors: Richard Deno, Cardiff, CA; Furniture: Kathy Burnham; Art: Richard Fitzpatrick, M.D.; Photographer: Kim Brun.*)

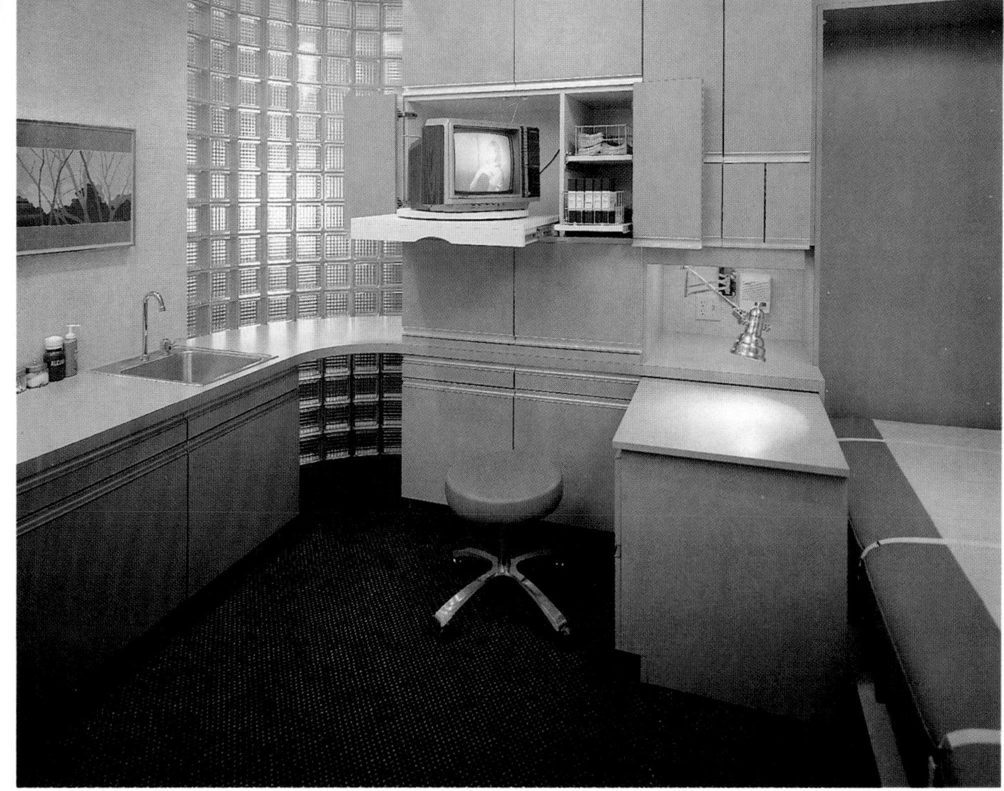

Figure 4-54. Plastic surgery examination room for hands, also serves as recovery room. (*Photo courtesy Sue Walling, SW Design, Inc., Minneappolis, MN; Photographer: P.R. Siegrist.*)

Plate 10

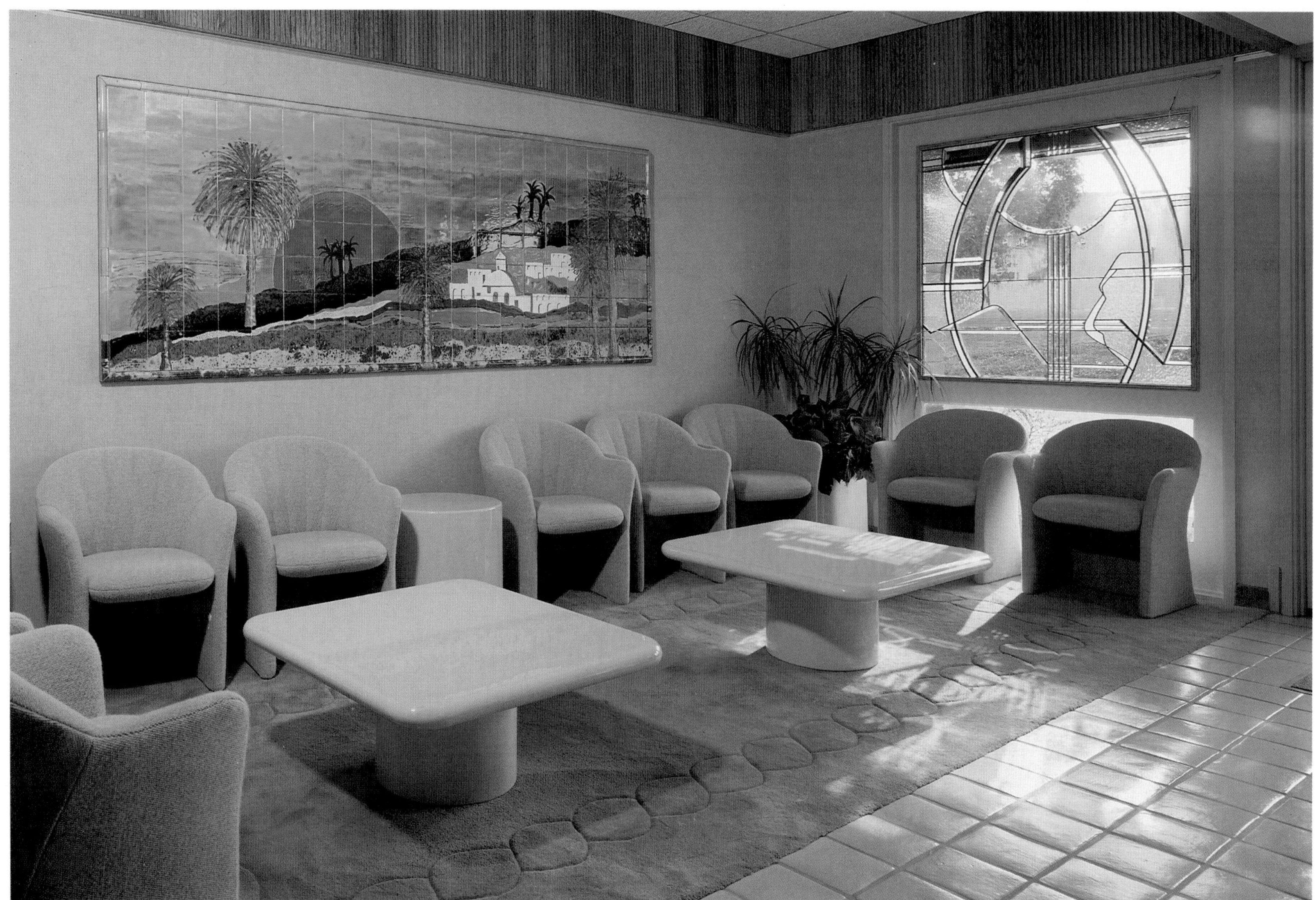

Figure 4-62. Waiting room, plastic surgery. (*Design: Jain Malkin Inc.; Photographer: Michael Denny.*)

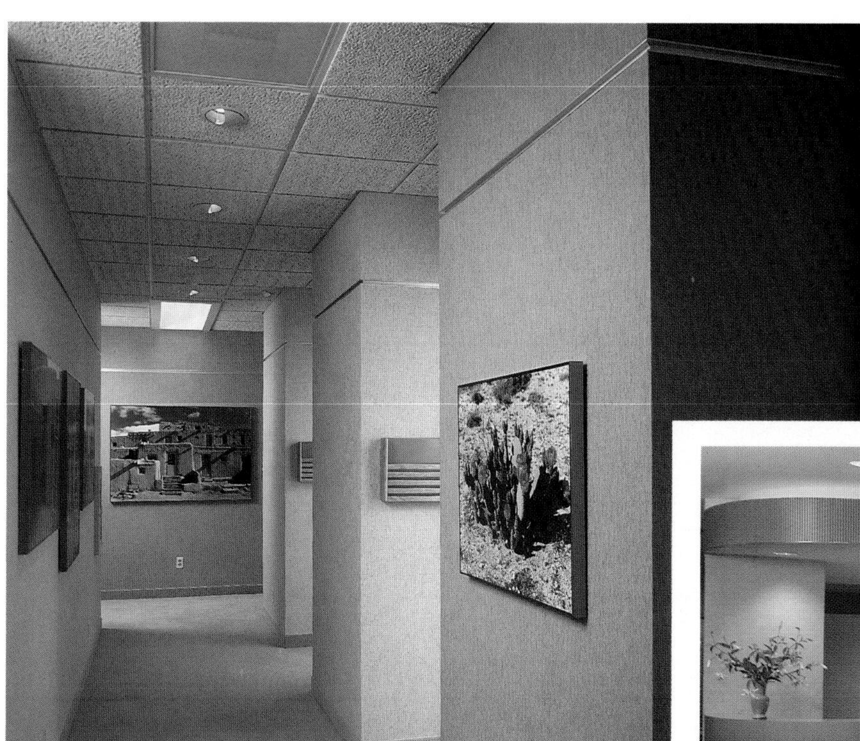

Figure 4-63. Corridor, plastic surgery suite. (*Design: Jain Malkin Inc.; Photographer: Michael Denny.*)

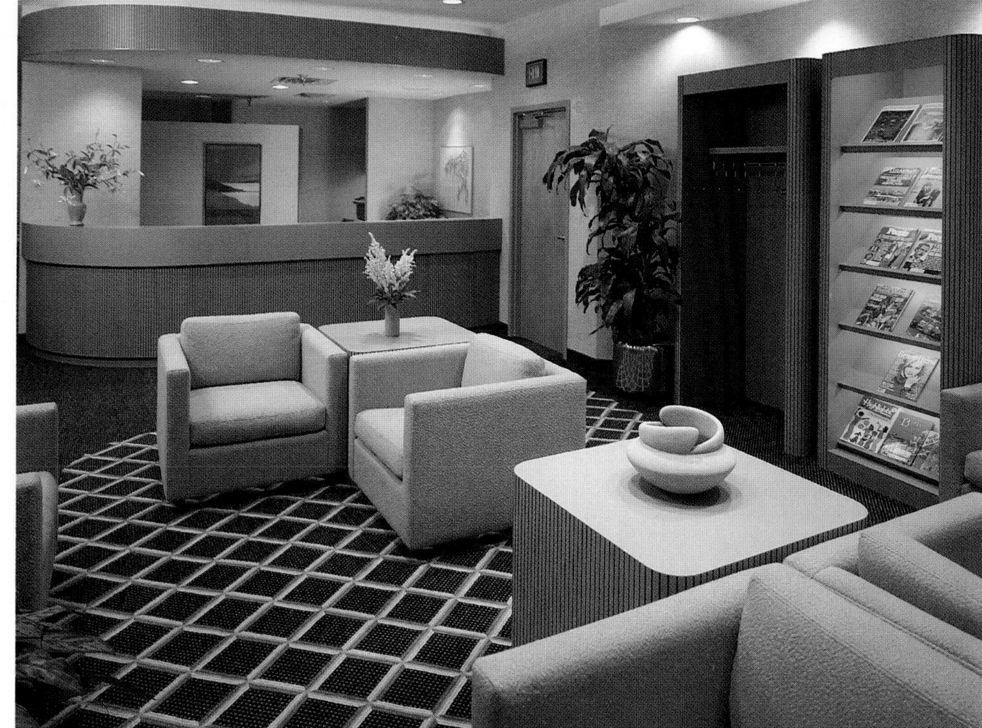

Figure 4-64. Waiting room, plastic surgery. (*Photo courtesy Sue Walling, SW Design, Inc., Minneapolis, MN; Photographer: P.R. Siegrist.*)

Plate 12

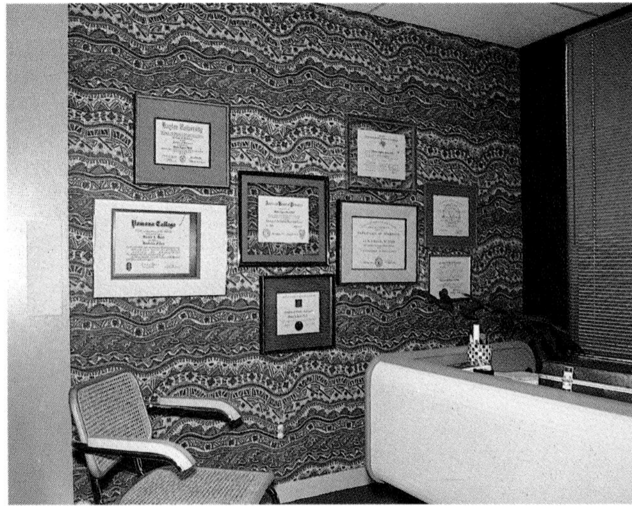

Figure 4-74. Diplomas, imaginatively framed. (*Design: Jain Malkin Inc.*)

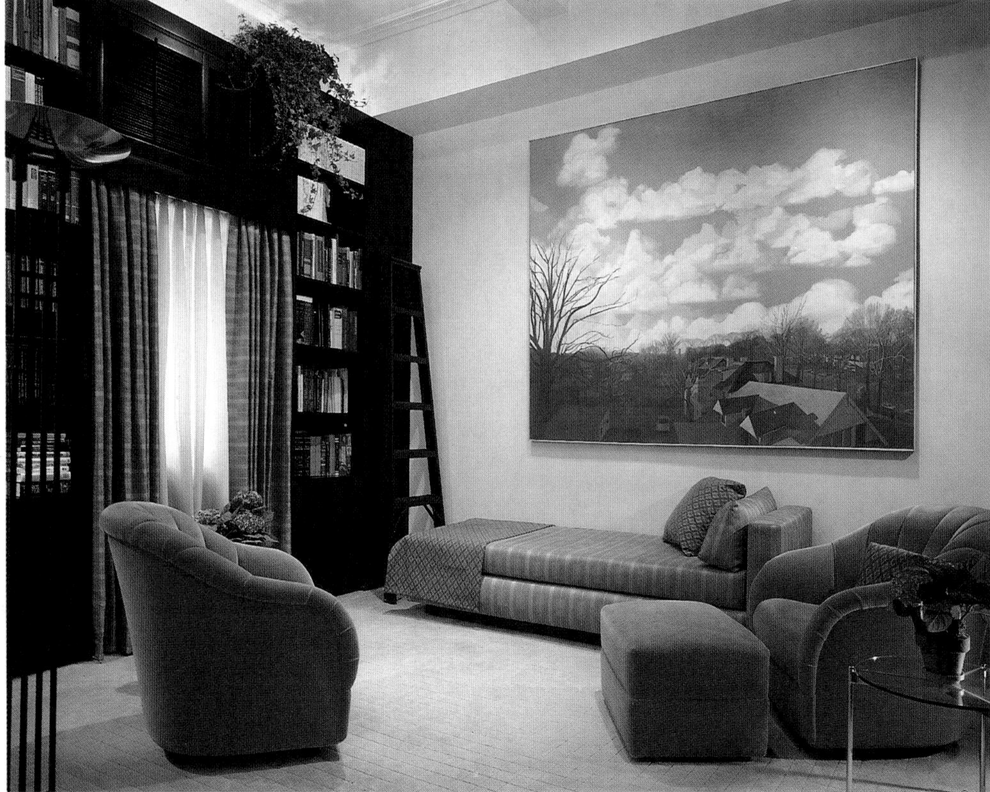

Figure 4-75. Consultation room, psychiatry. (*Photo courtesy Marna L. Sherman, Interiors, New York, NY; Photographer: Peter Vitale.*)

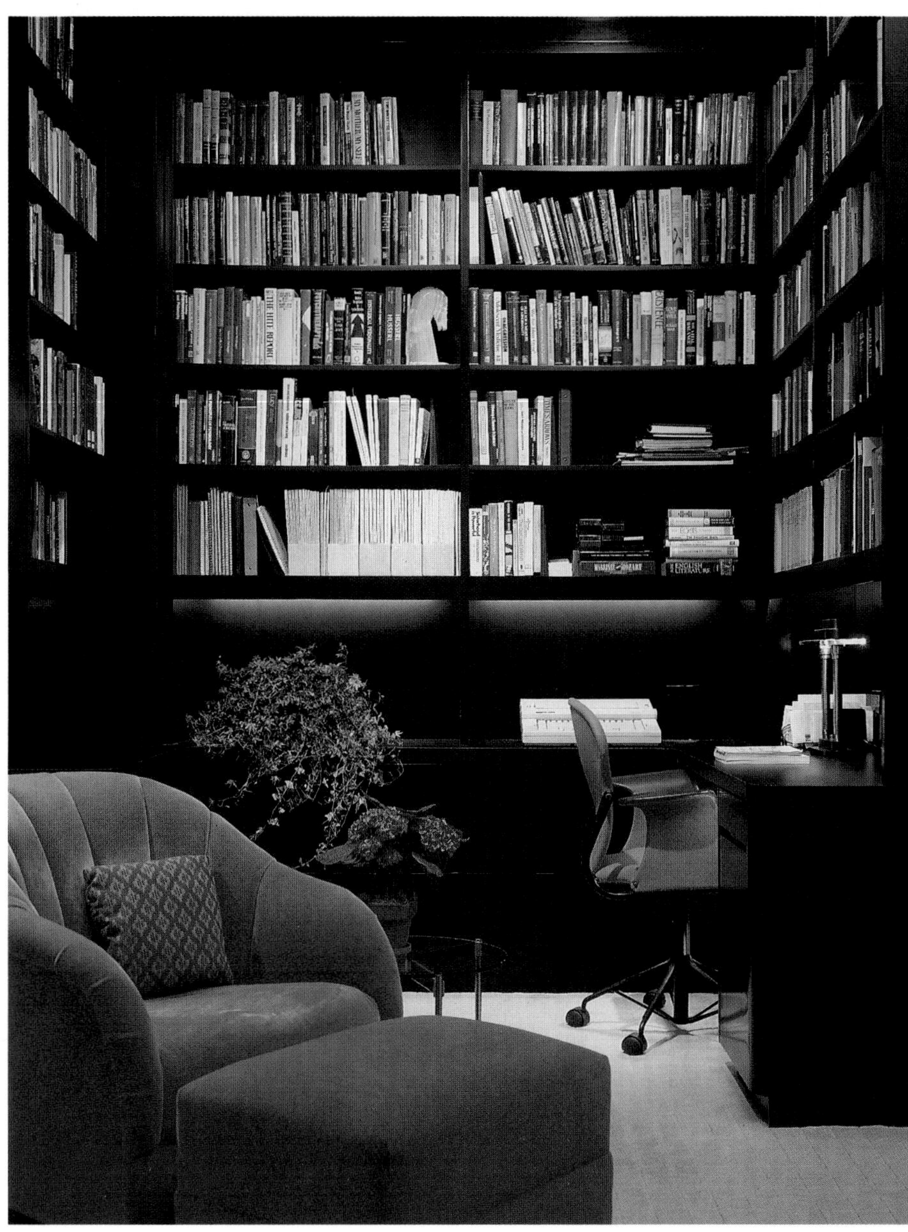

Figure 4-76. Consultation room, psychiatry (opposite view).

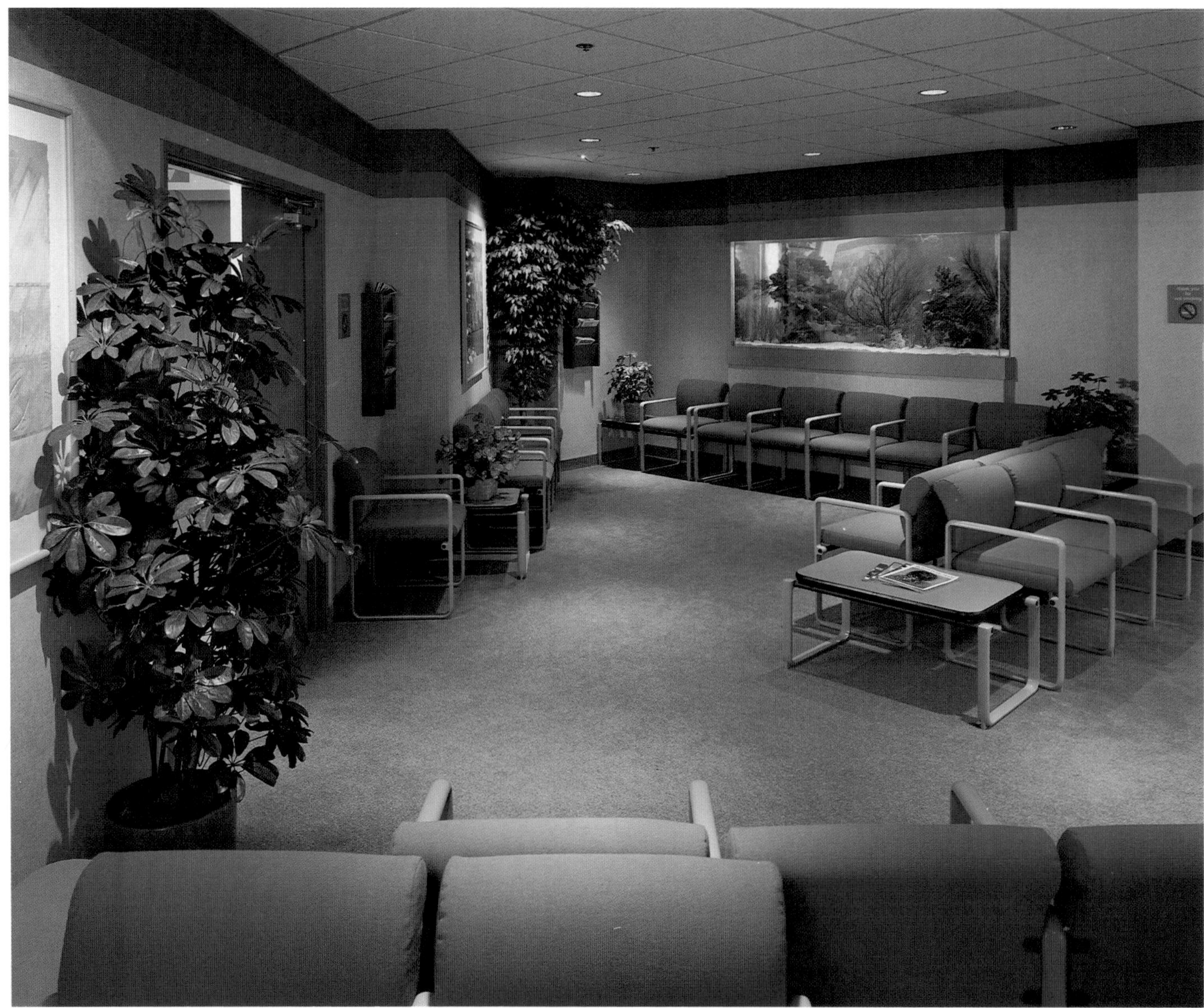

Figure 4-106. Waiting room, orthopedic surgery. (*Design: Jain Malkin Inc.; Photographer: Michael Denny.*)

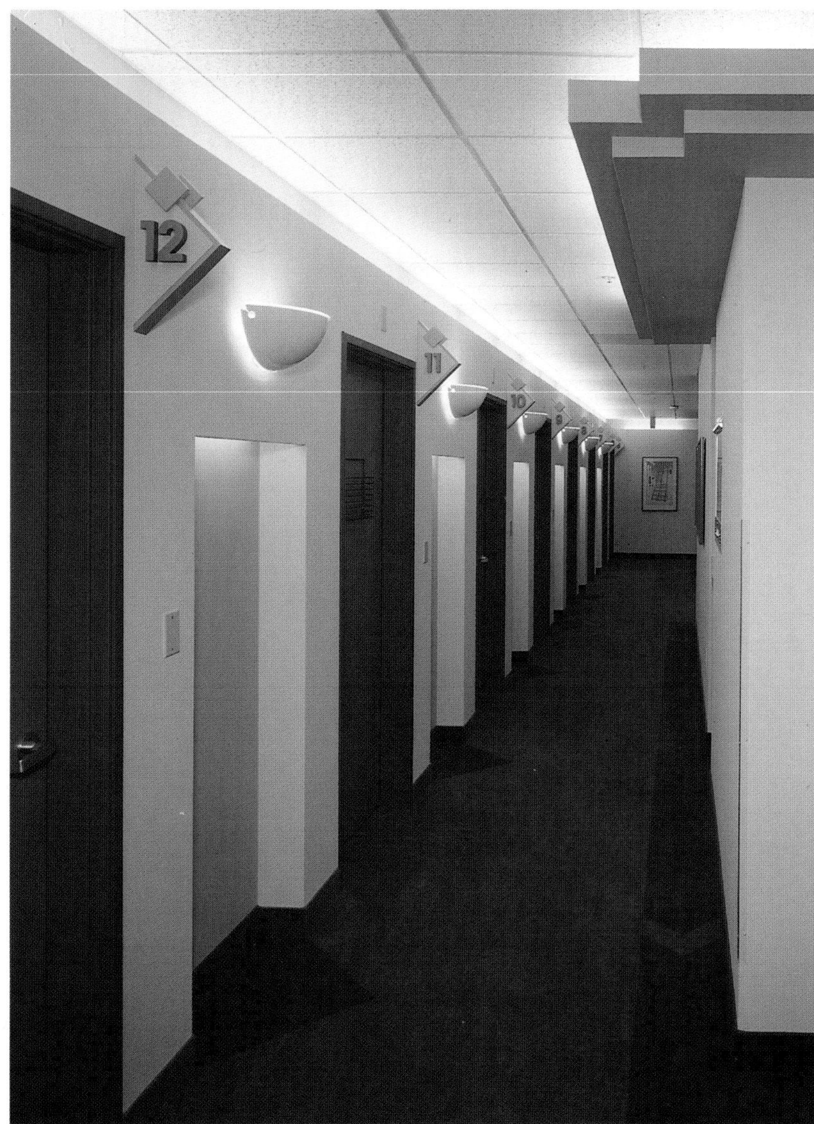

Figure 6-14. Corridor, group practice clinic. Note indirect lighting details and signage. (*Design Jain Malkin Inc.; Signage: McKinnon/Anderson; Photographer. Robinson/Ward.*)

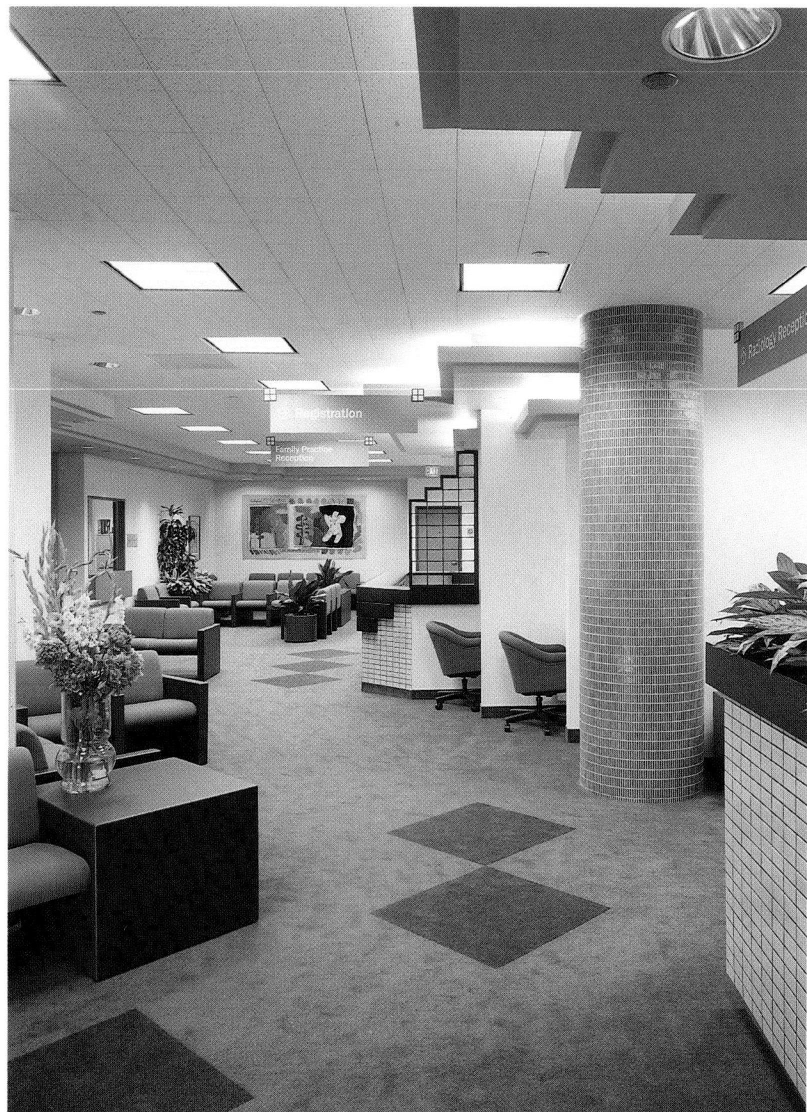

Figure 6-15. Waiting room, family practice module, group practice clinic. (*Design: Jain Malkin Inc.; Signage: McKinnon/Anderson; Photographer: Robinson/Ward.*)

Plate 16

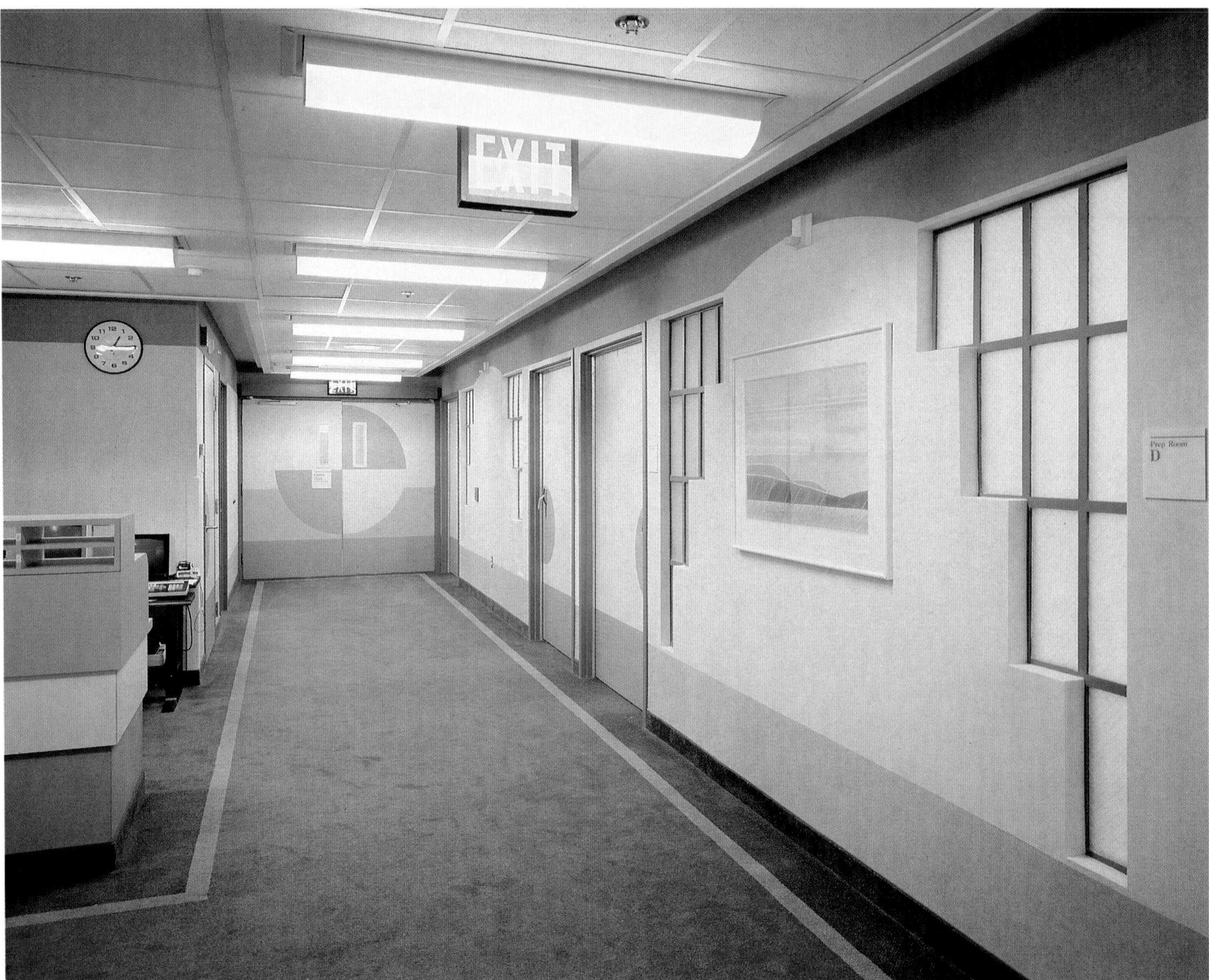

Figure 7-4. Patient prep corridor. Note use of frosted glass detail to add interest to corridor and visually open up examination rooms on other side of wall. (*Design: Jain Malkin Inc.; Photographer: John Christian.*)

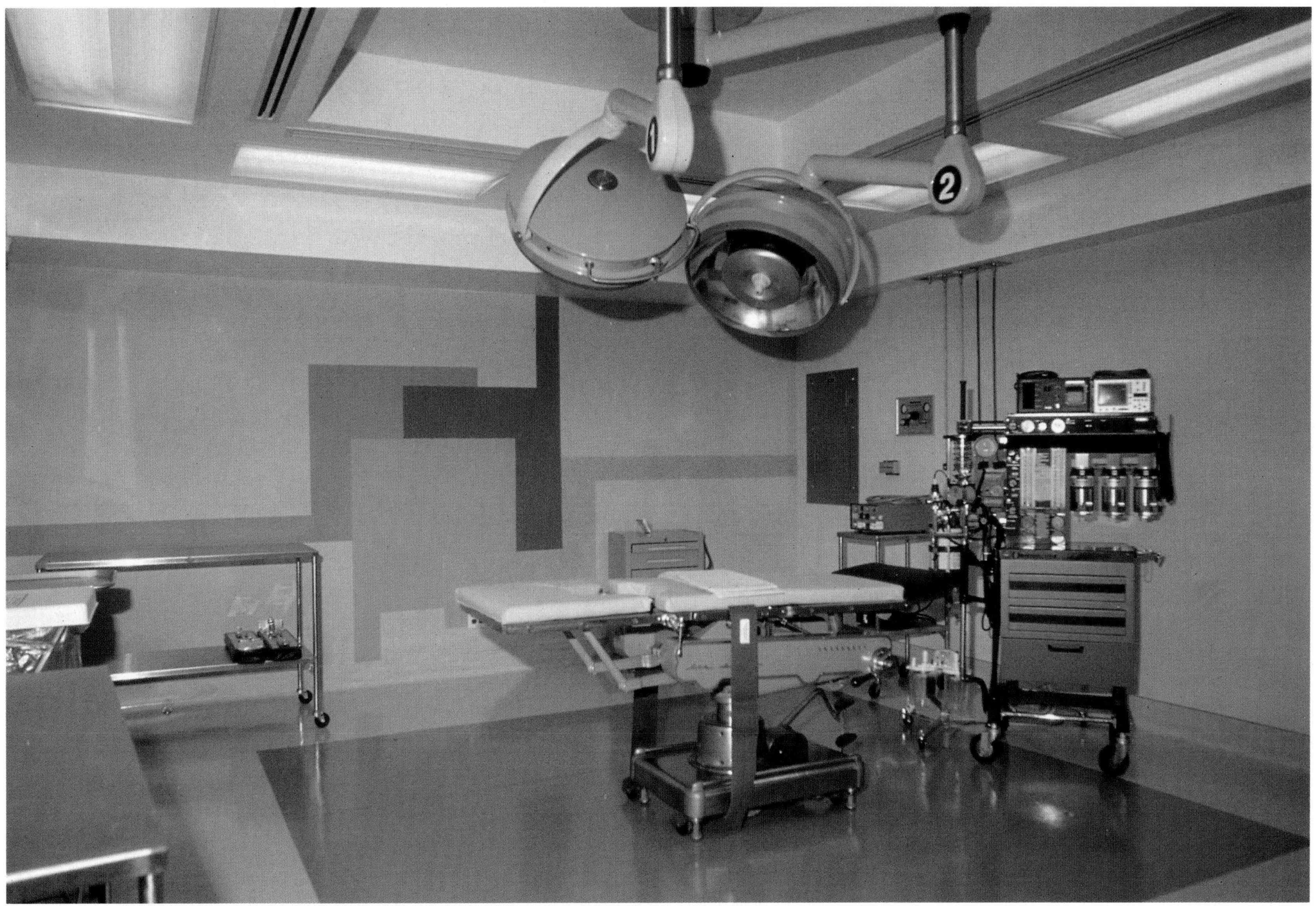

Figure 7-9. Operating room. Note vinyl inset wallgraphic. (*Design: Jain Malkin Inc.; Photographer: Jain Malkin.*)

Plate 18

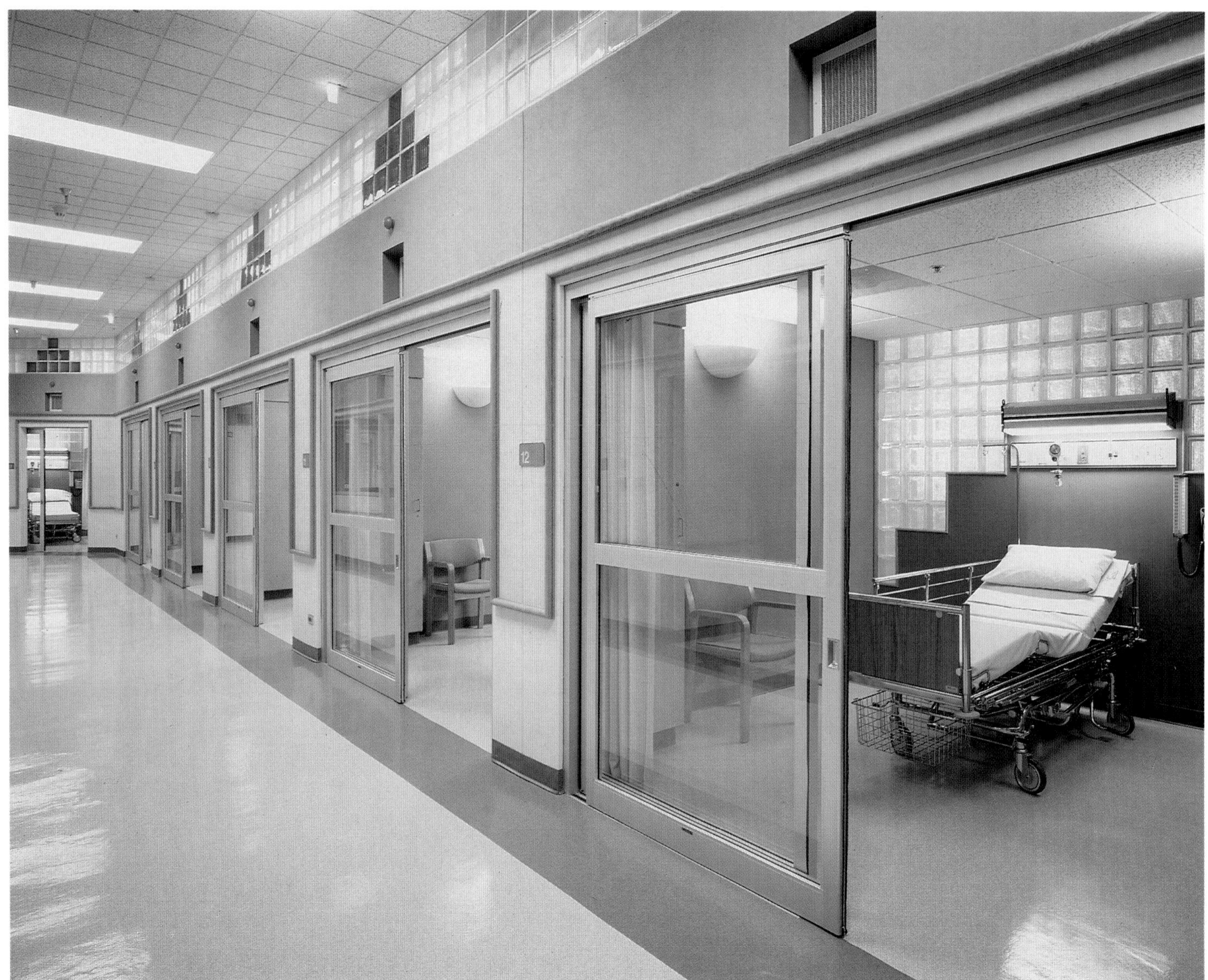

Figures 7-22 and 7-23. Recovery area with view into private recovery rooms. Note use of color, glass block and oak detailing. (*Photo courtesy Anderson Mikos Architects, Ltd., Oak Brook, IL; Photographer: Jay Wolke.*)

Plate 19

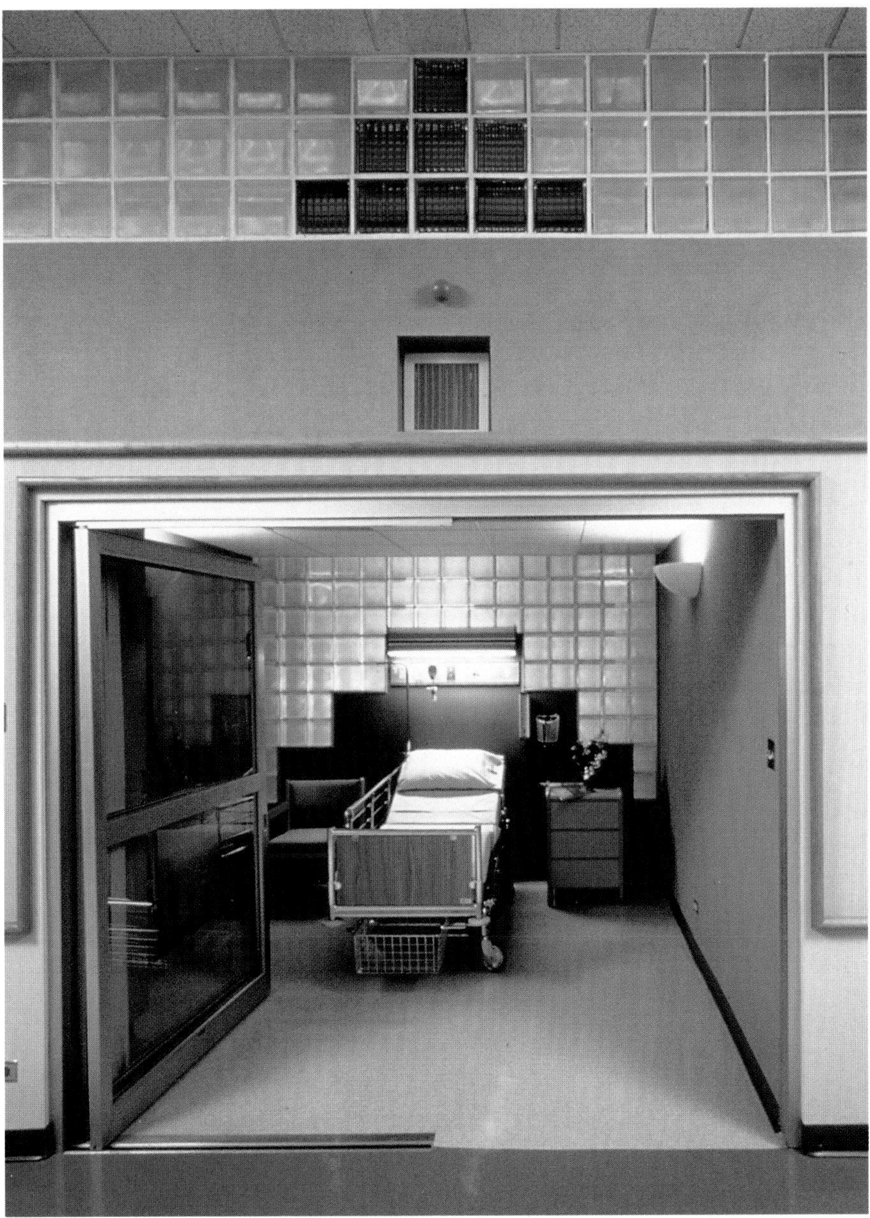

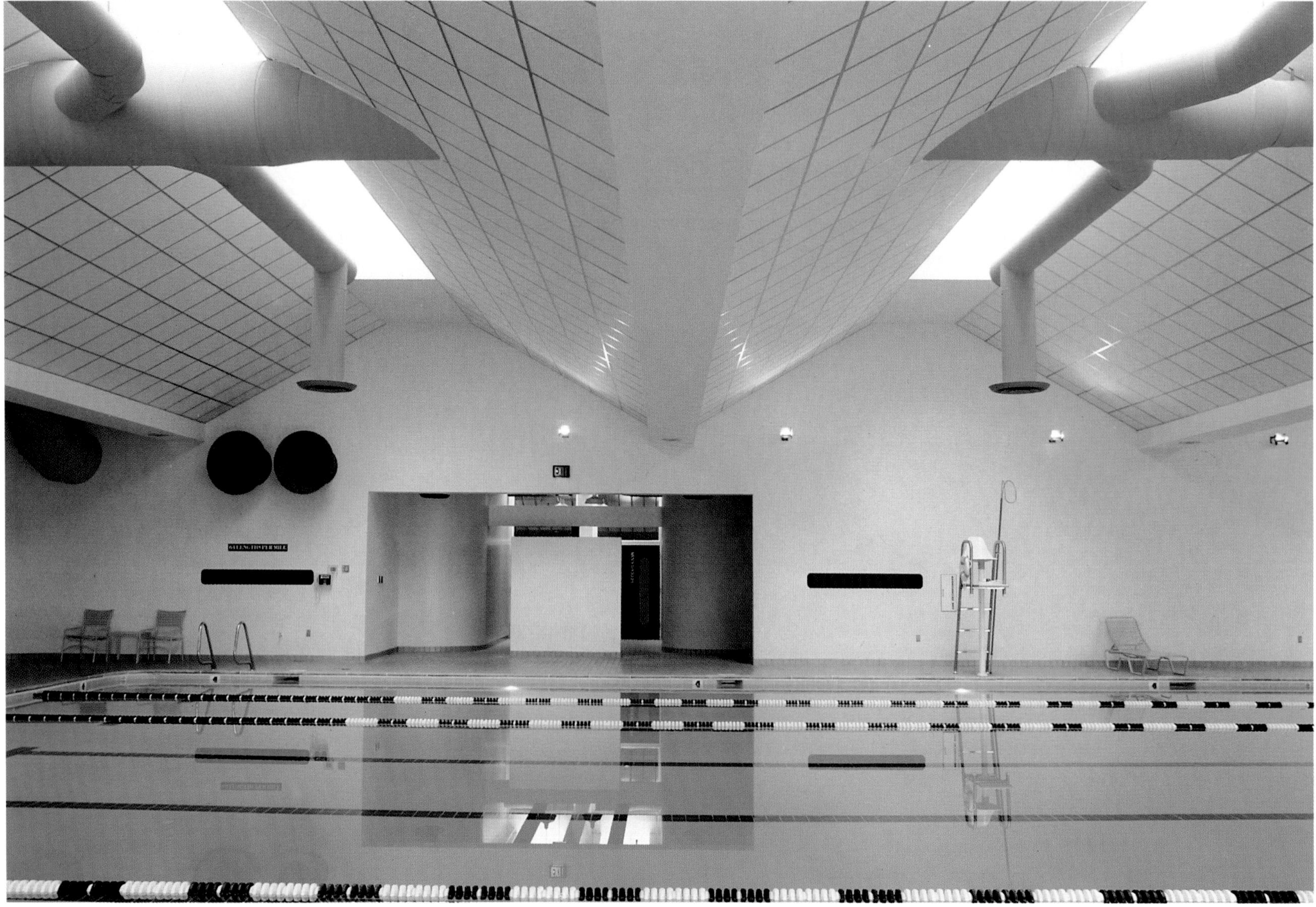

Figure 8-3. Pool and spa. Note interesting architectural features, lighting and use of color. (*Photo courtesy Eisenman & Enock, Inc., New York, NY; Photographer: Roger Bester.*)

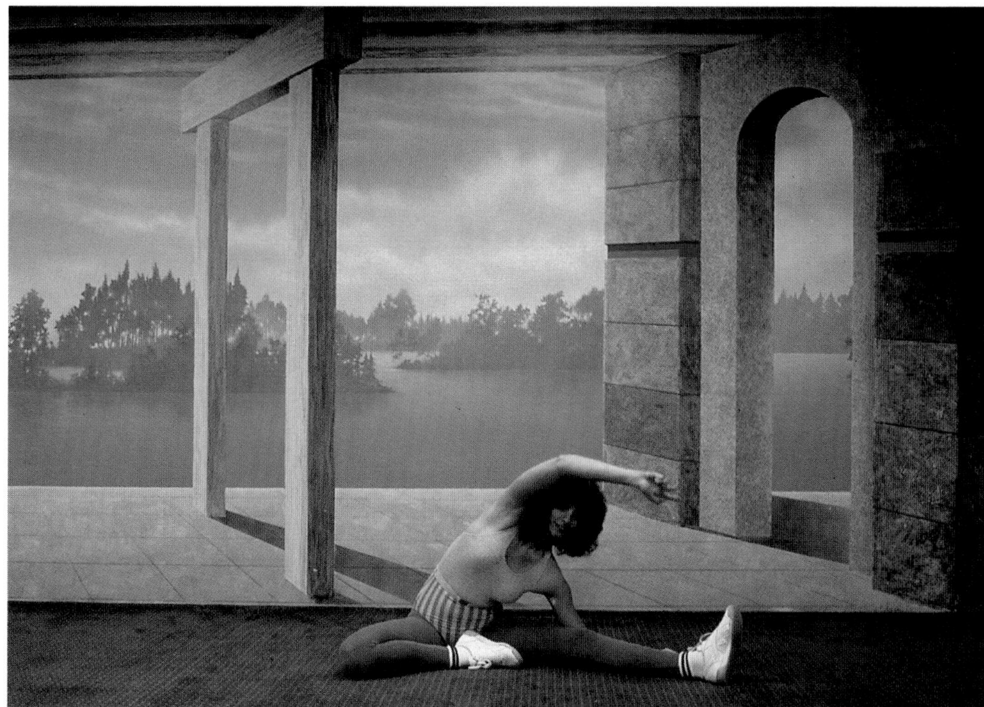

Figure 8-8. Trompe l'oeil mural expands, and adds dimension to the room. (*Photo courtesy Maxion Design, Sausalito, CA; Photographer: Peter Hendrix.*)

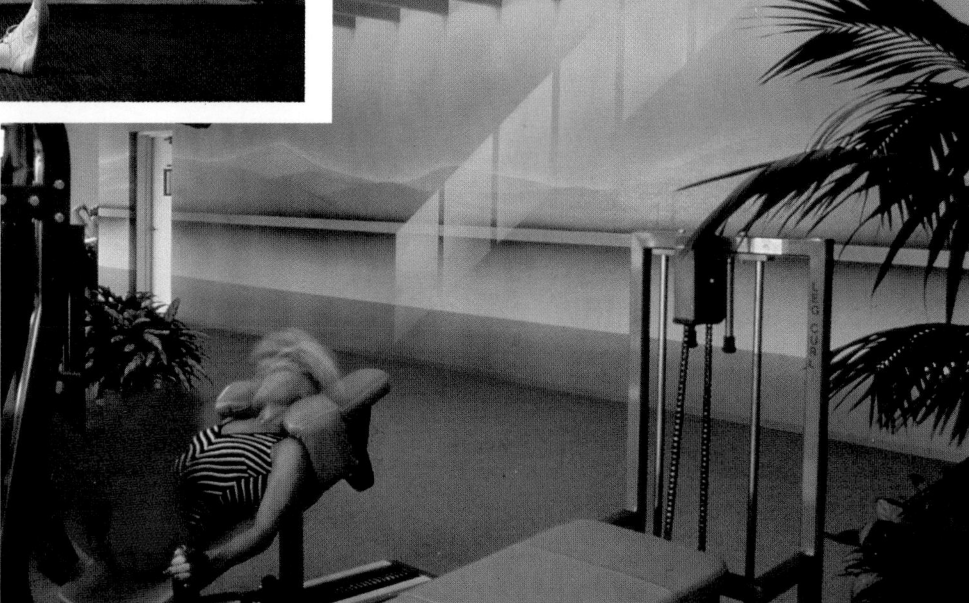

Figure 8-9. Sophisticated mural gives illusion of looking through panes of glass at the bay. (*Photo courtesy Maxion Design, Sausalito, CA; Photographer: Jeff Weissman.*)

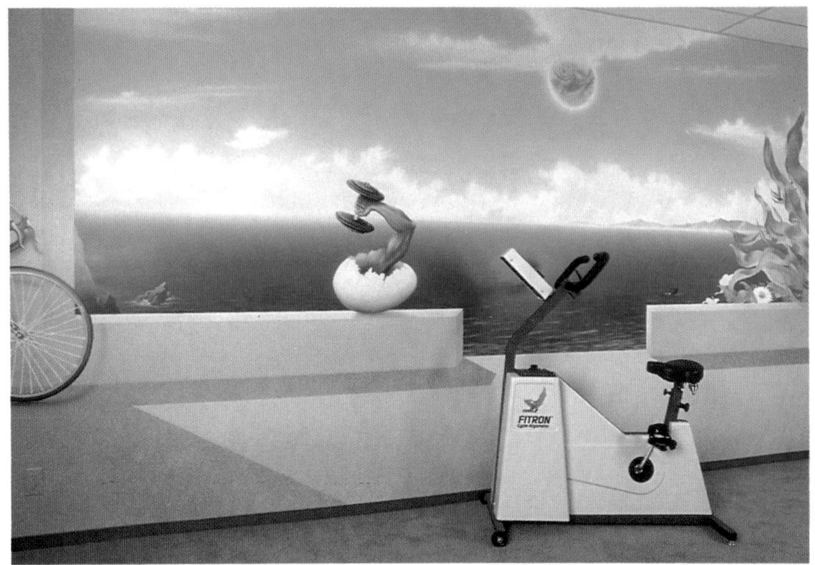

Figure 8-10. Skillfully executed trompe l'oeil mural gives person exercising the illusion of riding along the boardwalk. (*Courtesy Maxion Design, Sausalito, CA; Photographer: Joe Czop.*)

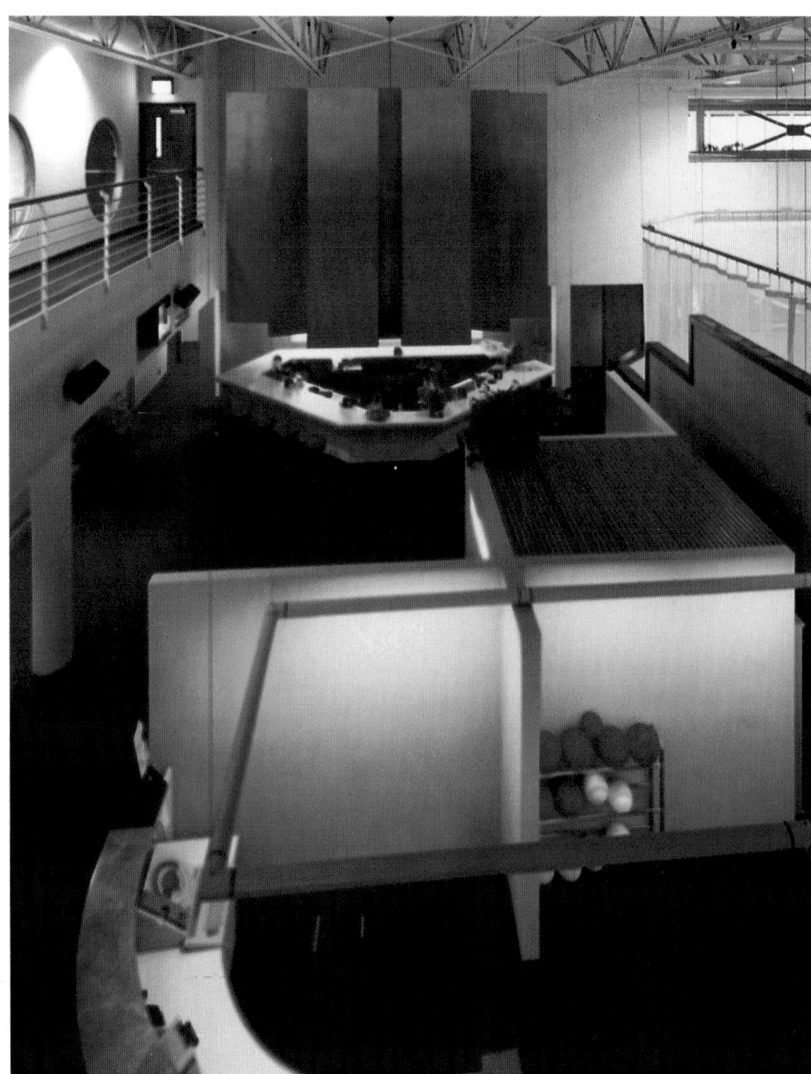

Figure 8-17. Snack bar/lounge, Western Montana Sports Medicine & Fitness Center. (*Courtesy Pamela Scharbauer, Missoula, MT; Photographer: R. Mark Bryant.*)

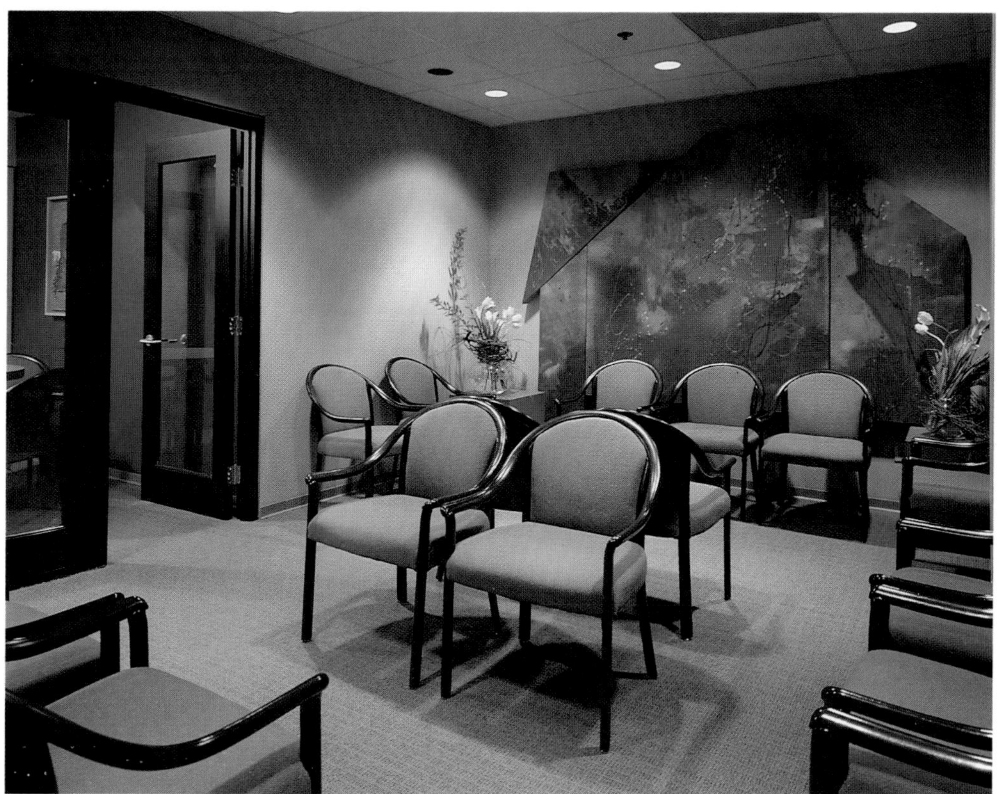

Figure 10-39. Waiting room, general dentistry office. (*Courtesy Carmel Repp Ltd., Interior Design Associates, San Diego, CA; Painting: Madeline Engle; Photographer: Kim Brun.*)

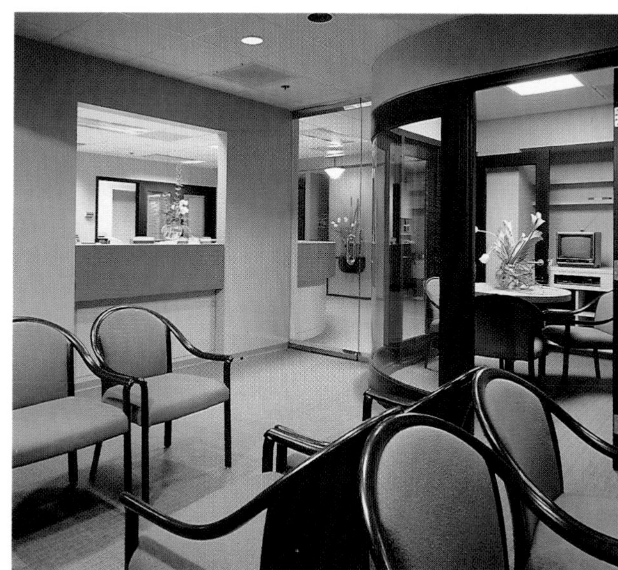

Figure 10-40. Reception area with patient education room. (*Courtesy Carmel Repp Ltd., Interior Design Associates, San Diego, CA; Photographer: Kim Brun.*)

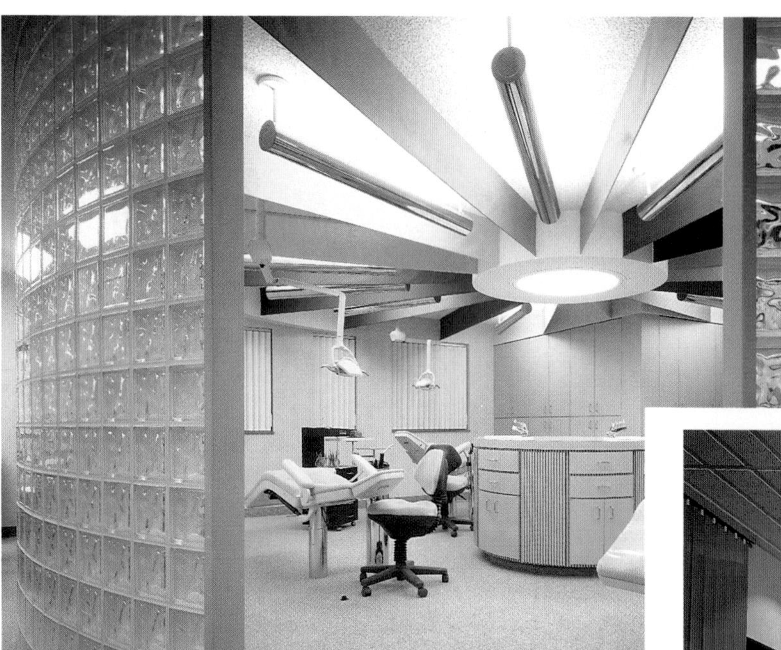

Figure 10-57. Orthodontic treatment bay. (*Courtesy Sue Walling, SW Design, Inc., Minneapolis, MN; Photographer: P.R. Siegrist.*)

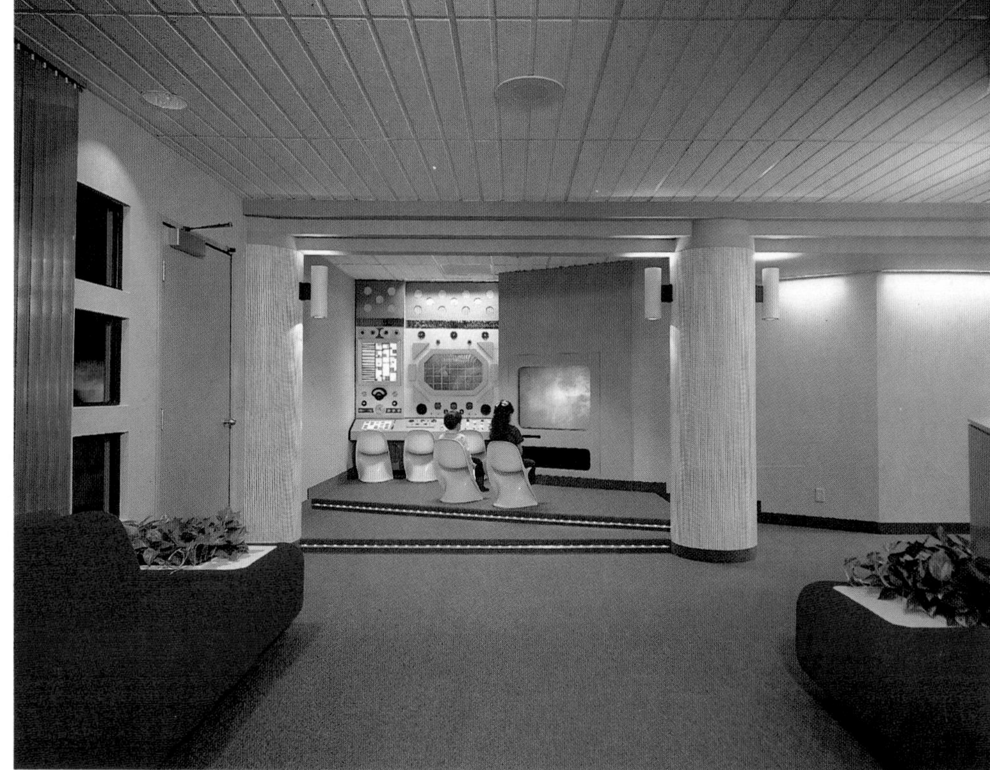

Figure 10-62. Waiting room, children's dental clinic. (*Architecture/ Interiors: Margo Hebald-Heymann, AIA and Associates, Santa Monica, CA; Photographer: Marvin Rand, Marina del Ray, CA.*)

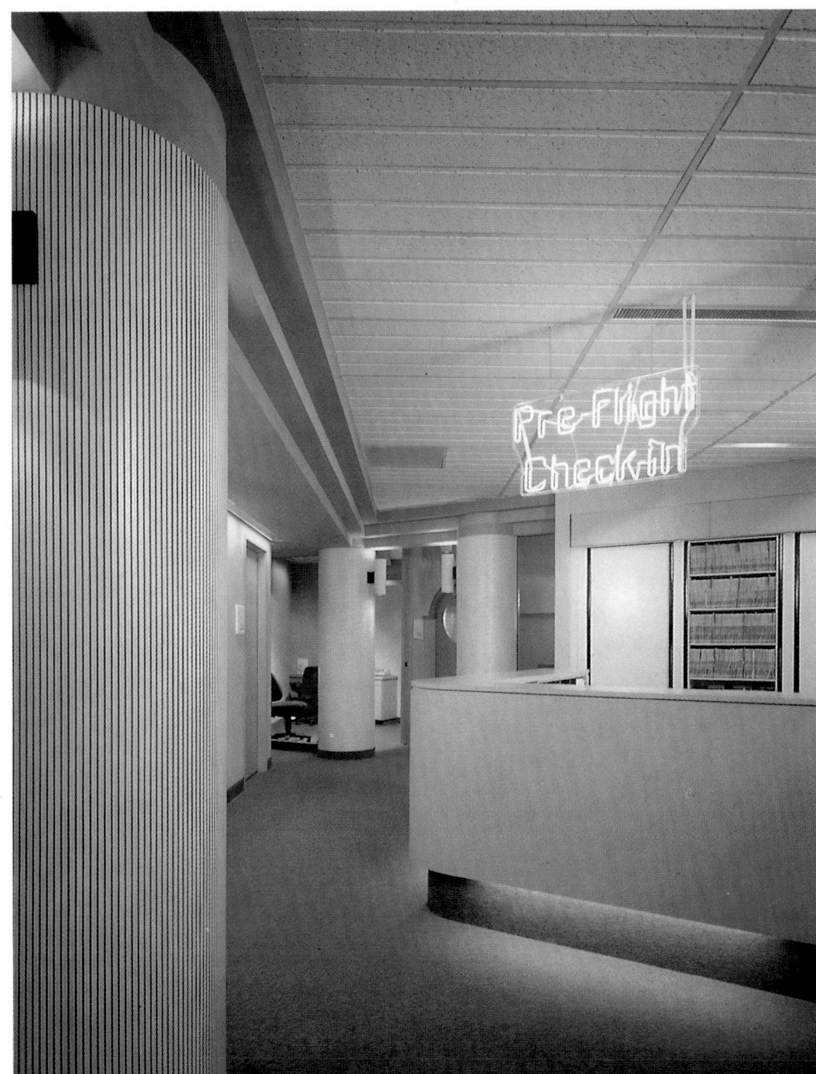

Figure 10-63. Pre-flight check-in, children's dental clinic. (*Architecture/Interiors: Margo Hebald-Heymann, AIA and Associates, Santa Monica, CA; Photographer: Marvin Rand, Marina del Ray, CA.*)

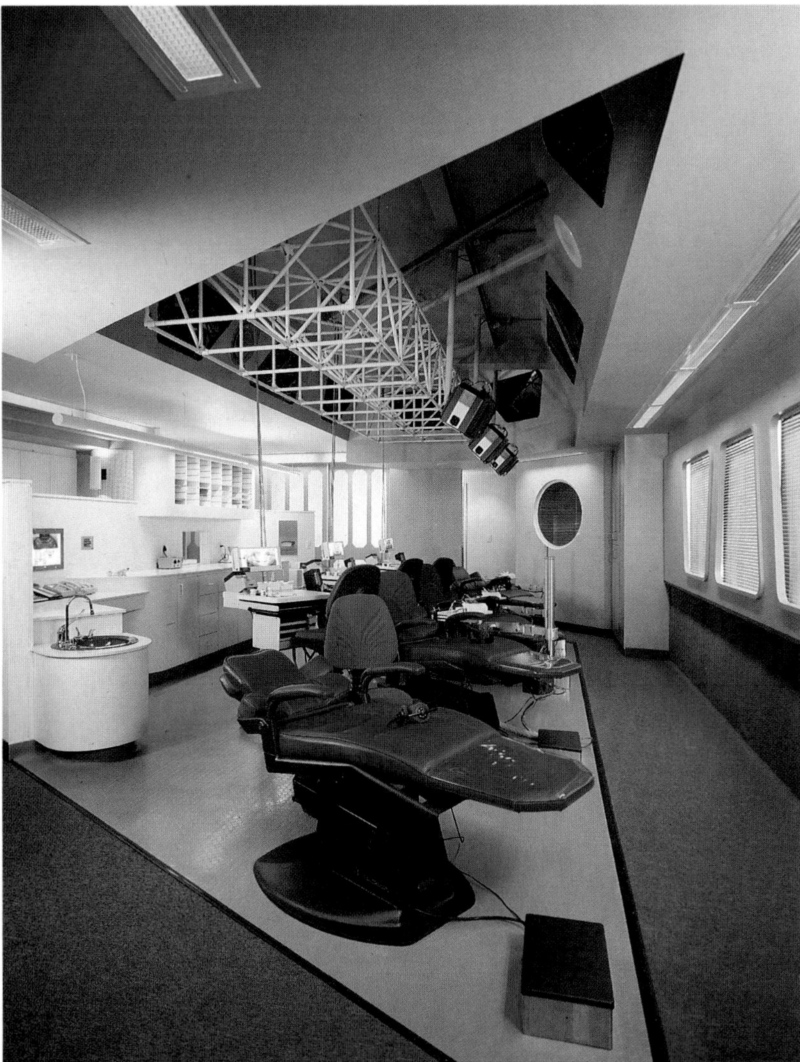

Figure 10-64. Pedodontic bay. (*Architecture/Interiors: Margo Hebald-Heymann, AIA and Associates, Santa Monica, CA; Photographer: Marvin Rand, Marina del Ray, CA.*)

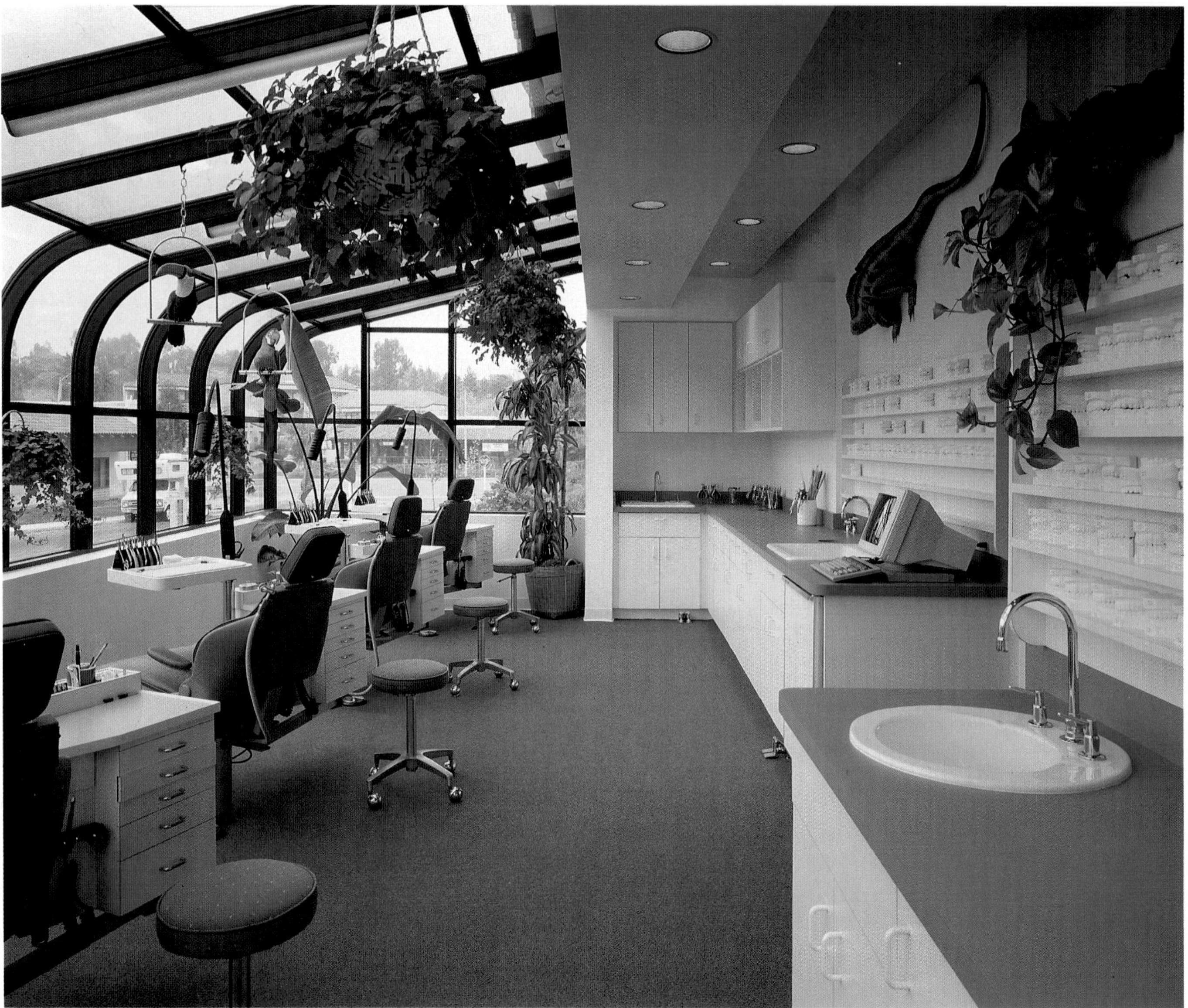

Figure 10-67. Operatory bay, orthodontics. (*Design: Jain Malkin Inc.; Photographer: John Christian.*)

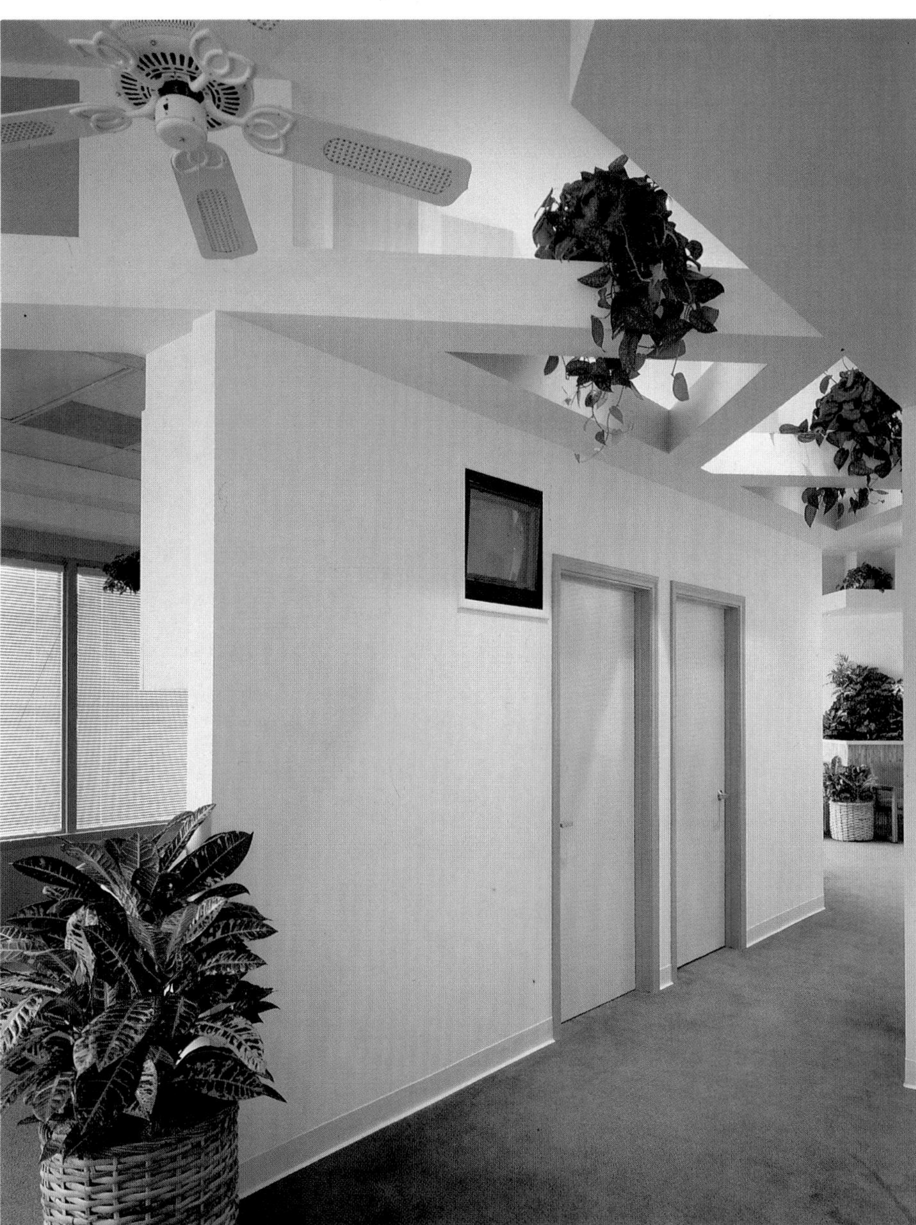

Figure 10-68. Corridor, orthodontic office. Note architectural detailing of ceiling. (*Design: Jain Malkin Inc.; Photographer: John Christian.*)

Plate 28

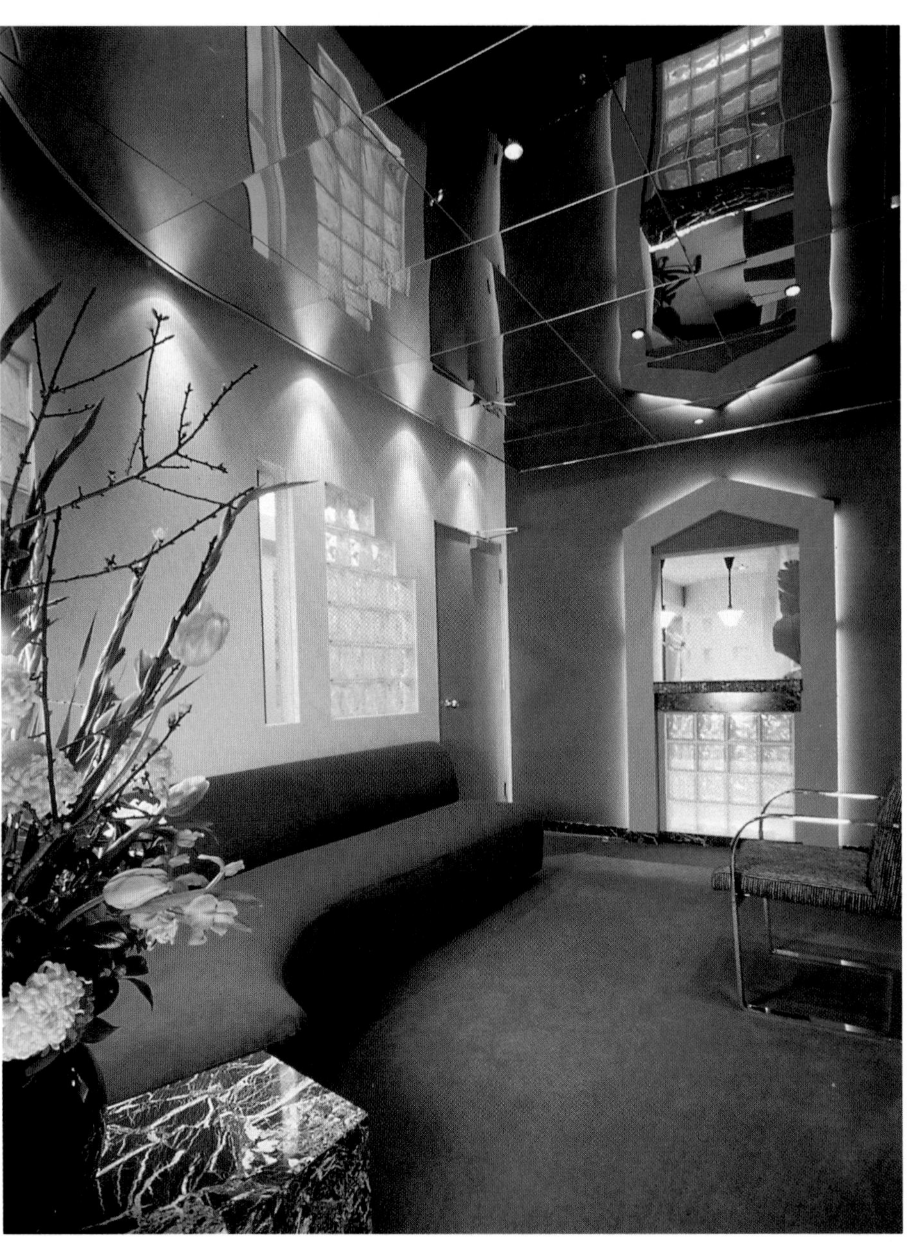

Figure 10-81. Waiting room, periodontics office. (*Courtesy Robert Ross, Robert Ross Inc., Culver City, CA; Photographer: David Glomb.*)

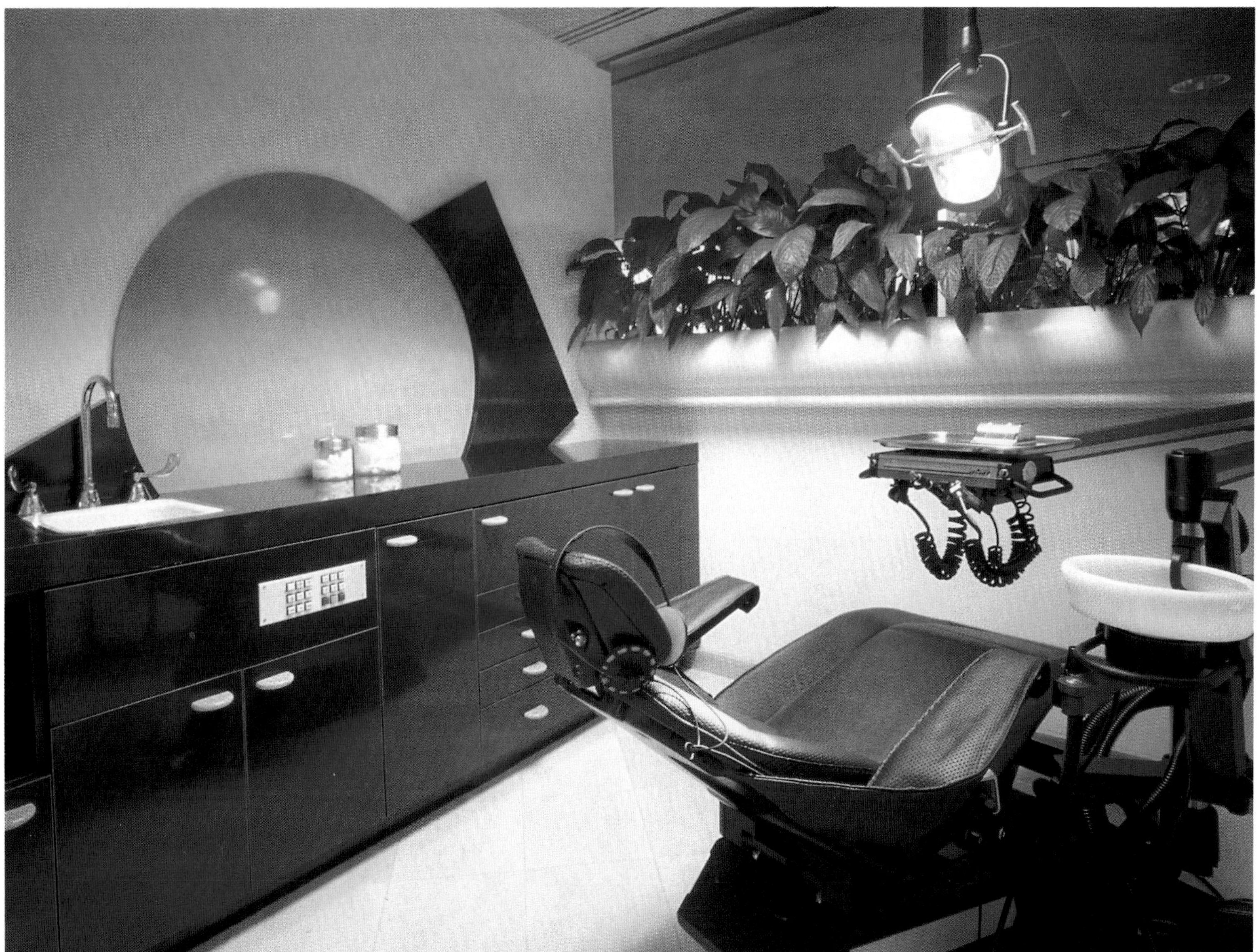

Figure 10-82. Operatory, periodontics. (*Courtesy Robert Ross, Robert Ross Inc., Culver City, CA; Photographer: David Glomb.*)

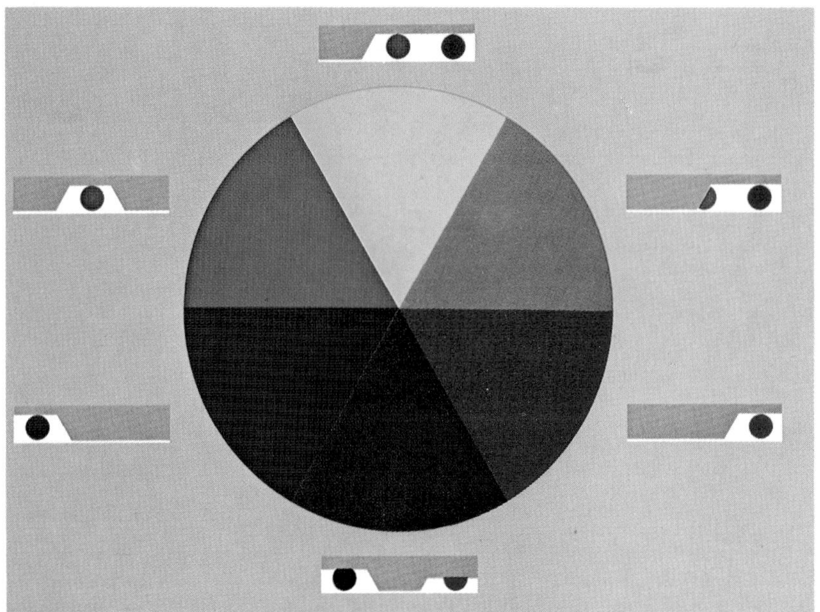

Figure 11-1. The old color wheel. (*Reprinted from The Theory and Practice of Color, by Frans Gerritsen, by permission of Van Nostrand Reinhold, New York, 1974, p. 172.*)

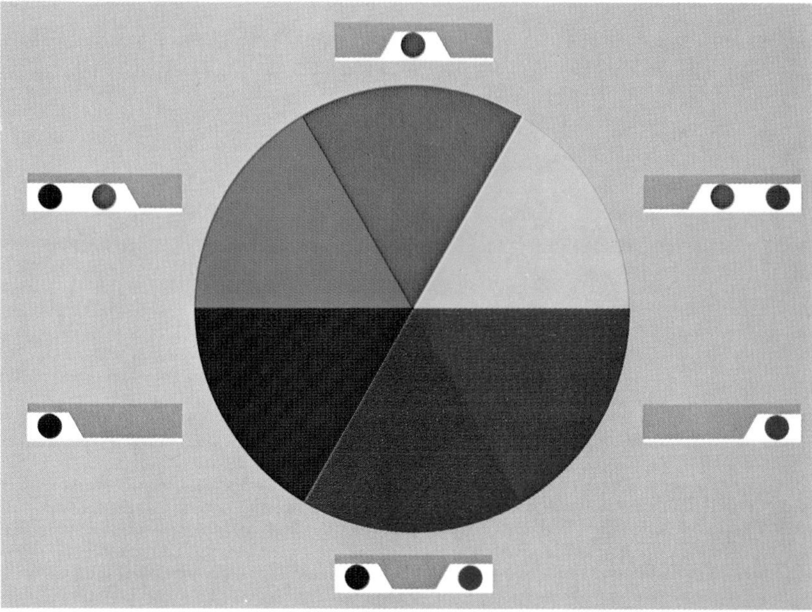

Figure 11-2. The new color wheel. (*Reprinted from The Theory and Practice of Color, by Frans Gerritsen, by permission of Van Nostrand Reinhold, New York, 1974, p. 173.*)

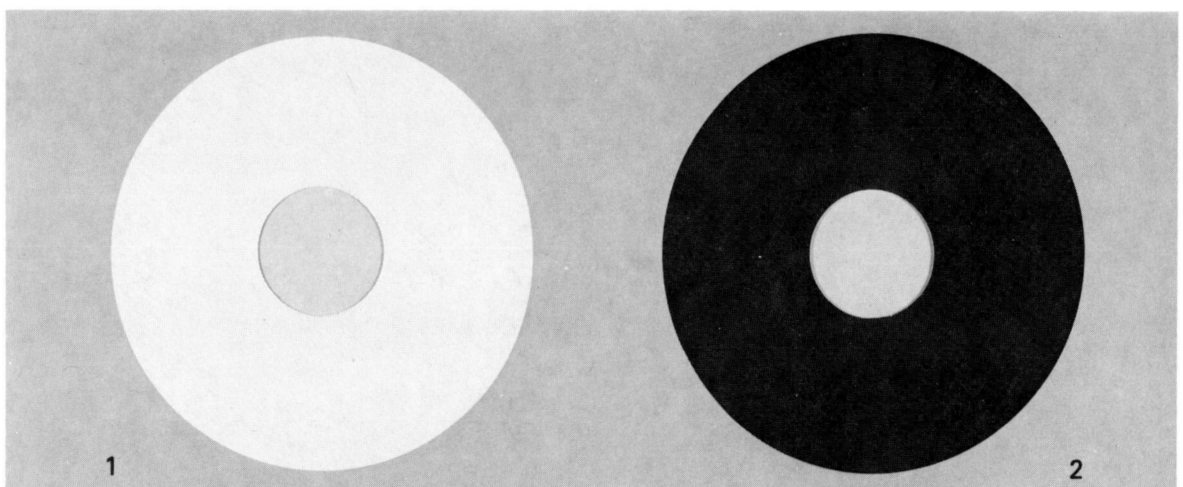

Figure 11-3. Simultaneous contrast. (*Reprinted from The Theory and Practice of Color, by Frans Gerritsen, by permission of Van Nostrand Reinhold, New York, 1974, p. 128.*)

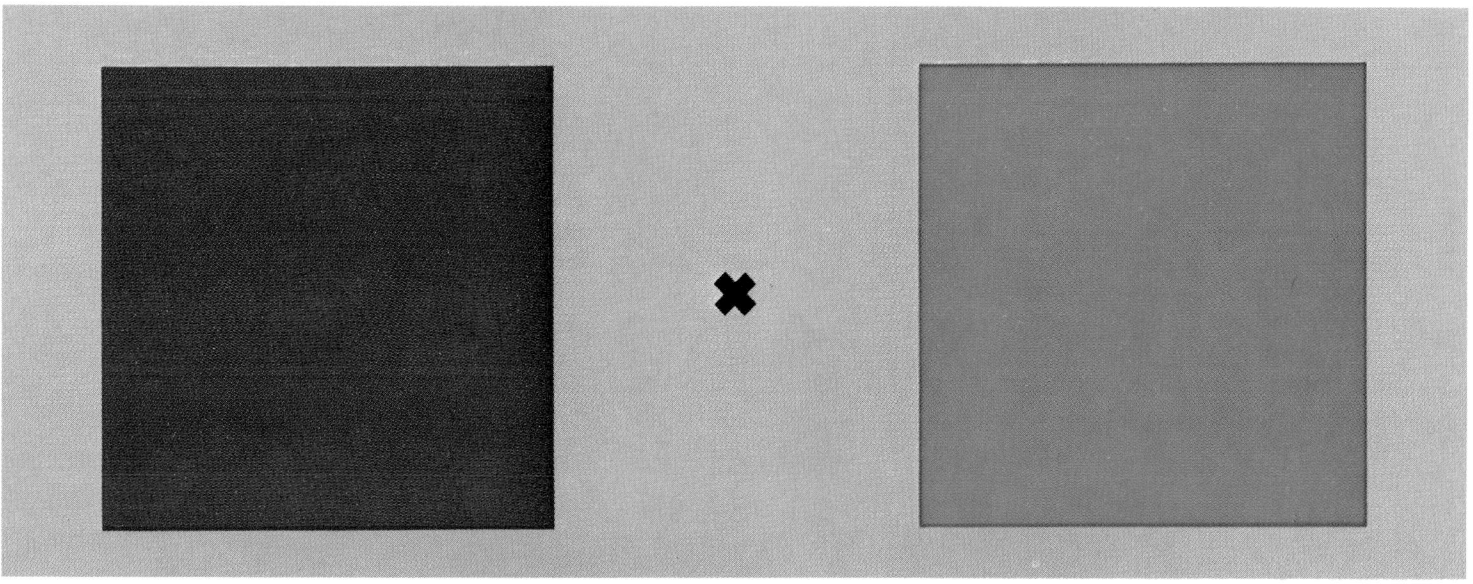

Figure 11-4. Successive contrast/afterimage. (*Reprinted from The Theory and Practice of Color, by Frans Gerritsen, by permission of Van Nostrand Reinhold, New York, 1974, p. 146.*)

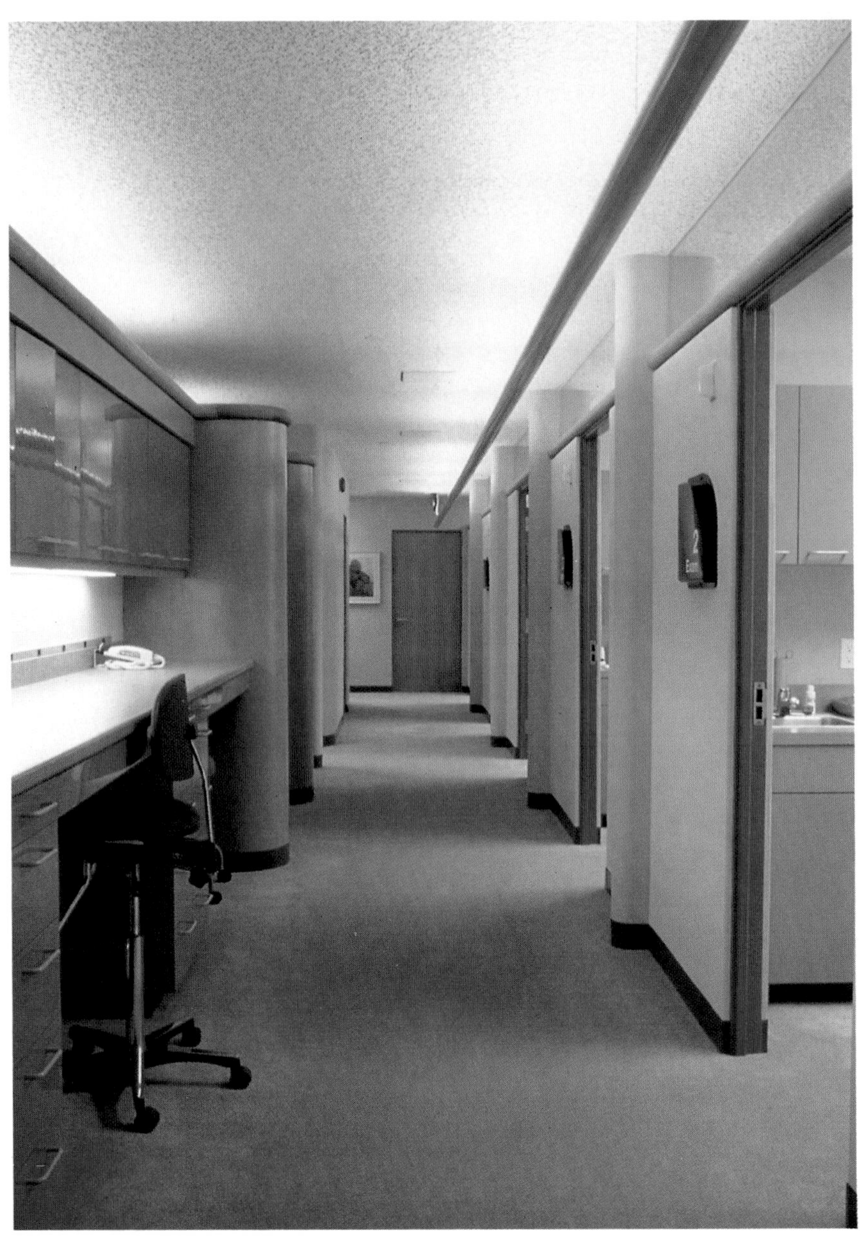

Figure 13-9. Corridor, dermatology suite, indirect lighting. (*Architecture/Interiors: Richard Deno, Cardiff, CA; Furniture: Kathy Burnham; Art: Richard Fitzpatrick, M.D.; Photographer: Kim Brun.*)

Some facilities, it should be noted, do the lab work on the day of surgery, which means patients may have to arrive a little earlier. The patient is next directed to a preparation area where street clothes are exchanged for surgical apparel. This may be handled in a number of ways. Some facilities have dressing rooms and lockers for storage of the patient's belongings, while others have the patient undress in a private prep/exam room, and belongings may be placed in a container that remains on the patient's gurney throughout the patient's stay. In the post-recovery room, belongings are returned to the patient prior to dressing for discharge.

Some facilities do not have individual patient prep rooms and, instead, use a large room (called Pre-op Holding) similar to the recovery room, with gurneys separated by cubicle drapes for privacy. In this situation, patients sometimes change clothes within this enclosure, or they may use a dressing/locker room.

After the patient is undressed, the operative site is scrubbed, shaved, and prepped for surgery. The anesthesiologist will generally talk to the patient in the prep area or in the pre-operative holding area, discussing the alternatives for anesthesia, and answering any questions the patient may have.

Most FASCs do not use pre-operative sedatives, as they increase recovery time. Therefore patients may read or chat with each other prior to being inducted into surgery. At the time of induction, the patient may walk or may be wheeled into the operating room. Some facilities prefer to have patients walk to enhance the patient's perception of himself or herself as a healthy individual.

Anesthetic induction almost always takes place in the operating room, although an intravenous fluid may be started in the pre-operative holding area. Following surgery, the patient is transferred to the post-anesthesia recovery area until he or she is conscious and stabilized. Many facilities use a second stage recovery area that has recliner chairs and lounge seating. Patients remain here after they are dressed, have some juice or tea, and leave when they feel well enough for discharge, or when their escort has arrived. Often, the escort is allowed to sit with the patient in the secondary recovery area. Instructions for post-operative care may be delivered here or in a private office, adjacent to the discharge area.

Facility Access

Handicap Requirements. Barrier-free access is a code requirement throughout the nation, and although patients are accompanied by staff in almost all areas of an ambulatory surgical center, the facility must be designed to accommodate the handicapped.

Vehicular Access—Patient Pick-up/Emergency. As the term ambulatory surgery implies, patients are able to walk into the facility without assistance. However, patient pick-up after surgery may become an issue. Patients often leave a facility in a wheelchair, due to protocols established by insurance carriers and regulatory agencies. The patient will be met by transportation at the facility's entrance or pick-up area, which is often a private driveway located near the surgical center's discharge area. Optimally, patients and families should never have to backtrack through the facility. As the patient progresses through the facility and ultimately to the secondary recovery and discharge area, the escort proceeds from the waiting room to the discharge area to greet the patient, and then goes to pull up the car at the patient pick-up exit.

When designing a medical office building with an ambulatory surgical center as a tenant, it is advisable to plan for a vehicular turnaround or drive-through, separate from the medical building lobby. This driveway must be large enough to accommodate an ambulance or a van.

Facility Entrance. The building or facility entrance and passage to the reception area should be easily identifiable, and should be pleasant and welcoming. If the patient has to hunt for the entrance, if signage is poor, or if the entry is poorly illuminated, it undermines the patient's confidence about the surgical experience.

The building lobby or the waiting room of the FASC must have a public telephone and a drinking fountain. Comfortable seating and current reading material should be provided for the patients' escorts. An outdoor courtyard or garden, accessible to the patients' companions, is a pleasant addition to the facility. If the FASC is located on an upper floor of the building, at least one of the elevators must be large enough to accept a gurney.

Physician/Staff Access. A physician/staff entrance should be provided near the staff lounge and locker area. Patients should not observe the coming and going of personnel. Dedicated physician parking close to the staff entry will be expected and appreciated by physicians.

Service Access. Thought must be given to service access for pick-up and delivery of laundry and for disposal of infectious waste and trash. Boxes of disposable supplies might be purchased in bulk lots and stored outside the surgical suite, replenishing the clinical area as needed.

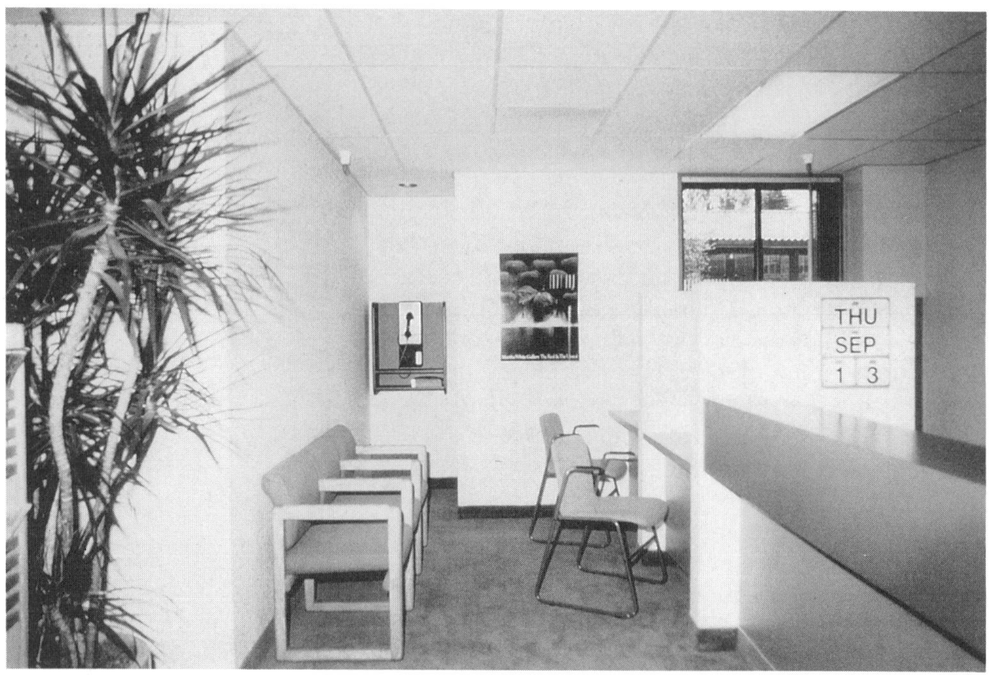

Figure 7-1. Registration area. (*Design: Jain Malkin Inc.; Photographer: Jain Malkin.*)

Individual Components of an FASC

Waiting/Reception Area. The patient's first impression of the surgical center will be formed in the waiting room. The patient should be able to reach the receptionist easily, and be able to speak with a certain amount of privacy. The registration area, where scheduling and financial arrangements are made, should be private, quiet, and comfortable. Figure 7-1 shows a registration area divided into privacy carrels. Note that a public telephone is provided for the convenience of patients and their families.

The design of the waiting room allows the surgical center to demonstrate visually to patients its concern for their comfort. Colors should be cheerful; furniture, comfortable; and lighting, appropriate for reading and/or relaxing. Natural light and views of the outdoors may be exploited whenever possible. Figure 7-2 shows a waiting room with a large picture window overlooking a fountain (opposite reception desk, out of view) and many live plants. Special artwork created for this facility adds texture and color.

Waiting Room Capacity. Waiting room capacity will be determined by the facility program. Most patients will be accompanied by a companion, and scheduling practices in an individual facility may cause last-minute rescheduling, necessitating a one- to two-hour patient wait in the waiting room. Turnover in an individual OR can be quite high, when taking into account that some procedures may only be 30 to 40 minutes in length. This means that a substantial number of patients and their companions may be in the waiting room at any one time, especially at peak scheduling periods. For example, patients who work often tend to schedule surgery on a Thursday or Friday so that they have the weekend to recover.

Sometimes a separate family waiting room is provided. It may be equipped with a television to help pass the time. The most convenient location for it would be near the secondary recovery area and discharge exit.

Business Office. The size of the business office will depend on the program established by the FASC. The reader is referred to Chapter 3 for a discussion of the business office and related areas. Medical record storage is minimal since the patient's chart is retained by

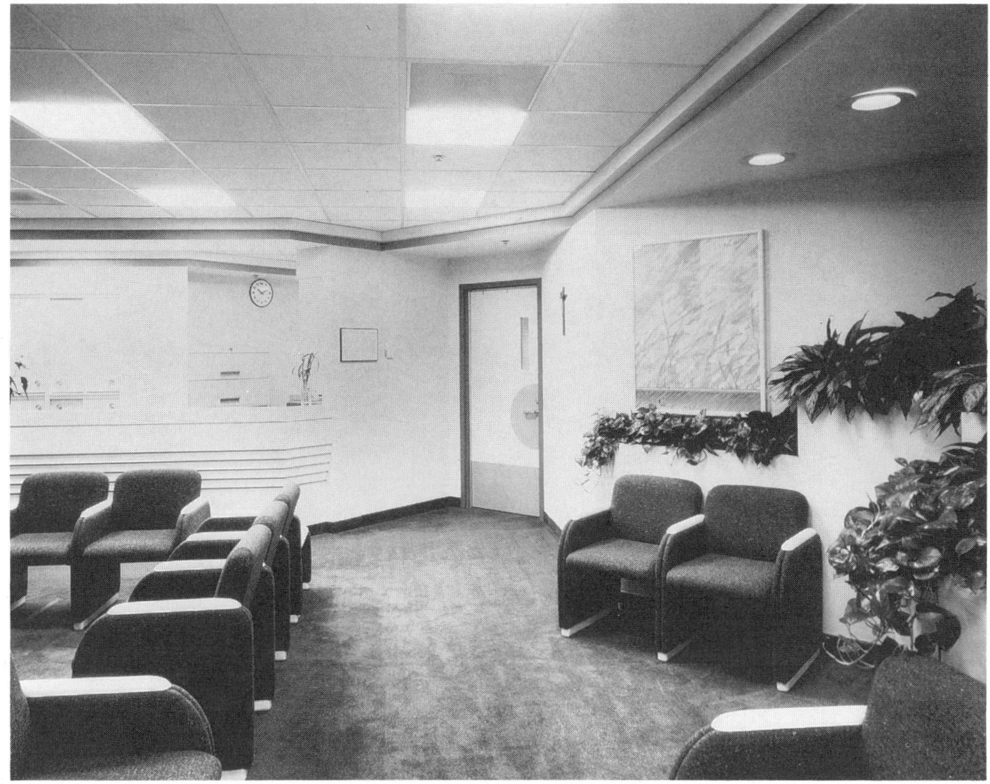

Figure 7-2. Waiting room. (*Design: Jain Malkin Inc.; Photographer: John Christian.*)

the referring physician, and only a brief medical history and a report of the surgical procedure is kept at the facility.

Scheduling is an important aspect of this type of facility. Scheduling staff may use sophisticated computer software that is linked to a physician referral network, whereby patients' histories and pre-admitting information are transmitted by computers, eliminating the need for the patient to be present prior to the day of surgery.

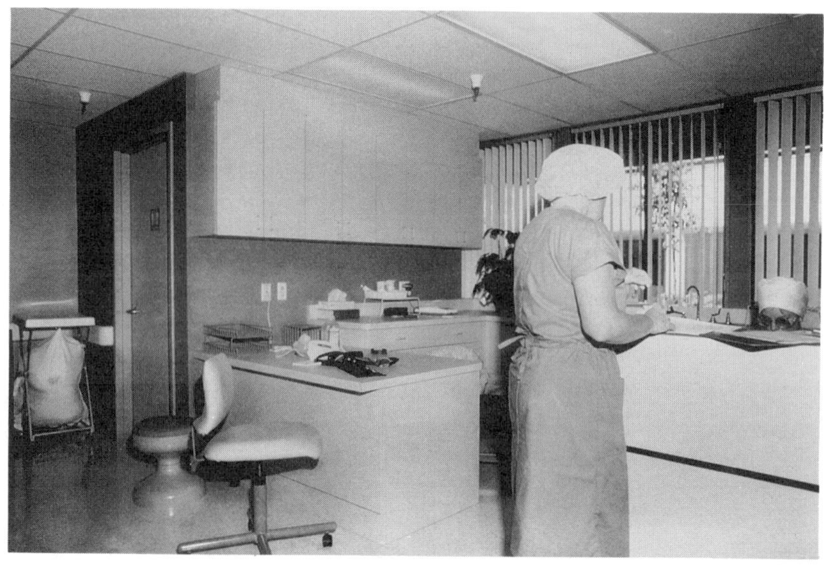

Figure 7-3. Nurse station, pre-op patient holding area. (*Design: Jain Malkin Inc.; Photographer: Jain Malkin.*)

Patient Examination/Prep Area. The patient examination and prep area should be close to the waiting room and have a direct path to the operating rooms. Patient prep areas generally have a nurse station nearby (Figure 7-3) where patients are weighed and their vital signs recorded. The patient will be supervised by the charge nurse, who reassures the patient during the preparation process and answers questions.

In many facilities, the patient prep corridor is clinical in appearance with portable medical equipment and gurneys stored there, all of which may contribute to the patient's anxiety. It is possible, however, to create a nonclinical ambience, devoid of medical equipment clutter and using textured vinyl wallcoverings, carpeting, and artwork (Color Plate 16, Figure 7-4).

A pre-operative or prep area needs a minimum of one bed per OR, varying as the facility program dictates. Individual prep rooms should be at least 8 × 10 feet in size. If a large room is used with privacy curtains dividing beds, 80 square feet of floor space, exclusive of circulation or storage, should be provided. Waiting for surgery is the patient's time of highest anxiety; therefore, a chair for a family member is desirable.

A nice touch in the prep and recovery areas is colored bed linens, accompanied by color-coordinated privacy curtains, wallcoverings, and upholstery. If natural light is not available, adding windows between the prep room and corridor (Color Plate 16, Figure 7-4), helps to expand the space visually.

In some facilities the pre-operative holding area is used, later in the day, for recovering patients. If such is the case, each bed should be equipped with oxygen and vacuum. If the prep room is not used for recovering patients, there are fewer restrictions with respect to finishes and materials that may be used to achieve a pleasant interior design.

Pediatric Patients. If the facility will serve a significant number of pediatric patients, a number of factors should be considered. It is important for the parent to be able to accompany the child through as much of the process as possible. Dedicated pre-op holding (Figure 7-5) and recovery areas assure that parents will not be infringing upon the privacy of adult surgical patients, nor will adult surgical patients be disturbed by the crying of children.

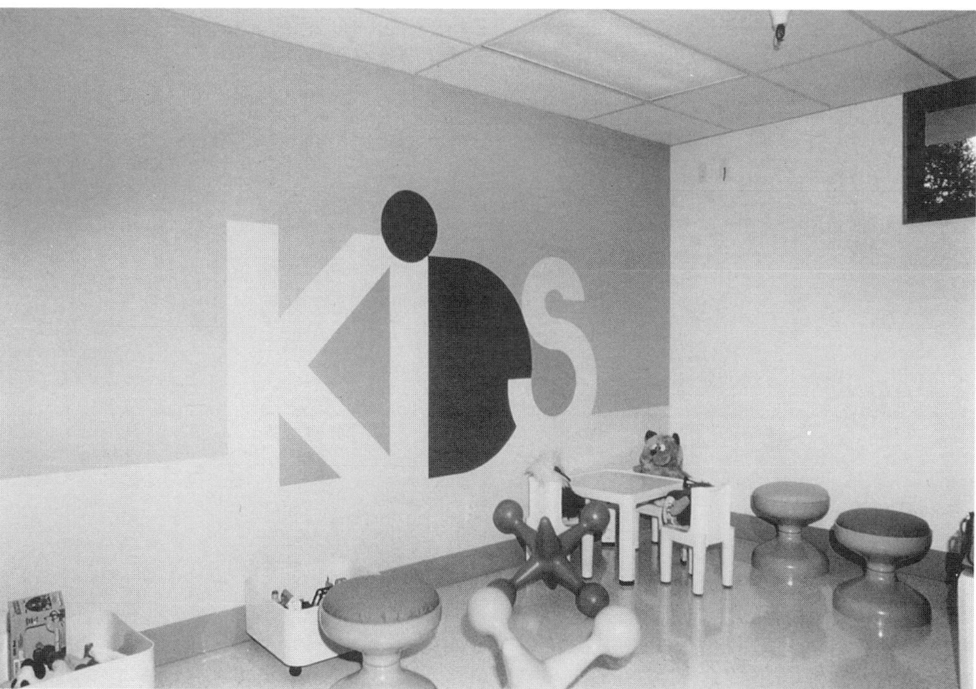

Figure 7-5. Children's play area, pre-op holding. (*Design: Jain Malkin Inc.; Photographer: Jain Malkin.*)

Surgical Core

Central Corridor/Scrub Area. The path to the operating rooms should be direct and as pleasant as possible, maintaining consistency with the prep area, which by now will have become familiar to the patient. Although a sterile zone is far more limited in terms of allowable finish materials, color and detailing may still reiterate the theme. Careful attention to detail and the use of oak molding in Figure 7-6 reinforce an image of quality.

The central corridor functions as a transitional buffer zone, separating operating rooms from patient prep and recovery. The sterile corridor should never be entered in order to reach another destination. Surgical apparel must always be worn in this corridor, and unprotected street clothes are not permitted.

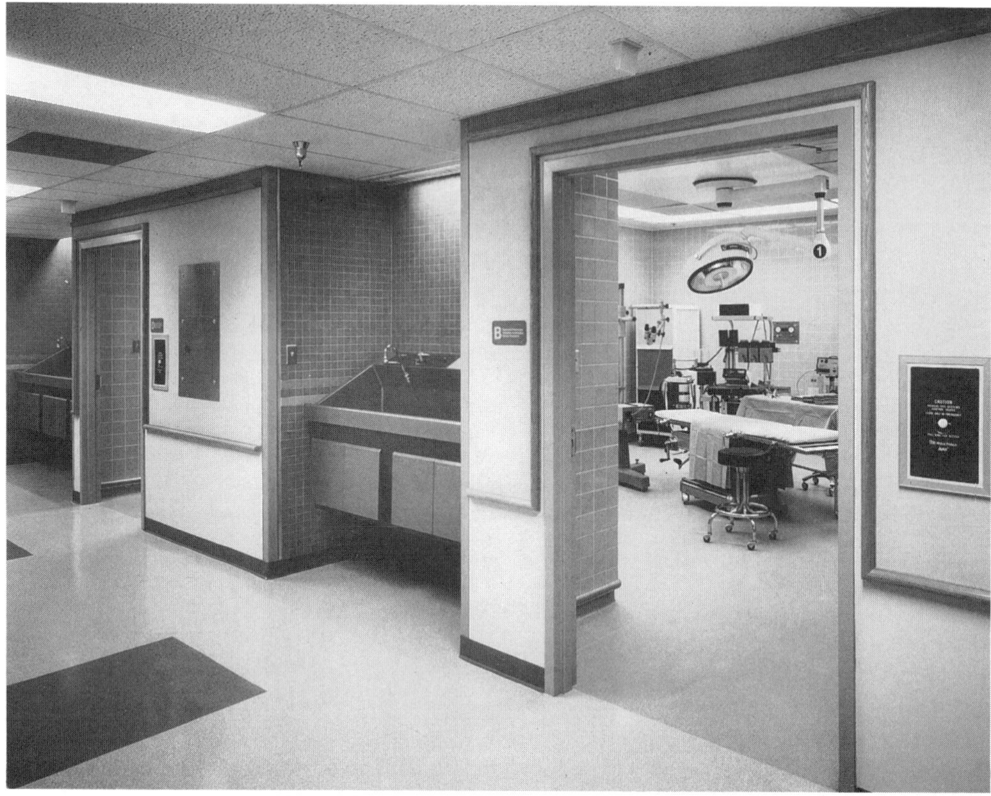

Figure 7-6. Scrub corridor. Beautiful detailing and unusual design features characterize this facility. Also see Color Plates, Figures 7-22 and 7-23. (*Photo courtesy Anderson Mikos Architects, Ltd., Oak Brook, IL; Photographer: Jay Wolke.*)

Scrub sinks are located near the entrance to each OR (Figure 7-6). State codes establish the specific number of sinks per OR. These should be positioned to prevent splashing of personnel or equipment. They are usually recessed in a niche lined with floor-to-ceiling ceramic tile, or other stain-resistant material. A clock must be visible from each scrub sink, and the OR door should push into the room to prevent personnel from using their hands to pull it open. Additionally, doors into ORs should be visible from the control or nurse station (Figure 7-7).

Operating Rooms. Operating room design requires the consideration of many factors, as described in the following sections.

Size. There seems to be a rule of thumb for economic viability of an FASC, which necessitates four ORs. With required support services, this translates to approximately 12,000 square feet. The minimum size of a minor OR is 270 net square feet, with a 15-foot minimum dimension across the room. The minimum size for a major OR is 350 net square feet, with an 18-foot minimum dimension across the room. It is prudent to size ORs larger than may have been anticipated in order to accommodate additional portable equipment such as microscopes for ophthalmic surgery, arthroscopes, lasers, C-arm X-ray, and other items of equipment that may become standard as ambulatory surgery takes on an expanded role.

As time goes on, more procedures will be done on an outpatient basis, such as cardiac catherizations. Pilot programs are in place nationally, to examine an intermediate level of FASC, where patients are allowed to remain overnight for extended care. This will allow more complicated types of surgery to be done in an FASC.

Hospital inpatient ORs are generally 400 net square feet. That size allows for great flexibility and space for a number of OR personnel and equipment. Room shape should be as close to square as possible for convenient placement of mobile and ceiling-mounted equipment around the table. (See *USDHHS Guidelines for Construction and Equipment of Hospital and Medical Facilities.*)

Sometimes a 12- × 12-foot minor procedure room may be included for procedures where minimal assistance is needed and where either no anesthesia or only local anesthesia is indicated. For example, this may be used for endoscopy procedures. Figure 7-8 and Color Plate 17, Figure 7-9, show typical operating rooms. Operating rooms in an FASC should be designed to the same exacting standards as hospital inpatient ORs. Precautions for infection control, fire safety, equipment performance, lighting design, air flow, and electrical backup power should all be carefully considered.

Planning Issues. Operating room features that affect turnaround time between procedures deserve careful examination. The typical inpatient OR may be used for three or four procedures per day, each of which may last two to three hours, whereas an FASC OR may be used six or seven times per day for procedures lasting 30 to 50 minutes. In an FASC, surgery generally terminates by 2 P.M., to allow patients to recover and leave by closing time.

In this regard, the route between the operating rooms and sterilization, and the manner in which instruments and sterile supplies are delivered to the room become significant. Some facilities have a separate sterile corridor (Figure 7-10) around the operating room for flash sterilization and for quickly supplying the operating rooms. This is a matter of individual consideration, based on the surgical program and available space. (Note that the facility in Figure 7-10 functions as an after-hours emergency care facility.)

Casework in operating rooms should be either recessed in the wall or, if freestanding, should have a sloped top to avoid a shelf that becomes a dust collector. Operating room casework often has glass doors for viewing the contents.

Electrical Systems. The electrical system must meet standards established by the National Electrical Code, NFPA 70; Essential Electrical Systems, NFPA 99; Use of Electricity in Patient Care, NFPA 99; and state codes. The USDHHS *Guidelines for Construction and Equipment of Hospital and Medical Facilities* gives a thorough description of requirements used as a model for most regional codes.

The electrical system in any facility where general anesthesia is used is very complex, and an electrical engineer experienced in health care design should be part of the design team. Code-mandated items include an alarm system, emergency power, ground fault protection, nurse call and communications systems, and possibly an isolated power system.

Electrical outlets in the OR should be mounted at waist height, when located on the wall. Outlets overhead are practical as cords are less likely to become tangled.

Mechanical System. Air handling systems (HVAC) in the OR and other areas of a surgical suite are very specifically regulated, and they require the technical expertise of a mechanical engineer experienced in health care design. Again, the USDHHS *Guidelines* gives a good description of requirements in various areas of the suite, and refers the designer to applicable NFPA codes that form the basis for regional requirements.

Simply stated, air flow in an OR should be from "clean" to "less clean" areas. Air should enter the room at the ceiling, above the patient, and be drawn off at

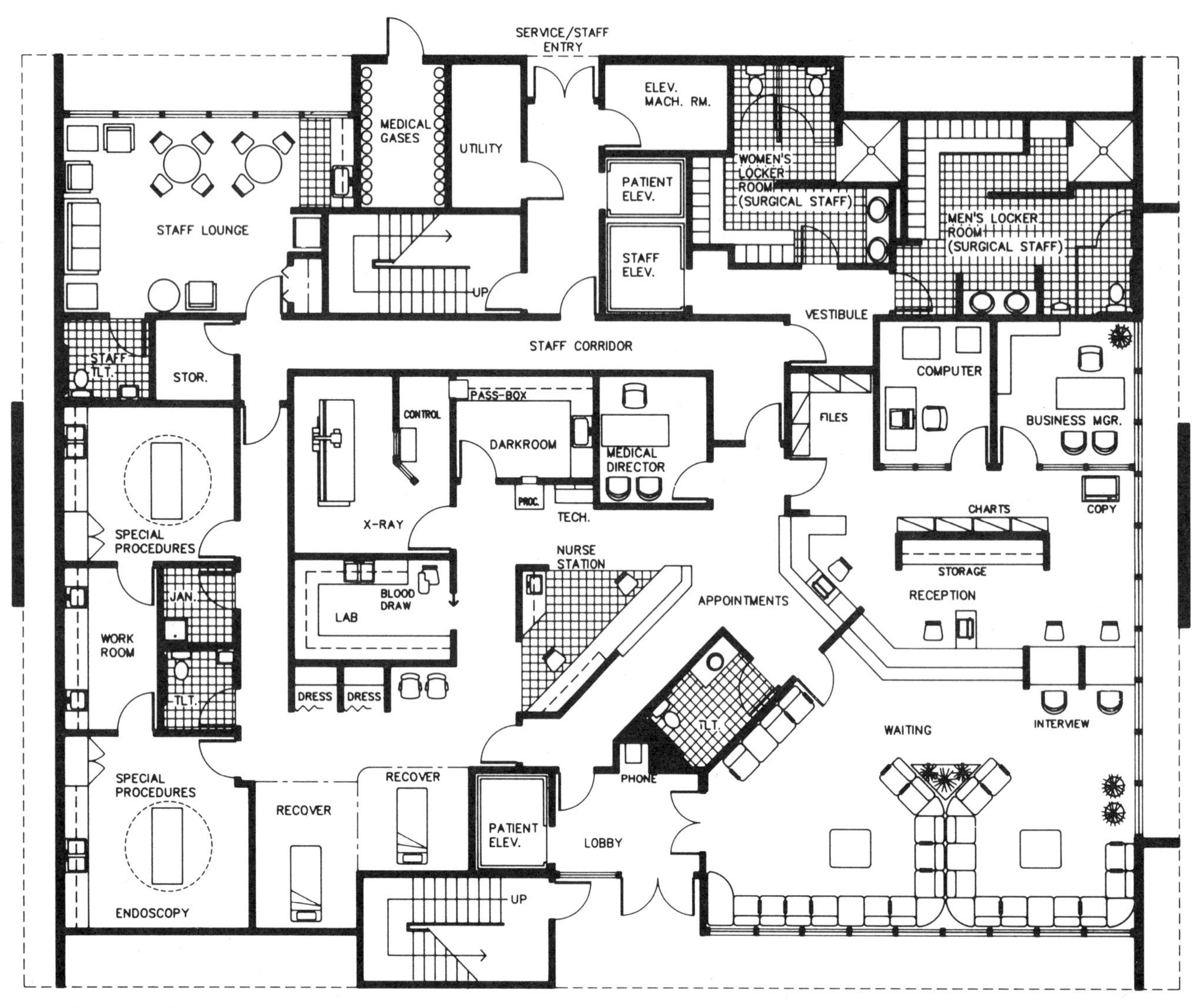

Figure 7-7. Suite plan for ambulatory surgical center on two floors, 12,744 square feet.

AMBULATORY SURGICAL CENTER
12744 SF

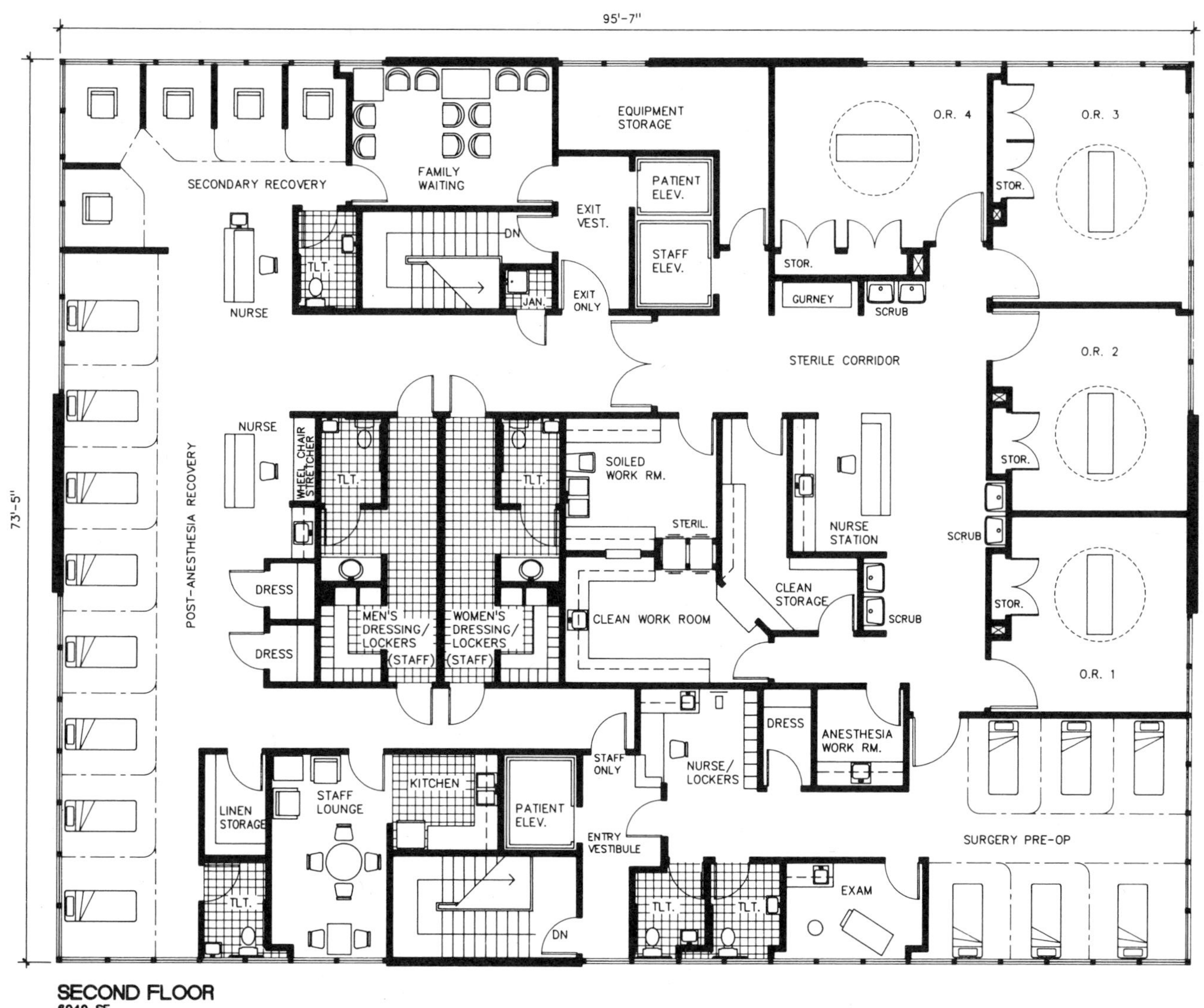

SECOND FLOOR
6949 SF

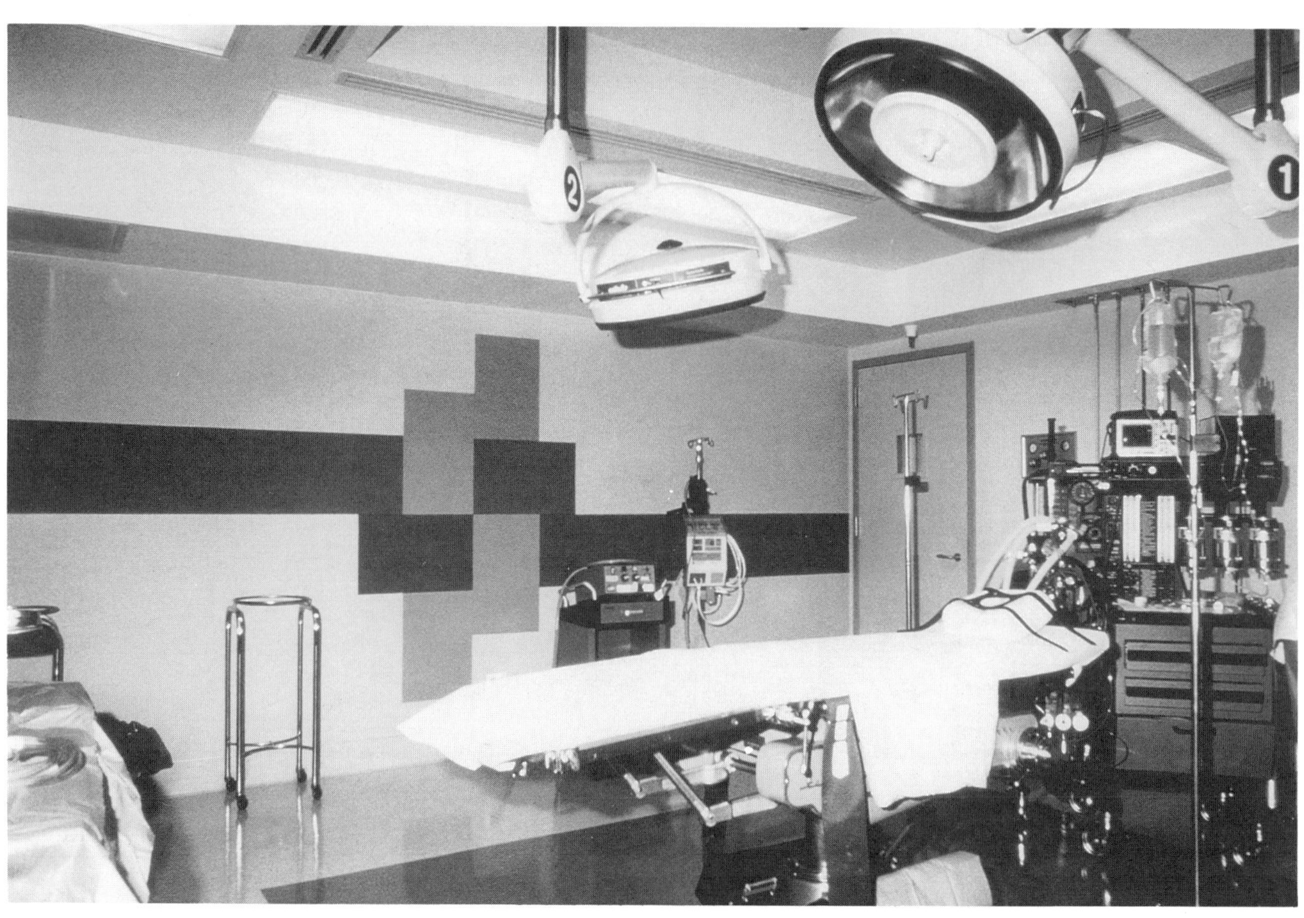

Figure 7-8. Operating room. Note vinyl inset wallgraphic. (*Design: Jain Malkin Inc.; Photographer: Jain Malkin.*)

two or more widely spaced locations near the floor. Filtration, number of air changes per hour, volume, humidity, and temperature are specifically mandated. In some circumstances, where the potential for infection is high, a laminar air flow system may be used. This system sends a large volume of slow-moving, nonturbulent, filtered air down over the patient and the operating team, preventing any particles from settling on the wound.

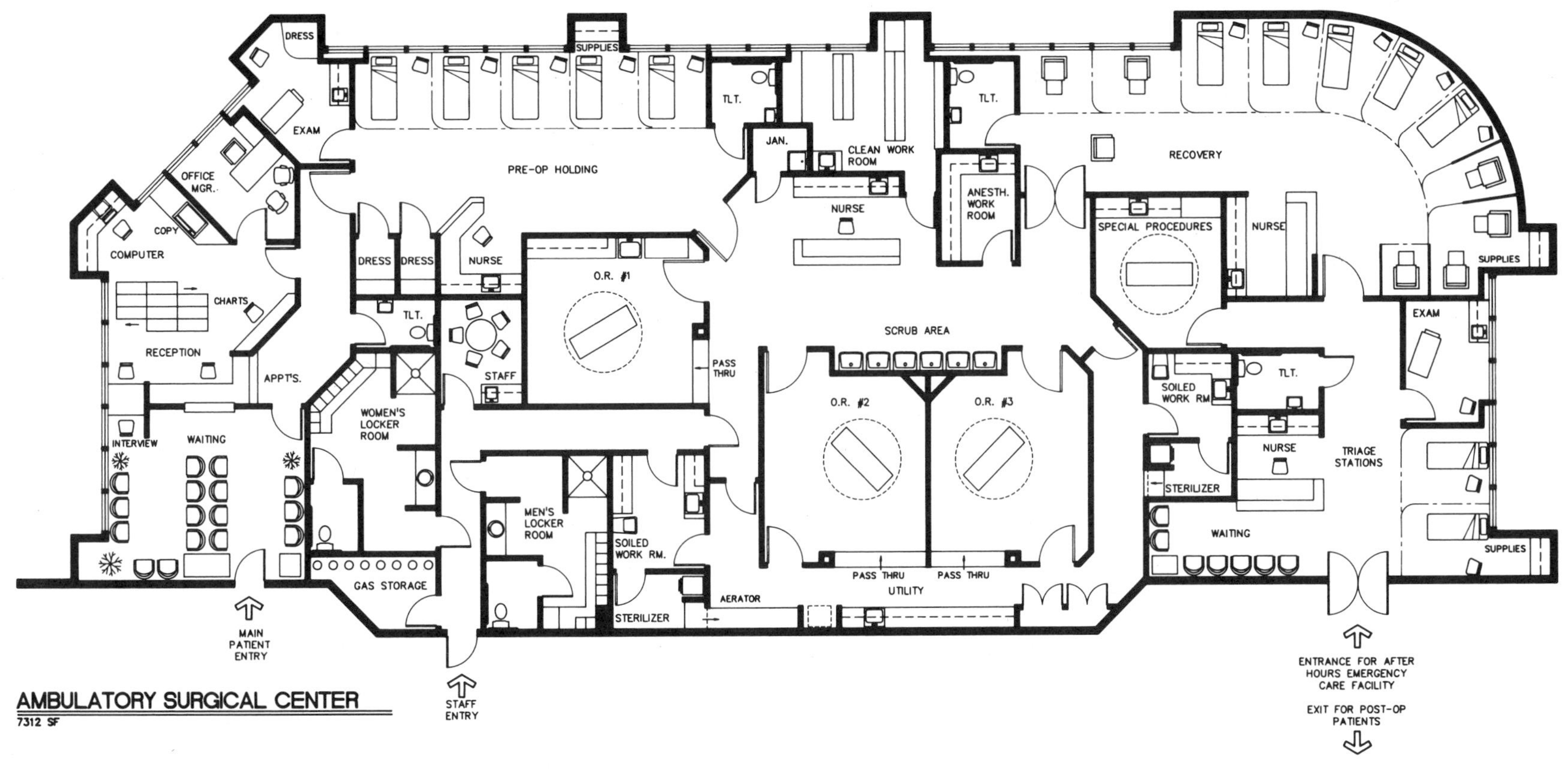

Figure 7-10. Space plan for ambulatory surgical center with emergency care facility, 7312 square feet.

An enhancement of this concept is the Steriflo® system by Krueger Manufacturing in Tucson, Arizona. Forced sterile air, which is comfort conditioned to specific surgical requirements, creates a cube from ceiling to floor surrounding the patient and the surgical team. Contaminated air between the actual operating area and the four walls of the operating room impinges, but cannot penetrate, the curtain of sterile air and is immediately exhausted through the return air system.

The curtain of sterile air is forced through pressure plenums and filtered downward through slot diffusers positioned in the ceiling, around the operating table.

Operating rooms must maintain positive air pressure to keep contaminants from being sucked into the room when the door is open. Air inputs at the ceiling, with exhausts at the base, ensure that contaminants from the floor are not carried up to the sterile field.

Room temperature and humidity affect each other and therefore must be reviewed accordingly. Relative humidity higher than 60 percent with a temperature in excess of 72°F can create condensation, while relative humidity lower than 50 percent at 72°F can create static electricity.

Lighting. Recommendations of lighting levels have been established by the Illuminating Engineers Society in its publication, CP29 *Lighting for Health Care Facilities.* In an operating room, general room illumination is provided by flush-mounted fluorescent fixtures (with dimmer controls), which give 200 footcandles of intensity at the work surface. Fluorescent lamp color should be full spectrum to render the patient's skin naturally. Ceiling-mounted surgical lights generally produce 2500 footcandles of illumination at a location approximately 42 inches from the lamp head.

Laser ORs must be equipped for blackouts controlled by the surgeon. When using microscope illumination, fluorescents and operating lights are turned off. (The surgeon should be able to control room lights with a foot switch.) Auxiliary downlights, located where they will not be distracting, provide lighting for nurses and the anesthesiologist during a controlled blackout.

USDHHS *Guidelines* is an excellent reference for tracing lighting requirements and for an explanation of design principles. The document emphasizes that quantity of light is of equal importance to quality of light, with reference to issues of glare, contrast, color rendering, surface reflectance, and dimming capacity.

Medical Gases. Medical gases include oxygen, compressed air, vacuum (suction), nitrous oxide, and nitrogen (used for power instruments). These are centrally piped to each operating room and may be delivered by an outlet in the wall, through a fixed column extending from the ceiling, or via a movable track. Medical gases are used by both the anesthesiologist and the operating team; separate outlets are needed for each.

Oxygen and suction are also required at each recovery bed. The endoscopy procedure room needs oxygen, compressed air, and suction. The endoscopy workroom needs compressed air and suction.

A gas scavenging system (to "clean" room air of any anesthesia gases) is required in any OR using inhalation anesthesia. USDHHS *Guidelines* lists requirements for each area of the surgical suite.

Use of Lasers. Lasers have become standard equipment in operating rooms. Different types of lasers, and how they function, are explained in Chapter 4, in the Ophthalmology section. The Nd:YAG laser in Figure 7-11 would be used for surgical procedures by a number of specialists including gastroenterologists, pulmonologists, urologists, gynecologists, and neurosurgeons. The laser in Figure 7-12 is a CO_2, commonly used by gynecologists, general surgeons, and plastic surgeons. The laser in Figure 7-13 is of the Argon/Krypton type, commonly used by ophthalmologists. (This unit requires water for cooling.)

The ability of lasers to cut precisely, vaporize tissue, and coagulate blood is truly remarkable and has revolutionized surgical techniques. Certain procedures that used to be done in an operating room can now be done in a physician's office, which illustrates that lasers are very much a part of ambulatory care. Valuable though they are, lasers do require thorough understanding and respect for associated occupational hazards.

Two major occupational hazards associated with lasers are exposure to the eyes and skin, and toxic fumes,

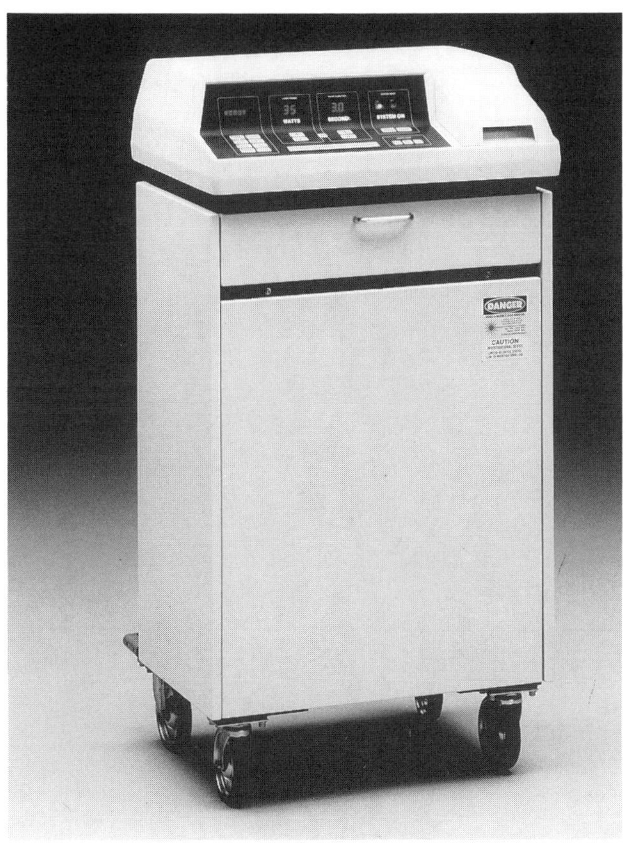

Figure 7-11. Nd:YAG surgical laser system, air-cooled. (*Copyright 1988 Heraeus LaserSonics, Inc., Santa Clara, CA.*)

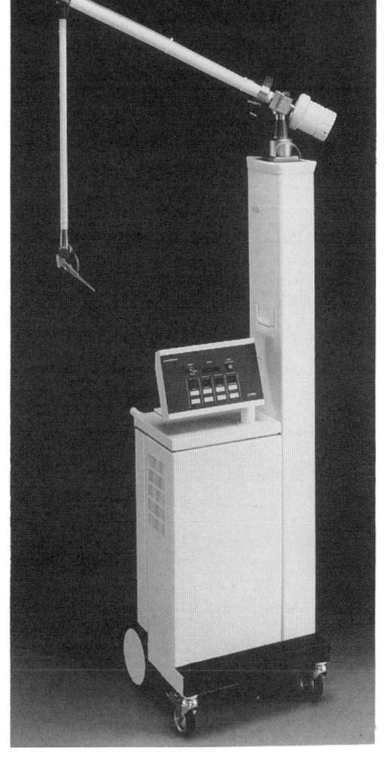

Figure 7-12. CO_2 surgical laser system, sealed-tube. (*Copyright 1988 Heraeus LaserSonics, Inc., Santa Clara, CA.*)

especially the CO_2 laser plume, about which much has been written. Standard surgical masks are ineffective as a precaution against inhaling the minute particulate matter in the laser plume. Surgical masks filter out particles down to 5 microns in size, whereas particulate matter in the laser plume goes down to 0.3 microns in size. Early scientific studies claimed that the CO_2 laser plume was harmless, but there is currently much controversy surrounding this issue and it has been demonstrated that viral infections have occurred in operating room personnel after laser surgery.

The laser smoke filtration system in Figure 7-14 suctions the laser plume and filters particles as small as 0.12 microns. It also helps to control the odor of vaporized tissue.

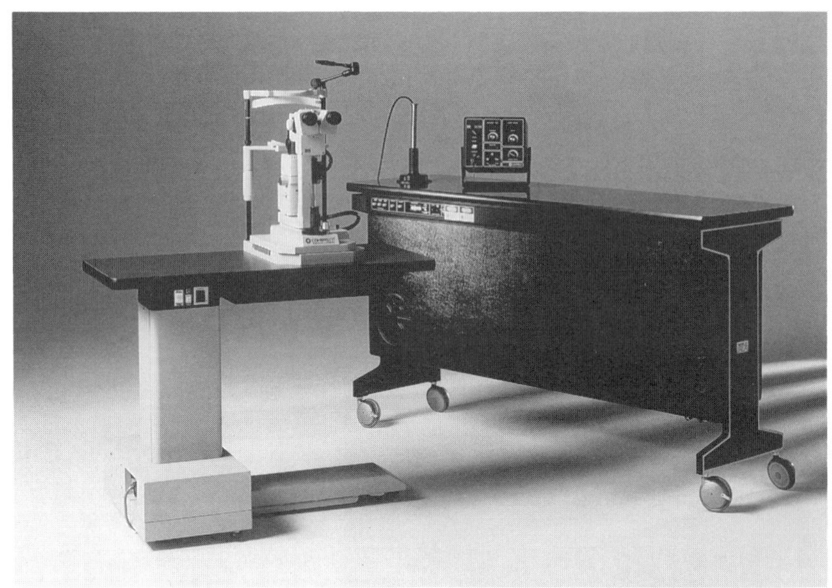

Figure 7-13. Argon laser system, water-cooled. (*Courtesy Coherent Medical Group, Palo Alto, CA.*)

The American National Standards Institute (ANSI) document Z-136.1 (1986) describes four basic categories of controls that should be employed in laser environments. These involve *engineering controls, personal protective gear, administrative and procedural protocols,* and *special controls.* Personal protective equipment includes goggles, clothing, gloves, and respirators, depending upon the type of laser and the amount of laser radiation emitted. Sometimes a temporary barrier screen is used in an operating room in front of the entry to the room, to prevent the laser beam from exiting the room. The barrier must be able to withstand direct or scattered laser light for a specified period of time without producing a fire hazard.

All windows in operating rooms or glazing in doors must be covered during laser procedures, as laser beams can pass through glass. Appropriate warning

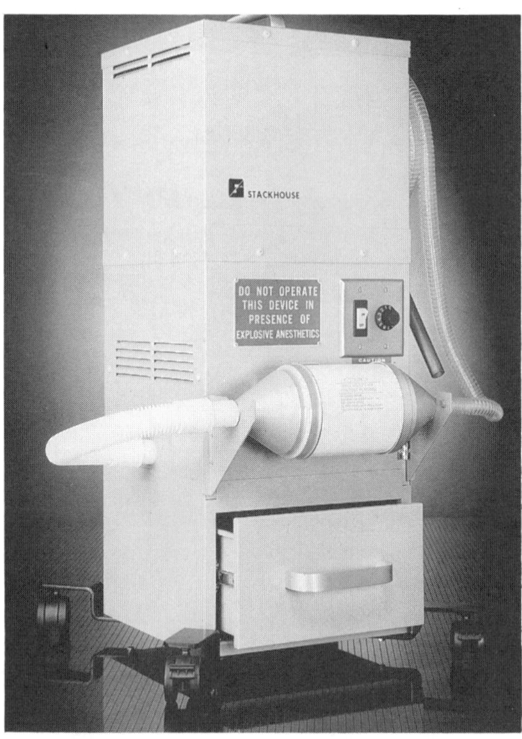

Figure 7-14. Laser smoke evacuation system. (*Courtesy Stackhouse Associates, Inc., El Segundo, CA.*)

signs must be placed on doors to ORs where lasers are in use. Nondefeatable entryway controls may be required on OR doors to prevent people from entering when lasers are in use. Safety interlocks that terminate the laser beam are standard on most laser systems. These allow an electrical connection to an emergency master disconnect (panic button) or to room, door, or fixture interlocks.

Special controls are often necessary for infrared and ultraviolet laser beams because of their invisibility. Such beams must be terminated in highly absorbent, nonspecular, nonreflective materials. Many surfaces that appear dull to the human eye actually act as specular reflectors at infrared wavelengths. A number of scientific studies have been performed to demonstrate the effects of the reflection of CO_2 laser radiation from typical surfaces encountered in the operating room. (Medical instruments themselves are usually specular and cause the beam to scatter.) A number of these studies have concluded that stray reflections of CO_2 laser radiation can present a potential hazard.

Even an unglazed wall tile, generally a poor reflector, was found to reflect up to 20 percent of laser radiation on it. Other materials reflected 50 percent of the light. One study recommended the use of ceramic tile coated with an acrylic resin as a way of dramatically decreasing reflectivity.

Some lasers have special power requirements (208 to 220 volt, three-phase power), but many function with standard current. Some lasers have two plugs, each needing dedicated circuits. It is important to mark, or code, for operating room personnel, which outlets are intended for lasers.

Operating rooms do not require a source of water unless it is required for cooling a laser system. In this case, valves should be located on the wall at waist height, with inflow and outflow labeled. A quick disconnect, such as that used on a garden hose, is convenient. A fold-down locking cover to seal off the water source, when the laser is not in use, may be provided. Generally, a filter system must be added to the water supply to protect the laser.

The American National Standards Institute document Z-136.3 (1988) specifically deals with the use of lasers in the medical environment. This is required reading for anyone designing facilities where lasers will be used.

Equipment Storage. Ideally, an equipment room convenient to the ORs would be provided for the storage of lasers. If they are stored in the OR, one has to plan well in advance to move them to the OR where they will be needed next. If they are all kept in one OR, dedicated strictly to laser surgery, scheduling and flexibility can become a problem. Since only one procedure can be done at a time, the other lasers in the room would be unusable. Other types of equipment might also be stored in this room, such as a C-arm X-ray machine.

Accessory Items. Operating rooms will have two clocks with second hands (one for tracking elapsed time) and a recessed X-ray film illuminator. An individual room may have a C-arm fluoroscopic X-ray unit with TV monitor; there may be a number of ceiling-mounted monitors, a ceiling-mounted microscope, and a number of portable pieces of equipment, including an emergency resuscitation cart. Each piece of equipment has specific power requirements, which must be carefully coordinated between the equipment suppliers and the electrical engineer. A structural engineer should be consulted to ensure that all ceiling-mounted equipment is adequately supported. A Unistrut system above the finished ceiling may be required.

Overhead Utilities. The designer must provide enough space above the finished ceiling to accommodate structural support, HVAC ducts, recessed fluorescent lighting, electrical conduits, and medical gas piping. The finished ceiling height in an OR should be 10 feet plus another 2 feet in the plenum above. It is sometimes difficult to achieve this height within the structure of the standard medical office building.

Interior Finishes. Finish materials used in the OR must be very durable and able to be cleaned with strong, germicidal agents. Materials should be as free of seams as possible. Frequent, harsh cleanings tend to open seams, which then harbor microorganisms.

Floors. ORs often used to have terrazzo floors. This is an excellent material, but in today's market, it is expensive and not adaptable to remodeling. A high quality cushioned sheet vinyl with heat welded or chemically welded seams is ideal for ORs. Attractive products are available that can be cut and inlaid with contrasting borders. Sheet vinyl should be installed with a self-coved, 6-inch-high base. Conductive flooring is not required unless flammable anesthetic gases are used.

Walls. For years operating rooms had ceramic tile walls, usually in surgical green color. Largely for cost considerations, epoxy paint and smooth, heavy-duty vinyl wallcoverings have become more common in recent years. Today, ceramic tile is once again the material of choice for ORs using lasers. However, the tile must have a nonreflective matte finish and should be of a medium color value, rather than light. Grout joints must be flush, and latex grout should be considered. Smooth vinyl wallcovering may be used as well, but it must have a dull finish and medium color value.

Ceilings. Operating room ceilings must be smooth and washable. Gypsum board with a washable, nonreflective paint in a medium color tone is recommended.

Endoscopy/Minor Procedure Rooms. Ambulatory surgical centers often have an endoscopy suite. Specific design details are discussed in Chapter 3 under Internal Medicine. Figure 7-7 shows an endoscopy suite. This room can be used for other types of minor procedures that require a clean, but not a sterile, environment.

Workrooms. The movement of clean and soiled instruments and materials through the surgical suite should be as efficient and economical as possible and must be carefully studied during the programming stage of design. There must be a continual flow of clean disposable supplies, linens, and instruments into and removal of soiled items from the OR.

Sterilization. To ensure quick instrument turnaround and availability of correct instruments and equipment, the decontamination and sterilization process is done as close to the OR as possible. Two basic arrangements are typically found: a central location servicing all ORs (see Figure 7-7), or a decentralized sterilization room either immediately off the OR (see Figure 7-10) or arranged between two ORs. The latter allows easy access for flash sterilization (pre-vac computerized sterilization takes only 3 to 10 minutes per cycle and is used between cases).

Whatever the configuration, the sterilization room would contain a large, high-speed autoclave, ethylene oxide sterilizer (depending on type of instruments used), sink, adequate countertop work surfaces, and storage of clean materials needed to restock the ORs. Wall finishes and flooring should be smooth and washable.

Soiled Workroom. Instruments leaving the OR go directly to a soiled workroom, where they are decontaminated prior to sterilization. Blood and debris will be washed off by hand or in a washer/sterilizer. This room requires a clinic (flush) service sink, deep utility sink, built-in washer/sterilizer, countertop work surface, and storage for sorting soiled materials (Figure 7-15).

A pass-through allows passage of instruments into the clean workroom, where they are put into peel packs for visualization or wrapped and labelled into kits prior to terminal sterilization. (Lighting level recommended by the Illuminating Engineers Society is 100 footcandles.)

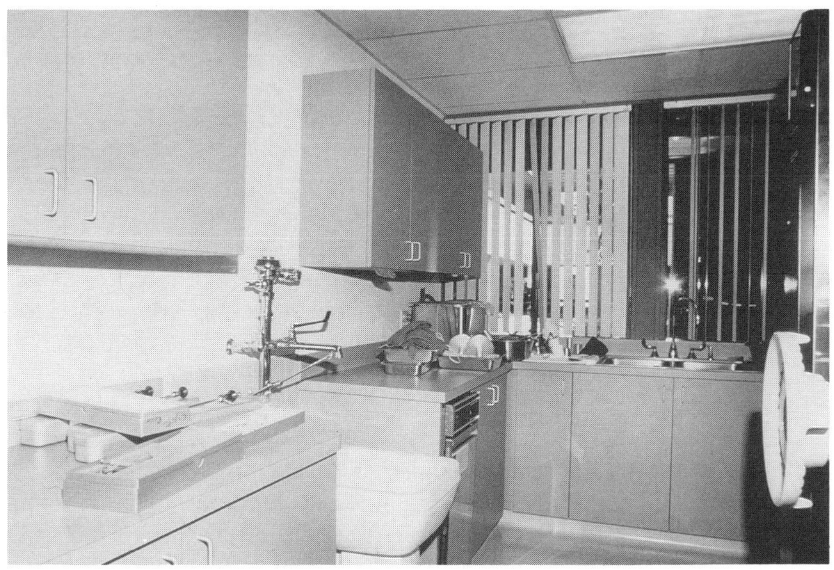

Figure 7-15. Soiled workroom, with clinic service "flush" sink and sterilizer.

Clean Workroom and Supply. This room is used for assembling and wrapping instruments after they have been washed and decontaminated. From here, the instrument kits proceed to sterilization. The sterilization function may be located in this room, depending on program needs and available space. This room requires a sink, adequate countertop work surfaces, and sufficient storage to accommodate supplies. Access should be convenient to the ORs. Smooth and washable floor and wall finishes are recommended.

Clean Storage. After instrument kits have been removed from terminal sterilization, they are allowed to cool before being stored in a clean environment convenient to the OR. Adequate open-shelf storage should be provided (Figures 7-16*a* and *b*), where humidity from the sterilizer is not a factor.

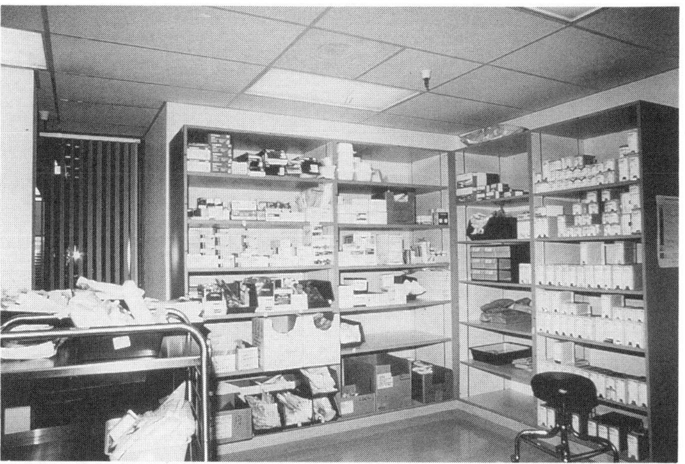

Figure 7-16a. Clean workroom and supply. (*Design: Jain Malkin Inc.; Photographer: Jain Malkin.*)

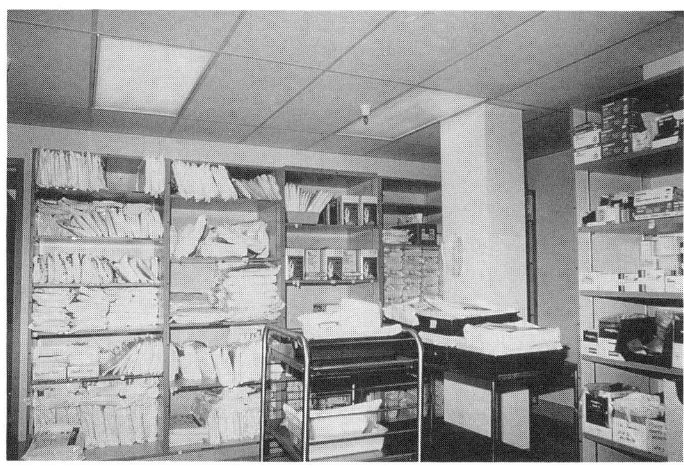

Figure 7-16b. Clean workroom and supply. (*Design: Jain Malkin Inc.; Photographer: Jain Malkin.*)

Anesthesia Workroom. Anesthesia equipment is cleaned and tested in this room. At least one compressed air and one oxygen outlet are needed at the work surface. A sink should be provided, as should sufficient storage for separating soiled from clean equipment. All surfaces must be easily cleanable.

Janitor's Closet. The surgical core must have its own janitor's closet, even if one is located elsewhere in the suite. It will need a service sink and storage for all cleaning supplies and materials.

Storage of Medical Gases. Storage of medical gases must be evaluated in terms of convenient access, separation from other areas (fire hazards), and security. A room near the service entry is generally convenient. Gas storage may be outside the facility, if securely protected from vandalism. Building codes normally require wall construction of at least one-hour fire rating around the room. Other requirements such as an alarm and automatic extinguishing equipment may be required, based on location and type of gases used. Fire codes are very specific with respect to the storage and handling of medical gases. The designer is referred to NFPA 99, Chapter 4, and NFPA 56F for more information.

Vacuum and Compressed Air. Vacuum (suction) and compressed air are provided by compressors located on site. These may be remotely located, limited only by flow resistance in the supply pipe. Sometimes a basement, a rooftop, or an outlying utility pen may be utilized. These compressors are very noisy and should be properly installed to isolate vibration and noise.

Staff Areas. The design of staff areas may vary. The main factors to consider are outlined in the following sections.

Dressing/Locker Rooms. Facilities for medical staff such as toilets and showers, dressing and gowning, and lounge/kitchen may vary widely, depending upon program requirements, available space, and expectations for licensure and/or accreditation. At a minimum, the facility should offer separate toilet and locker room facilities for male and female staff, with street-side and sterile-side access so that street clothes are never worn into the surgical core, nor surgical apparel into the uncontrolled area. Each locker room needs storage for surgical apparel, with bins for soiled garments separated from clean garments (Figure 7-17).

Lounge. A staff lounge with kitchen should be provided for surgical personnel to allow them to relax between procedures without having to regown (Figure 7-18). This area is not considered "clean" in terms of maintaining sterile conditions such as exist in the surgical core. Walls may have vinyl wallcovering, and a suspended acoustical ceiling may be utilized. Type of furniture in this area is not specifically addressed in codes or guidelines; however, the Association of Operating Room Nurses recommends upholstered furniture and carpeting, provided that a good maintenance program is enforced.

Sometimes the lounge has carrels to enable physicians to dictate and chart. These functions can also be accommodated in a small dictation room.

The lounge should be a comfortable, softly illuminated room, with space for dining as well as lounging. Telephones are necessary, as well as a tackboard for posting notices of clinical or social importance to the staff. If natural light is available, it should, by all means, be exploited. The surgical staff lounge in Figure 7-19 uses clerestory windows whose light is reflected by a mirror down into the room. The staff lounge is a high-traffic area used throughout the day.

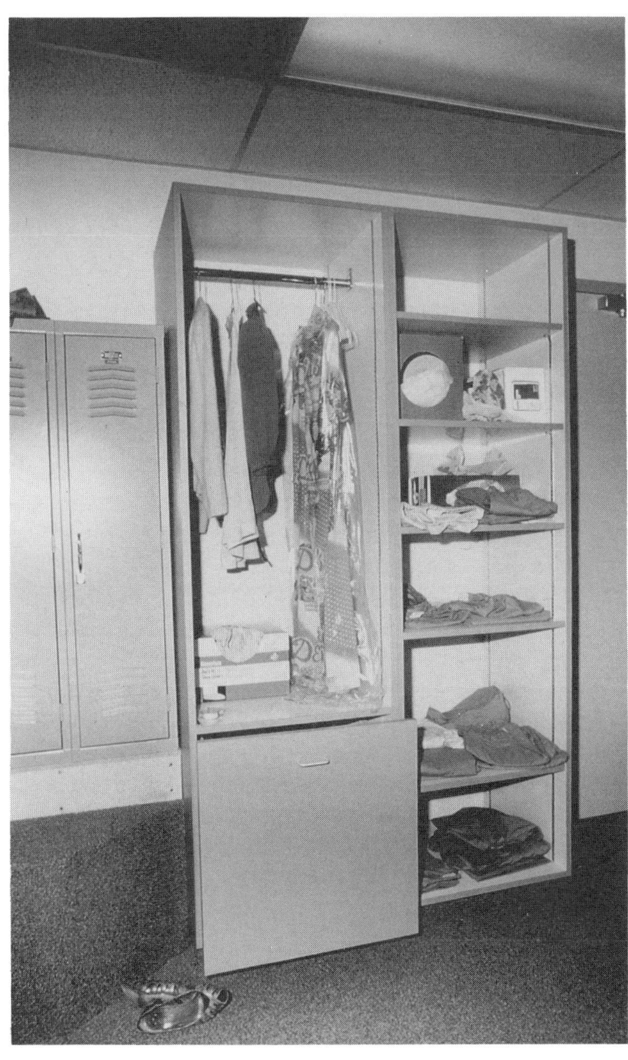

Figure 7-17. Staff dressing area with storage for surgical apparel and a bin for soiled garments. (*Design: Jain Malkin Inc.; Photographer: Jain Malkin.*)

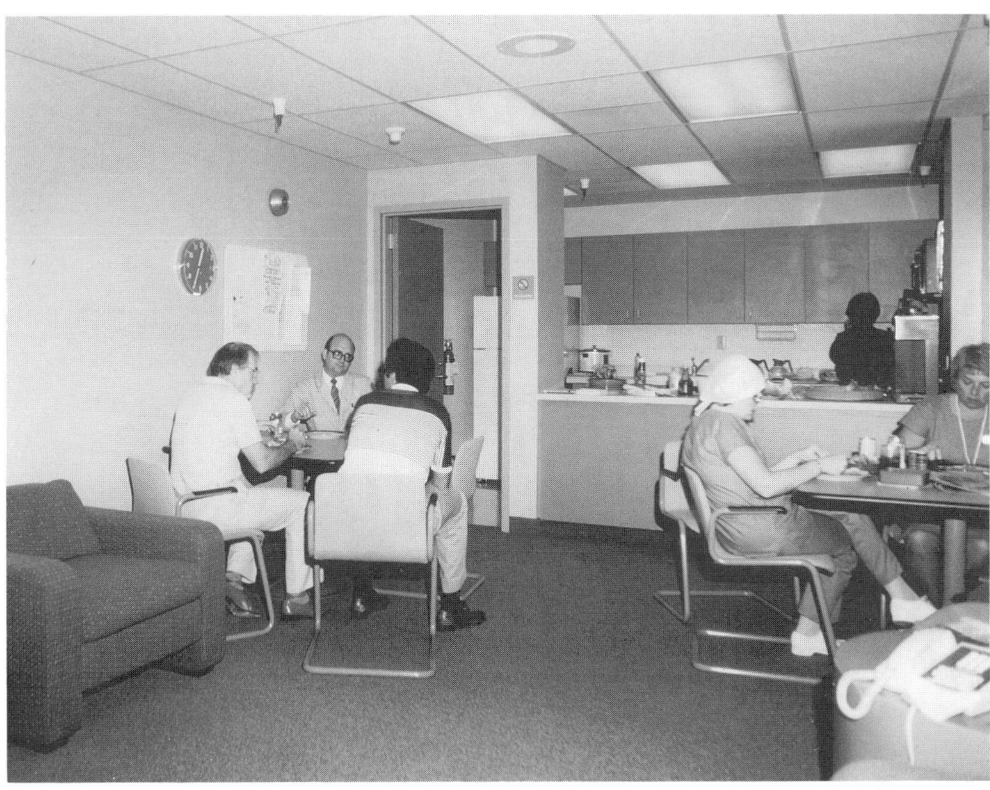

Figure 7-18. Staff lounge, with kitchen. (*Design: Jain Malkin Inc.; Photographer: Jain Malkin.*)

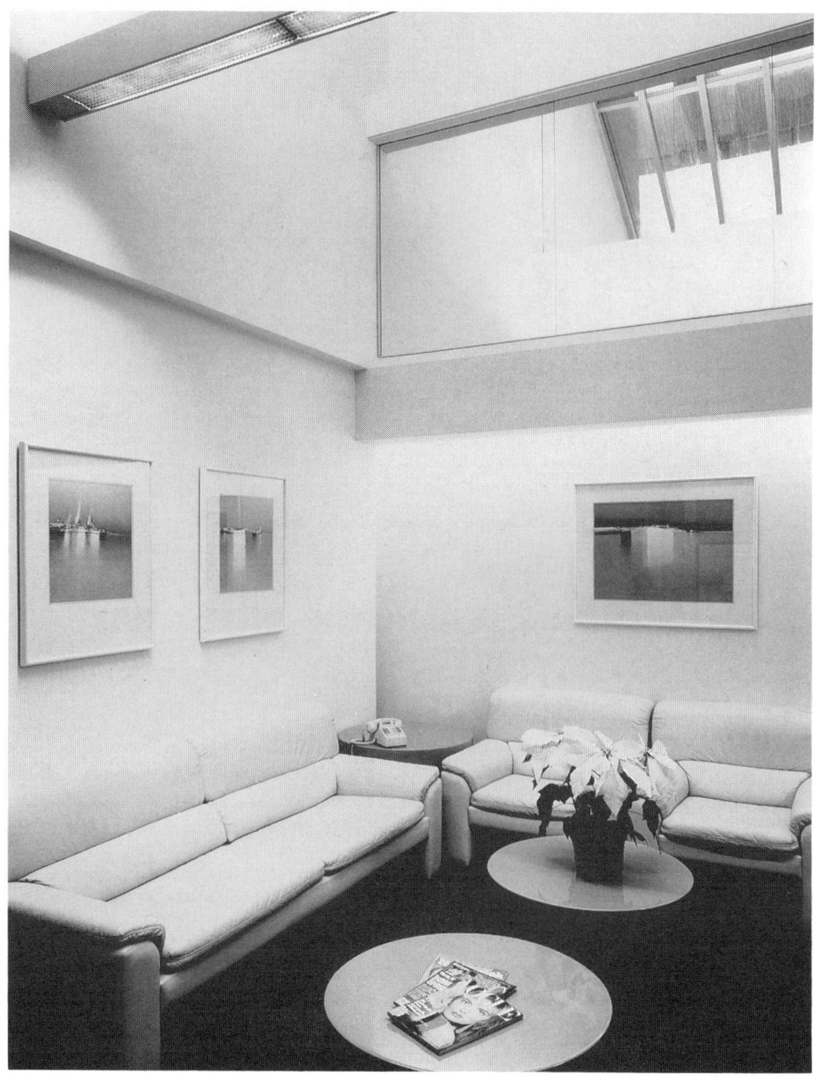

Figure 7-19. Staff lounge, with natural light from clerestory windows. Note use of mirror to reflect light. (*Interior Design: Jain Malkin Inc.; Architecture: Hope Consulting; Photographer: John Christian.*)

Nurse Station/Control. The nerve center of the surgical core is the nurses' control station, to which all information ultimately goes and from which it comes. The station commands total visual control of the area, including OR doors and surgical core access. There would also be a nurse station in the pre-op holding area and in the recovery room.

The nurse station should be large enough to allow adequate staff work space to monitor activities, should contain a built-in blanket warmer in the casework, and requires a sink and a locked drug storage cabinet. The area will contain a crash cart (emergency resuscitation), wheelchair, and gurney storage (Figure 7-20).

Waste/Trash Disposal. If space permits, a small room, perhaps 6 × 8 feet, should be provided directly accessible to the exit corridor or rear access for bagged trash and infectious waste.

Post-Anesthesia Recovery (Primary). The patient's destination from the OR is the post-anesthesia recovery room. This should be immediately accessible from the central sterile corridor. It should be noted that economies, with respect to staffing, may be achieved by designing the pre-op holding area immediately adjacent to the recovery room, with a single large nurse station overlapping the two areas.

To determine the size of the recovery room, allow two beds per OR. The area allocated for each bed, inside the cubicle curtain, should be a minimum of 80 square feet, allowing at least 3 feet on all sides of the bed for work space and/or circulation. A patient is generally alert enough to be moved to second stage recovery in about an hour. Theoretically, this would allow for two procedures per hour in each OR. Recovery room capacity may be adjusted higher or lower, depending upon the program and the experience of the medical staff.

The level of asepsis control measures applied in this area are based on licensing and accreditation guidelines. A sheet vinyl flooring is recommended for the high volume of wheeled traffic and also to facilitate clean-up if someone vomits.

Indirect lighting is ideal, adjusting light levels lower over recovery beds and higher at the nurse station. The area should be colorful, but avoid busy patterns or bold colors which may cause discomfort when a patient is nauseated. Cubicle drapes are probably the best vehicle for accent color, as they are easily changed. The color of fluorescent lamps in this area is a critical factor, as skin tone is an indicator of the patient's condition.

The nurse station must have good visibility of all beds (Figure 7-21), and must have a handwashing sink, emergency resuscitation cart, lockable drug cabinet, wheelchair storage, and a staff toilet.

It is unlikely that an isolation recovery room for a single occupant would be required in an FASC. However, the facility in Color Plates 18 and 19, Figures 7-22 and 7-23, has private recovery rooms. The architectural detailing, color, and amenities of these rooms express quality and an attention to detail.

Recovery Lounge (Secondary). As the patient becomes more alert, the staff evaluate his or her condition and, as soon as vital signs have stabilized and level of nausea subsided, the patient would walk to the recovery lounge. This room accommodates the final stages of recovery in a more comfortable setting, where companions may sit with the patient. When the staff observe that the patient has been stable for at least half an hour, discharge instructions will be given, and the patient will be formally discharged.

The recovery lounge, equipped with comfortable recliner chairs and lounge seating, should be immediately adjacent to post-anesthesia recovery. Observa-

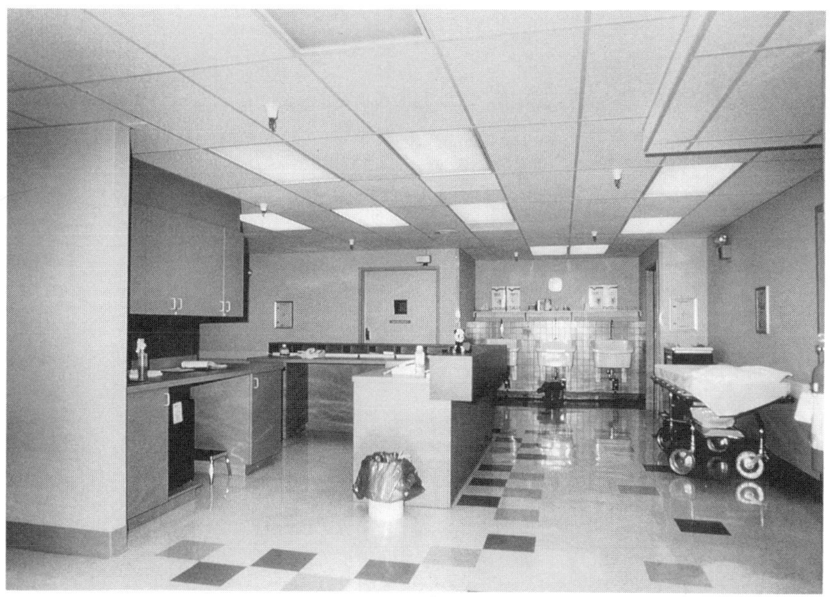

Figure 7-20. Nurses' station, in operating room core. (*Design: Jain Malkin Inc.; Photographer: Jain Malkin.*)

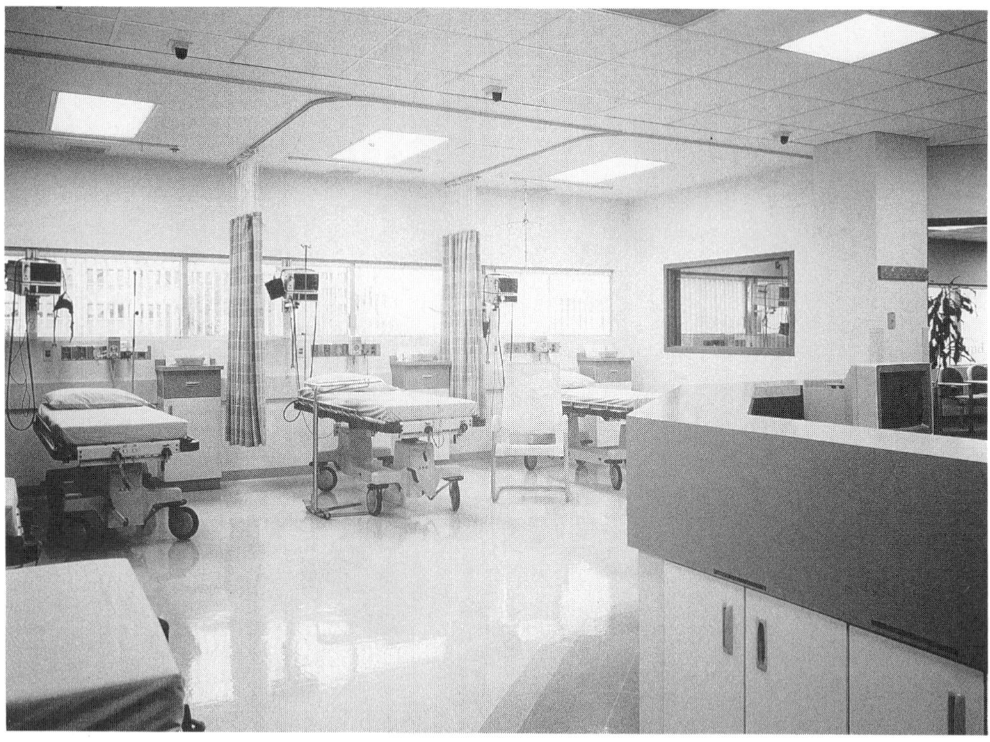

Figure 7-21. Recovery room, with nurse station. Note secondary recovery in background on the right. (*Design: Jain Malkin Inc.; Photographer: Jain Malkin.*)

tion by medical staff is still required, but it is far more casual.

The short duration of stay and the use of chairs, rather than beds, allows this area to be considerably smaller than post-anesthesia recovery. The number of chairs depends on individual program requirements. For example, patients undergoing ophthalmic surgery with a local anesthetic may proceed almost immediately from the OR to a recliner chair in secondary recovery. The dressing area will be immediately adjacent to secondary recovery.

There is no restriction on types of interior finishes that may be used in the recovery lounge, other than what good sense would mandate with respect to flammability and maintenance. Carpet is an appropriate floorcovering, and vinyl works well on the walls. This area can be designed like a residential living room, with indirect lighting or table lamps. Natural light and views are highly desirable.

Pediatric Recovery. When the FASC accommodates children on a regular basis, a pediatric recovery area should be provided that is separate from, but adjacent to, adult recovery. Space for a family member must be provided near each crib or bed, which means that more area per patient may be required than for adult beds. Sound control is very important here, as it is unpleasant for adults to hear children screaming and crying.

Pediatric recovery should receive the same interior finishes as the adult area, but might have a pediatric wallpaper border to make the environment a little less clinical.

Generally, this area would be monitored by the adult recovery nurse station. This can be accomplished by utilizing glass walls to enclose each pediatric bed, allowing good visibility from the nurse station.

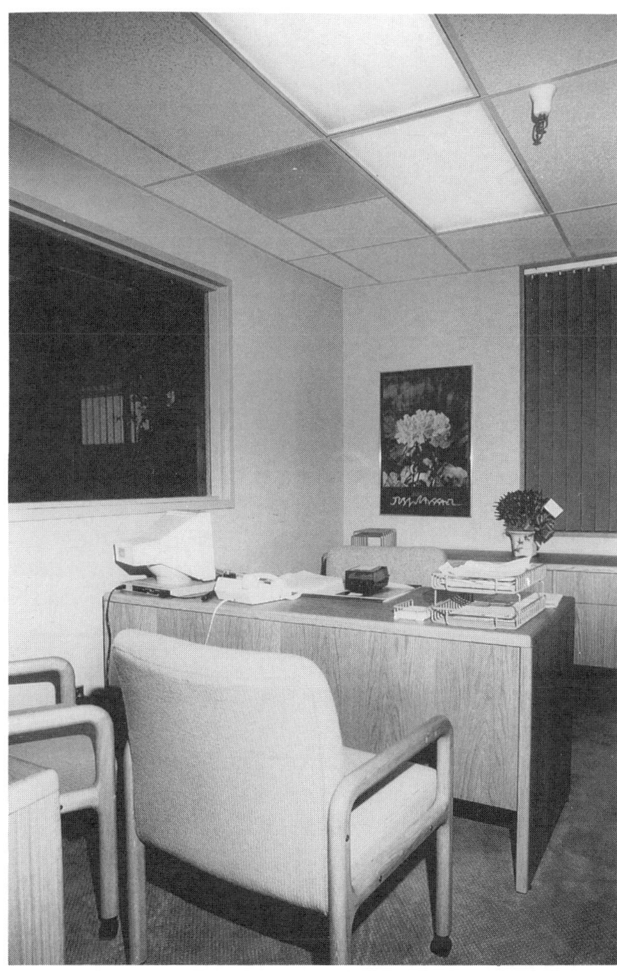

Figure 7-24. Office for director of operating room. Note one-way glass with view into OR nurse station. (*Design: Jain Malkin Inc.; Photographer: Jain Malkin.*)

Administration. An FASC will need private offices for the medical director, the director of nursing or the OR supervisor, and the business manager or clinic administrator. The director of nursing's office should be adjacent to the surgical core or to the recovery room, where he or she can keep an eye on operations. The office in Figure 7-24 has a one-way glass window overlooking the nurse station in the surgical core.

Summary

There are a number of basic models for designing ambulatory surgical centers. Each meets the goals of a specific program, and the final design of the facility is influenced by available space, the shape of the building, budget, and the personalities of the decision-makers. Success, however, can only be achieved by meeting the universal goals of ambulatory surgery: lower cost and convenience for patients and physicians.

CHAPTER 8

Sports Medicine

OVERVIEW

Sports medicine may be practiced from a sideline bench, a storefront therapist's office, or a multimillion dollar facility employing highly sophisticated techniques appropriate for highly paid professional athletes. Programs for these facilities vary widely depending upon the location of the facility, the client or patient population it serves, the treatment philosophy of those who have set up the practice, and the medical background or skills of those individuals. In spite of these disparate considerations, many issues and concerns are germane to all sports medicine facilities, large or small.

Sports medicine is a practice that focuses on the physiological health of athletes — professional, amateur, and recreational — and the problems and injuries athletes encounter. The medical practice most closely allied with sports medicine is orthopedics, and the medical director of these facilities is often an orthopedic surgeon. Physical therapy and fitness training are the other two disciplines integrated into this practice. Sports medicine endeavors to achieve four goals:

1. Maintenance of health and physiological function
2. Improvement of performance
3. Prevention of injuries through training and education
4. Treatment and rehabilitation from injuries

These goals are not unique to sports medicine, but the approach to achieving them may be. In the wake of ever-increasing investments in professional and collegiate sports and with technological advances in medical treatment capabilities, practitioners have developed techniques to allow athletes to recover from injuries more quickly and successfully. Treatment has gradually become more aggressive, and it is applied in a wholly integrated manner, taking into consideration the person's entire range of activities in relation to his or her strengths and deficits in body structure, musculature, and overall fitness. The objective is to transfer the responsibility and motivation for success to the athlete rather than to allow the person to be a passive recipient of treatment.

The success of these techniques has created public demand for access to testing, training, and treatment from sports medicine specialists. Practitioners have responded to this increasing demand by creating environments that offer services suited to the needs of a wide cross section of the public. A sports medicine facility may combine any number of services, including physical therapy, nutritional counseling, deep-tissue massage therapy, biomechanical analysis, and even prosthetic or reconstructive orthopedic surgery.

Marketing Plan

A sports medicine facility's marketing plan will have a direct effect on site selection and design. Location near a medical complex or hospital is very common for a source of patient referrals. Choice of facility, such as an existing space or a new building designed to suit, would be determined by the availability and flexibility of space and the complexity of the service program. Architectural detailing within the facility and interior design will be directly related to the desired public image.

User Mix

A sports medicine center's users are at any given time associated with one particular function of the center, be it physical therapy, fitness training, testing, or medical treatment. The client's activity may change from time to time from one function to another, such as from physical therapy to fitness, but normally users are focused on one major activity at a time. Thus, the same facility must accommodate a variety of needs simultaneously. As an example, a physical therapist rehabilitating a patient from an injury must be situated so as not to have difficulty communicating with the patient due to loud machine noise from the hydrotherapy area or disco music drifting in from the aerobics class around the corner. Each group of users expects to be treated with dignity and consideration, and designers must be aware and respond to these needs.

Providers of these services expect the facility itself — its physical layout — to support the goals they establish. The facility can do that successfully only if the designers clearly understand the practice program and if they meet users' expectations for a convenient, comfortable, and attractive environment.

Convenient Access

A center that is conveniently located, visible from the street, and easily accessible from the parking area will both enhance its marketing plan objectives and meet users' expectations for convenience. A physical therapy patient, who faces an intensive six- or eight-week course of treatment, may be discouraged by difficult access or parking that involves too long a walk to the building entrance. These facilities can attract very high volumes of users especially if they also sell memberships to the fitness gym and pool.

Internal Layout — Need for Visibility

In physical therapy, fitness, and medical treatment, visibility by staff is essential for safety and efficiency. In the physical therapy area, therapists may work with several patients, alternating from one to another. They may be applying a muscle stimulator to one person, cervical traction to another, setting up a patient on a Cybex machine, and placing another one in a hydrotherapy whirlpool. Each of these patients, once set up, needs no further assistance until the 8- to 20-minute cycle has ended. Therapists are constantly circulating among patients in an open plan area set up with physical therapy tables, exercise bikes, large mat tables, and private physical therapy rooms or cubicles partitioned with a curtain (Figure 8-1).

In addition to circulating among patients, therapists often return to a central charting desk to record events on each patient's record. Visibility is essential to controlling these activities. Therapists also must be able to watch the entry area to greet new patients who have arrived, and keep an eye on the hydrotherapy area, which is generally a separate room positioned so that visibility can be maintained. The reader is referred to Chapter 9 for a more detailed discussion of physical therapy facilities.

The fitness area should be entirely open, so that staff can monitor use of equipment and weights and so that socializing can take place if users desire (Figure 8-2). An open plan enables exercise equipment to be arranged efficiently. It is important to have mirrors on any walls in the exercise area that do not contain wall-mounted equipment. Mirrors are not for vanity or for the purpose of expanding the room visually; they allow people using weight training equipment to make corrections in their form.

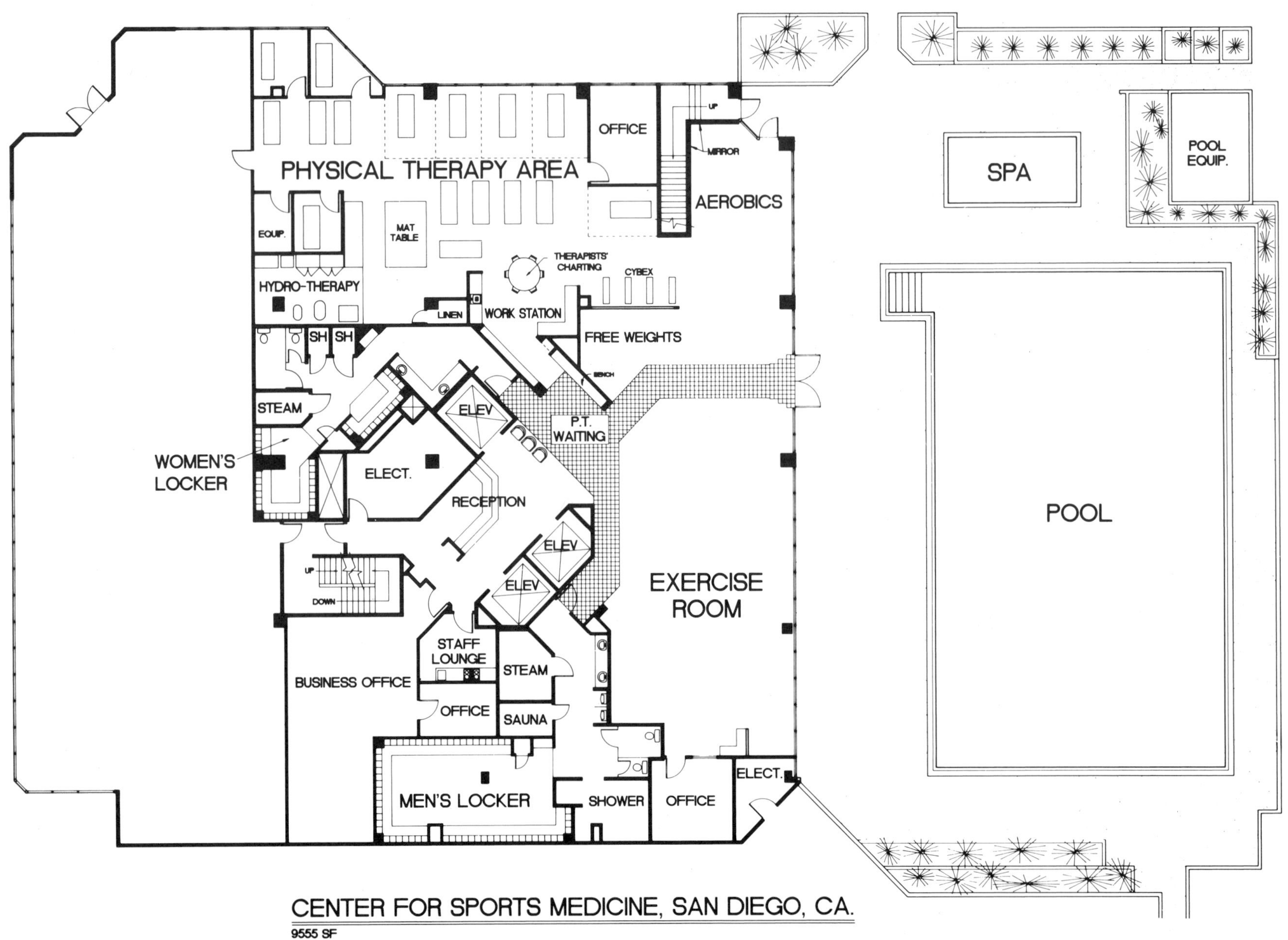

CENTER FOR SPORTS MEDICINE, SAN DIEGO, CA.

9555 SF

Figure 8-1. Suite plan for sports medicine, 9555 square feet.

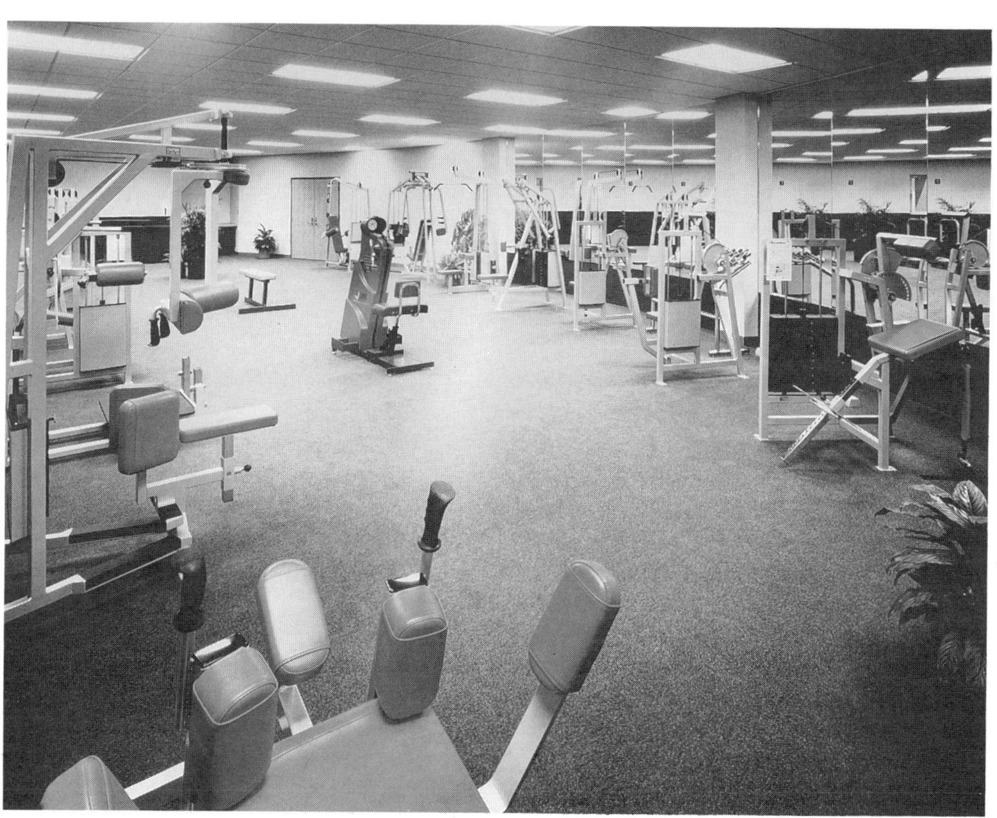

Figure 8-2. Fitness/therapy gym. (*Courtesy Pamela Scharbauer, Missoula, MT; Photographer: R. Mark Bryant.*)

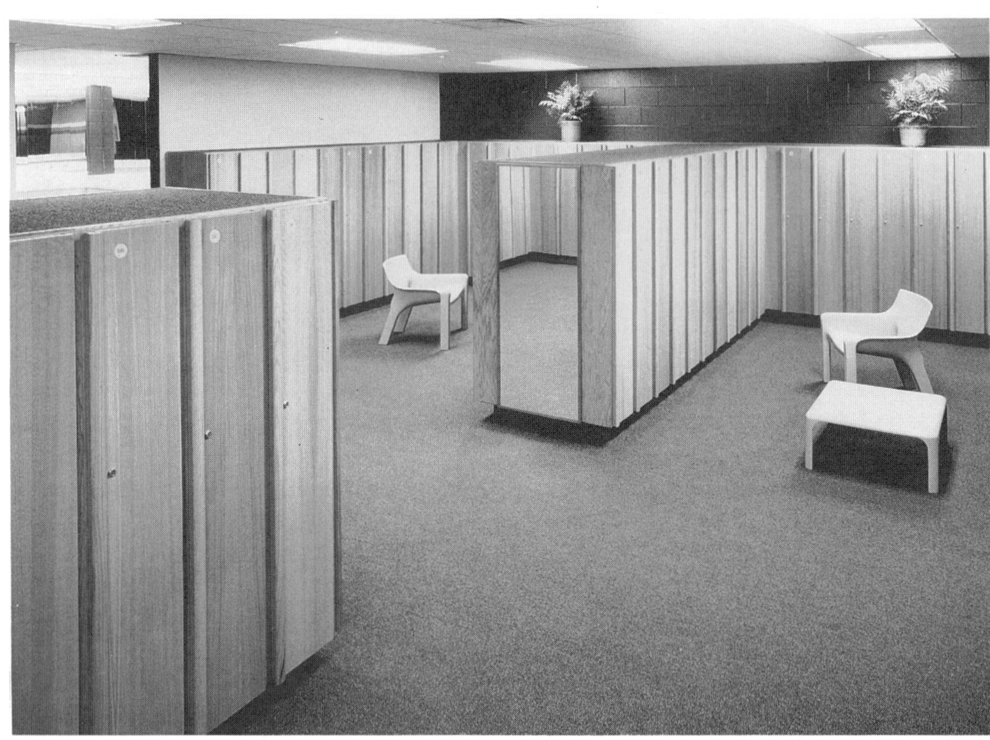

Figure 8-4. Attractive locker rooms are an amenity appreciated by patrons. (*Courtesy Pamela Scharbäuer, Missoula, MT; Photographer: R. Mark Bryant.*)

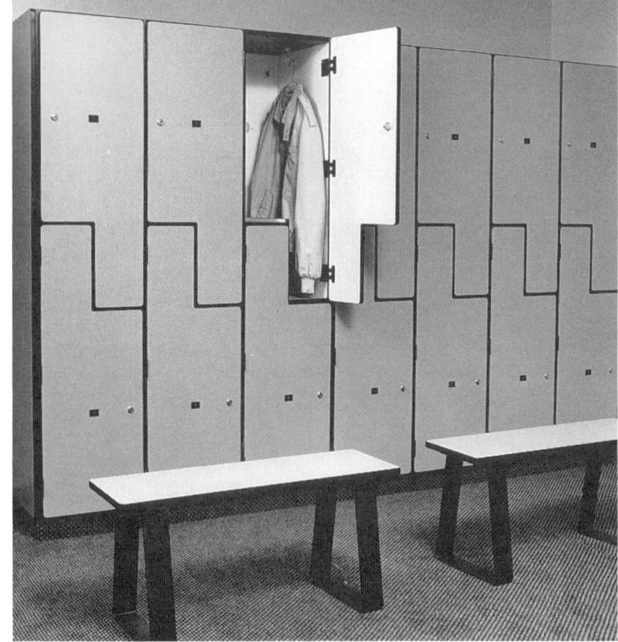

Figure 8-5. Space-saving lockers are designed to provide space to hang a suit. (*Courtesy Ideal Lockers, Brea, CA.*)

If there is a medical practice associated with the facility, the area would be partitioned into examination or treatment rooms, private offices or consultation rooms, a minor surgery room, and a nurse station which should be located so as to command surveillance over all treatment areas. The reader is referred to other sections of this book for a discussion of efficient layout and requirements of orthopedic suites, physical therapy units, and family practice suites.

A pool and spa, if provided, could be either indoors or outdoors, depending on the locale's climate. The pool and spa generally command a high visual profile from an image-building standpoint (Color Plate 20, Figure 8-3), and they should be adjacent to the fitness area and locker/shower facilities.

The aerobics area can be separated completely, needing no direct visibility from staff other than the instructor conducting the session. Visual separation will avoid user self-consciousness caused by onlookers. The aerobics floor should be well cushioned. There are specific products designed for this purpose, but success can also be achieved with a very dense thick foam rubber pad under an 88 ounce per square yard faceweight cut pile carpet. The pile need not be high, but must be dense.

Lockers and showers (Figures 8-4 and 8-5) will be used mostly by fitness and pool patrons, but should be convenient to other areas as well. These should be directly accessible from the lobby area to avoid unnecessary traffic through other activity areas.

The business office and reception desk need not necessarily be combined (Figure 8-6). As the reception area is so hectic, it is advisable to locate administrative and bookkeeping offices in a quieter area. Medical charts must be close to reception, but will still need to be accessible to the bookkeeping office for billing. In this or any medical practice, however, staffing does benefit from one person's ability to cover another's sta-

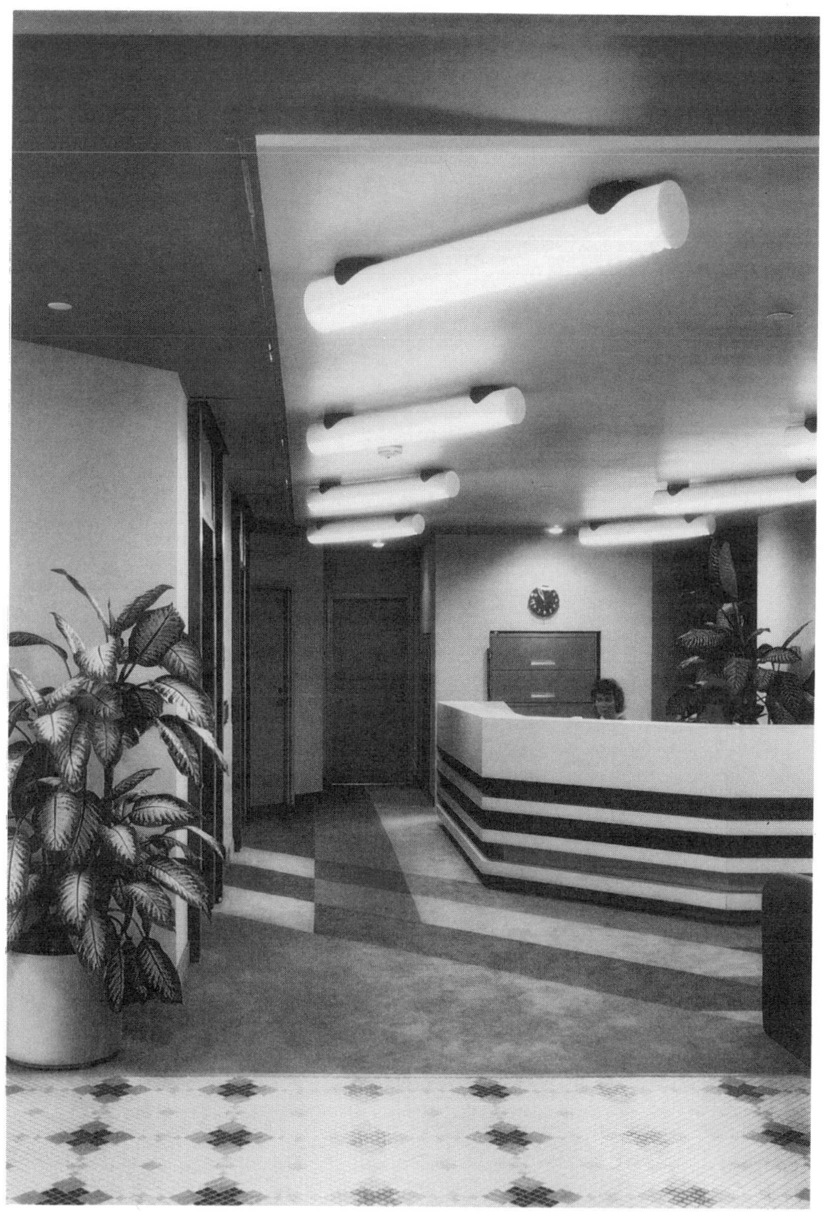

Figure 8-6. Elevator lobby/reception desk. (*Courtesy Jain Malkin Inc.; Photographer: Robinson/Ward.*)

tion if an absence is required. Depending upon the size of the facility, there may be a need for anywhere from 6 to 12 seats in the reception area for those awaiting a physical therapy appointment, for a family member who accompanied a physical therapy patient, or for someone waiting for a friend, although those who plan to use the pool or work out in the gym generally go immediately to the locker room and change clothes.

Noise

Several functions cause considerable noise and should be separated by distance or mass (walls) without unduly restricting visual access where needed. Hydrotherapy generates some noise. This area may be separated by partially glazed partitions to reduce noise transmission to the adjacent physical therapy area. Jacuzzi pump noises can be reduced by surrounding pumps with an isolation closet.

The aerobics area should be fully separated by well-insulated partitions that run above the finished ceiling, since exercisers usually enjoy feeling the beat of the music. If the facility is not on the first floor, the designer must consider the effect of the aerobics activity on the tenants immediately below. The vibration caused by jumping and extremely loud music can be unbearable.

Aesthetics

The aesthetic character of a sports medicine facility depends upon the marketing philosophy, target population, locale, and budget. A facility that draws patients from within a controlled environment, such as member-physicians, contracted service to sports teams or corporate clients, or from referrals within a tightly knit medical office environment, would not generally need to invest in a high-profile design or use expensive materials to be successful.

On the other hand, a facility that concentrates on providing highly specialized services, which would draw from outside the immediate geographic area, or one that emphasizes memberships or establishes an exclusive character would be more likely to require an image-setting design treatment. Health clubs, for example, depend entirely on membership sales, and image is very important to their marketing effort. Generally, the higher the membership fee, the more elaborate the design treatment.

Wet Areas

Areas within the suite where significant moisture or wet activity is present should be carefully considered for moisture control, cross traffic, and noise. Obvious areas where moisture is present are spa areas, hydrotherapy, shower rooms, and steam rooms. Not so obvious, but significant, are the fitness gym and aerobics area, where high concentrations of vapor will occur due to heavy exertion and breathing. Without adequate ventilation, greater than needed for normal use, the area will seem "stuffy," and mildew odors are likely to occur over a period of time in carpets and in areas where cleaning is difficult.

With the exception of hydrotherapy, wet areas should be adjacent to one another or be connected by paths of moisture-resistant, slip-resistant flooring. Wet bodies or bare feet should not cross carpeting or areas of nonrelated activity. An outdoor pool may not be immediately adjacent to the locker/shower rooms, but a path of nonskid ceramic tile or slip-resistant rubber flooring can connect them and provide spatial definition between areas of different functions without wall separations (Figure 8-6).

Users of hydrotherapy usually are dry and dressed before leaving that area, so isolation may not be a problem. This must be evaluated on an individual basis to ensure proper adjacencies and traffic flow.

All wet areas, including locker and dressing rooms adjacent to showers, toilet rooms, spa, and hydrotherapy, should be supplied with floor drains. A slight, almost imperceptible slope of ⅛ inch per foot towards strategically located floor drains may prevent a broken pipe or stuck valve from flooding carpet in adjacent areas.

Shower and steam rooms should have threshold water stops or dams of ½-inch maximum height on the wet side of the entry, with a floor slope that directs water away from the entry. Some shower or steam room doors have water troughs at the bottom to prevent water from dripping off the door. This water must be delivered somewhere and usually winds up at the hinged edge, where floor slope is very difficult to control. At this point, water will go everywhere, including to the dry side, getting trampled into public areas by outgoing feet. One must pay special attention to wet doors.

Rooms housing steam equipment should be well drained and ventilated, since steam generators create heat and present a hazard of leaking. Ventilation of these same areas should be sized to prevent heat and moisture build-up.

Linen Storage

A designer must be aware of the copious amounts of linen used in the daily routine of a sports medicine facility. Clean and soiled towels must be accommodated in locker rooms (Figure 8-7), as well as the hydrotherapy area. The physical therapy area uses linen sheets on the tables, pillowcases, and towels. All of this linen must be delivered, stored before and after use, and later picked up by the linen service. The designer must be sure to provide adequate storage space for linen, plus additional ventilation to keep soiled, damp linen from becoming a nuisance. However, ventilation alone cannot overcome an environment that is not kept clean and orderly with soiled linen stowed in the proper location.

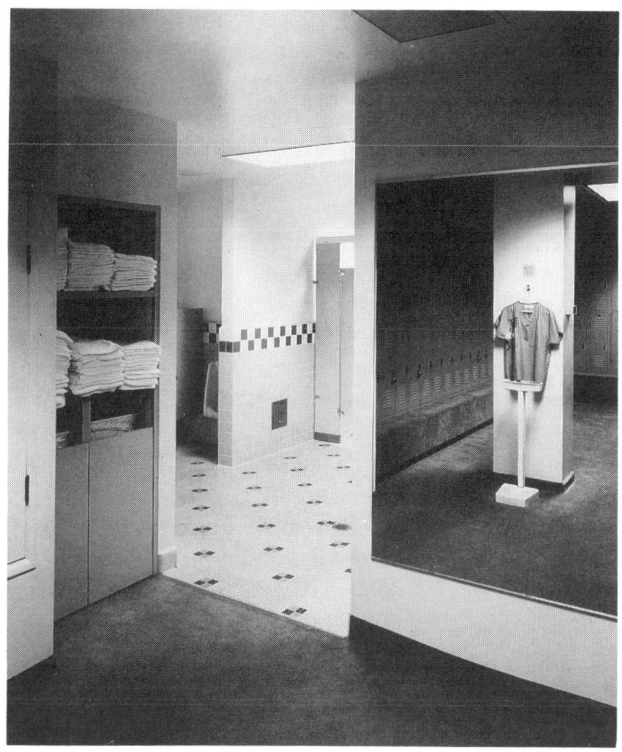

Figure 8-7. Clean and soiled linen storage, in locker room. (*Design: Jain Malkin Inc.; Photographer: Robinson/Ward.*)

Interior Finishes

The floor surface in wet areas should be slip-resistant and consistent in texture. The user should not be challenged with changing from one material to another, because he or she will not be concentrating on the difference. The change could provide a hazardous surprise.

For wet areas, ceramic tile is the most favored flooring for design application, durability, and surface texture. However, contrary to public perception, ceramic tile is not always easy to clean. Sheet vinyl is an option of compromise to be used in damp areas when budget is a consideration. In hydrotherapy, sheet vinyl is quite suitable, preferably with a self-coved base. The designer should note whether heavy portable tanks will be used. They could compress and destroy a flooring material not designed for heavy loads. Vinyl composition tile, because of its many seams, is undesirable in high-moisture areas.

Vinyl wallcovering is ideal in a sports medicine facility because it offers great variety in texture as well as ease of cleaning. If paint is used, it must be semi-gloss or eggshell enamel, fully washable. Painted wallgraphics can be especially appealing in this type of facility. The reader is referred to Color Plates 21 and 22, Figures 8-8, 8-9, and 8-10.

Lighting

Treatment areas within the facility normally require broadly distributed lighting of 30 to 50 footcandles. Under ideal conditions, the physical therapy area would have indirect or ambient lighting. Fixtures might be suspended from the ceiling, with the light shining on and bouncing off the ceiling, creating an overall high level of diffused illumination without casting glare in the eyes of patients lying on physical therapy tables. In the hydrotherapy area, fitness gym, and aerobics room, on the other hand, the standard 2- × 4-foot fluorescent troffer with a parabolic low brightness lens would be appropriate. The reception area, lobby, or corridors might benefit from accent lighting focusing on wallgraphics, special artwork, or educational exhibits. Other chapters of this book provide detailed information on lighting medical spaces such as exam rooms, minor surgery, and nurse stations.

CASE STUDIES

Several examples of sports medicine facilities serve as case studies to illustrate the concepts outlined above. Each illustrates a different approach to the practice of sports medicine. Their facilities are clear reflections of their individual goals.

San Diego Sports Medicine Center: San Diego, California

The San Diego Sports Medicine Center has built its practice on high volume and a well-developed general referral system. Located near a 214-bed National Medical Enterprises hospital, it occupies a ground floor location in one of a group of medical office buildings. It is surrounded by parking and has immediate access from a major freeway.

This 11,000-square-foot facility is operated by a group of osteopathic physicians with offices immediately adjacent to the center. These internal referrals, as well as those from practitioners in adjacent medical office buildings, contribute to the volume of this facility. In addition, contracts with local schools (athletic programs), municipalities, and corporations provide the largest source of referrals for both physical therapy and fitness programs. Of the four case studies, this facility most actively markets the fitness and testing program to a wide cross section of the public. As family practitioners, the osteopathic physicians encourage outside specialists' referrals for physical therapy relatively free of competitive conditions.

The Center's programs focus on wellness — maximizing one's level of physical fitness and minimizing individual health risk factors. This involves assessment of one's fitness, education about wellness, and lifestyle evaluation. The Center also offers worksite evaluation to employers, incorporating site walk-throughs to assess high risk opportunities for injury.

Features include a 5500-square-foot physical fitness gym, separate aerobics room, physical therapy treatment area, and a four-lane lap pool, all contained within a large square surrounding a central locker and spa area. From the entry, one has immediate access either to the medical offices or the sports center administration area, through which one must pass to reach the locker rooms. Across the parking lot is a one-half mile winding running track.

The 4000-square-foot medical office accommodates a staff of ten physicians and clinicians, including radiology and a physiology testing lab. This area functions independently of the sports center.

The central location of the locker/spa area allows convenient access to other areas. Access control is easily maintained by staff in the business/administration area. Access to the track is located outside the immediate control of the center. The track is used frequently by staff from nearby medical offices, and this relationship facilitates outside use without unnecessary traffic in the sports center lobby.

The design character is low-key and simple. The center prefers to project an understated image that allows the facility to remain low profile compared to the high-profile service provided. Since clients and patients represent a wide cross section of the population through referrals from a variety of sources, a straightforward unimposing appearance was considered most appropriate.

Center for Sports Medicine and Orthopedics: Phoenix, Arizona

The second case study incorporates many of the basic elements of other sports medicine facilities, but it is unique in that it is virtually self-sufficient, relying very little on outside physician referrals or recreational memberships to support it. The Center for Sports Medicine and Orthopedics is a $3 million, 40,000-square-foot medical treatment and diagnostic center which sits on a tiny site in the middle of a major metropolitan hospital campus (Figure 8-11). The freestanding building was raised one story to provide parking and to provide shelter for entry during periods of inclement weather. Since it opened in February 1985, the facility has been a great business success and won a "Facility of Merit" award in 1985 from *Athletic Business* magazine.

The Center is the creation of three Phoenix orthopedic surgeons and a sports medicine specialist who, together, are team physicians to 18 professional and amateur sports organizations.

This facility provides contract services to local professional athletes and purposely integrates amateur and recreational athletes in the same treatment program. From a marketing standpoint, being able to converse with professional athletes during rehabilitation is a powerful attraction. The physical therapy program and fitness gym are designed to operate directly in conjunction with treatment and diagnostic programs, rather than retain the more traditional independent relationship. The 4000-square-foot physical therapy department is managed by the Baxter Healthcare Corporation, Physical Therapy Division. All together, medical treatment, diagnostic testing, the physical therapy program, and the fitness area generate enough referrals to one another to make the center economically self-sufficient, relying little on outside physician referrals or recreational memberships in the gym.

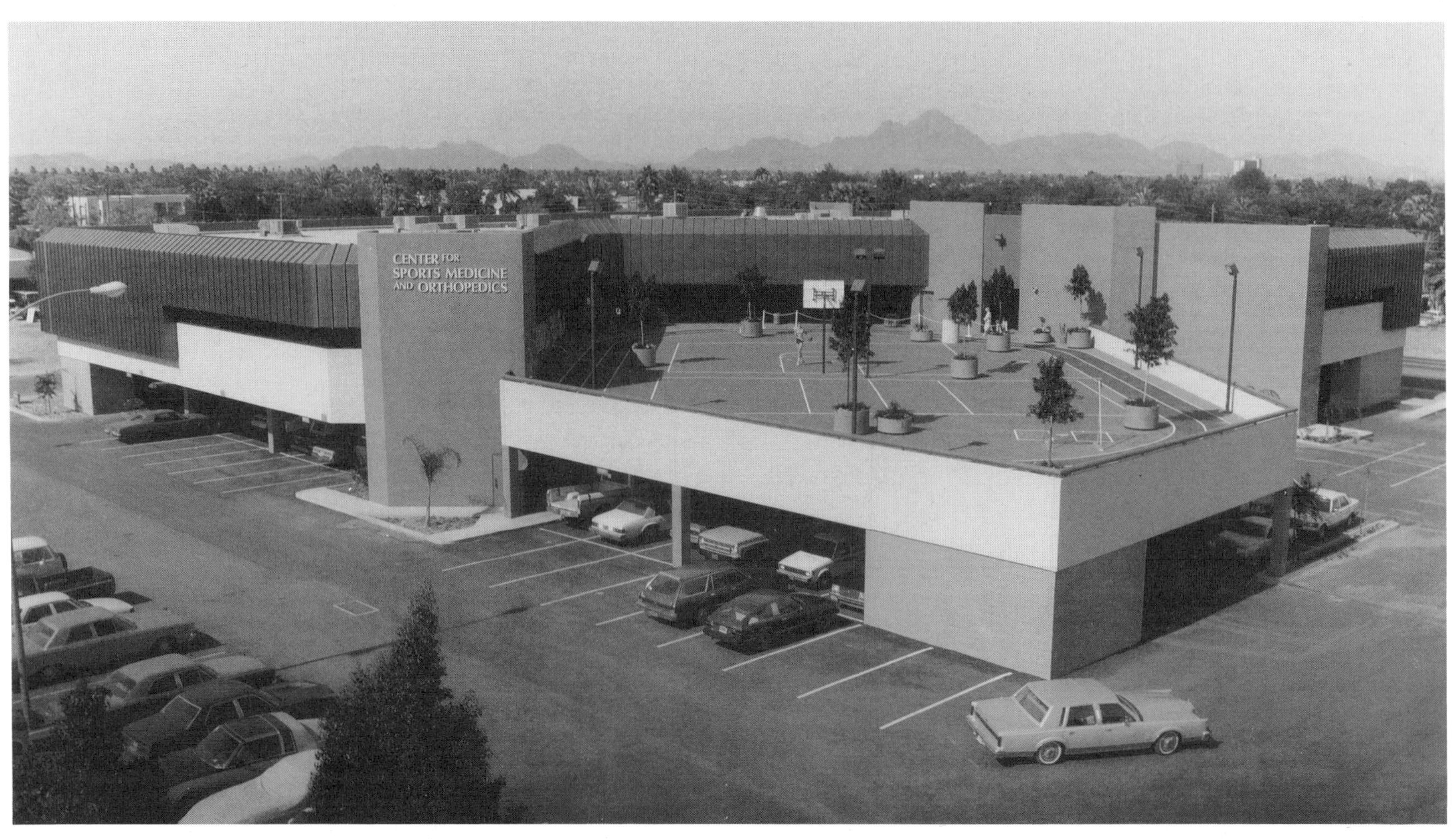

Figure 8-11. Center for Sports Medicine and Orthopedics, Phoenix, AZ. (*Courtesy Devenney Associates, Ltd., Phoenix, AZ; Photographer: Michael Much.*)

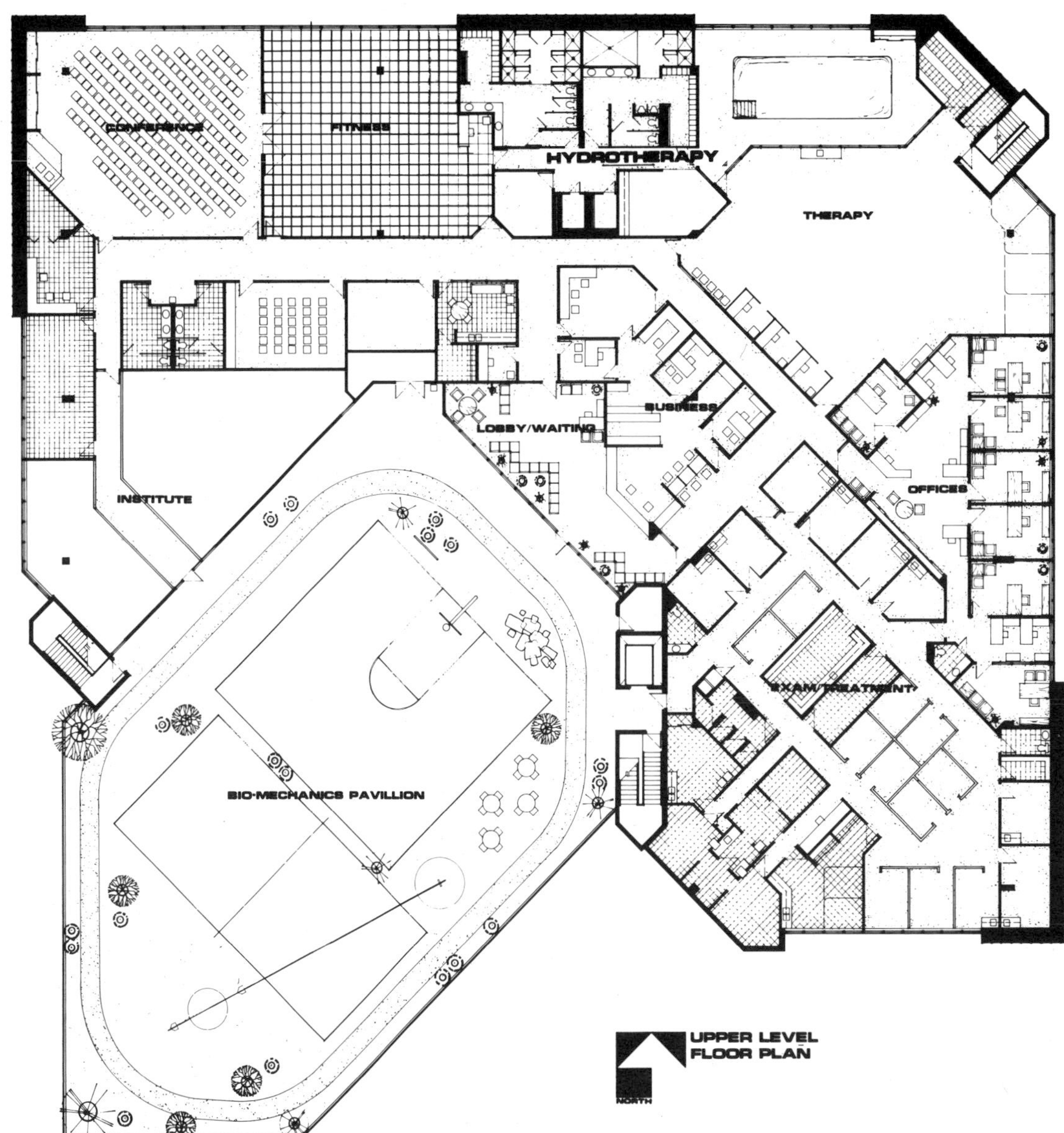

Figure 8-12. Floor plan, Center for Sports Medicine and Orthopedics, Phoenix, AZ. (*Courtesy Devenney Associates, Ltd., Phoenix, AZ.*)

The center also markets to local employers a successful work hardening program called the "Industrial Athlete." It is designed to train workers for the type of tasks they are doing and to rehabilitate injured workers quickly to get them back on the job.

The overriding concept of the facility, according to executive director Peter Altieri, is that it is a medical facility first and foremost, as opposed to a membership fitness facility. The image is tailored to a center specializing in sports medicine treatment. As a result, an ever-increasing number of patients have been attracted to the facility from beyond the local service area.

As the facility is newly built and freestanding, it was possible to express the program's concepts through the architecture, sculpting various activities around the 10,000-square-foot biomechanics pavilion.

What appears to be an open-air park (Figure 8-11) located above the covered parking area is, in fact, a sophisticated training field that allows athletes' motions to be captured on high-speed video so that experts can observe defects in technique that might lead to injuries. A basketball court, pitcher's mound, running track and volleyball court are included, each with the type of flooring material typically found in a professional setting.

The entry and reception area form the facility's center to allow direct access to all areas, similar to the previous case study (Figure 8-12). The medical treatment center, fitness gym, administrative offices, physical therapy area, lockers, and swimming pool radiate around the reception station for visual control and convenient access.

Directly beyond the fitness area is the conference center, which includes a large auditorium, classrooms, separate restroom facilities, and entrance from the parking area below.

Athletic activity is the theme of an extensive collection of artwork displayed throughout the building, including a prominent life-sized bronze sculpture of a gymnast. Interior finishes and furnishings are color-coordinated right down to the staff uniforms, to emphasize the discipline devoted to all details of the facility, reflecting consistency between the physical setting and manner of treatment. This sports medicine facility displays the design continuity that can be achieved when all objectives and goals are gathered together into one program and expressed between the client and designers as an integrated whole.

The Center for Sports Medicine: San Diego, California

The third case study is an example of a facility that has become the centerpiece of an older, well-established medical office complex. The site consists of five sizable medical office buildings, the newest of which is a 90,000-square-foot, high-profile building with glass elevators. Located on the lower or plaza level of this building, just across the street, are a regional children's hospital and a 415-bed community hospital with a tertiary program in cardiac surgery. The site is accessed by two converging freeways.

The 9500-square-foot facility includes a physical therapy program, fitness gym, aerobics room, administrative and business offices, locker rooms, an NCAA-sized lap pool and large outdoor spa (see Figure 8-1).

The physical therapy area serves patients referred by physicians in adjacent medical buildings as well as by others off-site. The fitness gym is used by physicians and staff of nearby medical offices who participate through private memberships. Some physicians offer employees memberships to the facility as an employment benefit.

This sports medicine facility was developed partly as a marketing feature to attract physicians to the medical buildings, to generate revenue for the physicians and others who own stock in the corporation, and to provide convenient treatment for patients at the same location as their physicians' offices. Design image was established as a high priority. Intricate ceramic tile designs were created for locker rooms and the path connecting the locker rooms to the pool (see Figure 8-6). Colorful soffitted ceilings, wallgraphics, and inset carpet borders were used to create an upbeat, stylish environment.

Decorative lighting is used in the reception lobby. From the lobby, all other areas of the facility are directly accessible, arranged somewhat like spokes around a hub. The locker rooms, physical therapy area, administration offices, and fitness gym are accessible without any cross traffic. The aerobics area (Figure 8-13) is open and accessible from both the gym and the physical therapy area for overflow needs as one or the other becomes more or less busy throughout the day. Occasionally, there is some interference between the aerobics use and physical therapy due to loud music being played during the aerobics sessions. Early in the programming, however, it was determined that the availability of space to physical therapy would justify the occasional periods of possible conflict in the early morning and late afternoon, when therapy activity is light. The staff report that the tradeoff has proven worthwhile.

Through a team effort of the Center's staff, the building owners, and local building officials, the designers were able to transform some rather unusual and challenging existing building conditions into assets. The resultant design was functional, flexible, and affordable, allowing the center to expand by 25 percent without remodeling existing features or suspending ongoing activities.

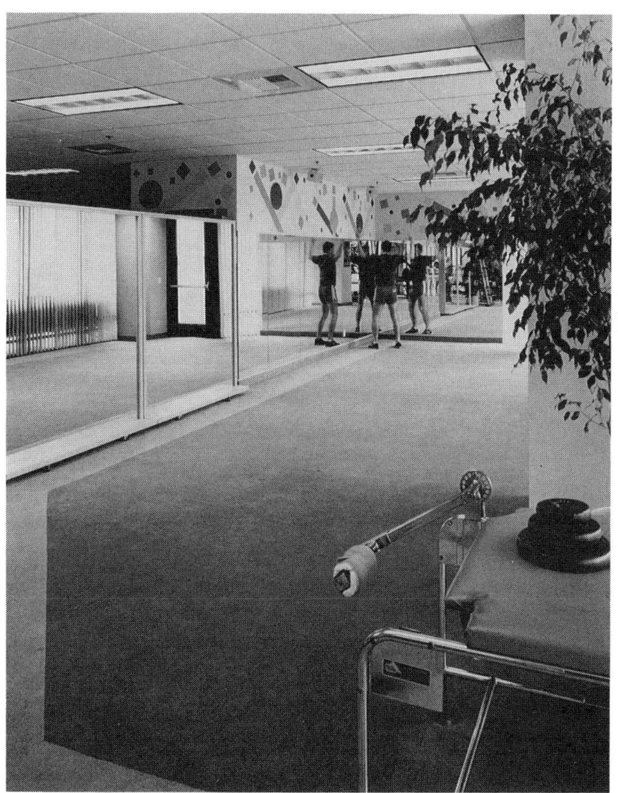

Figure 8-13. Aerobics area. (*Design: Jain Malkin Inc.; Photographer: Robinson/Ward.*)

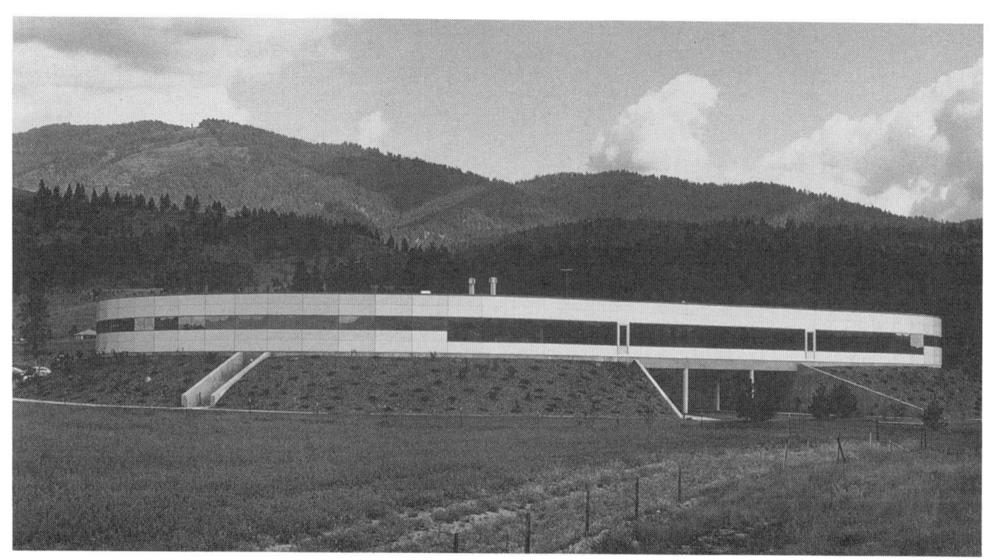

Figure 8-14. Western Montana Sports Medicine & Fitness Center, Missoula, MT. (*Courtesy William Merci; Kessler, Merci and Associates, Chicago, IL; Photographer: Gregg Merci.*)

Western Montana Sports Medicine & Fitness Center: Missoula, Montana

Appearing to grow out of the earth, nestled in the mountains (Figure 8-14), this $4.6 million high-tech facility has a three-fold mission. It functions as a health club, a physical therapy clinic for the rehabilitation of sports injuries, and it supplies certified athletic trainers, on contract, to local schools and recreational sports teams.

The facility markets corporate memberships to employers as a perk for employees. A new Cardiac Phase III and Phase IV rehabilitation program addresses the large senior citizen population the Center serves. Administrator Pamela R. Scharbauer states that physician referral accounts for 70 percent of its physical therapy business.

Owned by a woman with a degree in pre-physical therapy services, the facility employs an exercise physiologist as well as physical therapists and certified trainers. The indoor competition-sized track (Figure 8-15) was an important component of the design program, biomechanically designed to reduce the runner's potential for injury and to increase speed by as much as 3 percent. Windows offer runners a panoramic view of the valley. The 1500-square-foot physical therapy area includes a separate hydrotherapy room (Figure 8-16). Large locker rooms (see Figure 8-4), a fitness gym, basketball court, pool, spa, snack bar/lounge (Color Plate 22, Figure 8-17), pro shop, conference room, classrooms, and administrative offices are arranged with great care in a layout that is both functional

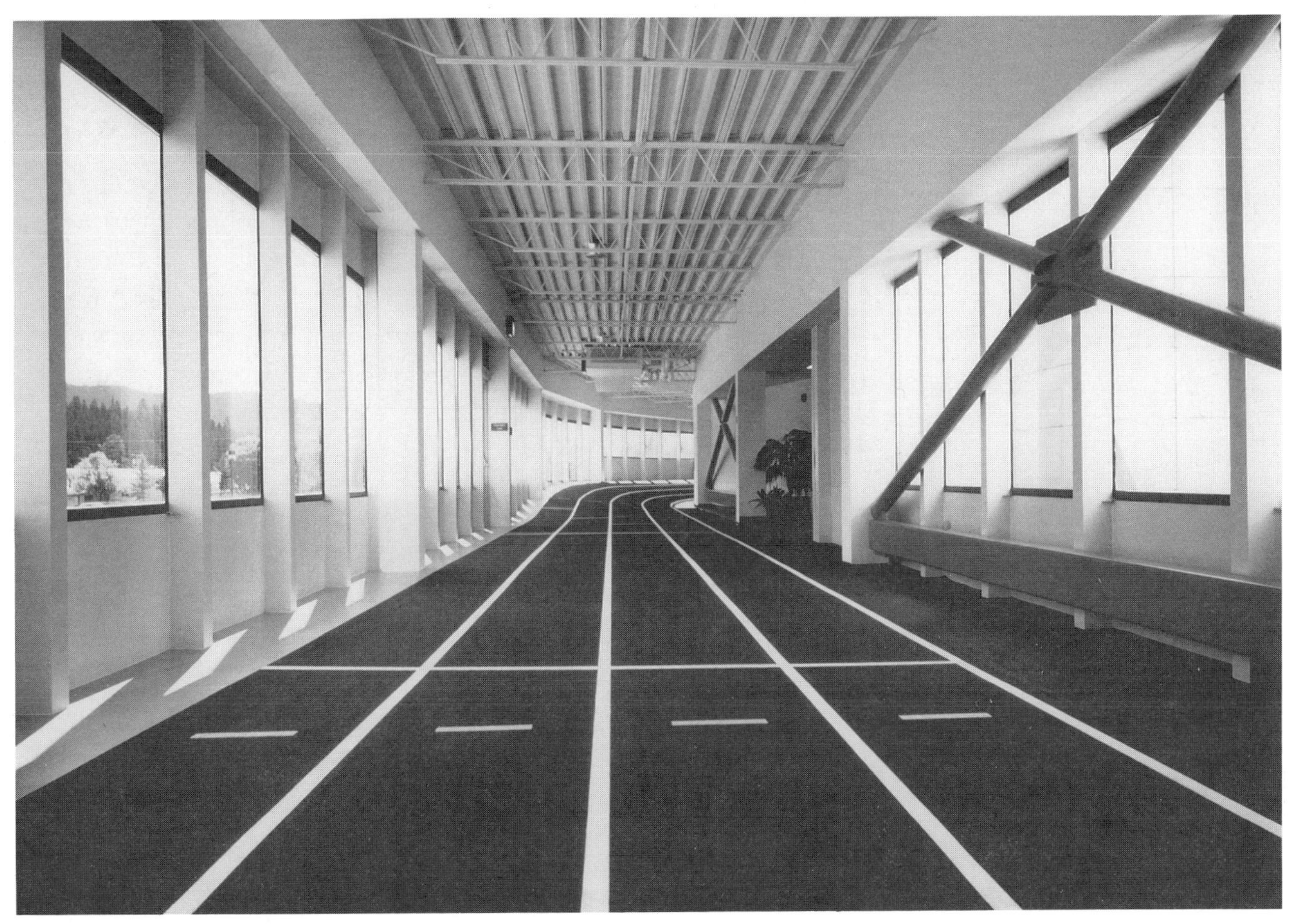

Figure 8-15. Indoor track, biomechanically designed to reduce runner's potential for injury and to increase speed. Windows offer panoramic view of valley. (*Courtesy Pamela Scharbauer, Missoula, MT; Photographer: R. Mark Bryant.*)

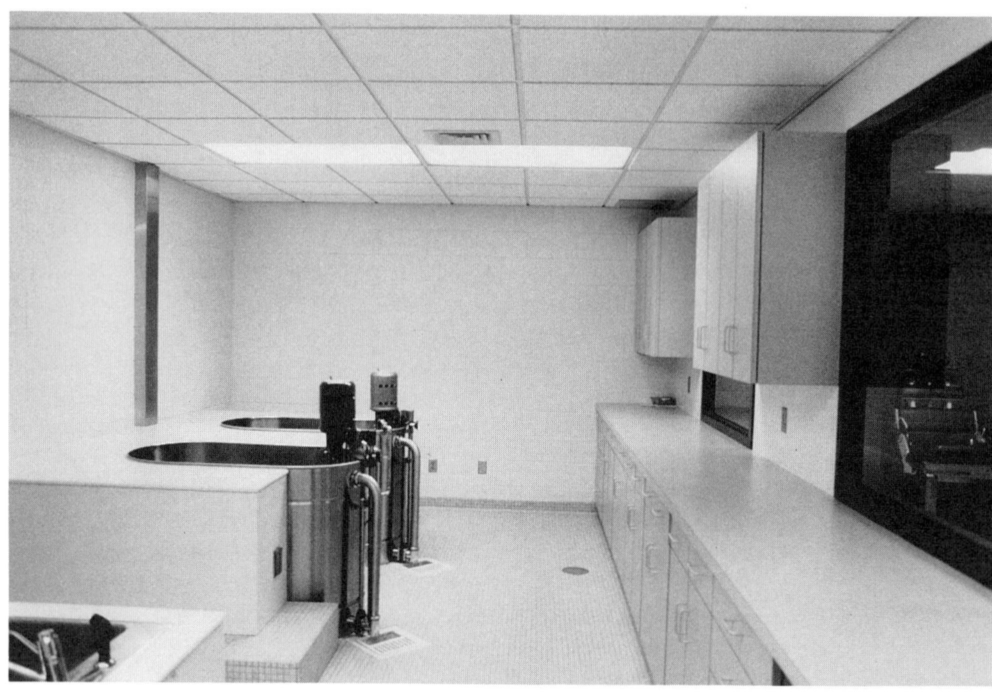

Figure 8-16. Hydrotherapy room. Note that whirlpools have been built in. (*Courtesy William Merci; Kessler, Merci and Associates, Chicago, IL; Photographer: Gregg Merci.*)

and aesthetically appealing (Figures 8-18, 8-19, and 8-20). Architecturally, this facility merits high marks for its high-tech design and careful detailing not often found in facilities of this type. It is easy to see why it was named a "Facility of Merit" by *Athletic Business* in 1987.

One of the innovations of the design involves the mechanical system which integrates, through a highly sophisticated computer, all the HVAC components of the building in order to achieve energy conservation. The pool, for example, serves as a heat dump for the rest of the building.

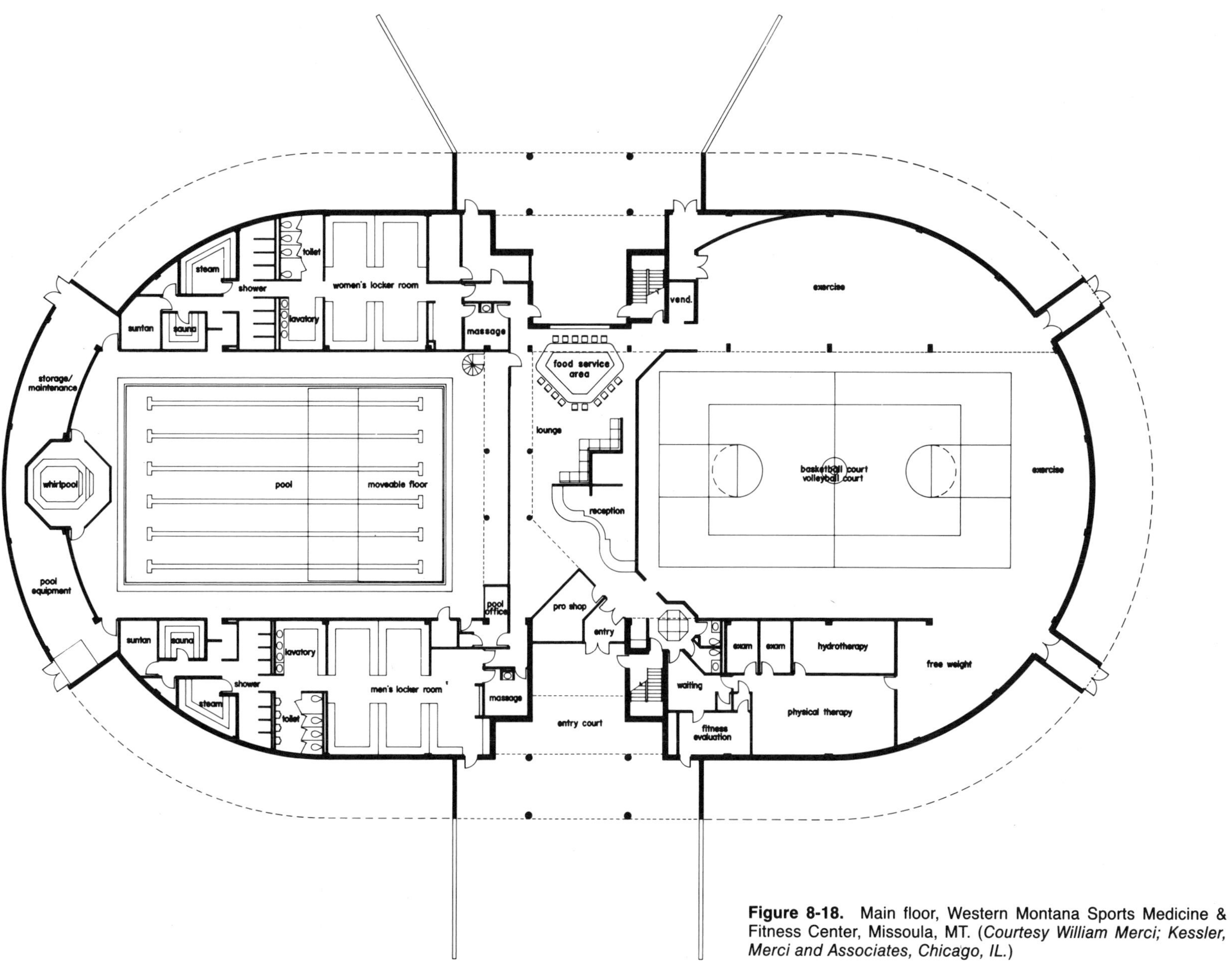

Figure 8-18. Main floor, Western Montana Sports Medicine & Fitness Center, Missoula, MT. (*Courtesy William Merci; Kessler, Merci and Associates, Chicago, IL.*)

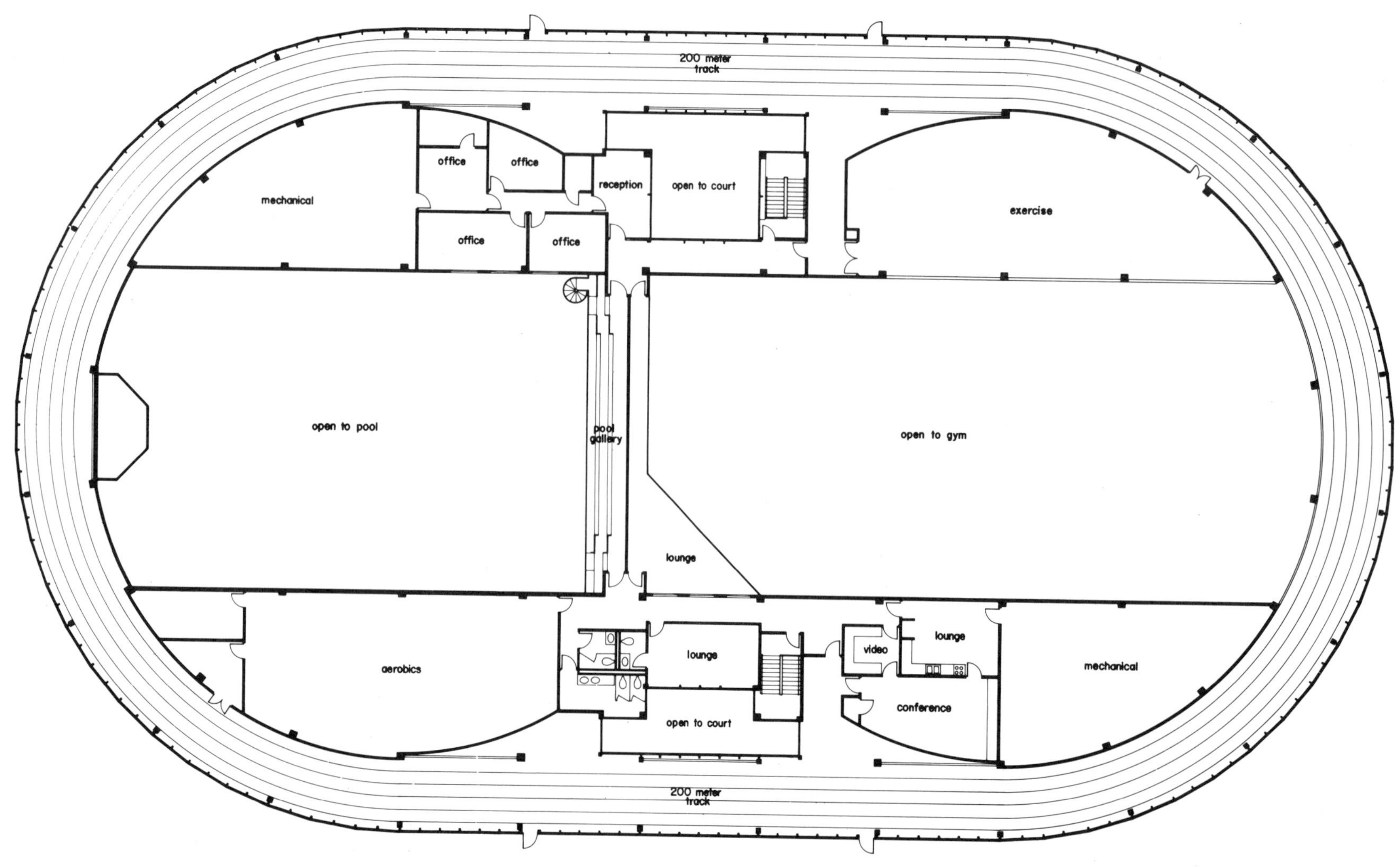

Figure 8-19. Second floor, Western Montana Sports Medicine & Fitness Center, Missoula, MT. (*Courtesy William Merci; Kessler, Merci and Associates, Chicago IL.*)

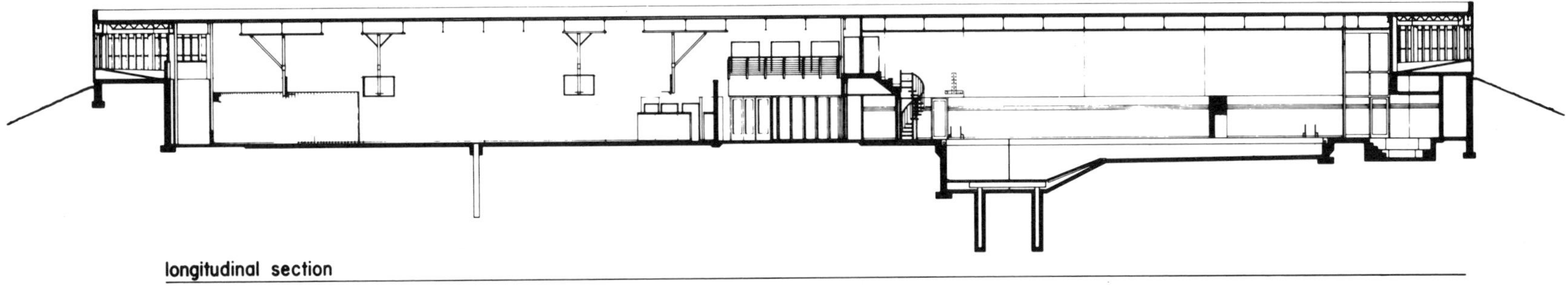

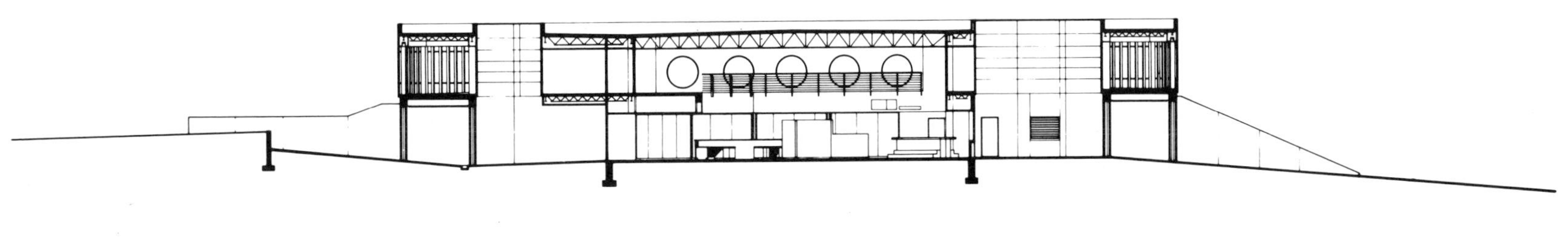

Figure 8-20. Sections through building, Western Montana Sports Medicine & Fitness Center, Missoula, MT. (*Courtesy William Merci; Kessler, Merci and Associates, Chicago, IL.*)

CHAPTER 9

Paramedical Suites

Two types of paramedical suites, physical therapy and pharmacy, will be discussed in this chapter.

PHYSICAL THERAPY

There are eleven basic methods of physical therapy:

1. Hydrotherapy
2. Heat or Cold
3. Massage
4. Exercise
5. Ultrasound
6. Traction
7. Electrical Stimulation
8. Transcutaneous Electrical Nerve Stimulation (T.E.N.S.)
9. Iontophoresis
10. Continuous Passive Motion
11. Mobilization

Hydrotherapy

Hydrotherapy involves immersion of a limb or, at times even the entire body, in water. The tank may be a portable whirlpool or a full-body Hubbard tank (Figure 9-1). The latter is more apt to be found in a hospital physical medicine department. Mobile whirlpool tanks (Figure 9-2) may be filled and drained with a hose. The patient sits in a high chair such as that shown in Figure 9-4 and swings a leg over into the whirlpool. The full-body whirlpool in Figure 9-3 requires permanent water and waste connections. Since large amounts of hot water release a lot of steam, the walls of rooms with large tanks should have at least a five-foot high ceramic tile wainscot with commercial vinyl wallcovering above. The preferable flooring material is ceramic tile, or else commercial quality sheet vinyl.

Occasionally physical therapy suites have built-in whirlpools, but most will have a couple of small portable tanks suitable for an arm or a leg. Floor sinks must be provided for portable tanks, which have to be drained and filled for each patient. A hose connection to a nearby tap may suffice for filling the tank. Whirlpool rooms or enclosures are usually 5 × 8 feet in size and may be closed off on the open side by a cubicle drape.

There are several ways of designing the hydrotherapy area.

1. A large hydrotherapy room can be designed to accommodate several portable whirlpools, plus the Hydrocollator* units (steam packs), the cold pack unit, and ice machine.
2. Individual privacy cubicles can be created as in Figure 9-11, each having a sloped ceramic tile floor

*Hydrocollator is a registered trademark of Chattanooga Corp.

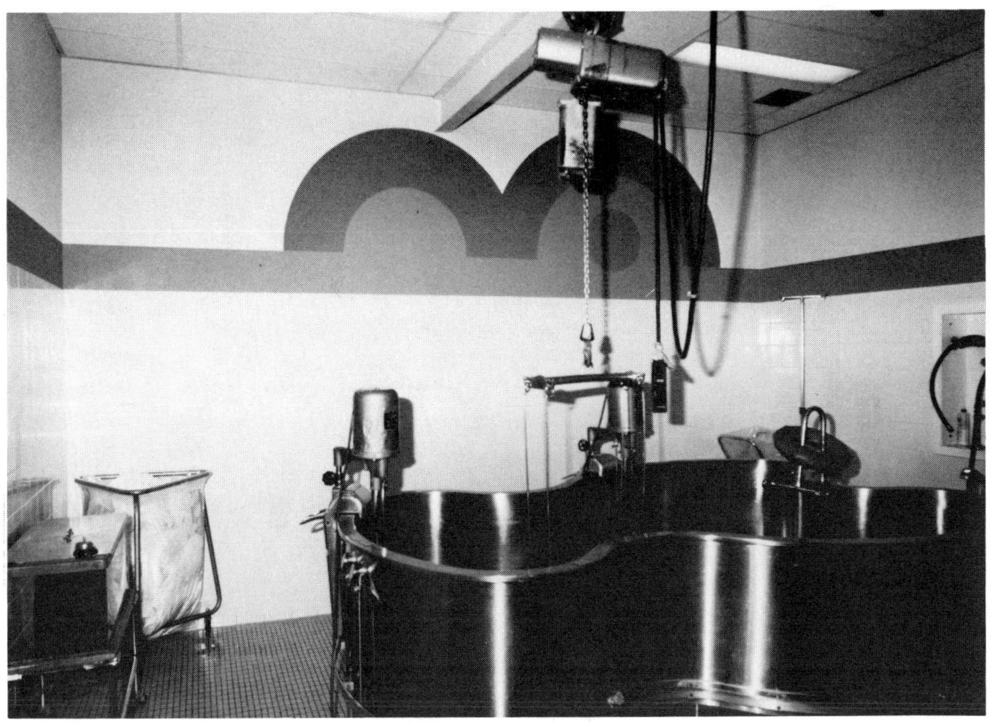

Figure 9-1. Full-body immersion hydrotherapy tank. (*Courtesy Jain Malkin Inc.*)

Table 9-1. Analysis of Program. Physical Therapy

Gym	15 × 27 =	405
Whirlpool Rooms	3 @ 5 × 8 =	120
Nurse Station	6 × 9 =	54
Treatment Rooms	5 @ 6 × 8 =	240
Waiting Room	14 × 16 =	224
Business Office	10 × 16 =	160
Toilet	6 × 8 =	48
Laundry	11 × 12 =	132
Private Office	11 × 12 =	132
Storage	6 × 8 =	48
Subtotal		1563 ft^2
15% Circulation		235
Total		1798 ft^2

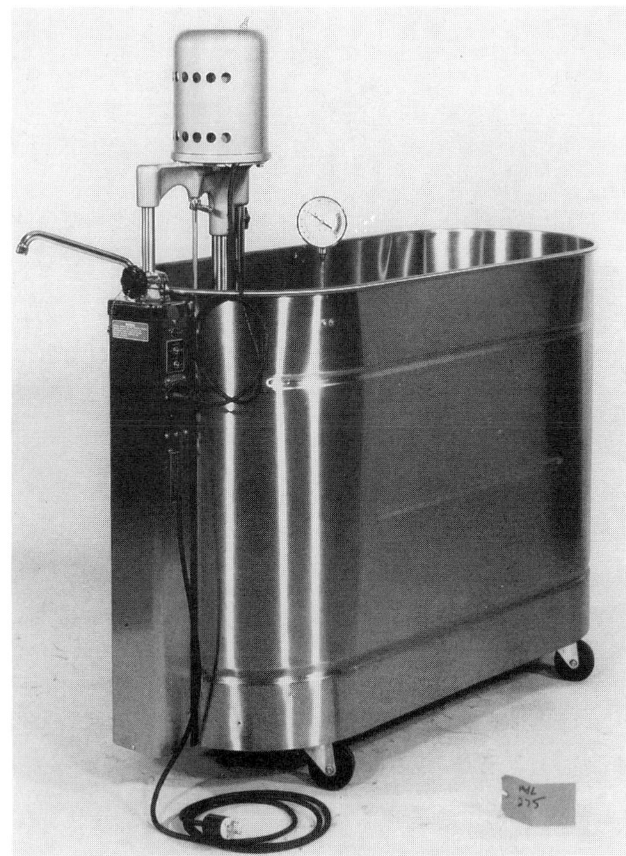

Figure 9-2. Mobile arm, foot, and knee whirlpool. (*Courtesy Ferno Ille, Wilmington, OH.*)

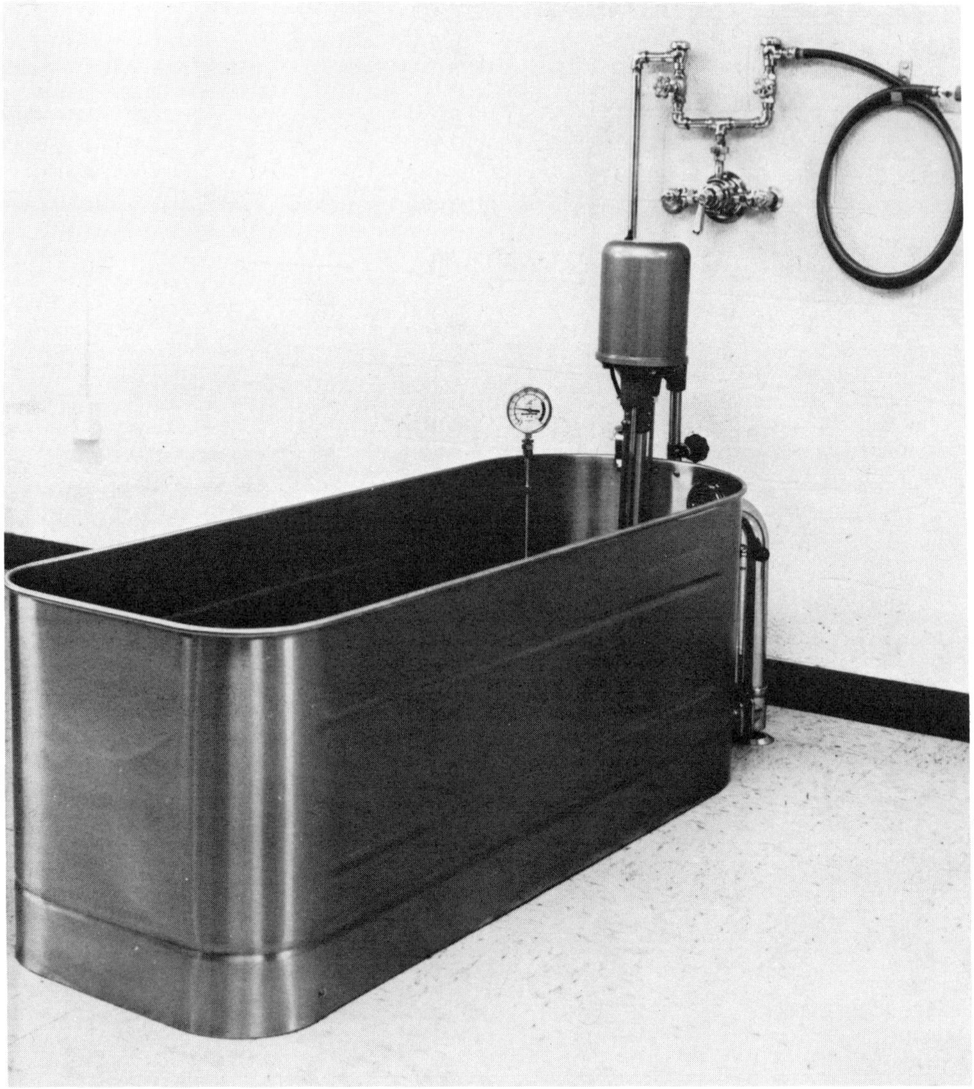

Figure 9-3. Full-body stationary whirlpool. (*Courtesy Ferno Ille, Wilmington, OH.*)

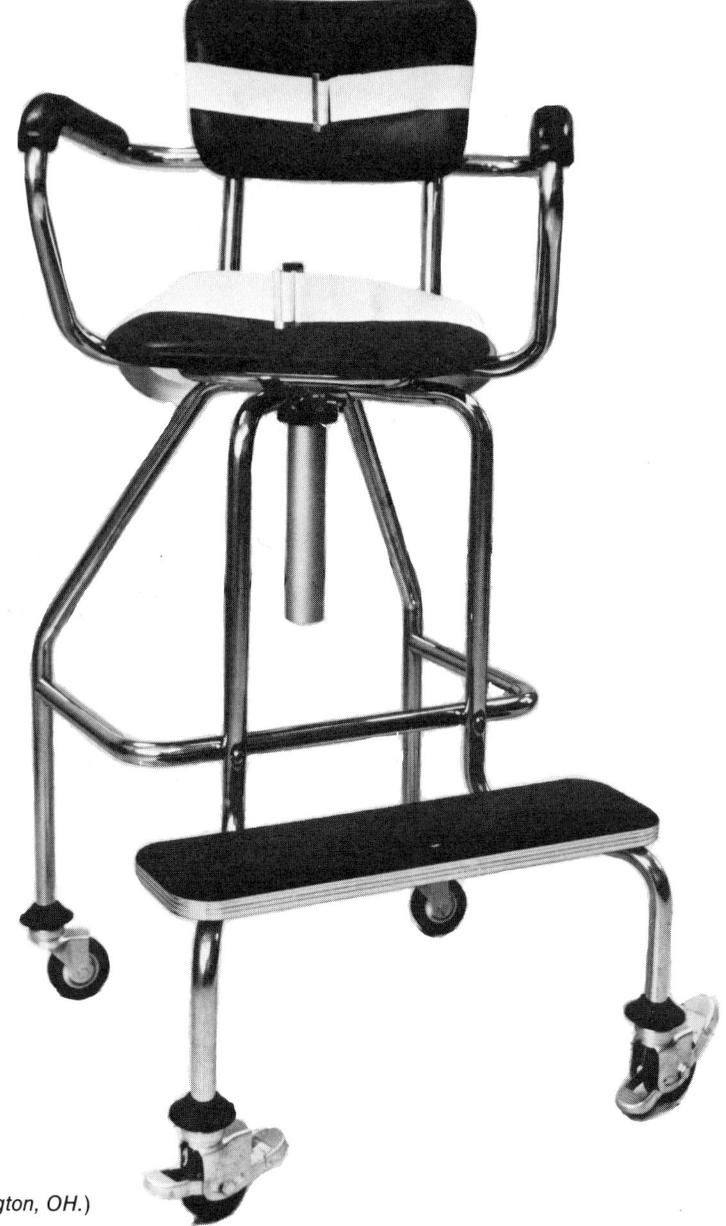

Figure 9-4. Mobile adjustable high chair. (*Courtesy Ferno Ille, Wilmington, OH.*)

with drain and plumbed for hot and cold water to fill the mobile whirlpool tank.

3. Fiberglas or stainless steel mobile whirlpool tanks may be enclosed to appear built-in as in Figure 8-16. This may be done either in the large open room or the individual privacy cubicles.

If whirlpool tanks are put in privacy cubicles, walls of these enclosures should have a 3- or 4-foot-high wainscot of ceramic tile, and the wall above the tile must have a waterproof enamel finish or commercial vinyl wallcovering.

Heat or Cold

Heat is produced by a variety of methods from a simple electric heating pad to hot steam packs, to soaking the affected part of the body in hot water. Figure 9-6 shows two models of heating units. The unit must be filled with water by a hose from a nearby faucet. It plugs into a standard 120-volt AC grounded outlet. Figure 9-7 shows what the steam packs look like, and Figure 9-8 shows optional terrycloth covers for wrapping the steam packs. If these covers are not used, the steam packs must be wrapped in several layers of terrycloth towels.

A good deal of laundry is generated here. Suitable storage must be provided for clean linen, a large hamper for soiled linen, and a drying rack in a ventilated louver-door closet for drying wet towels until the linen service picks them up.

Cold is normally produced by cold packs or ice, which are applied to the affected part of the body. Figure 9-9 shows various sizes of chilling units. Figure 9-10 shows what the cold packs look like. These units have the same electrical requirements as the steam pack units. Both the cold pack and steam pack units may be positioned immediately adjacent to built-in cabinetry in order to provide a large countertop area for wrapping steam packs. The average height of these units is 33 inches.

The steam pack and cold pack units, along with an ice machine (Figure 9-10a), may be located in the hydrotherapy room with the portable whirlpools or may be located in a separate equipment room, as shown in Figure 9-11. This equipment room might also contain a storage area for small pieces of portable equipment when not in use, such as muscle stimulators, the ultrasound cart, continuous passive motion devices, and the T.E.N.S. unit.

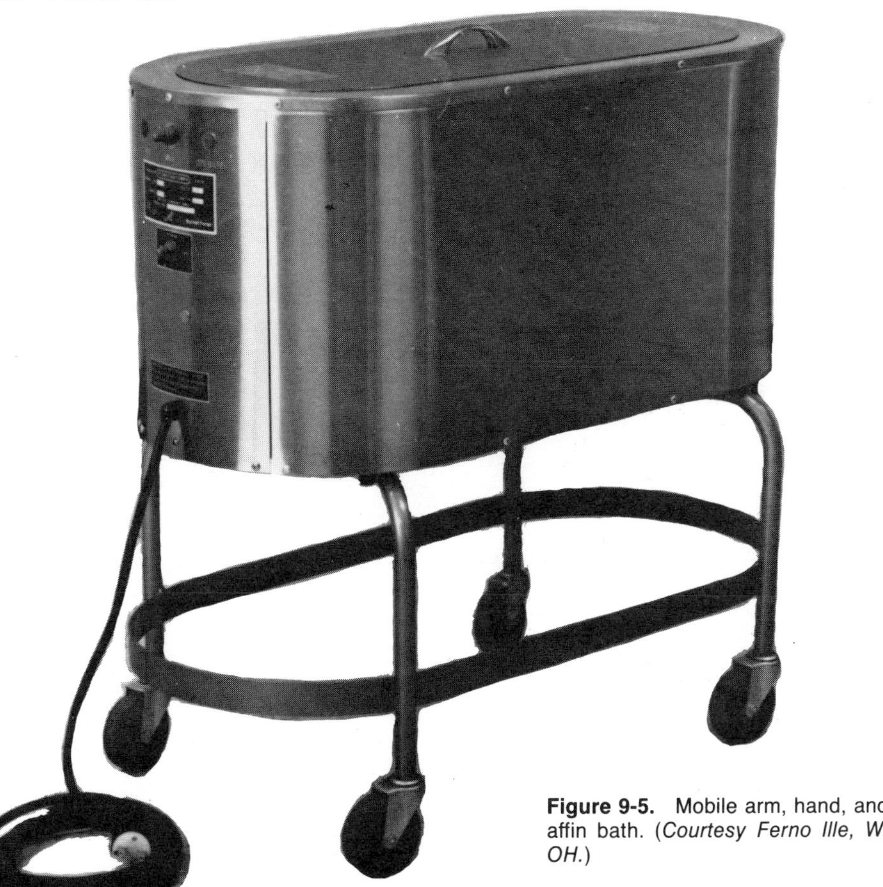

Figure 9-5. Mobile arm, hand, and foot paraffin bath. (*Courtesy Ferno Ille, Wilmington, OH.*)

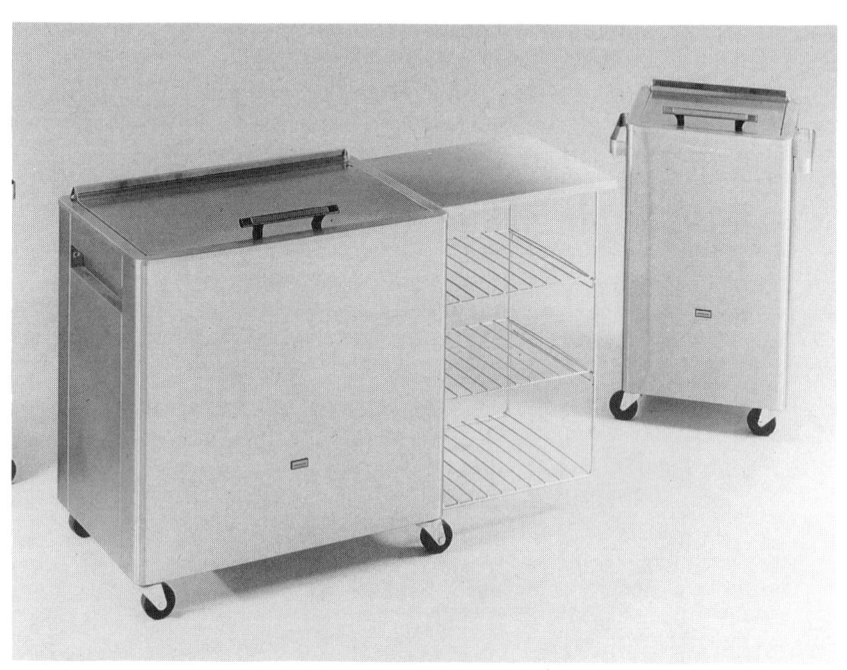

Figure 9-6. Hydrocollator® (hot pack) unit. (*Courtesy Chattanooga Corp., Chattanooga, TN.*)

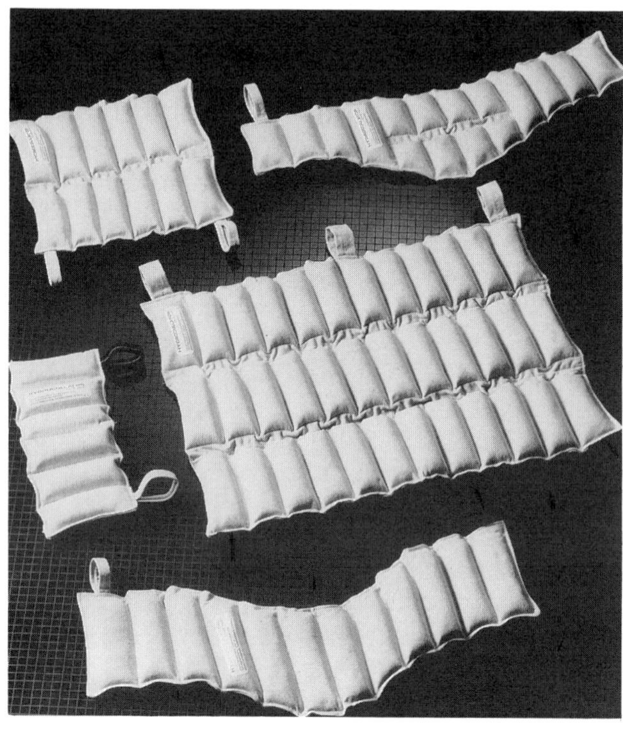

Figure 9-7. Steam packs. (*Courtesy Chattanooga Corp., Chattanooga, TN.*)

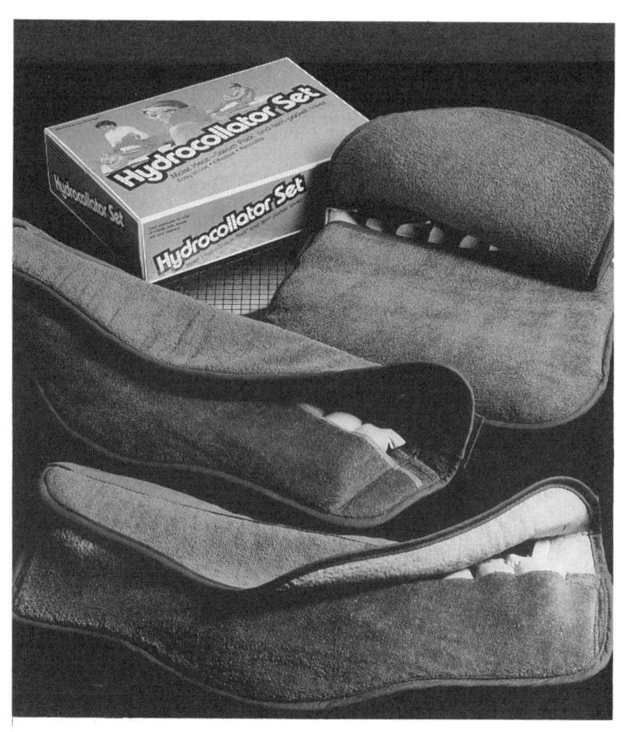

Figure 9-8. Terrycloth covers for steam packs. (*Courtesy Chattanooga Corp., Chattanooga, TN.*)

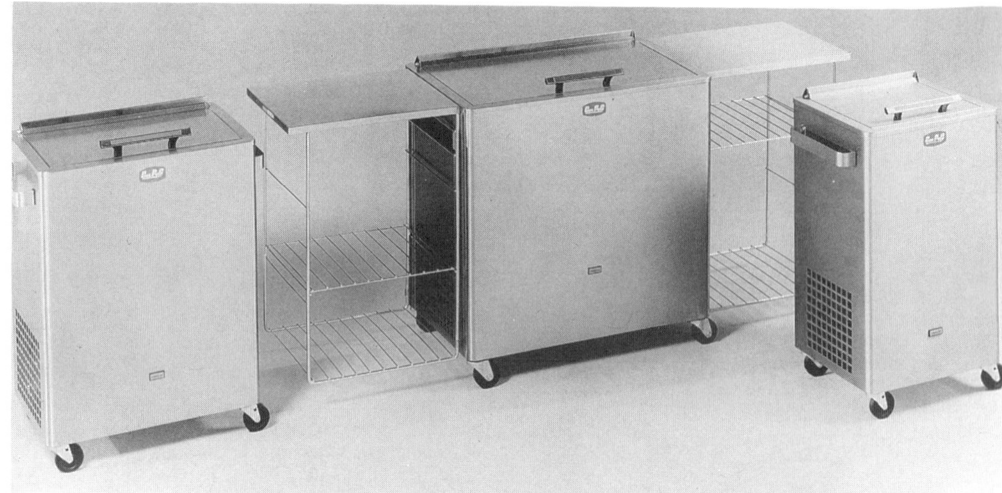

Figure 9-9. Chilling units. (*Courtesy Chattanooga Corp., Chattanooga, TN.*)

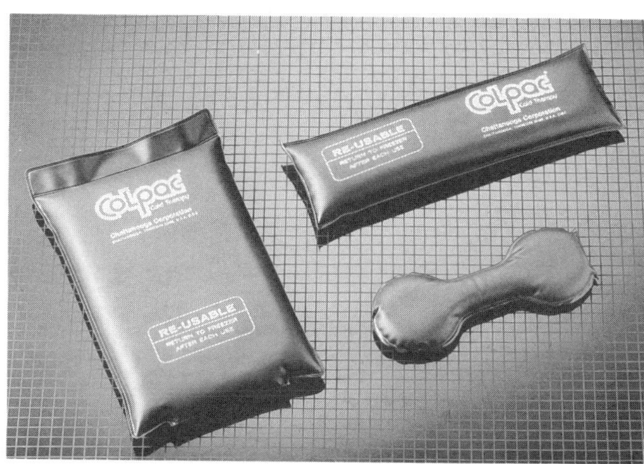

Figure 9-10. Cold packs. (*Courtesy Chattanooga Corp., Chattanooga, TN.*)

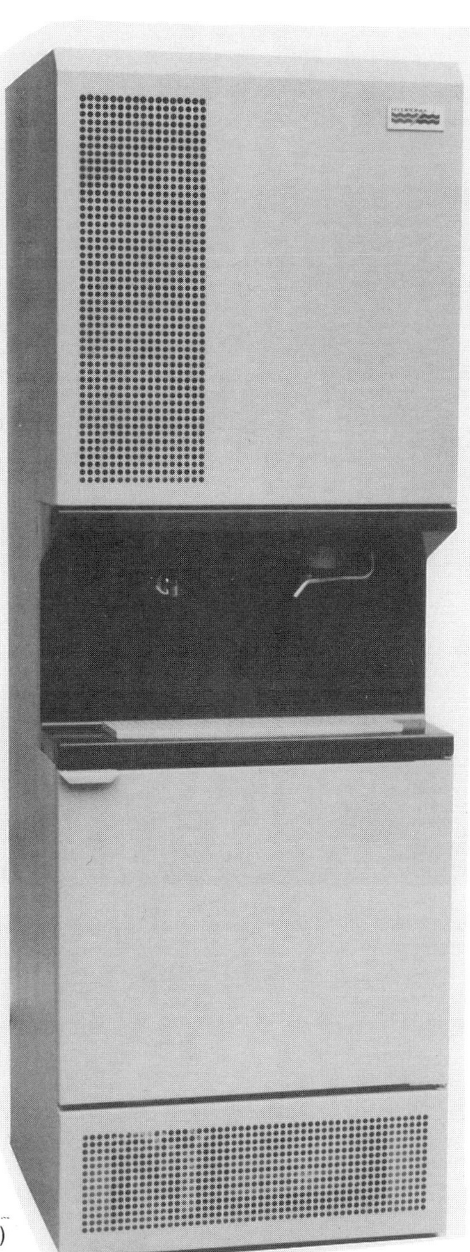

Figure 9-10a. Ice machine. (*Courtesy Ferno Ille, Wilmington, OH.*)

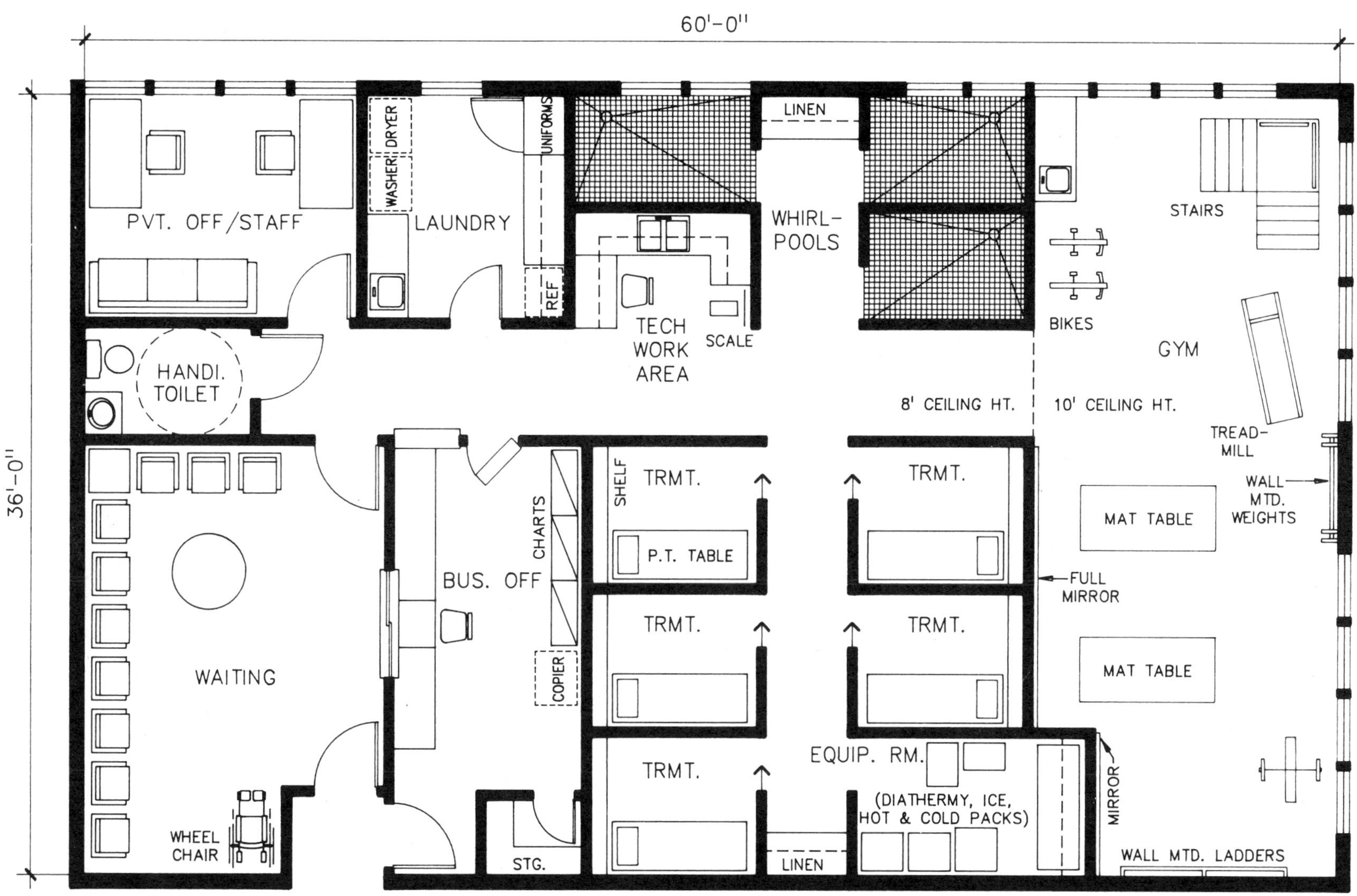

PHYSICAL THERAPY

2160 SF

Figure 9-11. Suite plan for physical therapy, 2160 square feet.

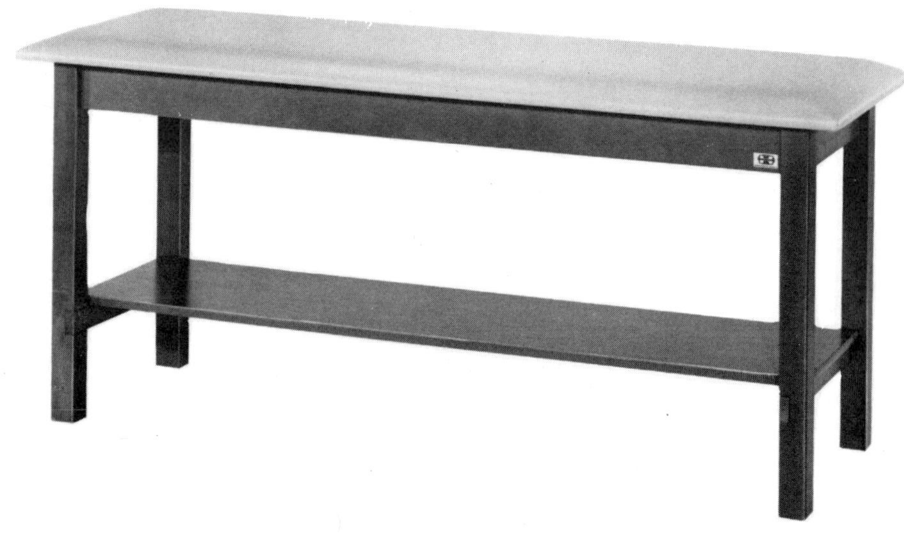

Figure 9-12. Physical therapy treatment table. (*Courtesy Hausmann Industries, Northvale, NJ.*)

Massage

Massage is the oldest form of physical therapy. It is generally performed in private cubicles, which may be constructed of standard gypsum board partitions on three sides with a ceiling-mounted cubicle drape on the fourth side (Figure 9-11), or treatment cubicles may be contained in one large room, each one separated from the others only by ceiling-mounted cubicle drapes. In either case, the treatment modules need to be approximately 6 feet wide by 8 feet long. A physical therapy treatment table (Figure 9-12) is 27 to 30 inches wide and 78 inches long. It would be placed in the center of the room. The room may also have a chair, wall mirror, hooks for a patient's clothing, and a shelf for creams and ointments that may be used during the massage. Various types of portable equipment, such as a muscle stimulator or ultrasound unit, may be wheeled into the cubicles as needed (Figure 9-13).

Subdued, indirect lighting is optimal for these rooms. One would not want to subject the patient to the glare of overhead lighting. The interior finishes and color of these rooms should be soothing and restful, not stimulating.

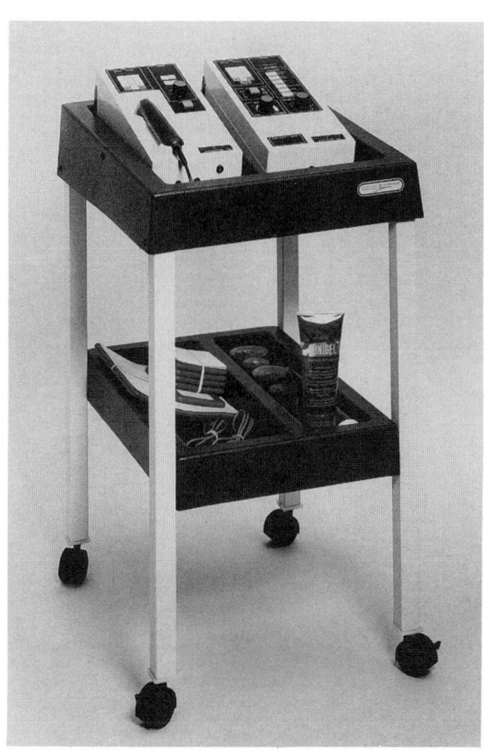

Figure 9-13. Ultrasound unit and muscle stimulator, Sonicator® 706 and Sys*Stim® 206, on mobile cart. (*Courtesy Mettler Electronics, Anaheim, CA.*)

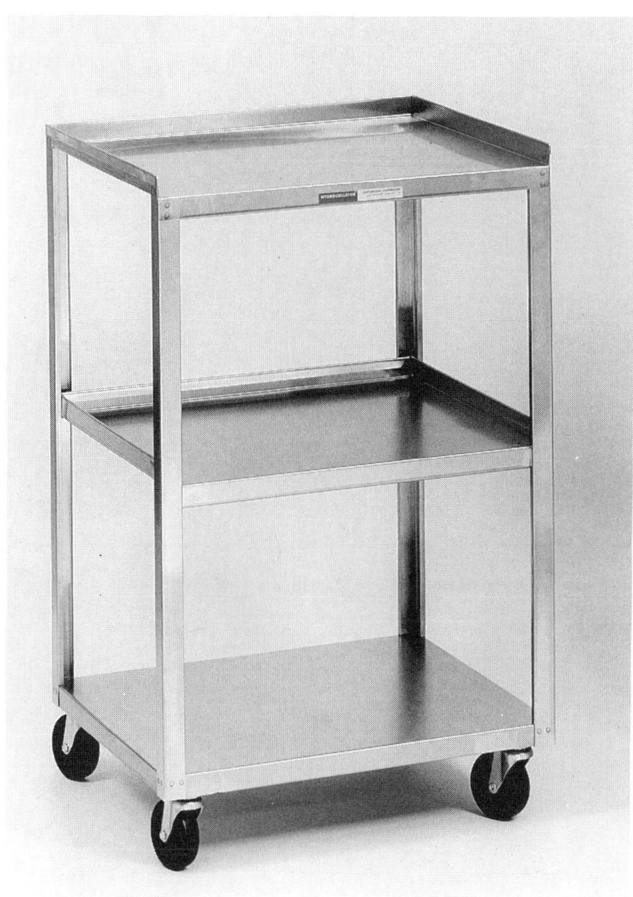

Figure 9-13a. Standard physical therapy mobile equipment cart. (*Courtesy Chattanooga Corp., Chattanooga, TN.*)

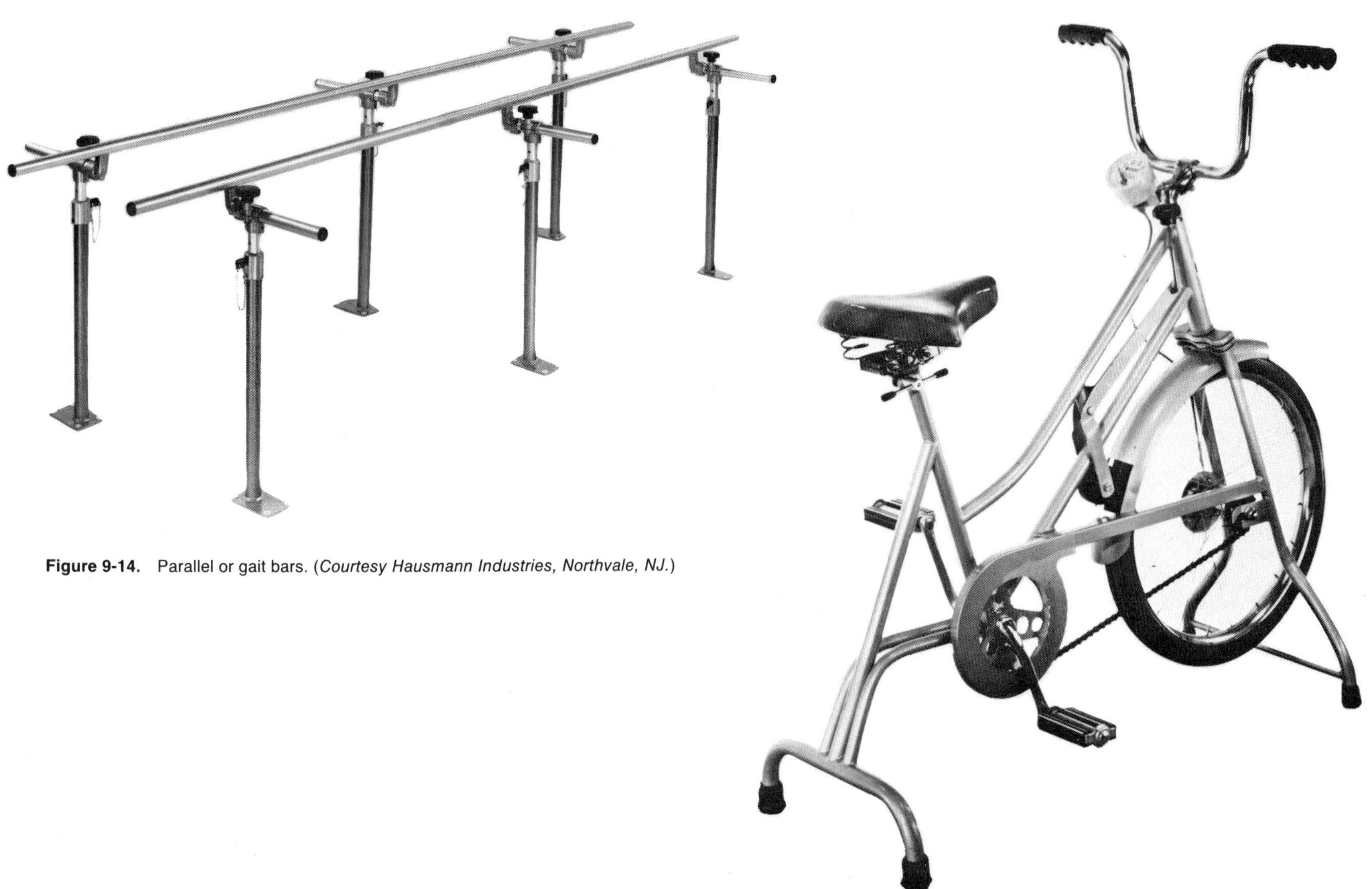

Figure 9-14. Parallel or gait bars. (*Courtesy Hausmann Industries, Northvale, NJ.*)

Figure 9-15. Exercise bike. (*Courtesy Hausman Industries, Northvale, NJ.*)

Exercise

A good deal of physical therapy involves the use of gym equipment. A large exercise room should be provided for exercise equipment, some of which is wall-mounted and some of which stands on the floor. Although windows and a nice view make exercising very pleasant, considerable wall space will be required for positioning wall-mounted equipment such as stall bars, weights, and pulleys.

The room may also have gait bars (Figure 9-14), exercise bicycles (Figure 9-15), barbells, an ambulation staircase (Figure 9-16), and a shoulder wheel (Figure 9-17), as well as other gym equipment. Wall-mounted equipment must be located before construction begins, since the walls will require plywood reinforcement to support the additional weight. The room should have a 9-foot ceiling height and large mirrors, which must be positioned so that people can see themselves using the equipment. Stylized wallgraphics of people exercising add vitality to the room (Figures 9-18 and 9-19). Color Plates 21 and 22, Figures 8-8 through 8-10, are examples of a sophisticated mural treatment. Carpet is a nice addition to the gym. Functionally, it softens the blow if weights are dropped, and, visually, it softens the geometry of the equipment. Carpet should be very dense, low pile and should be directly glued to the slab, without pad.

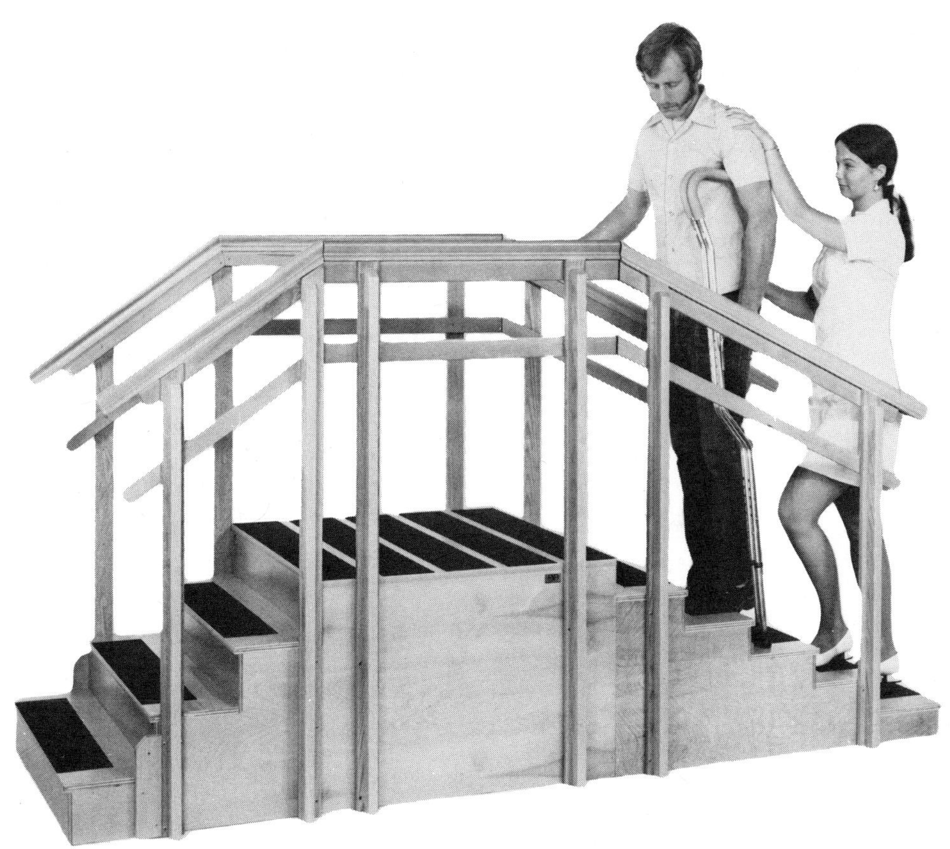

Figure 9-16. Ambulation staircase. (*Courtesy Hausmann Industries, Northvale, NJ.*)

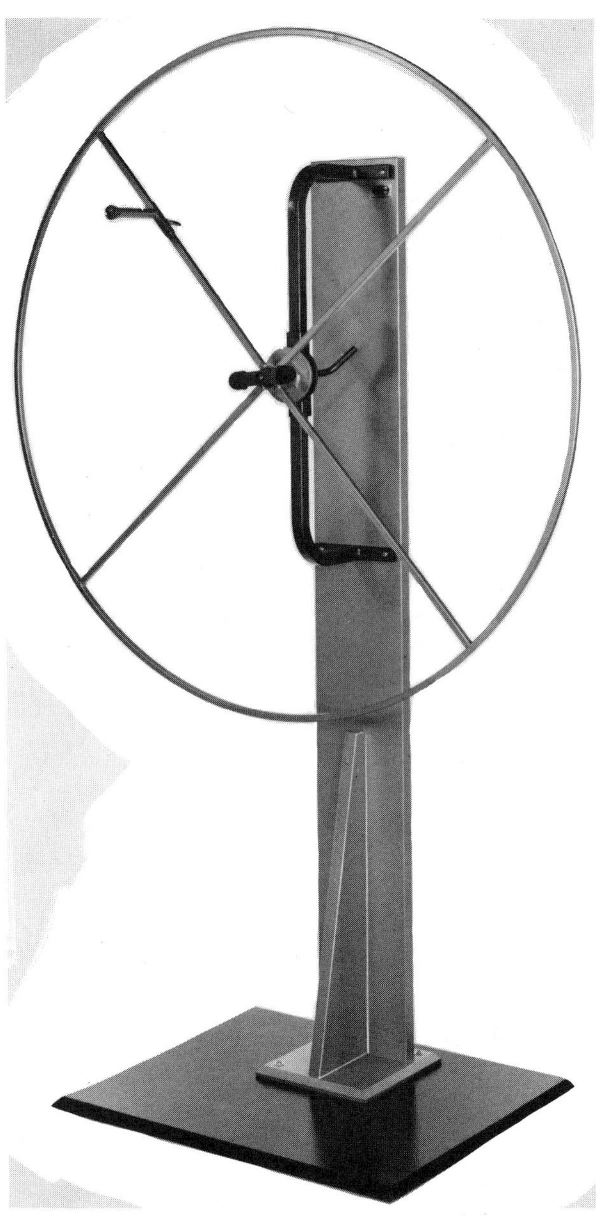

Figure 9-17. Shoulder wheel. (*Courtesy Hausmann Industries, Northvale, NJ.*)

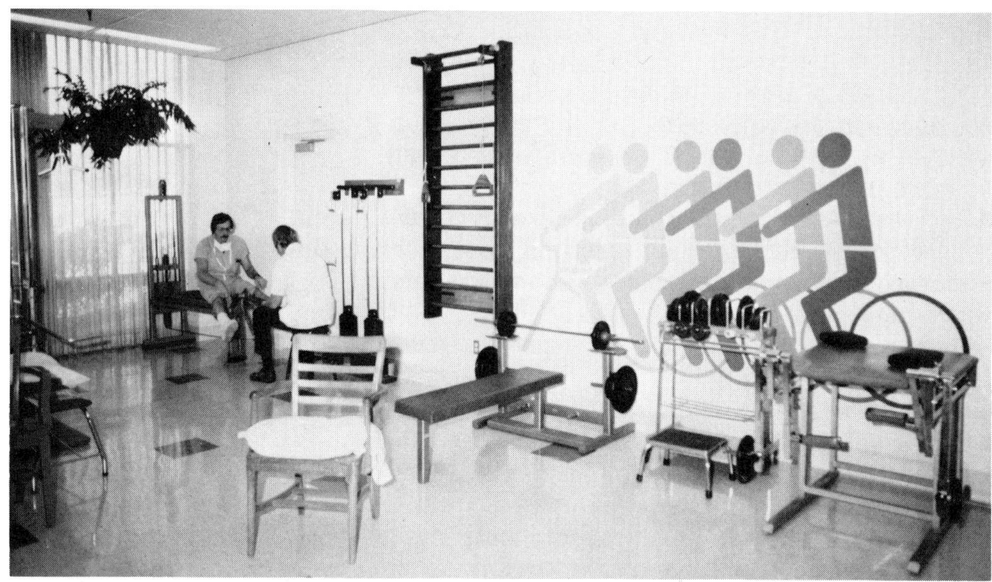

Figure 9-18. Physical therapy gym. (*Courtesy Jain Malkin Inc.*)

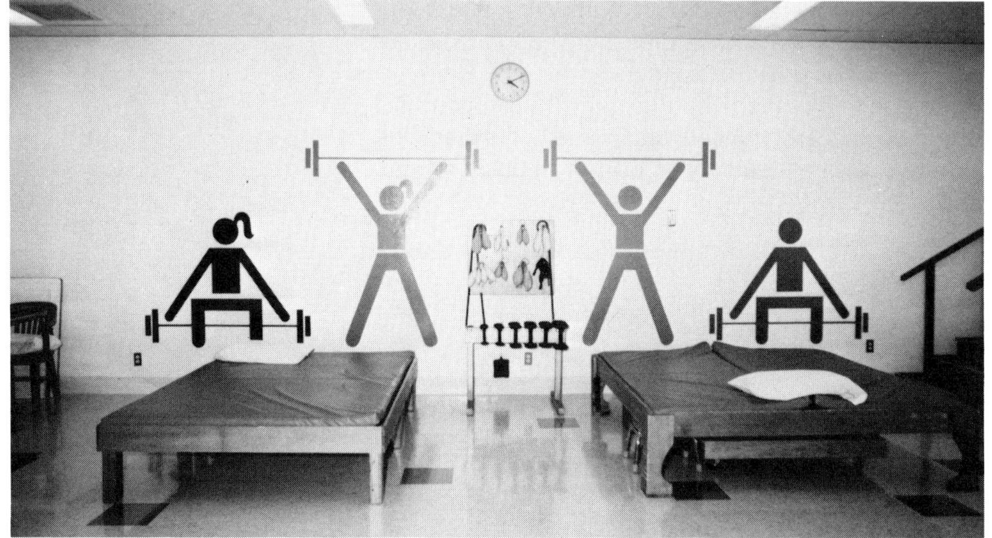

Figure 9-19. Physical therapy gym. (*Courtesy Jain Malkin Inc.*)

Ultrasound

Ultrasound involves an acoustic high-frequency vibration that is used to produce deep heat in muscle tissues. The ultrasound unit is small (see Figure 9-13) and can be wheeled on a mobile cart to a room as needed. It requires no special accommodation.

Traction

Traction can be applied to various parts of the body. The procedure removes pressure from the muscles, ligaments, and tendons of the area being treated to allow the return of proper nerve flow and blood flow through the area, as well as to promote normal joint mobility patterns. A traction table is shown in Figure 9-20. The electronic control unit is affixed to the end of the table.

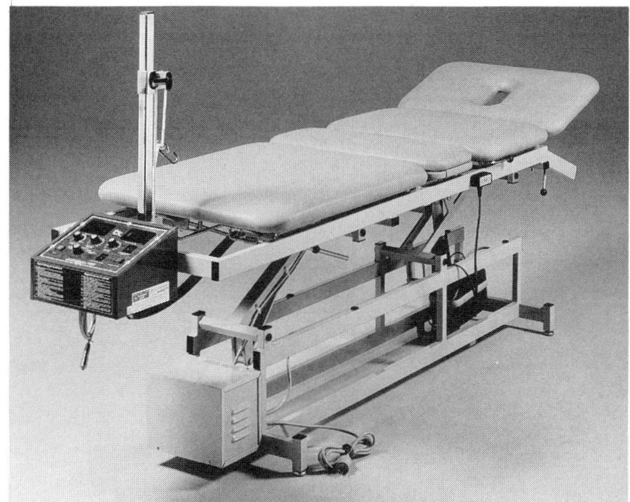

Figure 9-20. Table used for mobilization adjustments, with traction device attached. (*Courtesy Ferno Ille, Wilmington, OH.*)

Electrical Stimulation

Electrical impulses in milli-amperages are delivered into the muscles to elicit external control of the muscle. Ranges of control extend from slight muscle tension to complete and extended muscle contraction. This may be used to fatigue a muscle for treating spasm, for muscle re-education, to strengthen muscles, to stimulate debilitated muscles, and for pain management. Figure 9-13 features a neuromuscular stimulator on a mobile cart.

T.E.N.S.

Transcutaneous Electrical Nerve Stimulation is the procedure of applying controlled, low-voltage electrical impulses to the nervous system by passing electrical current through the skin via electrodes placed on the skin. T.E.N.S. therapy has been shown to interrupt or break the pain cycle, which facilitates control of spasms, inflammation, and pain. The T.E.N.S. unit is shown in Figure 9-22.

Iontophoresis

Iontophoresis is the process of driving medication topically through the skin by means of an ion transfer device. This is a small unit that may be stored in a cabinet.

Continuous Passive Motion

Continuous Passive Motion (CPM) is a technique for rehabilitating a joint or muscle group that has become inhibited, weak, tight, or otherwise injured. Figure 9-23 shows a CPM device designed for the hand. Figure 9-24 shows a CPM device that sits on a physical therapy table and is used for the lower extremities.

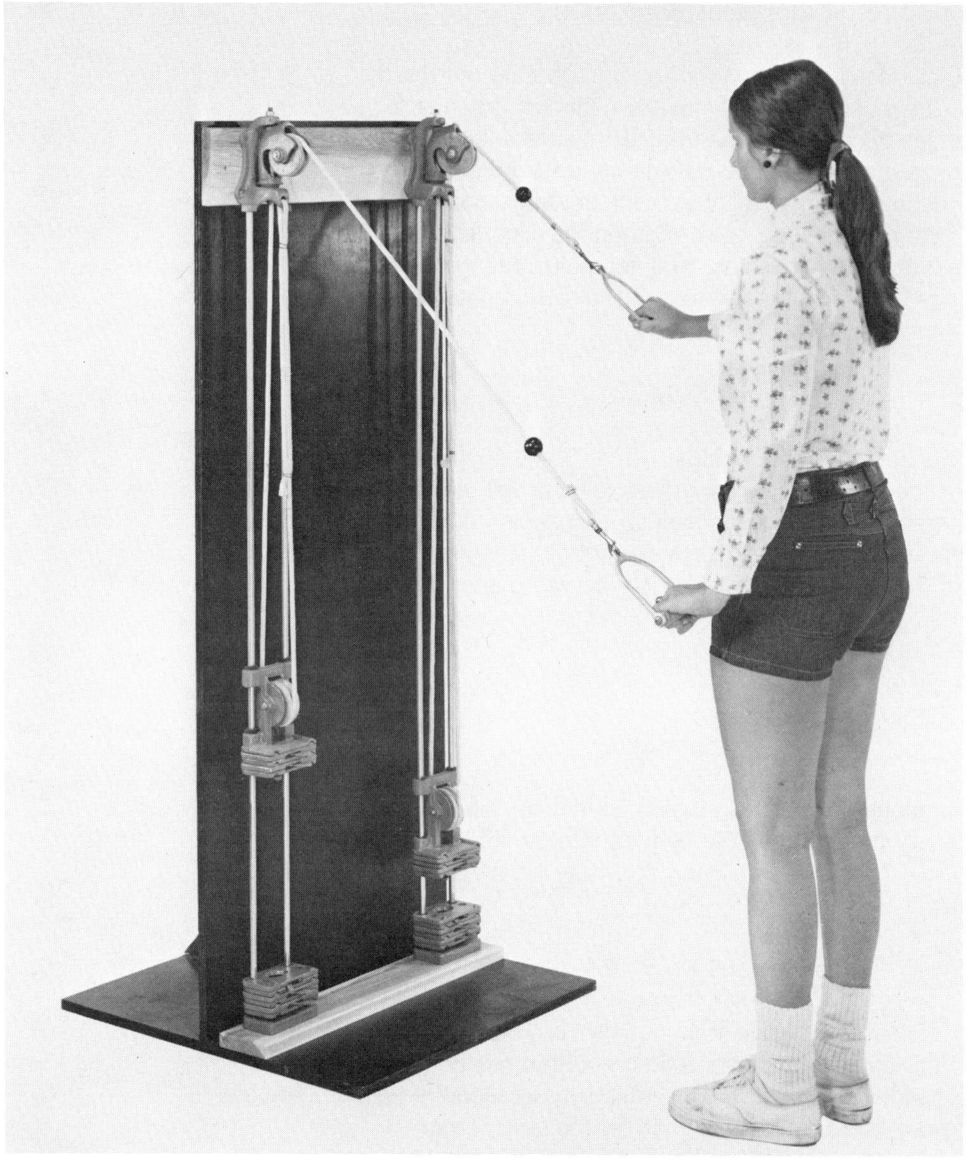

Figure 9-21. Chest pulley weights. (*Courtesy Hausmann Industries, Northvale, NJ.*)

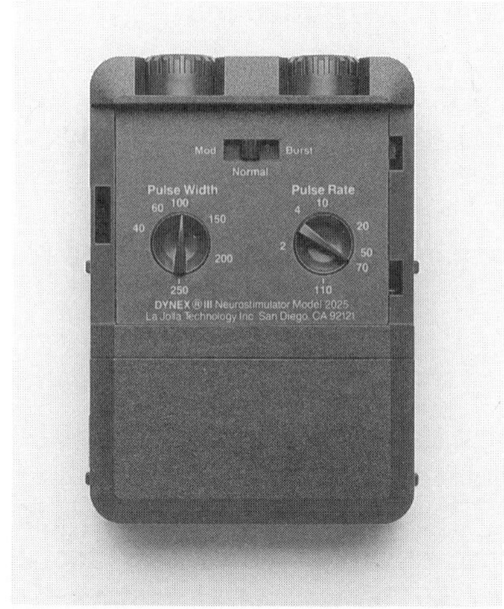

Figure 9-22. T.E.N.S. unit neurostimulator. (*Courtesy La Jolla Technology Inc., San Diego, CA.*)

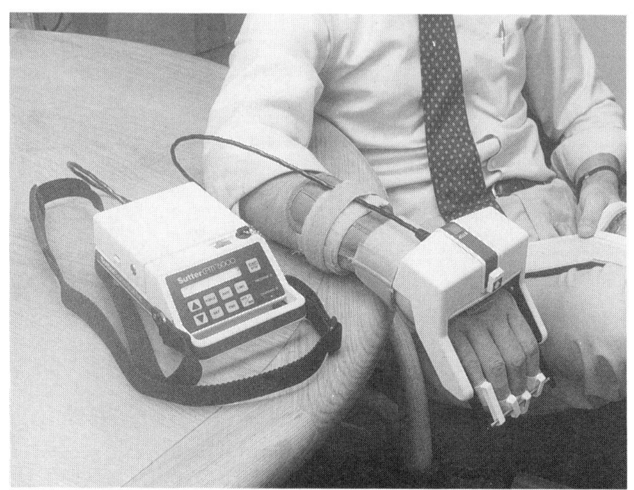

Figure 9-23. Continuous passive motion device. (*Courtesy Sutter Biomedical, Inc., San Diego, CA.*)

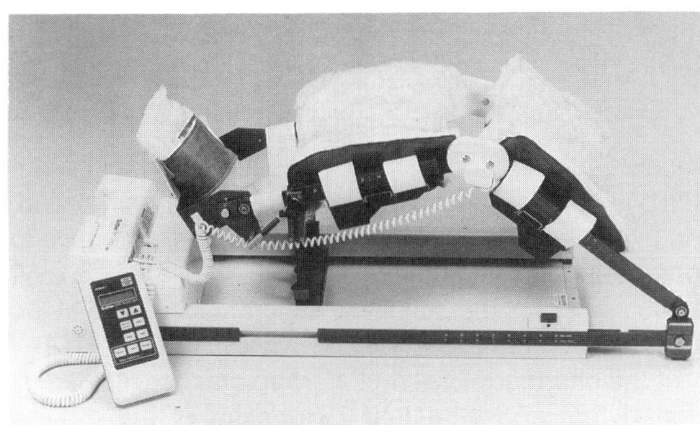

Figure 9-24. Continuous passive motion device for lower extremities. (*Courtesy Sutter Biomedical, Inc., San Diego, CA.*)

Mobilization

Mobilization is a chiropractic-type manipulative therapy that mobilizes vertebral segments and other joints of the body to realign them to proper positioning and to restore normal joint motion. These procedures are sometimes called *adjustments.* A special segmented, adjustable table is used (see Figure 9-20) for these treatments.

Other Areas

A physical therapy suite will also contain a business office, a waiting room that will accommodate a wheelchair and people on crutches, a toilet that will serve the handicapped, one or more private offices for administration, a staff lounge, perhaps a laundry room with washer and dryer, convenient storage for clean and dirty linens, and a therapists' charting station.

The charting station may be a large circular table with four or five chairs on casters for the therapists. It should be placed in the large exercise room so that therapists may keep an eye on patients while completing paperwork and also have a good view of all treatment areas.

Physical therapy treatment is such that one therapist may be treating three or four patients at once. A muscle stimulator device may be placed on one patient for 20 minutes, while a cold pack is placed on another for half an hour, and a third patient receives 10 minutes of cervical traction. There are many activities going on simultaneously, and each therapist may be working with three or more patients at any one time, making the treatment area very hectic.

A small men's and women's locker room/bathroom may be provided to facilitate patients changing into shorts prior to their treatment.

All electrical outlets must be grounded, and local codes may require ground-fault interrupters on whirlpool tanks.

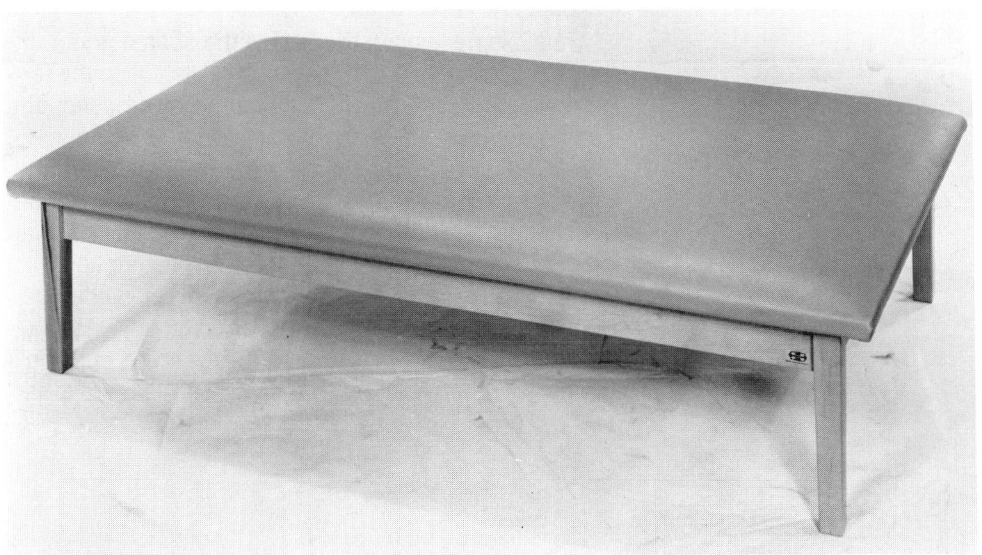

Figure 9-25. Exercise mat table. (*Courtesy Hausmann Industries, Northvale, NJ.*)

PHARMACY

This discussion will be limited to pharmacies located in medical office buildings. Since the pharmacy's primary (and in some cases, total) source of business is the tenants in the building, it is wise not to plan the pharmacy's space until the tenants and their respective specialties are known. If the medical office building is isolated and not adjacent to neighborhood foot traffic, the pharmacy's referrals will come exclusively from the medical office building. However, if the pharmacy was in business in the neighborhood before moving into the new medical building, chances are a certain amount of outside business will follow the pharmacist to the new location due to loyalty or to prior business arrangements.

Thus it is necessary to analyze the source and number of prescriptions, both new and refills. Once the tenant population is known, the volume of prescriptions can be analyzed. A general practitioner or internist will see 25 to 35 patients per day, and perhaps two-thirds of those patients will be given a prescription. Certain specialties tend to generate more prescriptions than others. When the estimated total of prescriptions (or "scripts") to be derived from the tenant population has been determined, one must speculate on what percentage of those scripts will end up at the building's pharmacy. If physicians in the building like the pharmacist, if the pharmacist provides a comfortable place for patients to wait while a prescription is being filled, and if the pharmacy is located so that patients have to pass it upon exiting the building, one may anticipate 50 to 65 percent of the building's scripts will be filled at the building's pharmacy.

If the pharmacy is part of a group practice, it is anticipated that approximately 75 percent of the group's prescriptions will be filled at its own pharmacy. If the pharmacy happens to be located in a medical complex, but it is in a separate building and the patient has to walk outdoors to reach it, perhaps less than 40 percent of the building-generated prescriptions will reach it. Some patients will remain loyal to local pharmacies near their homes or use ones that will deliver.

After the volume of prescriptions is determined, display space must be defined. If the pharmacy will sell prosthetic devices (crutches, braces, artificial limbs, colostomy supplies, etc.), a fitting room and a large storage room should be provided. Undoubtedly a certain amount of display space will be required, even in a professional pharmacy, for toothpaste, special soaps, first aid items, personal hygiene supplies, non-prescription drugs, candy and chewing gum, and perhaps a limited line of cosmetics.

One pharmacist can usually fill 50 prescriptions in a day, including compounding, packaging, and dispensing. If he or she can prepackage certain frequently used medications, scripts per day can be boosted to 70 per pharmacist. That is, certain physicians who are major sources of scripts may routinely prescribe certain medications in standard dosages. If the pharmacist knows this, he or she can, in slack periods, prepackage these items and store them on a shelf. When a patient requests them, only a label need be typed, and the script is complete.

Each pharmacist requires 4 to 5 feet of countertop work surface for compounding and another 2 to 3 feet of countertop for typing and labeling. Each workstation needs a phone. A full-size refrigerator and a built-in cabinet with a double sink should also be provided. Adjustable open shelving 8- to 10-inches deep is all that is required for storage of pharmaceuticals. Twelve lineal feet (6-feet high) of shelving is a minimum, with an additional 4 lineal feet per pharmacist.

The dispensing area often has a raised platform floor (8 inches above the display and sales area floor), a required 5-foot-high security wall separating the dispensing and sales area, a required bathroom, and a bulk storage room. Sometimes a small private office is included. The bathroom is a code requirement based upon the reasoning that the pharmacist should never have to leave the store unattended to use a public restroom. A professional pharmacy will occupy anywhere from 800 to 1200 square feet of space (Figure 9-26).

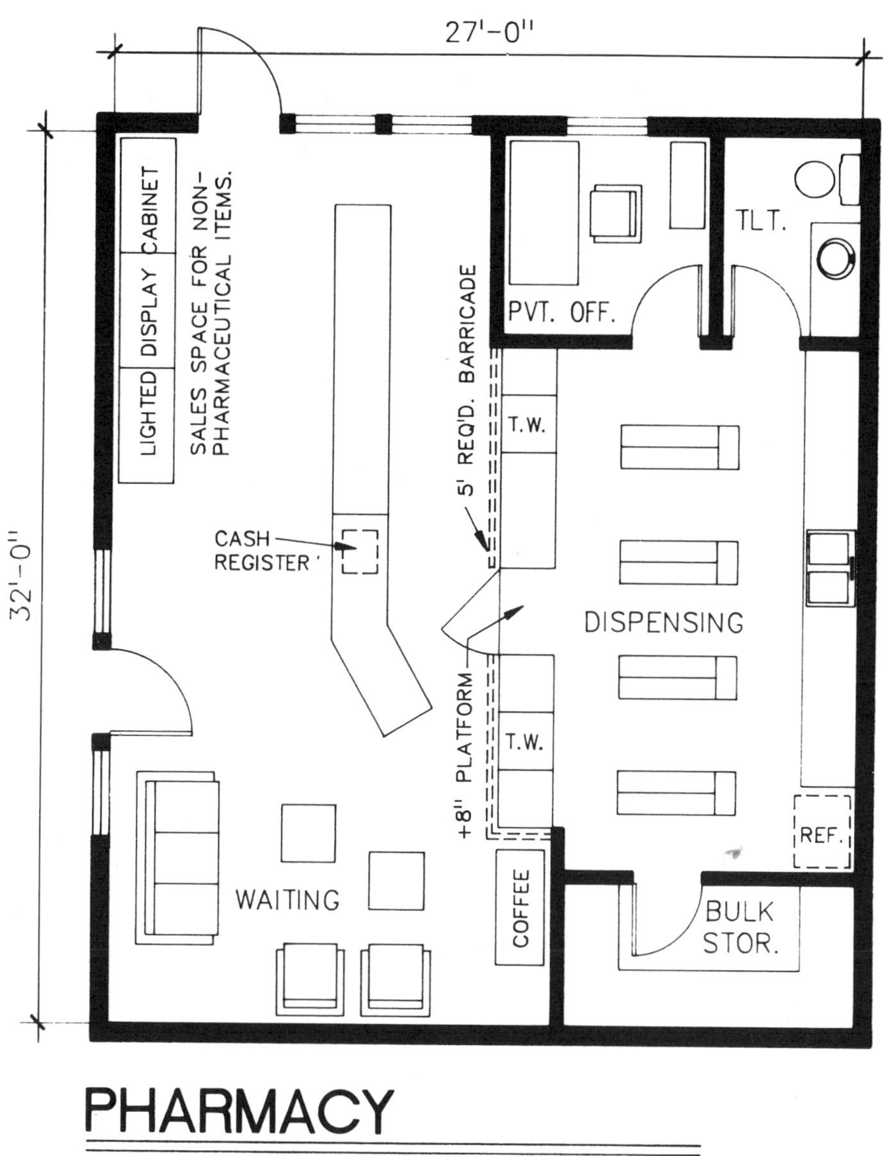

Figure 9-26. Suite plan for pharmacy, 864 square feet.

CHAPTER 10

The Practice of Dentistry

Dentists, as a group, have been well attuned to marketing and customer satisfaction. This may be due to the fact that many dental procedures are becoming elective in nature as the incidence of tooth decay and gum disease decreases, unlike medical procedures, which do not tend to be elective. In dentistry, with the exception of oral surgery, endodontics (root canal), and sometimes periodontics (gum surgery), many treatments are not done so much for curing disease and restoring health as for *quality of life.* Therefore, marketing and design tend to reflect these health and treatment trends.

Dentists were among the first to advertise, use color-coordinated uniforms, open offices in shopping malls, and attend seminars on office design, stress reduction, and the psychology of dealing with patients.

Some dentists have what is called a *values-driven practice,* in which the staff has been trained to redefine their roles. The practice philosophy of drill, fill, and bill is replaced with one of bringing wellness to patients and improving the quality of their lives. The staff is trained to listen to patients, interpret behavior, and respond positively to confrontation and problems. Employees learn pleasant telephone manners and how to discuss financial arrangements without offending patients. Dental teams are aware of their self-image. They practice time management and stress reduction, and they set goals together. A values-centered staff makes it easier for patients to accept and want fine dentistry.

Progressive dentists with finely tuned management skills are a source of many satisfying design jobs. These dentists will want both their personnel and physical plant to make people feel comfortable and confident about receiving care. In order to satisfy these dentists, the dental design specialist must be continually educated in changes in dental practice management.

Dentistry allows for highly personalized practice methods which must be set by the dentist before the space planner can begin. Some dentists moving into modern new offices will bring their outdated dental equipment with them, which might necessitate a less-than-optimal operatory layout. Others will buy sleek, state-of-the-art equipment that will allow the designer to create a most efficient operatory. This chapter will acquaint the designer with the equipment and general requirements for the evolving practices of general dentistry, pediatric dentistry, orthodontics, periodontics, oral surgery, and endodontics.

While guidelines will be given, remember that the organization of dental offices is somewhat less standardized then that of medical facilities, owing to the number of options in size and design of the operatory. The equipment, location of casework, and the preferred style of delivery of instrumentation (rear, over-the-

The author wishes to thank Stuart Isler, D.M.D., for his generous assistance in editing this chapter.

patient, or side), will determine the size and layout of the operatory.

Therefore, although there is an optimal design of an operatory, other choices will also be presented. That which is common to all dental suites will be discussed under General Dentistry. Modifications required for other dental specialties will be discussed thereafter. First, however, it is apropos to understand a phenomenon that is looming and will affect changes in dental design for years to come.

INFECTION CONTROL

1988 will be remembered as the year that the United States Occupational Safety and Health Administration (OSHA) began enforcing mandatory compliance with CDA/ADA (Centers for Disease Control/American Dental Association) asepsis control recommendations. Failure to comply results in heavy penalties. This aggressive position arose from a desire to protect dental patients and employees from the risk of contracting HIV or hepatitis B virus from one another.

People in a dental setting are exposed to a wide variety of infectious microorganisms in the blood and saliva of patients. Proper infection control procedures used in both the operatory and dental laboratory prevent cross-contamination that may affect patients, dental office staff, and dentists.

While it is true that much attention is currently focused on AIDS, the dental team is much more at risk for hepatitis B. In 1982, the Council on Dental Therapeutics adopted a resolution recommending that all dental personnel be vaccinated against this virus. As it is difficult to determine whether a patient is a carrier of one of these dangerous viruses, each patient must be considered potentially infectious, and the same infection control procedures must be repeated at all times. The dental team is expected to wear protective eyewear, masks, gloves, and sometimes, gowns, to create a protective barrier between themselves and contact with blood, saliva, debris spatter, or aerosols. Head covers are recommended during invasive procedures that are likely to result in splashing blood or other body fluids. Laundry service or in-office washer/dryers should be considered, since it is recommended that gowns or lab coats not be worn home due to the possibility of transporting microorganisms to one's children or house.

All surfaces within the operatory must be able to be thoroughly cleaned and disinfected. The design of cabinetry should be simple and easy to clean, with few crevices. Wallcoverings should be smooth, and floors should not be carpeted.

Dentists are asked to cover any surfaces that may be contaminated by blood or saliva (such as the handle of the dental light or the X-ray head) with aluminum foil or clear plastic wrap. This wrapping should be changed between every patient. Surfaces that cannot be covered or removed for cleaning and sterilization must be scrubbed and disinfected between each patient. It is anticipated that these procedures will reduce the dentist's productivity, increase the cost of doing business, and, most likely, result in higher dental fees.

Thinking of dental design in the latter part of the twentieth century, consider the effect material selection has on asepsis and, secondarily, on intra-office cross-contamination. Dental offices are increasingly becoming hospital-like in their appreciation of asepsis. Crumbs on countertops, lunches stored in the refrigerator in sterilization, and a common sterilization/lab are viewed with disfavor.

Upholstery fabrics, window coverings, wallcoverings, and flooring must be selected with asepsis in mind. The new vinyl upholstery fabrics that look and feel like fabric are advised for patient treatment areas.

Flooring in operatories may be smooth sheet vinyl, vinyl composition tile, or perhaps vinyl-coated wood. Any smooth, nonporous, easy-to-clean flooring material would be acceptable. Washable paint or vinyl wallcoverings (smooth textures) would be fine for operatory walls. Polyvinylchloride (PVC) vertical louver blinds are an easy-to-clean window treatment. The reader is referred to Chapter 12 for a more detailed discussion of finishes.

The newest dental chairs and equipment are designed with asepsis in mind. The patient chair is devoid of fabric, with seamless, easy-to-clean design (Figures 10-1, 10-2, and 10-3). High-speed evacuation (wet vacuum system), dry, oil-free compressed air system, and proper patient positioning (made easier by having the right chair) all help to control infection. Sterilization of handpieces and air/water syringe attachments is recommended between each patient. This amounts to a lot of "spare parts" for each piece of equipment in each operatory. Ample storage must be provided for disposables, and space for special waste containers must be planned in the operatory. These containers are lined with plastic bags that can be sealed before being removed from the operatory for disposal.

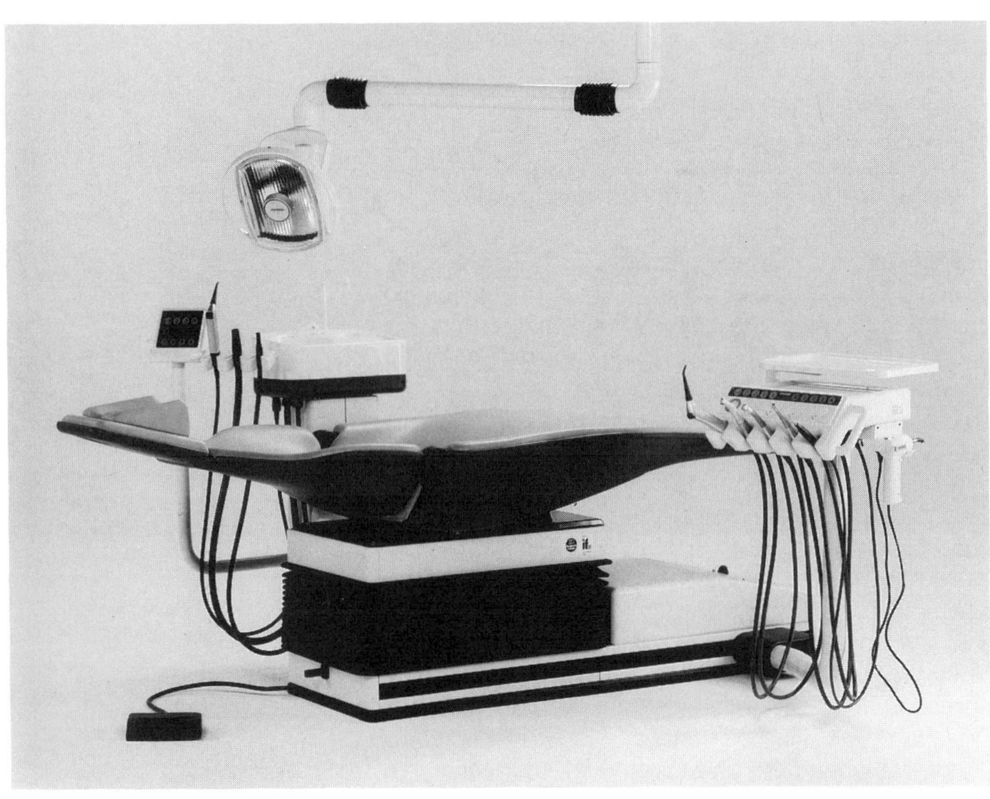

Figure 10-1. *Sirona* dental chair. (*Courtesy Pelton & Crane, a division of Siemens Corporation, Charlotte, NC.*)

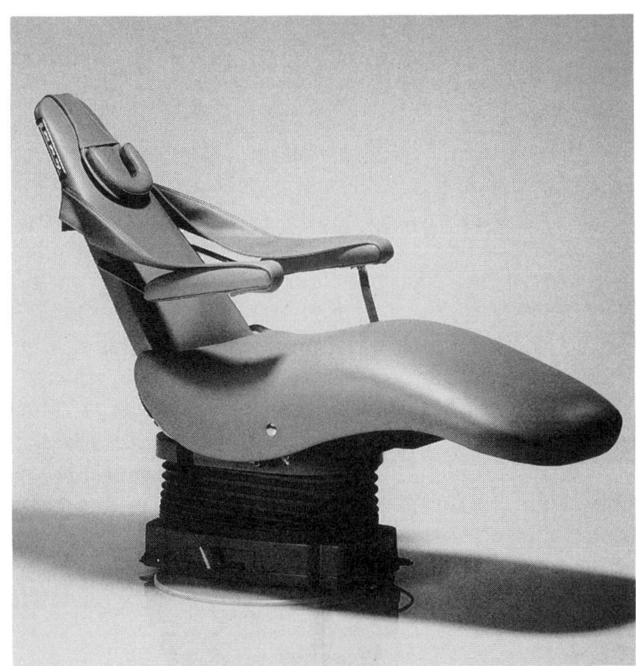

Figure 10-2. Dental chair. (*Courtesy Den-Tal-Ez, Bay Minette, AL.*)

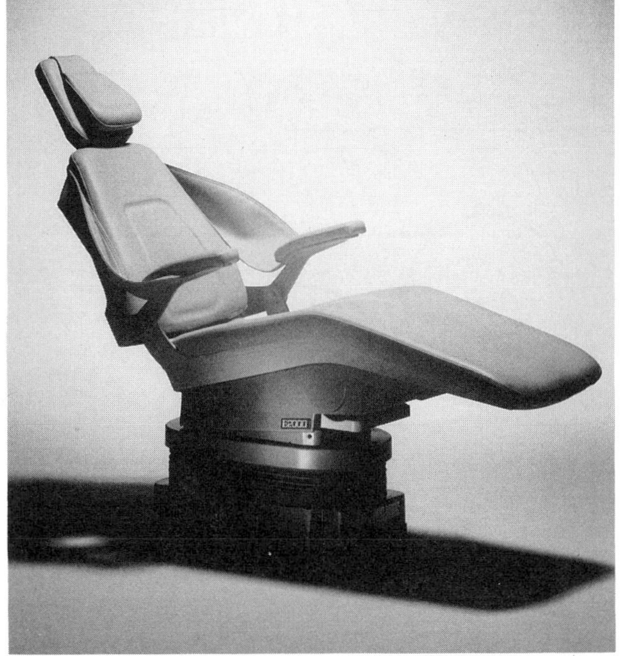

Figure 10-3. Dental chair. (*Courtesy Den-Tal-Ez, Bay Minette, AL.*)

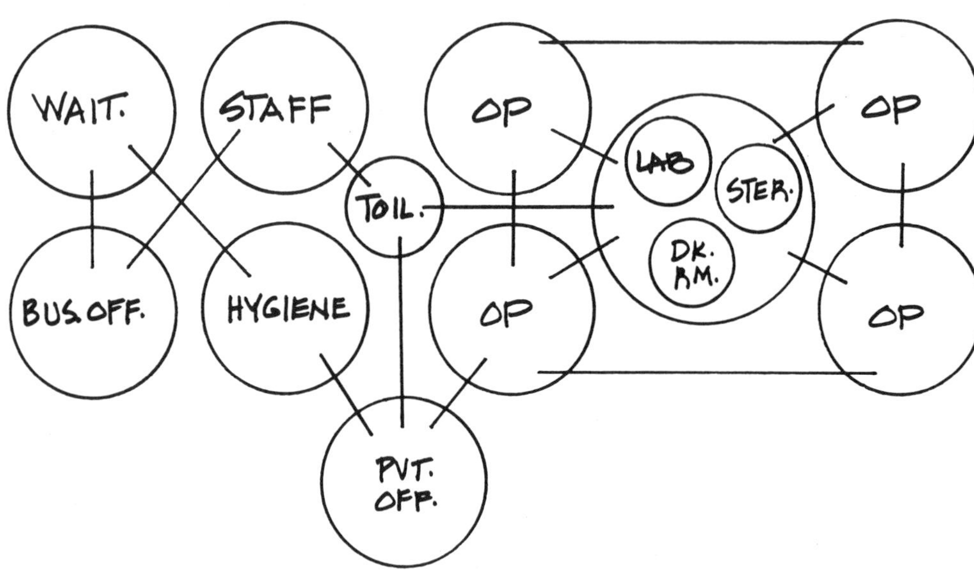

Figure 10-4. Schematic diagram of a general dentistry suite.

GENERAL DENTISTRY

Office Circulation Patterns

Traffic flow within a dental office is from waiting room to X-ray (either a special room for this purpose or located in a standard operatory) to operatory for a new patient examination or for a periodic re-check. For subsequent visits during the course of treatment, X-ray may not be required. The patient should be able to enter the operatory and sit down on the right side of the chair (for a right-handed dentist) without walking around the chair or through the assistant's work area (Figure 10-5). At the end of the procedure, the patient walks to the reception area, repairs makeup or combs hair at the vanity niche in the corridor or in the restroom, books a future appointment if required, and pays for services. Proper flow prevents exiting patients from interrupting the reception of incoming or new patients (Figure 10-6).

The dentist's circulation is from private office to operatory and between operatories. He or she should be able to enter the operatory without having to walk around the chair or through the assistant's work area, wash hands, and be seated on the patient's right (if he or she is right-handed), as in Figure 10-5. The assistant's path is from the sterilizing area to the operatories, darkroom, and occasionally, the lab.

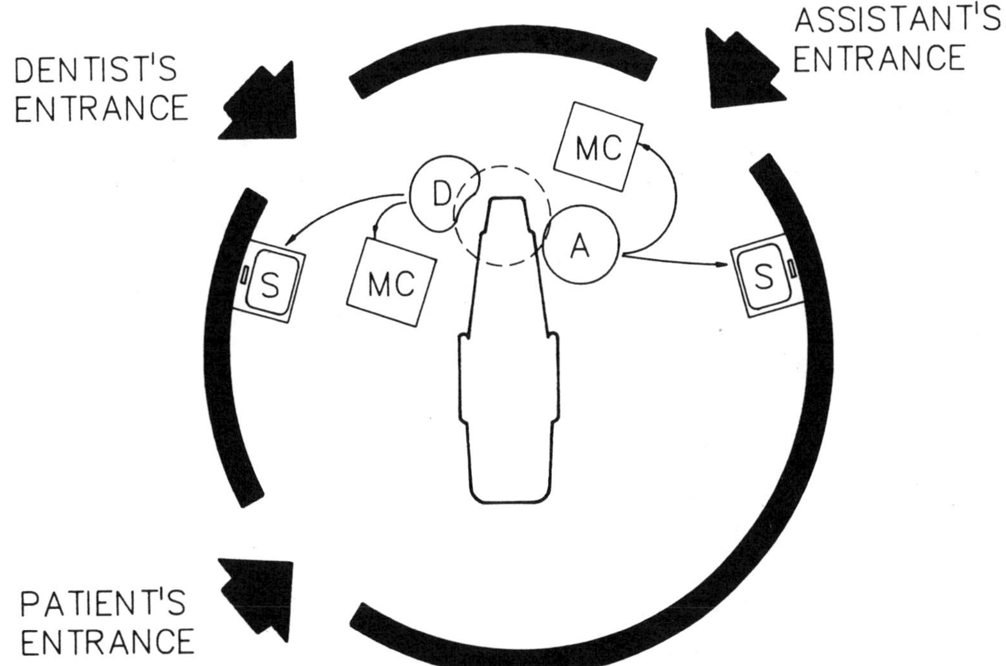

Figure 10-5. Optimum traffic flow pattern.

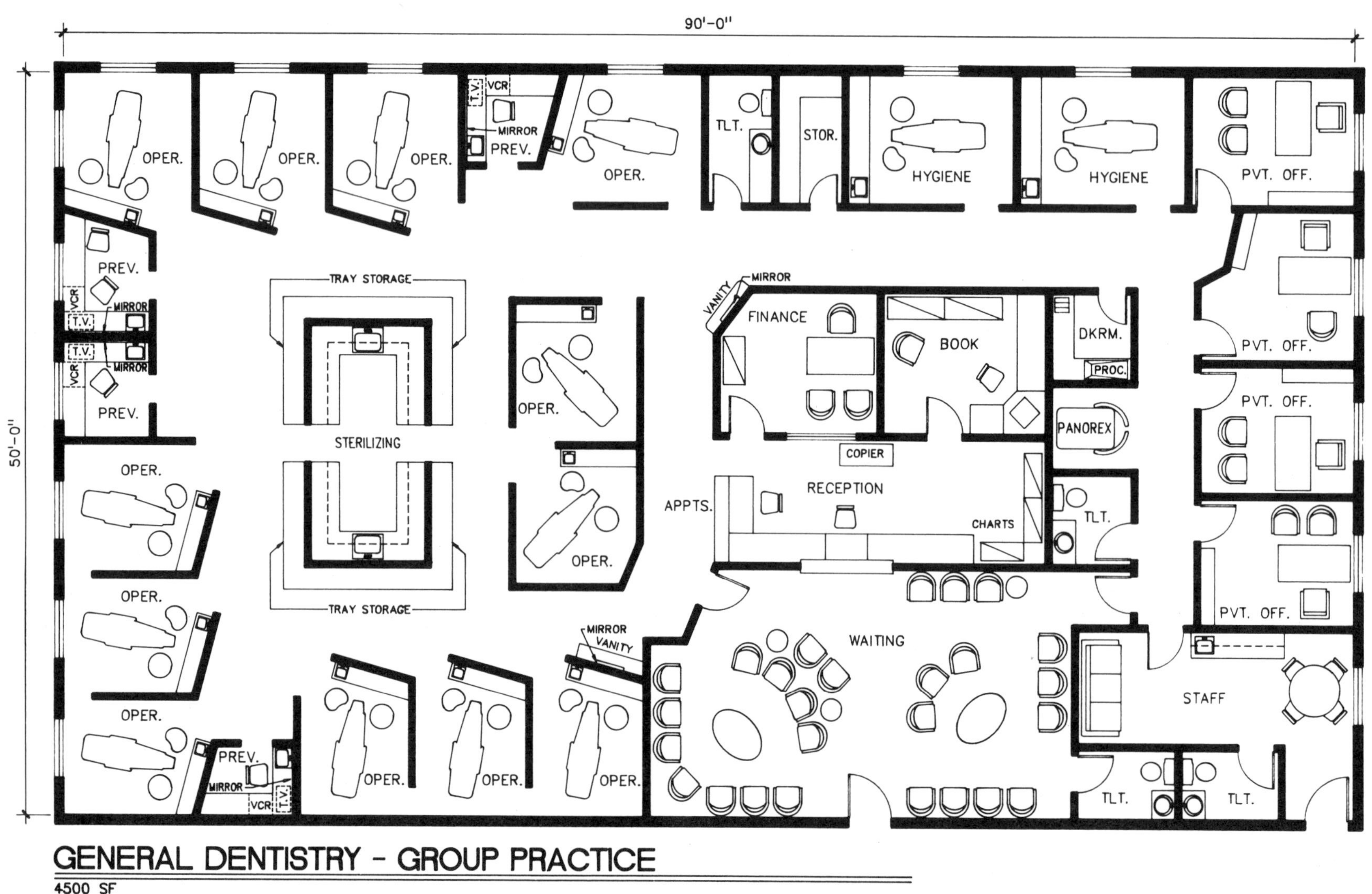

Figure 10-6. Suite plan for group practice, 4500 square feet.

The chairside assistant (also called the auxiliary) in most cases will have to walk the greater distance in order to reach his or her work area since it is more important, to maximize production, for the dentist to have the shortest route (Figure 10-7, Plan C, and Figure 10-8). However, the operatory in Figure 10-9 has two entrances, one for the auxiliary and one for the dentist. This eliminates stress by making it easy for the assistant to enter and leave the room without walking behind the chair. Since the dentist and assistant are working in such confined areas, it is critical that these spaces be well planned and efficient. As with a medical office, a dental office should have a private entrance/exit for the staff and dentist so that they do not have to pass through the waiting room.

The Dental Assistant

The dental assistant or auxiliary performs many duties. Among them are cleanup of operatories; seating patients in the dental chair; preparing tray setups; taking X-rays; sterilizing instruments; loading anesthetic syringes; pouring impressions, mixing amalgams; charting and numbering teeth; handling suction, air, and water syringes; and assisting the dentist in dozens of restorative and surgical procedures.

Some dental practices use licensed expanded-duty assistants who perform tissue retraction, suture removal, take impressions, change periodontal packing, and sometimes, depending upon state practice laws, perform the more routine aspects of completing a procedure, thereby freeing the dentist to move to the next patient.

Table 10-1. Analysis of Program. General Dentistry

No. of Dentists:	**1**	**2**
Waiting Room[a]	12 × 14 = 168	16 × 18 = 288
Business Office/Recept.	12 × 14 = 168	12 × 16 = 192
Operatories[b]	2 @ 9-1/2 × 11-1/2 = 218	5 @ 9-1/2 × 11-1/2 = 546
Lab	8 × 10 = 80	8 × 12 = 96
Sterilization Alcove	6 × 8 = 48	8 × 8 = 64
Darkroom	4 × 6 = 24	4 × 6 = 24
Staff Lounge	8 × 10 = 80	10 × 12 = 120
Toilets	2 @ 6 × 7 = 84	2 @ 6 × 7 = 84
Hygiene Operatory	9-1/2 × 11-1/2 = 109	9-1/2 × 11-1/2 = 109
Panoramic X-ray	5 × 8 = 40	5 × 8 = 40
Audiovisual/Patient Education	8 × 8 = 64	8 × 8 = 64
Private Office	10 × 10 = 100	2 @ 10 × 10 = 200
Storage	5 × 6 = 30	6 × 8 = 48
Mechanical Equipment Room	6 × 8 = 48	6 × 8 = 48
Subtotal	1261 ft²	1923 ft²
15% Circulation	189	288
Total	1450 ft²	2211 ft²

[a]A rule of thumb for estimating the number of seats in the waiting room is to allow 18 ft² per person.

[b]Size of operatories varies with doctor's practice preference for delivery of instrumentation and location of casework.

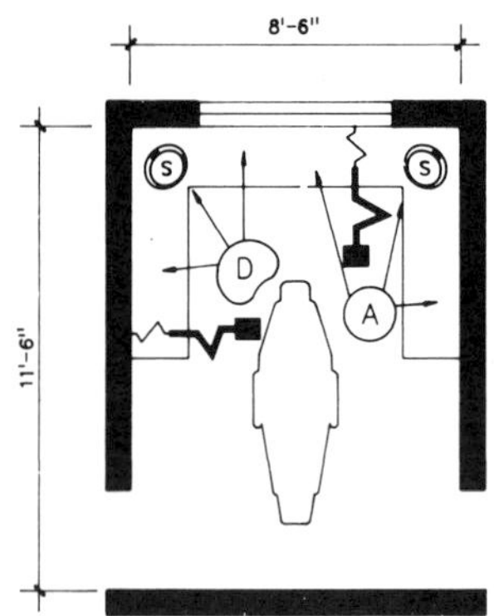

PLAN A · SIDE DELIVERY

"U" DESIGN OPERATORY DENTIST AND ASSISTANT WORK OFF OF FIXED CABINETS. CABINET MOUNTED INSTRUMENTATION PULLS OUT ON A FLEXIBLE ARM.

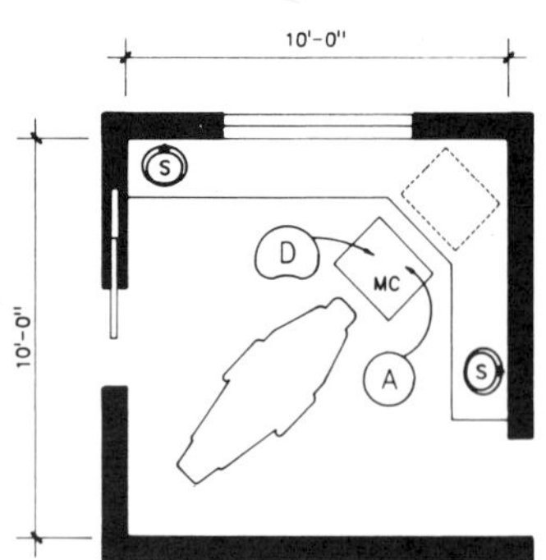

PLAN B · REAR DELIVERY

DIAGONAL CHAIR PLACEMENT WITH SINGLE DUAL-PURPOSE MOBILE CART BEHIND PATIENT'S HEAD. DENTIST AND ASSISTANT WORK OFF THE SAME CART.

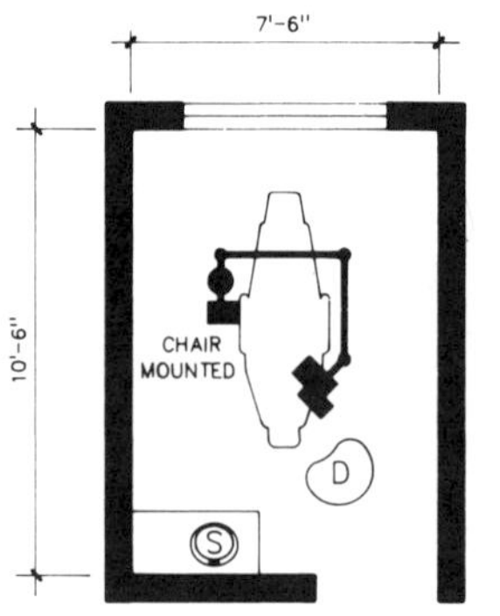

PLAN E · OVER-THE-PATIENT

AN OPERATORY FOR A DENTIST WHO WORKS WITHOUT AN ASSISTANT.

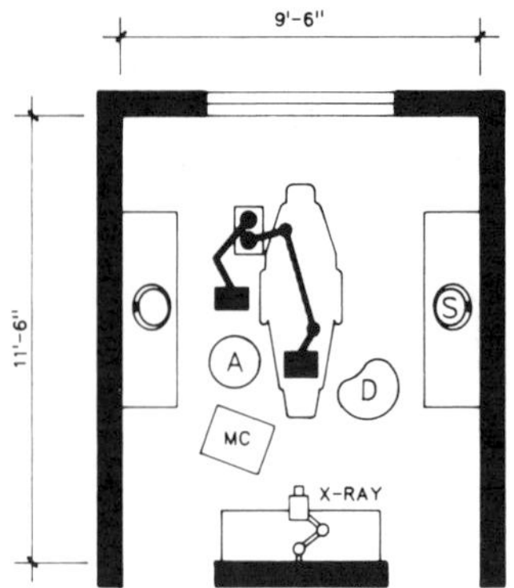

PLAN F · OVER-THE-PATIENT

DENTIST AND ASSISTANT WORK OFF OF POST-MOUNTED INSTRUMENTATION. MOBILE CART HOLDS TRAYS AND TUBS

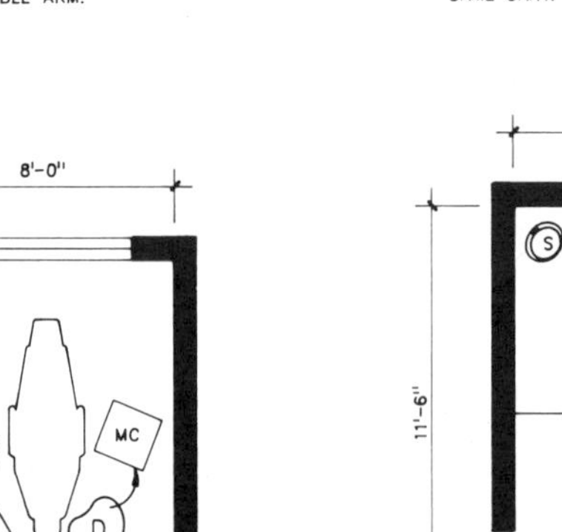

PLAN C · SIDE DELIVERY

ASSISTANT AND DENTIST WORK OFF OF SPLIT (SEPARATE) MOBILE CARTS. NO FIXED CABINETRY IN ROOM.

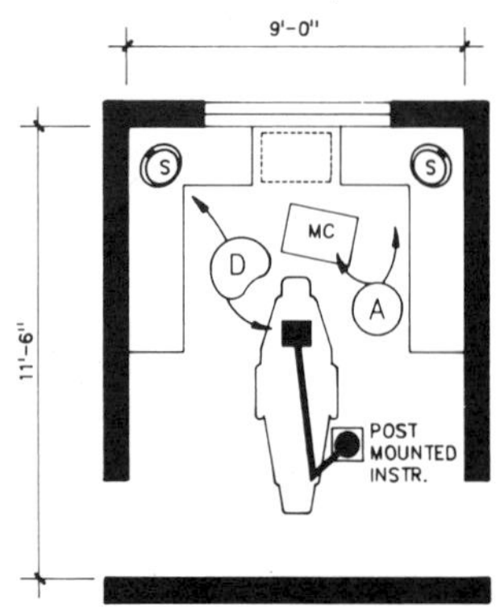

PLAN D · OVER-THE-PATIENT

MODIFIED "U" ARRANGEMENT FOR STORAGE OF MOBILE CART. ASSISTANT WORKS OFF OF MOBILE CART BEHIND PATIENT AND DENTIST RECEIVES DYNAMIC INSTRUMENTS OVER THE PATIENT'S CHEST (INSTRUMENTS ARE POST MOUNTED).

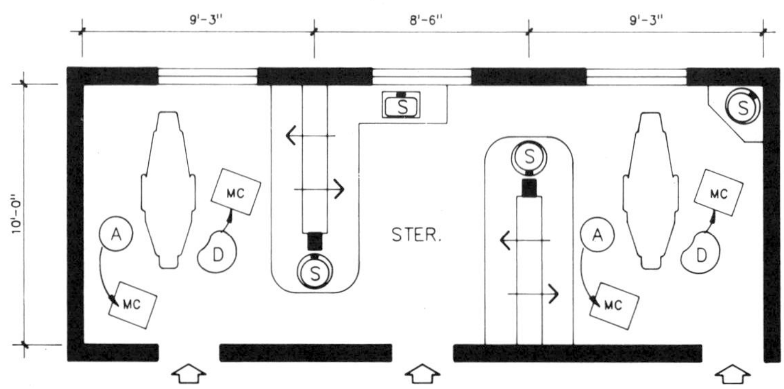

PLAN G · SIDE DELIVERY / SPLIT CART

DENTIST AND ASSISTANT WORK OFF MOBILE CARTS. BOTH OPERATORIES HAVE PASS-THROUGH FEATURE WITH STERILIZATION AREA WHICH PERMITS CLEAN TRAY SET-UPS TO BE PLACED IN OPERATORY (AND DIRTY ONES REMOVED) WITHOUT ENTERING THE ROOM.

ALTERNATIVES FOR OPERATORY LAYOUT

Figure 10-7. Alternatives for operatory layout.

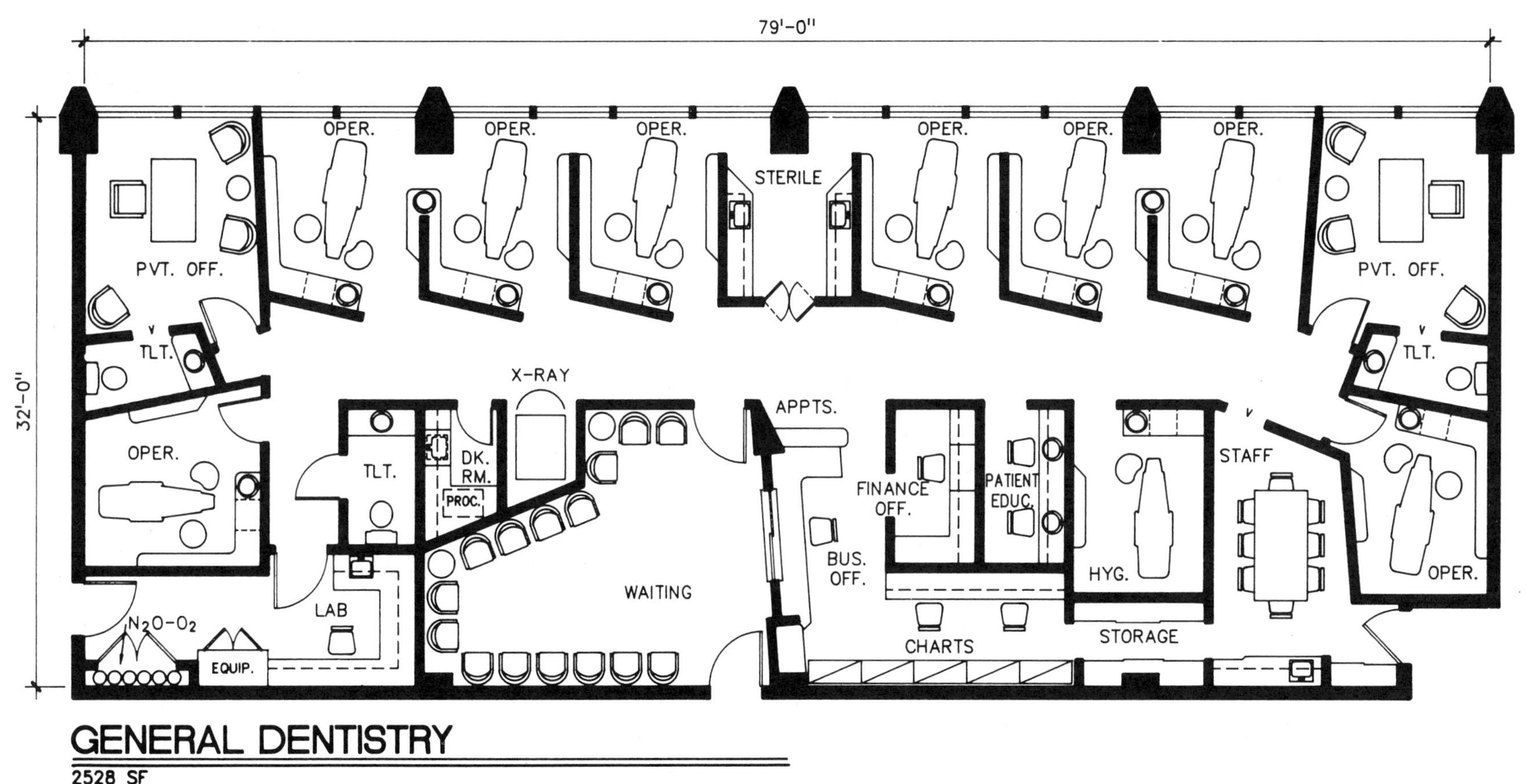

Figure 10-8. Suite plan for general dentistry, 2528 square feet.

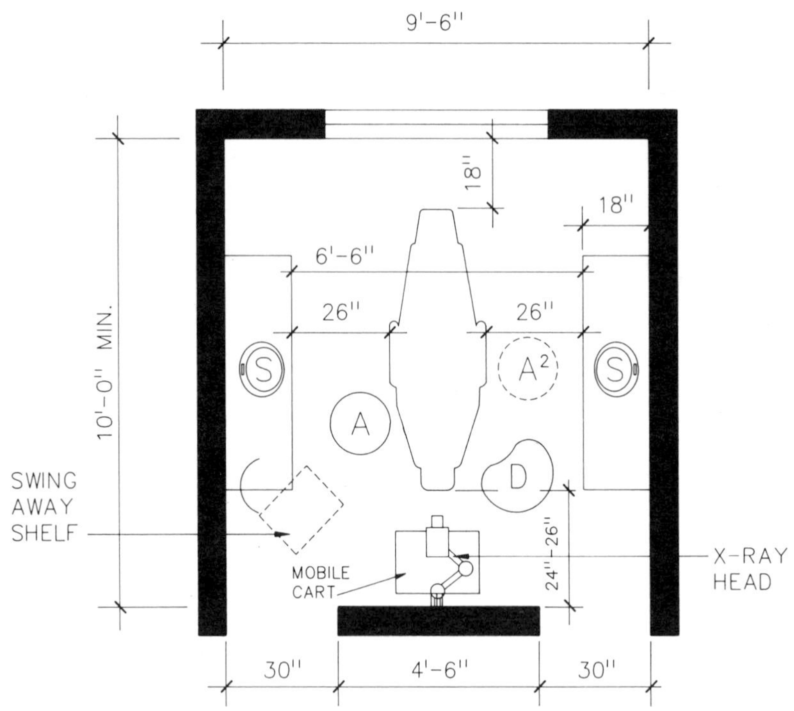

OPTIMAL OPERATORY LAYOUT

ALLOWS FREEDOM OF MOVEMENT FOR STAFF AND MAXIMIZES EFFICIENCY. BOTH CHAIRSIDE ASSISTANT AND DENTIST WORK OFF OF A SINGLE CART AT REAR OF PATIENT. CART IS LOCATED OUT OF THE PATH OF PATIENT AND STAFF. THIS WOULD ALSO ACCOMMODATE THE DENTIST WHO PREFERS EITHER OVER-THE-PATIENT OR SIDE DELIVERY OF INSTRUMENTATION. NOTE THAT THE OPTIONAL SECOND ASSISTANT (A^2) WORKS TO THE RIGHT OF THE DENTIST.

Figure 10-9. Optimal operatory layout.

Design Operatories for Flexibility

A right-handed dentist will work to the patient's right and a left-handed dentist to the patient's left. Traditionally, operatories were designed either for a right-handed dentist or a left-handed one. Today, flexibility is the key. New equipment is designed to accommodate change. In a practice composed of right-handed and left-handed dentists, an ambidextrous operatory can be designed (Figure 10-10) in which the utilities are brought up under the toe of the chair and are mounted near the chair on a swing-away bracket that is designed to swing to either the left or the right of the chair. The X-ray head should be mounted on the rear wall over the fixed cabinet, and the hoses for water, compressed air, and suction would come from the wall behind the fixed cabinet or from a swing-away bracket on the chair, arising from a junction box on the floor under the toe of the chair.

Size of Operatories

Operatories may be as small as 8 × 10 feet (Figure 10-7, Plan C) or as large as 10 × 12 feet, but 100 square feet is the average size. Figure 10-9 shows the minimum distances between the dental chair, cabinetry, and perimeter of the room. There was a time when dentists worked alone and preferred small operatories (Figure 10-7, Plan E), so that while seated (or standing) they could reach everything they needed. Now that dentists use a chairside assistant and the trend is toward longer appointments (it is more efficient to do a lot of work at one sitting), many dentists feel more comfortable working in a larger operatory. However, the size is related to the use and location of fixed cabinets and to the number and location of sinks and/or mobile carts.

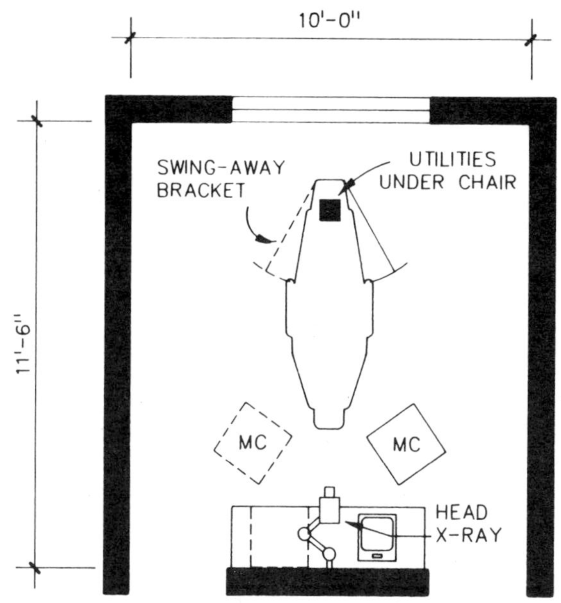

AMBIDEXTROUS OPERATORY

THIS ARRANGEMENT SERVES A PRACTICE COMPOSED OF RIGHT-AND-LEFT-HANDED DENTISTS. THE X-RAY HEAD IS MOUNTED BEHIND THE PATIENT. UTILITIES ARE UNDER THE TOE OF THE CHAIR AND THE ASSISTANT'S MOBILE CART CAN MOVE TO EITHER SIDE. DENTIST'S INSTRUMENTATION IS OVER-THE-PATIENT.

Figure 10-10. Ambidextrous operatory.

Plans A through G, Figure 10-7, and Figures 10-9 and 10-10 are but a few of the possibilities. The total number of options is related to the number of possible combinations of the following elements:

Dentist's Instrumentation. Instruments may be delivered *over-the-patient,* from the *side* (either from a mobile cart, mounted onto a fixed cabinet, or wall-mounted on an adjustable arm) or from the *rear* (sharing a mobile cart with the assistant), or mounted to a fixed cabinet behind the patient.

Assistant's Instrumentation. Instruments may be delivered *over-the-patient,* post-mounted from the *side* (post-mounted on a scissor arm, attached to a post-mounted cuspidor, or from a mobile cart or wall-mount), or from the *rear* (a dual-purpose cart shared with the dentist or built into fixed cabinetry).

Work Surfaces. These may be mobile carts, fixed cabinets, or shelves that slide out of fixed cabinets to hold the tray of instruments and medicaments used during the procedure. For example, if the assistant's instrumentation is being delivered post-mounted over the patient, the assistant will need an additional work surface, which would probably be a mobile cart placed near the head of the patient. Mobile carts can be selected with both instrumentation and a work surface combined.

Number of Doors. An operatory may have one or two entrances.

Number of Sinks. An operatory may have one or two sinks, wall-hung or built into fixed cabinets.

Casework. Drawers are rarely needed in an operatory: Standard practice with respect to infection control dictates that everything used for a procedure should be stored on sterilized tray setups, brought into the room. Reaching into drawers during a procedure is considered to compromise infection control. Cabinets need be only 18 inches deep, and, if they are going to be used as work surfaces while seated, should be at a 30-inch height. The most common use for upper cabinets in a dental operatory is for tray and tub storage and for boxes of disposable gloves, face masks, and patient bib towels.

There are advantages and disadvantages to each style of delivery of instrumentation and to each option listed above; nevertheless, change is difficult, and most practitioners will continue to work in the manner to which they have become accustomed, even if another method seems more efficient.

Modular Casework. Some dentists prefer to buy prefabricated casework that takes the place of stud and gypsum board partitions, integrates utilities, and also accommodates whichever style of delivery the dentist and assistant prefer. The theory is that the "walls" and casework can be moved with the dentist to a new location. This cuts construction costs somewhat, but this type of system is not inexpensive. It has a much more open appearance because the units are not full height. Some dentists like this, and others find there is a lack of acoustical privacy with a patient in one operatory being able to overhear the other patient's description of a toothache. Modular systems such as that shown in Figure 10-11 have always been popular in Europe, where space is at a premium. People who don't own their own buildings may not want to make a large investment in a rented office. For them, modular partitions and casework would be a solution.

Number of Operatories

There is no rule governing the number of operatories per dentist since the dentist's temperament and practice methods dictate size and design. A dentist who works slowly or does a lot of restorative work with long appointments may be comfortable with two operatories. A dentist with many short appointments will need four operatories in order not to lose time during the change of patients and the preparation or cleanup of operatories. *A rule of thumb is three operatories per dentist in a general practice.*

Design of the Dental Operatory

This is the most important room in a dental office. Although analogous to the physician's examination room, it is far more critical to a dentist's practice than the medical exam room is to a physician's, as the physician has ancillary rooms for diagnosis, testing, and treatment, but the dentist has only the operatory. In terms of economics, the physician has the opportunity to enhance his or her income from laboratory tests, X-ray films, and the use of medical aides to give injections, administer EKGs and EEGs, or to do physical therapy. But the dentist has only the operatory plus the laboratory and X-ray work from which to derive income. For this reason, many time and motion studies focusing on operatory efficiency have been published in dental journals.

Over the years, changes have evolved as a result of these studies. Patients now recline in a contoured chair with the dentist working from a seated position at the side of the patient. If right-handed, the dentist will be seated to the right of the patient and work in an area that could be designated as from 9 o'clock to 12 o'clock, imagining the patient's face as the clock, with 12 o'clock as the forehead and 6 o'clock as the chin. Most dentists use an assistant, which is called *four-handed dentistry.* Some dentists use two assistants, which is called *six-handed dentistry.* While Figure 10-5 illustrates optimum traffic flow pattern for an operatory, structural features of the space, the location of windows, and other immutable factors have an impact on the layout of the space and may yield compromises in circulation.

Optimal Operatory Layout

In recent years, concern for infection control, reduction of stress on chairside assistants and dentists, as well as optimum efficiency, have resulted in the operatory shown in Figure 10-9. This allows for total freedom of movement for the staff and comfort for the patient since nothing is delivered over the patient's chest. The instrumentation is behind the patient and therefore out of sight, and the auxiliary has a minimum of twisting and turning. The auxiliary faces forward working off a mobile cart which, when pushed back against the wall, is completely out of the path of the patient and staff.

Additionally, there are no unsightly utility umbilicals in view of the patient; thus, a clean, uncluttered appearance in the operatory is created. Some dentists might want a countertop on the rear wall over the mobile cart to place an ultrasonic scaler or other occasionally needed equipment. If this is the case, the length of the operatory would have to be extended to 11 feet, or possibly 11 feet 6 inches. The X-ray head in this operatory would be mounted on the rear wall, usable by a right- or left-handed person. Each operatory will require a view box illuminator, located to allow easy visibility by a seated dentist.

The critical distances shown in Figure 10-9 are based on ergonomic data regarding proper positioning of both the dentist and assistant to avoid back strain, fatigue, bending, twisting, turning, and reaching beyond limits. Everything the dental team needs is within easy reach.

It should be noted that the operatory in Figure 10-9 would also accommodate a dentist who prefers either over-the-patient or side delivery of instrumentation.

Instrumentation. There are four categories of instrumentation.

Handpiece Delivery System. This is composed of the drills (rotary tools) with drill bits that are used to cut and shape teeth.

Evacuation System. Blood, debris, and water are removed from the mouth, usually by suction. The vacuum system preferred for infection control is a "wet" system that empties into a waste pipe. The evacuation system typically has high-speed suction for rapid debris removal and a low-speed saliva ejector positioned in the patient's mouth. Both are the responsibility of the dental assistant.

Handheld Instruments. These tools include probes, scalers, forceps, etc.

Three-way Syringe. Used by both the dentist and the assistant for spraying water, compressed air, or a combination thereof. The assistant will have her own three-way syringe for drying or moistening preparations as well as for washing debris from the patient's mouth. She will also handle the saliva ejector.

Methods of Delivery. The dynamic instruments (drills, suction, syringes) can be delivered to the oral cavity of the patient by three methods.

Side Delivery System. This can be accomplished through the use of separate or *split carts* for the doctor and assistant or with cabinet or wall-mounted doctor's (see Figure 10-22) and assistant's units (see Figure 10-7, Plans A, C, and G). The dentist's cart has the handpieces and three-way syringe, while the assistant's cart has the three-way syringe and suction.

Advantages: Good patient access to chair; dynamic instruments out of patient's view; mobile carts permit flexibility of movement; wall-mounted units require minimal floor space.

Disadvantages: Reduces auxiliary's access to dynamic instruments; placement of umbilicals must be properly planned; most split carts require a wider operatory.

Figures 10-11, 10-12, and 10-13 show side delivery of instrumentation.

Rear Delivery System. Both the doctor's and the assistant's instrumentation are delivered from behind the patient's head either from a fixed cabinet (with the systems built into the face panel of the cabinet) or from a dual-purpose mobile cart (Figures 10-7, Plan B, 10-9, 10-14, and 10-15). Rear delivery can also be accomplished with what is called a *12 o'clock column* (Figures 10-16 and 10-17).

Advantages: Good patient access to chair; keeps dynamic instruments out of patient's view; dual cart gives assistant excellent access to dynamic instruments and a good work surface; ease of installation; requires minimal floor space. 12 o'clock column also works for two-handed dentistry, has excellent work surface for assistant, and has controls integrated into the cabinet.

Disadvantages: Limited to sit-down use; integration into fixed cabinet may increase installation time or cost; hand fatigue due to handpiece tubing pullback.

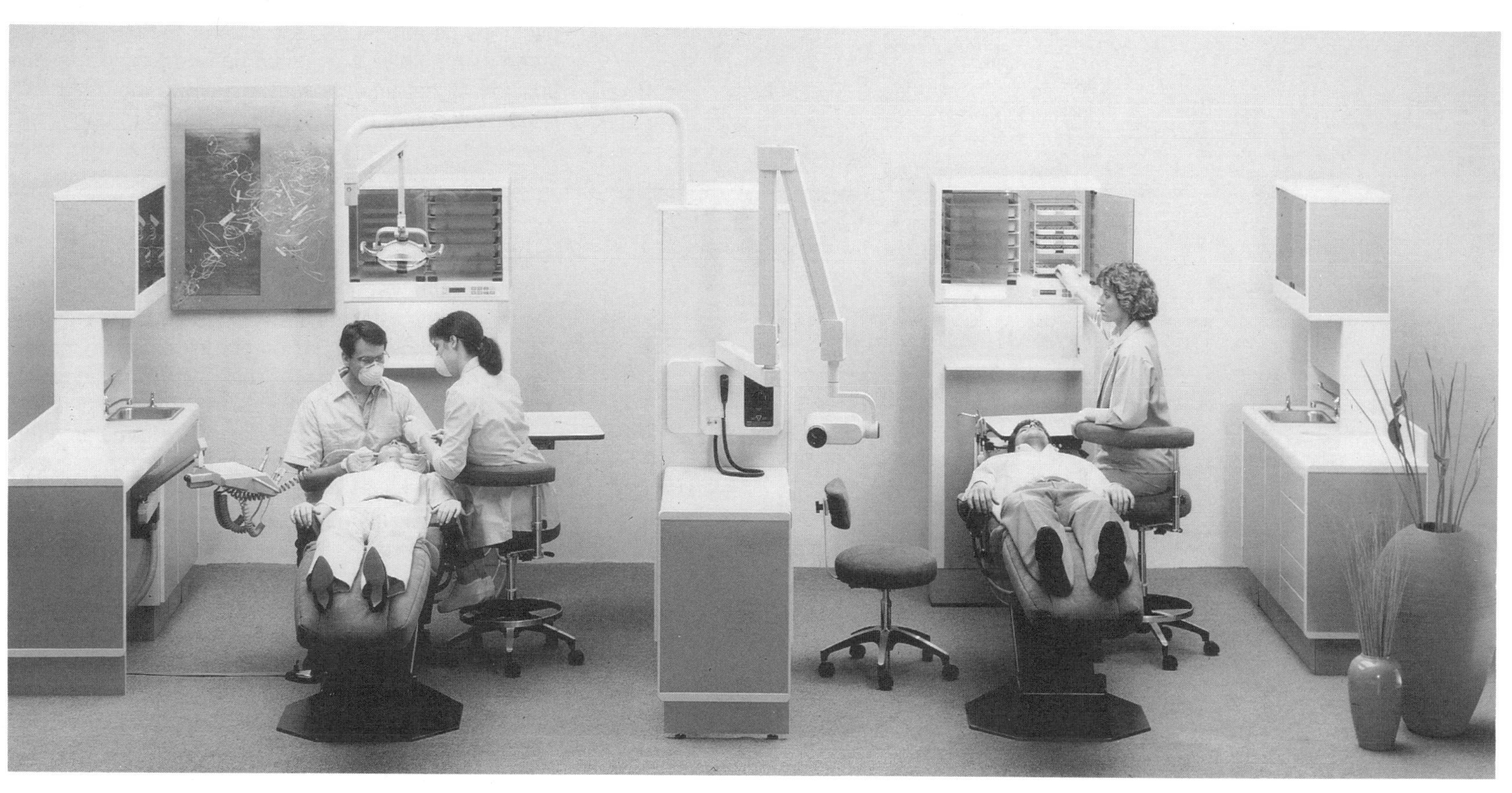

Figure 10-11. *Preference II* modular dental casework. Note intraoral X-ray shared between two operatories. (*Courtesy A-dec, Inc., Newberg, OR.*)

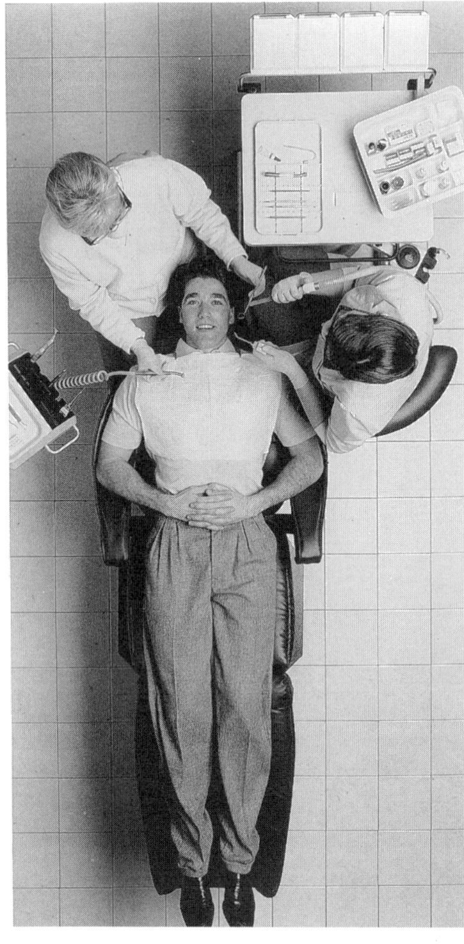

Figure 10-12. *Side delivery* of dynamic instruments. (*Courtesy A-dec, Inc., Newberg, OR.*)

Over-the-Patient Delivery System. Dynamic instruments are delivered either over the patient's chest or from the patient's left or right side. The systems are mounted on an arm, which is attached to a post. The post may be attached to the floor or to the chair. If the latter, as the chair is adjusted up or down, the relative position of instruments with respect to the oral cavity remains constant (Figure 10-7, Plans D, E, and F, and Figures 10-18 and 10-19). Statistics show that over-the-patient delivery is the most popular system, favored by nearly half of all practicing dentists.

Advantages: Functions for two- or four-handed stand-up or sit-down dentistry; requires minimal floor space; offers ambidextrous option; reduces eye fatigue as minimal adjustments in focus are necessary; handpieces are presented with easy access to the oval cavity and little handpiece tubing pullback; maximum flexibility in positioning instruments. (Tubing pullback occurs more often with coiled tubing than with noncoiled tubing.)

Disadvantages: Instruments are in patient's view; assistant's access to dynamic instruments is reduced.

With the three types of delivery systems available to the dentist, the chairside assistant may work with instrumentation that is post-mounted (Figure 10-19), a mobile cart (Figure 10-20), a dual cart (Figure 10-21), or wall-mounted instruments and work surface (Figure 10-22).

Cuspidors (Figure 10-23) were out of fashion for a while, but are increasing in popularity. They are available with or without attached assistant's instrumentation (suction, three-way syringe, and saliva ejector). Vacuum drain cuspidors are available for use with central vacuum systems.

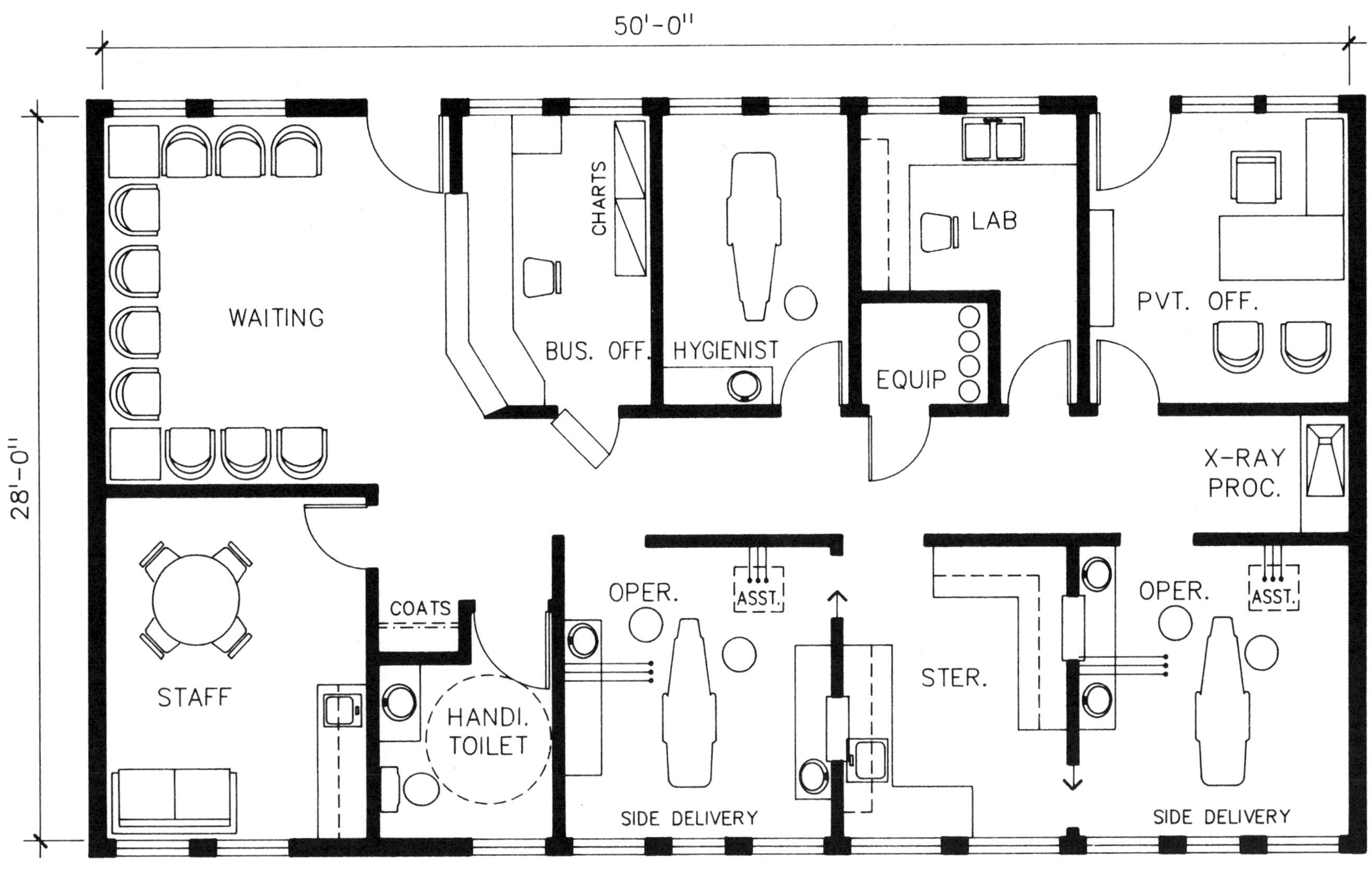

Figure 10-13. Suite plan for general dentistry, 1400 square feet.

Figure 10-14. *Rear delivery* of dynamic instruments, dual cart. (*Courtesy A-dec, Inc., Newberg, OR.*)

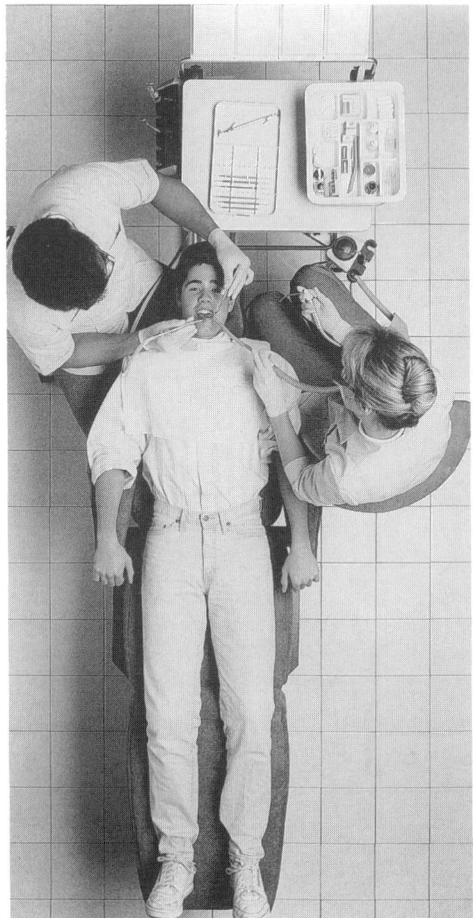

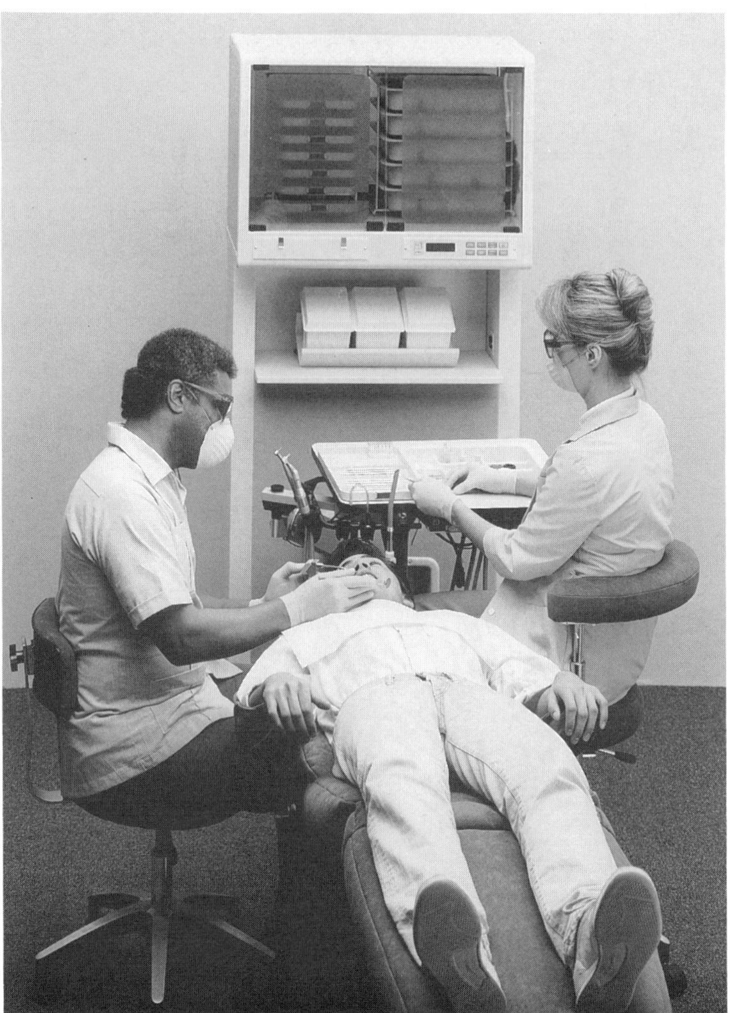

Figure 10-15. Cabinet-mounted *rear-delivery* system. Doctor's and assistant's instrumentation combined on arm-mounted unit. (*Courtesy A-dec, Inc., Newberg, OR.*)

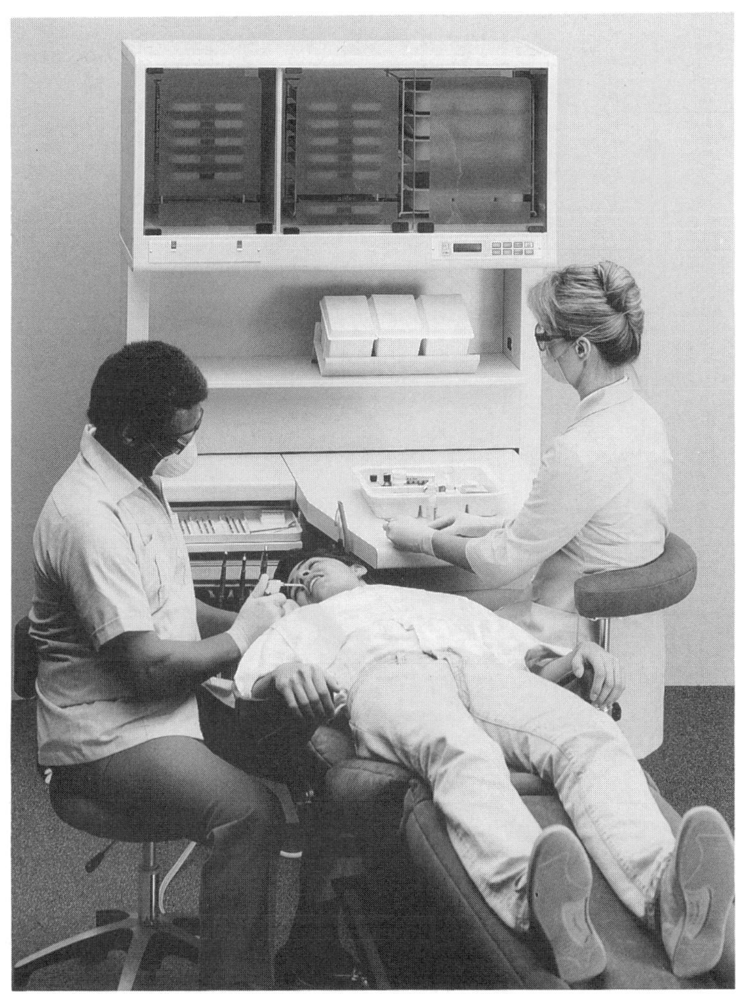

Figure 10-16. Cabinet-integrated *12 o'clock rear-delivery* system. Saves space because controls are integrated into the cabinet. (*Courtesy A-dec, Inc., Newberg, OR.*)

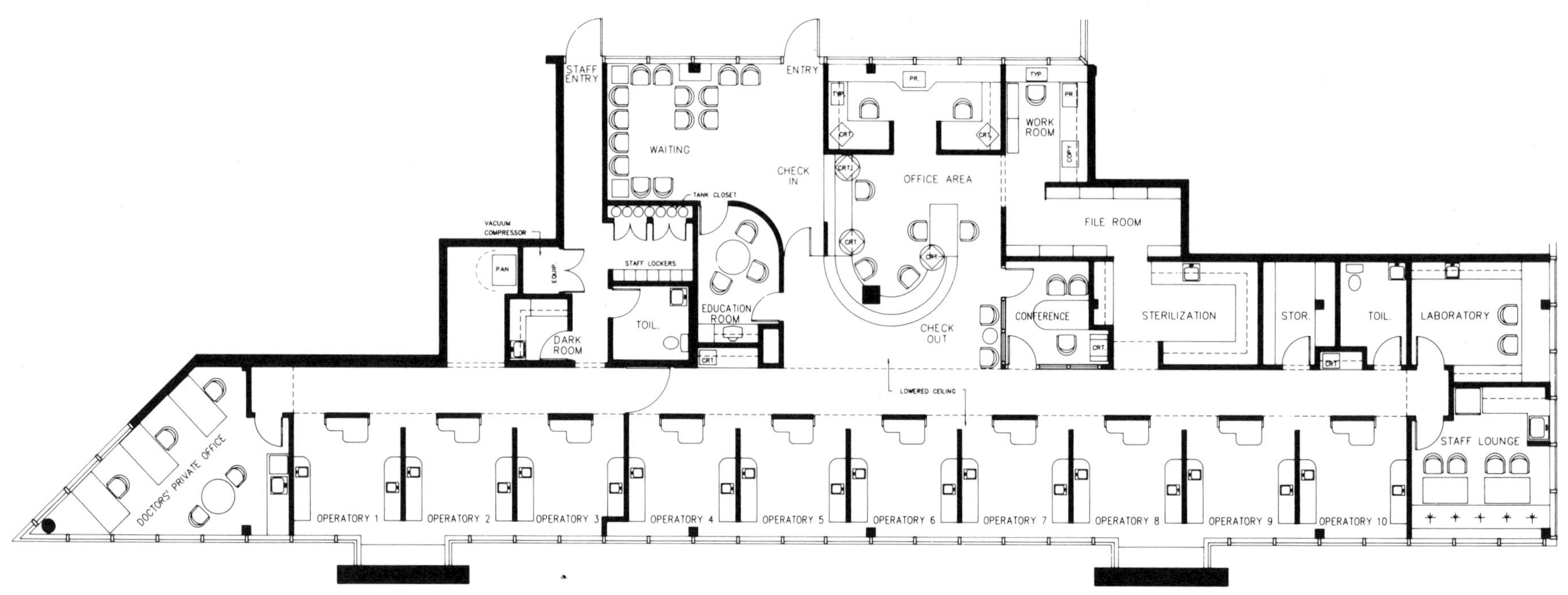

GENERAL DENTISTRY

3680 SF

Figure 10-17. Suite plan for general dentistry, 3680 square feet. (*Courtesy Carmel Repp Ltd., Interior Design Associates, San Diego, CA.*)

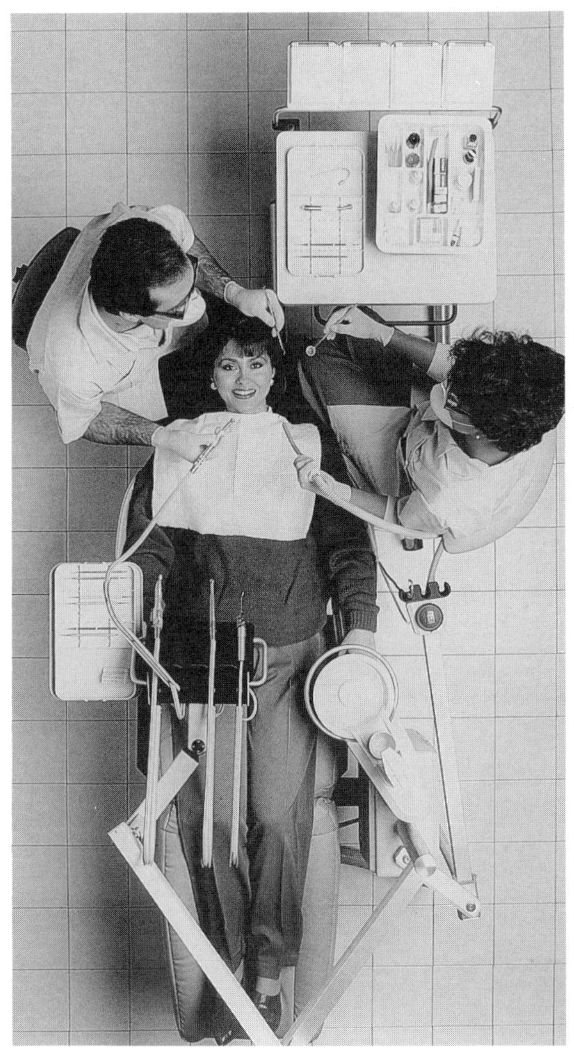

Figure 10-18. *Over-the-patient* delivery of instrumentation. (*Courtesy A-dec, Inc., Newberg, OR.*)

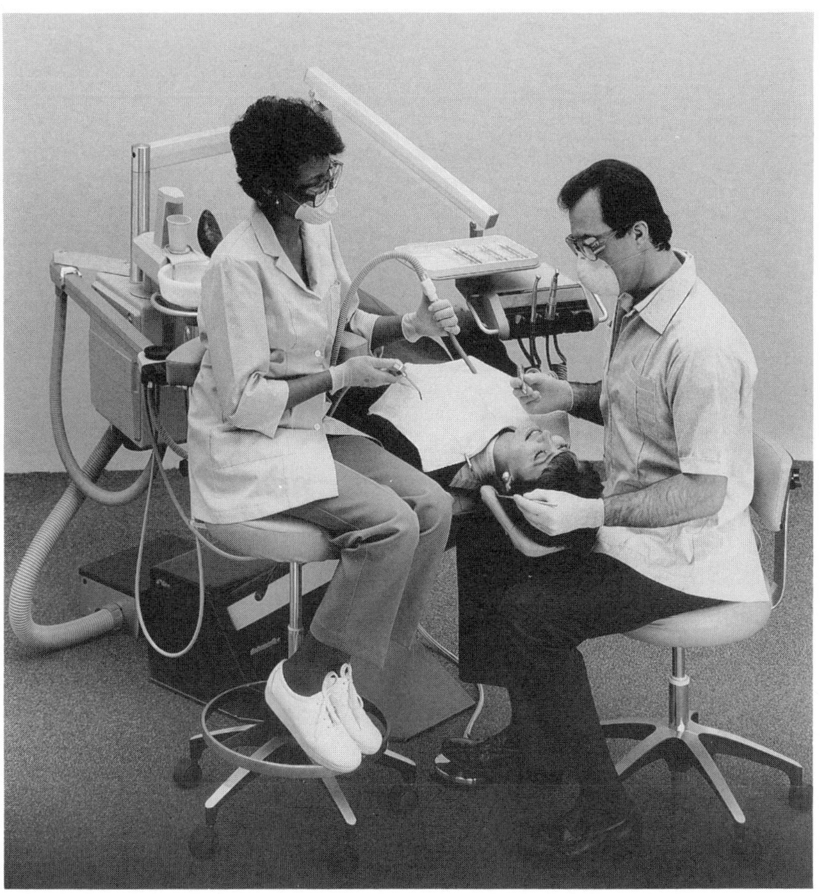

Figure 10-19. Over-the-patient delivery of instrumentation, chair-mounted doctor's and assistant's units. (*Courtesy A-dec, Inc., Newberg, OR.*)

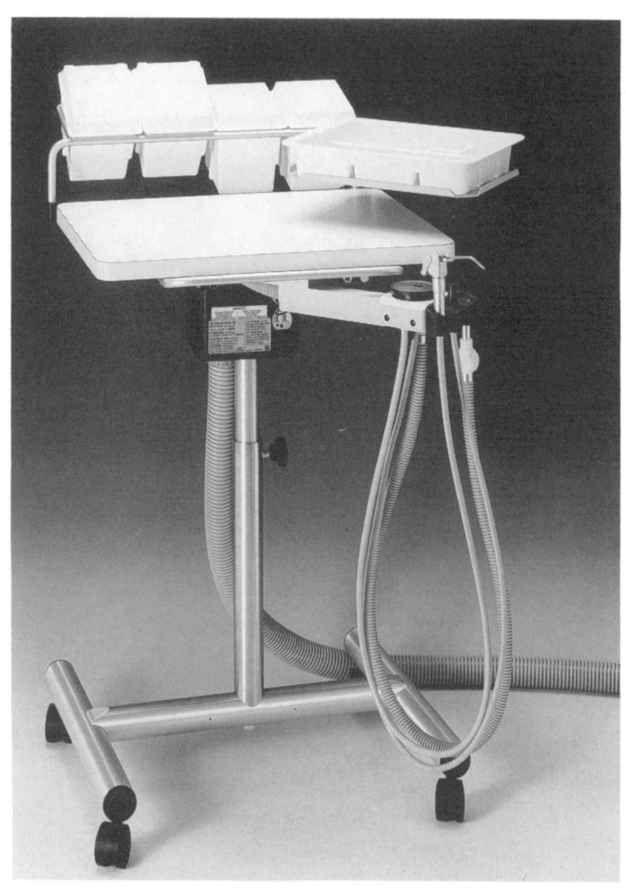

Figure 10-20. Assistant's mobile cart. (*Courtesy A-dec, Inc., Newberg, OR.*)

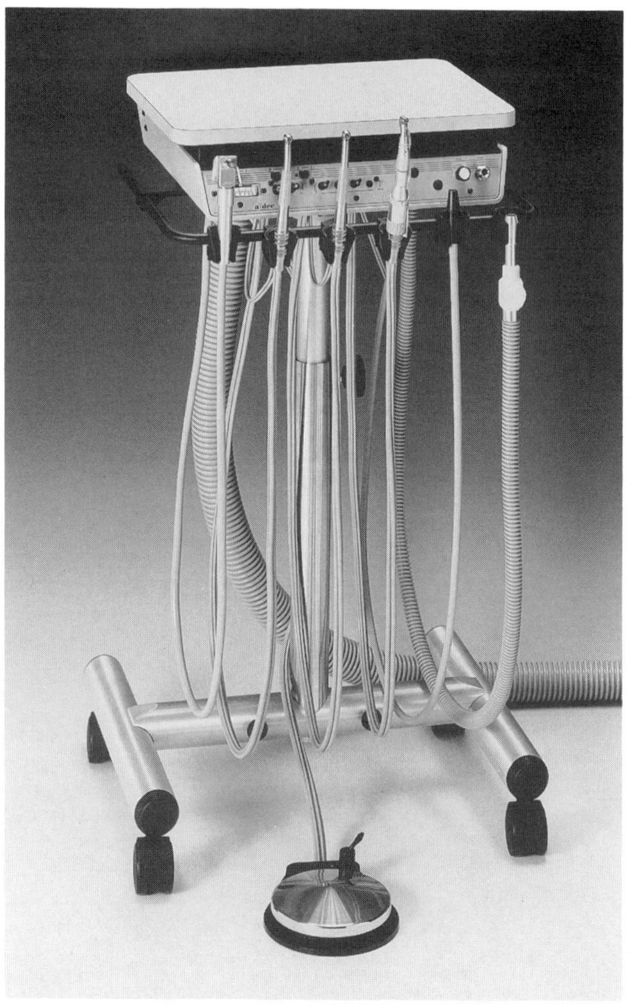

Figure 10-21. Dual cart, for doctor and assistant. (*Courtesy A-dec, Inc., Newberg, OR.*)

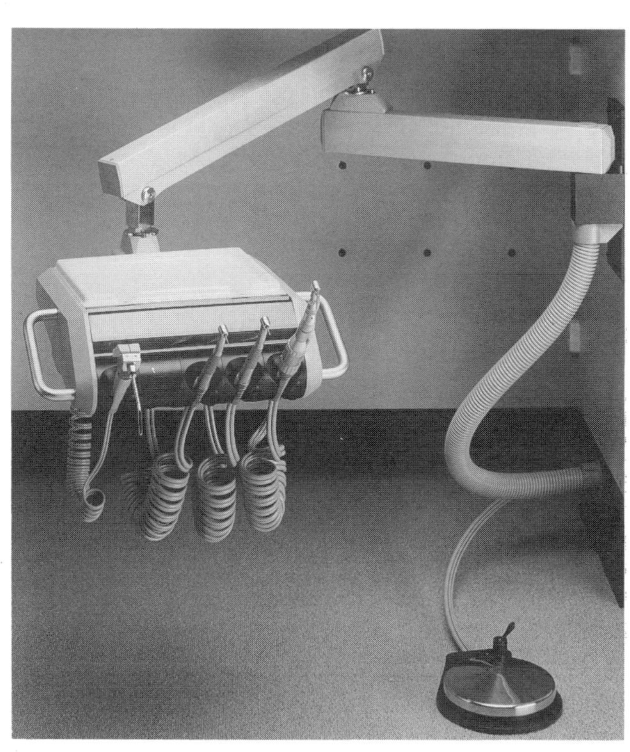

Figure 10-22. Wall-mounted doctor's unit. (*Courtesy A-dec, Inc., Newberg, OR.*)

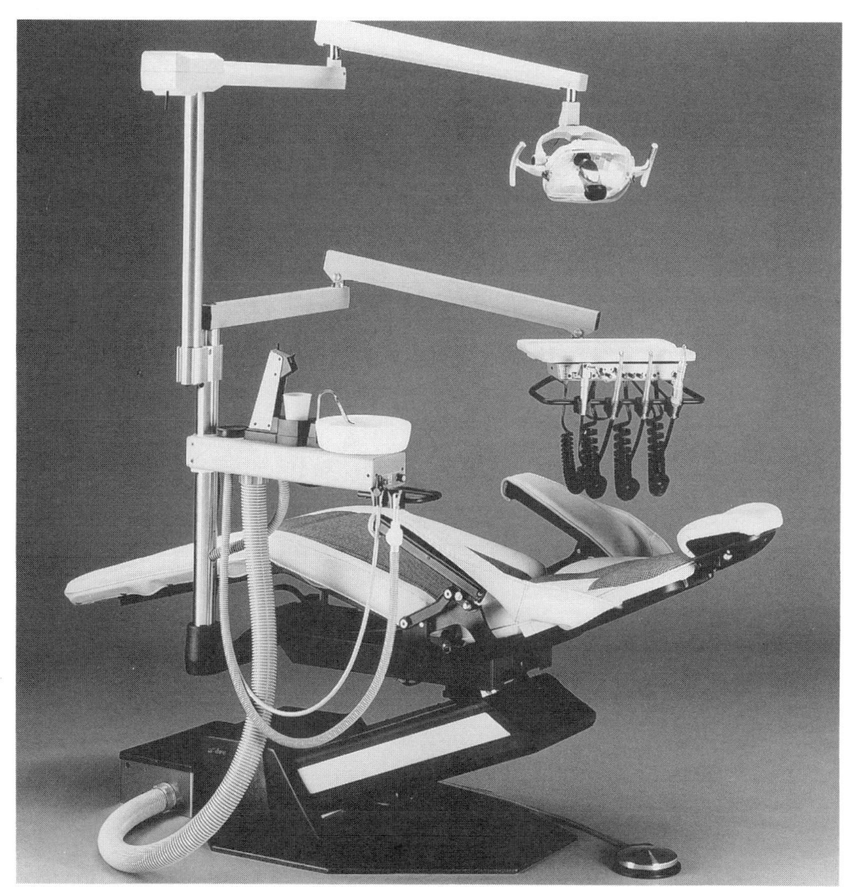

Figure 10-23. Chair with chair-mounted dental light and cuspidor with attached assistant's instrumentation. (*Courtesy A-dec, Inc., Newberg, OR.*)

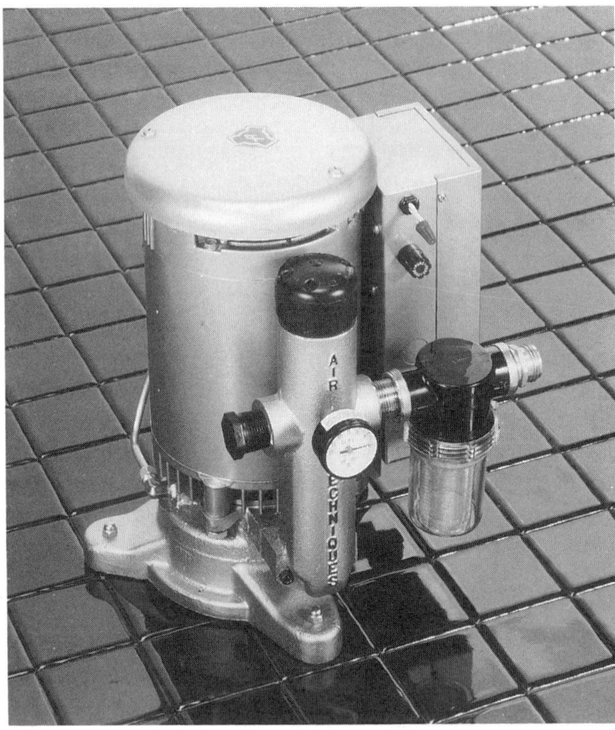

Figure 10-24. *VacStar 5* dental vacuum system. (*Courtesy Air Techniques, Inc., Hicksville, NY.*)

Central Suction

The suction at each operatory works off a central vacuum pump located in an equipment room, not too far from the operatories. The vacuum pump should not be located overhead, above the ceiling, because the additional amount of lift needed to pump overhead would reduce the efficiency of the system. The vacuum system shown in Figure 10-24 will accommodate up to three high-volume evacuators (HVE) plus up to six saliva ejectors, all in simultaneous use. The vacuum system is sized according to the number of HVE and saliva ejectors that might be in use at any one time. The space planner is advised to check with the manufacturer to verify recommended maximum distances for vacuum piping and diameter of vacuum lines, so as not to reduce efficiency. Additionally, it is desirable to enclose the vacuum pump and air compressor in a sound-insulated cabinet or room, as they can be quite noisy.

Quality vacuum systems provide consistent high-volume flow even when multiple users are on line, and they control infection by evacuating the pathogenic "cloud" surrounding the oral cavity. As stated previously, the "wet" system is preferred to the "dry" system for infection control.

Compressed Air

As with vacuum systems, compressed air systems must be sized according to the number of users. The unit in Figure 10-25 is appropriate for five simultaneous users. Air compressors need more sound insulation than do vacuum pumps, and they can generally be located at a greater distance from the operatories then can vacuum pumps; however, it is common to find both located in the same equipment room. Some manufacturers offer a sound-reducing cover for the air compressor that promises to reduce noise by 70 percent. The best air compressors are oil-free, because oil-lubricated compressors distribute oil aerosols through the air syringe, which may jeopardize dental techniques that require an uncontaminated air stream.

It is important to monitor the amount of moisture in compressed air because a humid condition promotes the growth of bacteria and fungi, which increases the risk of infection, when sprayed into the patient's mouth through the air syringe. Moisture can also prevent proper cohesion of composite restorative materials, cause premature failure of handpiece (drill) turbines, and cause water vapor damage to equipment. Figure 10-26 shows a remote control panel for switching on compressed air, the vacuum pump, and the moisture monitoring system.

Twin-headed compressors are popular as they allow the office to continue to operate when one compressor head fails to function.

Operatory Sinks

An operatory must have at least one sink, since the dentist and assistant must wash their hands upon entering the room. Some dentists may prefer a foot-lever or wrist-action faucet, but many use a single-lever type faucet. Operatories may have an additional sink for the assistant in order to save steps and keep the assistant out of the dentist's path. Regardless of number, operatory sinks may be quite small and may be round or oval in shape. Stainless steel bar sinks may also be used.

A new faucet that automatically turns on when hands are placed under it may achieve popularity as a method of enhancing asepsis.

Operatory Doors

Another variable in the operatory is the number and placement of doors — or whether to have doors. A solid-core hinged door would help to block the sound of high-speed drills, but is rarely used because it makes it difficult for the dentist and assistant to rotate quickly between operatories. Thus many operatories have sliding doors that remain open most of the time, but which can be closed for visual privacy (they offer little sound attenuation) when necessary.

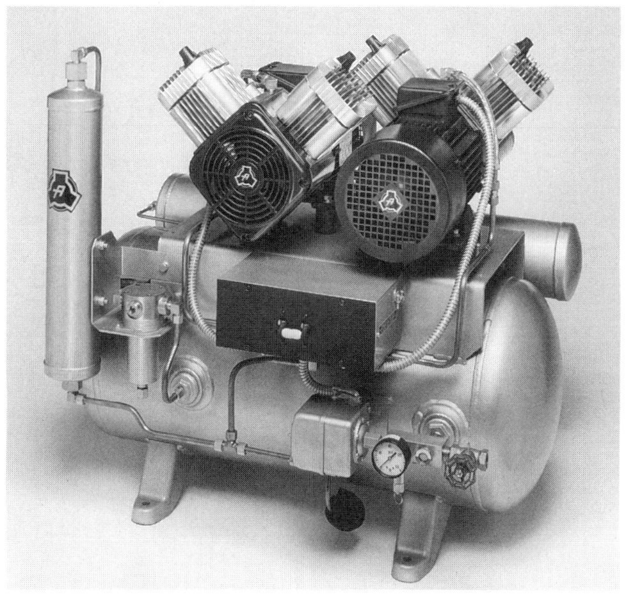

Figure 10-25. *AirStar 5* compressor. (*Courtesy Air Techniques, Inc., Hicksville, NY.*)

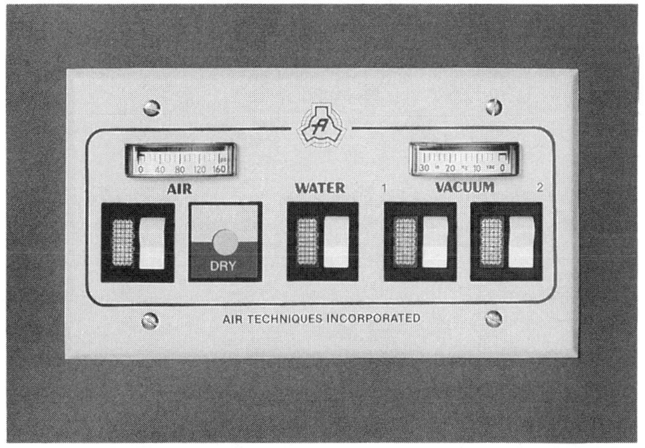

Figure 10-26. Remote control panel for air, water, and vacuum. (*Courtesy Air Techniques, Inc., Hicksville, NY.*)

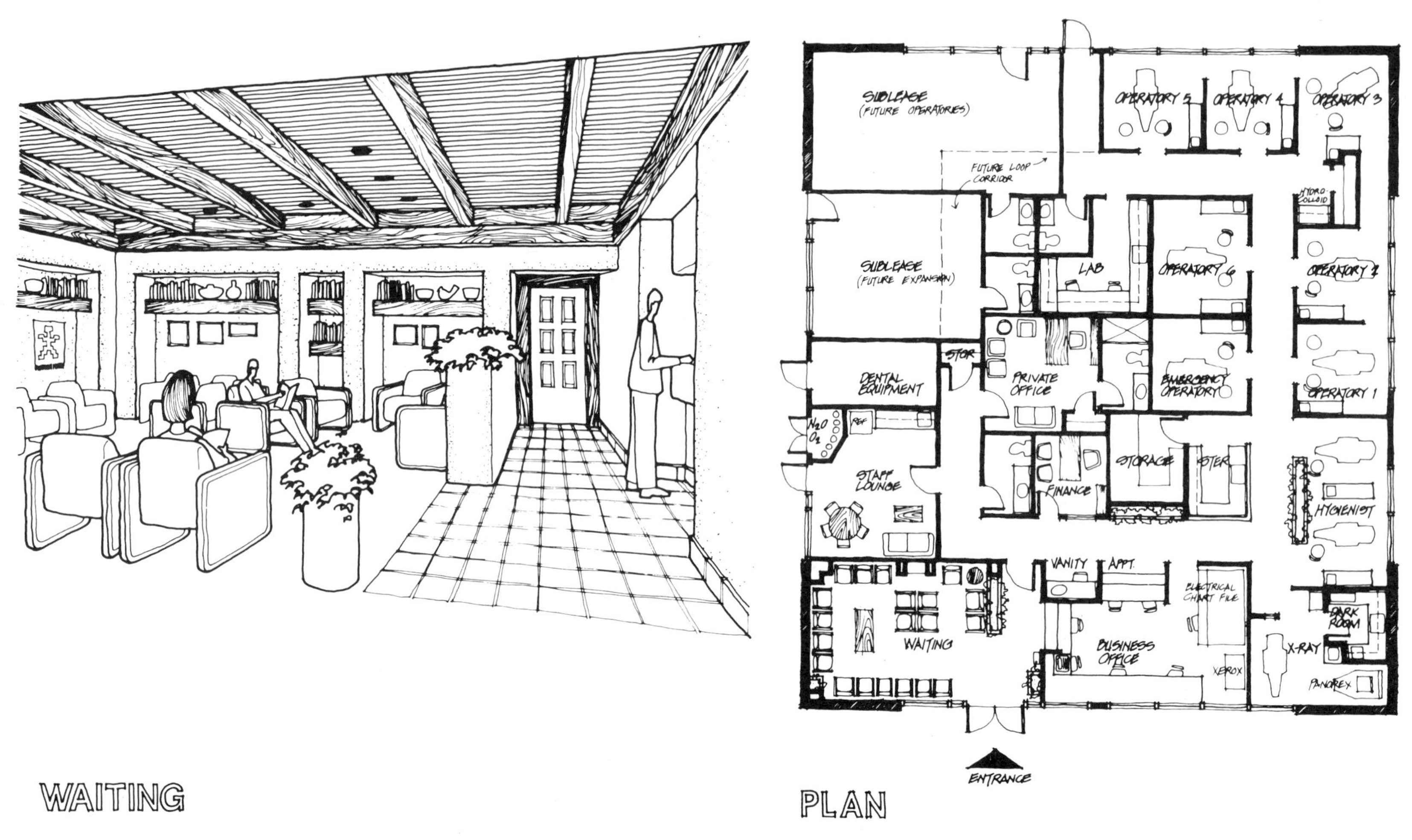

Figure 10-27. Suite plan for general dentistry. (*Courtesy T. Michael Hadley & Associates, AIA, Irvine, CA.*)

Many dentists, however, prefer openings without doors (see Figure 10-9), and some like openings between operatories (Figures 10-8 and 10-27) so that they and the assistants can quickly move back and forth between the rooms. An opening near the toe of the chair can make the patient feel a lack of privacy, but if there is no window in the room, it may actually decrease the feeling of being closed-in.

Tray Setups

Instruments are sterilized and then set up in advance on trays for various procedures. These trays vary in size from 7 × 10 to 10 × 15 inches, with 9½ × 13½ inches being the most common size. They may be stored in a central location (see Figure 10-6) or may be stored in each operatory (see Figures 10-15 and 10-16) for that day's work. Operatories that are contiguous with the sterilizing area (see Figure 10-7, Plan G) may have upper cabinets that open from both sides (pass-throughs), permitting trays of sterile instruments to be placed in an operatory without someone actually entering the room (see Figure 10-13). Dirty instrument trays can be removed from the operatory by the same procedure. The upper cabinet would have a clean side and a dirty side.

Tubs, an organizational vehicle, may also be used with tray setups. Tubs are generally 9½ × 11½ × 2½ inches deep. Both trays and tubs stack on racks (Figures 10-29 and 10-30), that in turn fit into cabinets for storage. These cabinets often have gray-tinted glass doors or glass etched with a design. Trays and tubs are color-coded by type of procedure for which they are set up, making it easy for staff to select the proper tray or tub. During the procedure, the instrument tray is placed on the mobile cart or other work surface convenient to the assistant. The tub, containing medicaments and other supplies necessary for the procedure, is also located near the assistant.

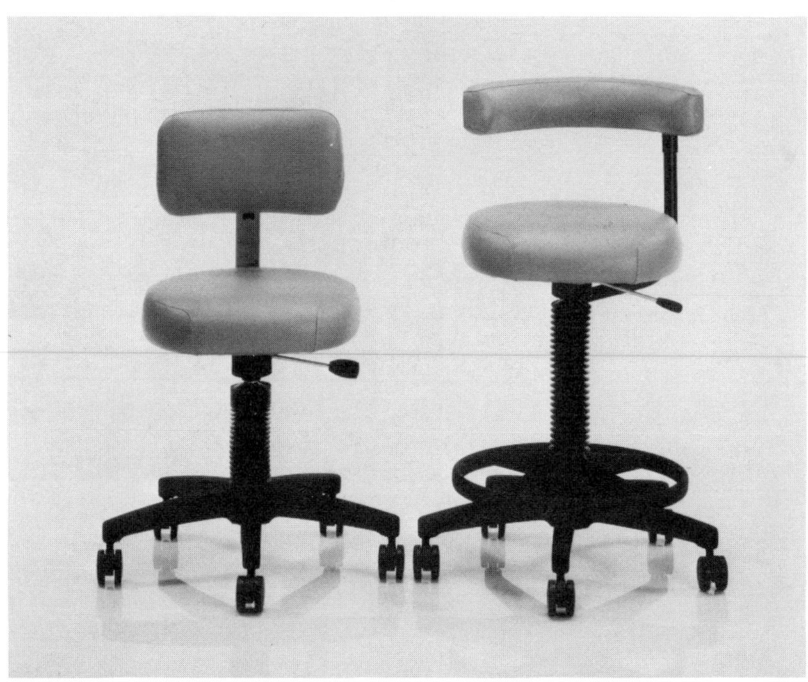

Figure 10-28. Dentist's and assistant's chairs. (*Courtesy Den-Tal-Ez, Bay Minette, AL.*)

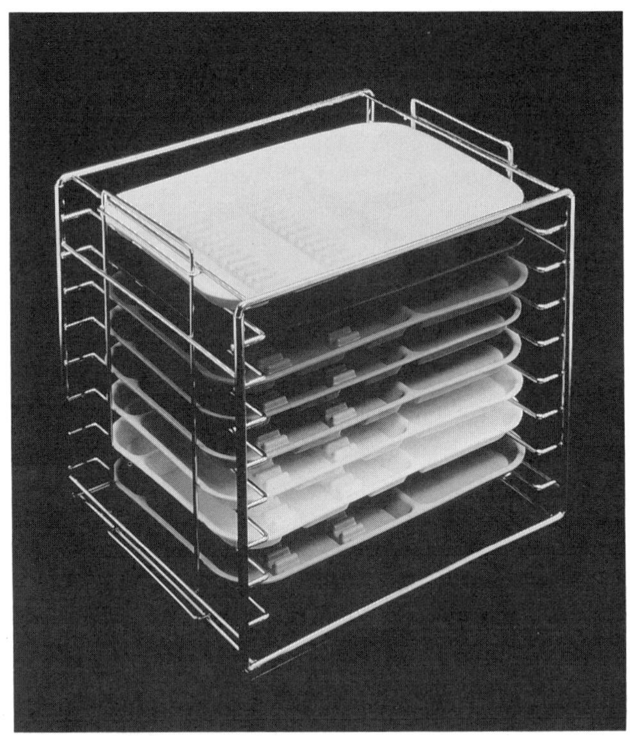

Figure 10-29. Tray rack. (*Courtesy Clive Craig Co., Los Angeles, CA.*)

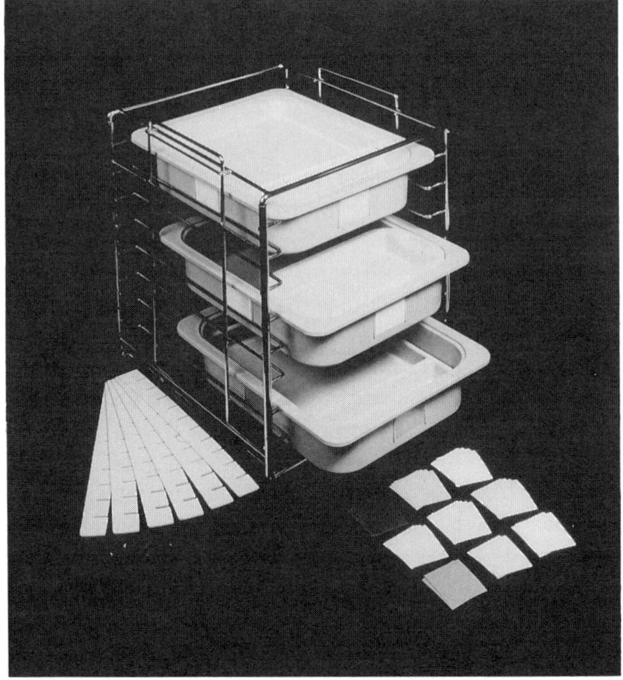

Figure 10-30. Tub rack. (*Courtesy Clive Craig Co., Los Angeles, CA.*)

Design Considerations

In addition to functional requirements, the operatory should meet certain psychological needs of the patient. A window is always desirable to give patients a psychological escape route and a pleasant view. In lieu of a window, a landscape mural or other wallcovering might be installed. A mobile suspended from the ceiling, which the patient can see while reclined in the chair, is a diversion. The dental chair and fixed casework and mobile carts should be selected in colors that coordinate with the room's interior design. Light, neutral colors used for cabinetry and dental units make them blend into the background and be less obtrusive.

Other amenities in the operatory are a hook for a handbag (located where the patient can see it), a tissue box accessible to the patient, and a waste receptacle. The choice of carpet versus hard-surface flooring is a matter of preference. Current concern about asepsis dictates a hard-surface floor; however, apart from that consideration, operatories can successfully be carpeted with a level-loop commercial nylon carpet glued directly to the floor. The flooring material should be in place and all decorating complete before the dental equipment is installed. Carpet used in dental operatories must have a synthetic backing (not jute), so that it does not rot in the event of a plumbing leak. (Jute has a vegetable dye that leaches to the surface of the carpet and stains it after exposure to moisture for a period of time.) The reader is referred to Chapter 12 for additional information.

Live plants and artwork add a nice touch to the operatory, but are an additional concern in terms of asepsis. Artwork, of course, can be framed between two pieces of Plexiglas that are sealed around the edges to make a totally smooth, cleanable surface with no frame.

Sterilization

The sterilization area should be close to the operatories and, if space permits, may be an island arrangement (see Figures 10-6 and 10-79), with access from two sides. It should be large enough for two or three people to work in it simultaneously, depending upon the number of operatories served. An area that is too small will cause stress for those who have to work there. In a small suite, sterilization can be performed in an alcove off the corridor (Figures 10-31 and 10-32).

A double sink (with a plaster trap), space for sterilization equipment, and sufficient countertop area for both a dirty and a clean side are needed. The dirty side of the sterilization area would be where trays are brought after a procedure. Disposable items would be removed and discarded, then the instruments rinsed in the sink to rid them of blood, debris, or extraneous material, after which they would be soaked in a holding solution, later rinsed in warm water, cleaned by an ultrasonic cleaner (Figure 10-33), removed and rinsed in cool water, patted or air-dried, and then wrapped or packaged for processing in a chemical sterilizer (Figure 10-34) or autoclave (Figure 10-35).

The clean side of the sterilization area would be used for setting up trays of sterilized instruments and for storage of tray setups. The sink would most commonly be located on the dirty side, and it should have a sprayer attachment. The clean side should have a 3-foot-wide kneespace desk at a 30-inch height to allow the assistant to make phone calls to order supplies or to do paperwork. One file drawer for forms and orders should suffice. Additionally, storage must be provided for clean and dirty linen, for supplies and disposables.

Tray setups can be stored in pass-through upper cabinets that open from both sides, making it unnecessary to enter the sterilization area in order to pick up

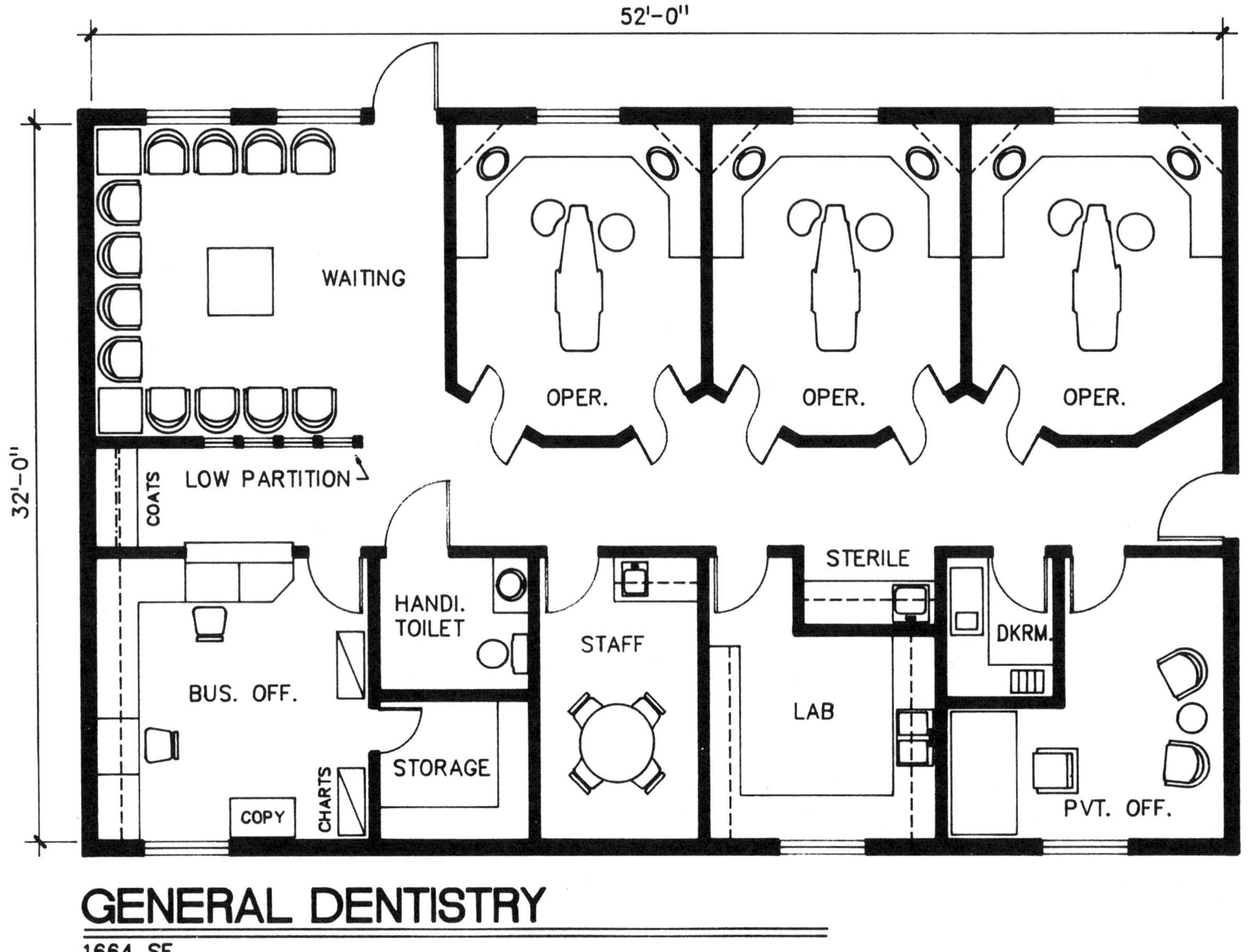

Figure 10-31. Suite plan for general dentistry, 1664 square feet.

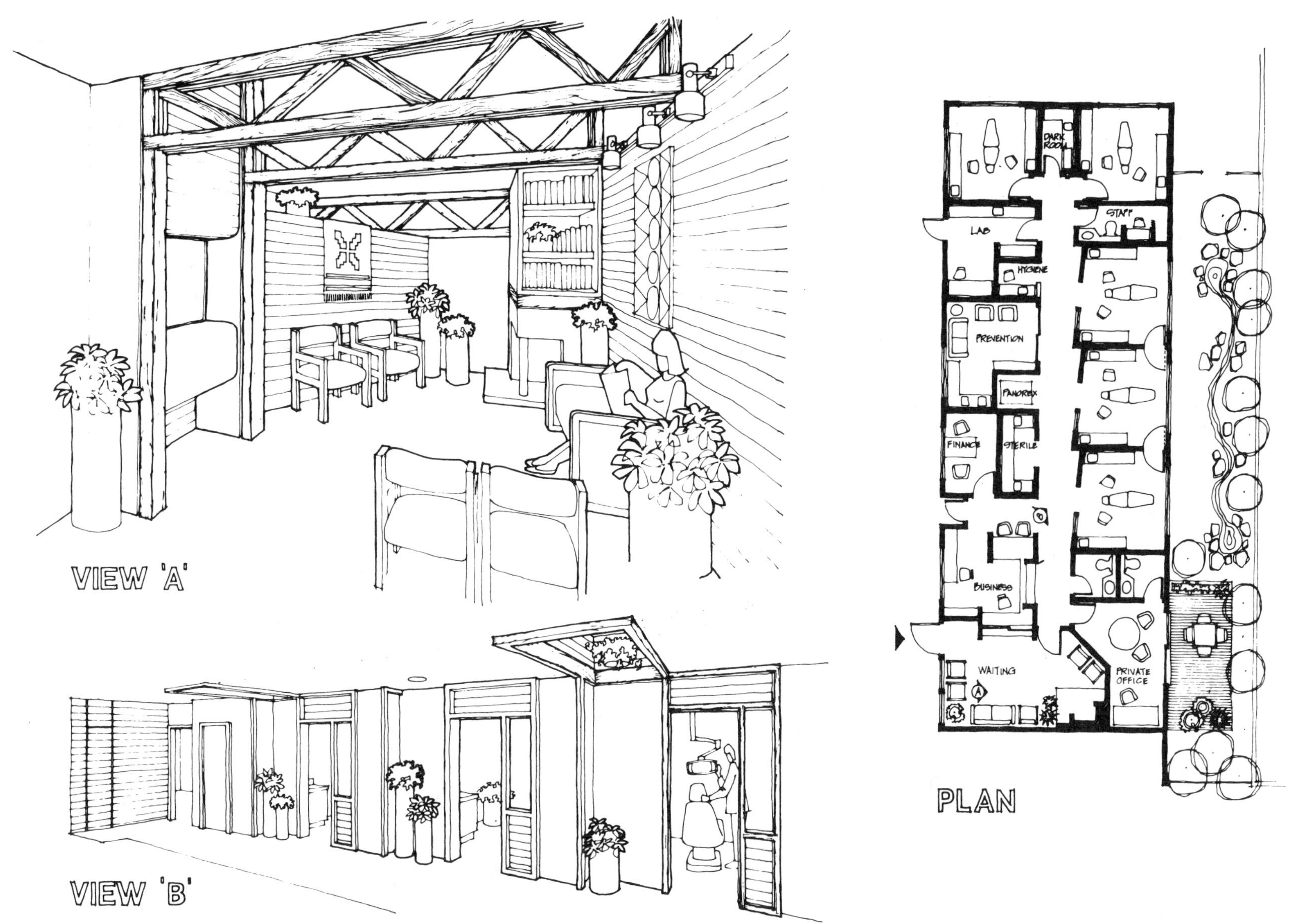

Figure 10-32. Suite plan. (*Courtesy T. Michael Hadley & Associates, AIA, Irvine, CA.*)

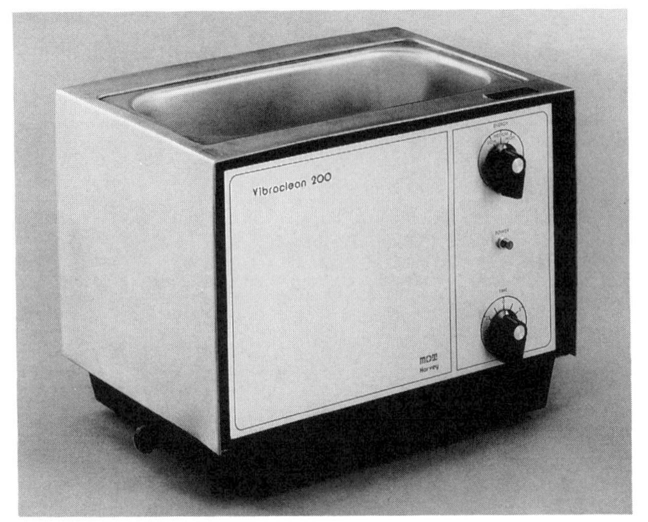

Figure 10-33. Ultrasonic cleaner. (*Courtesy MDT Corporation, Gardena, CA.*)

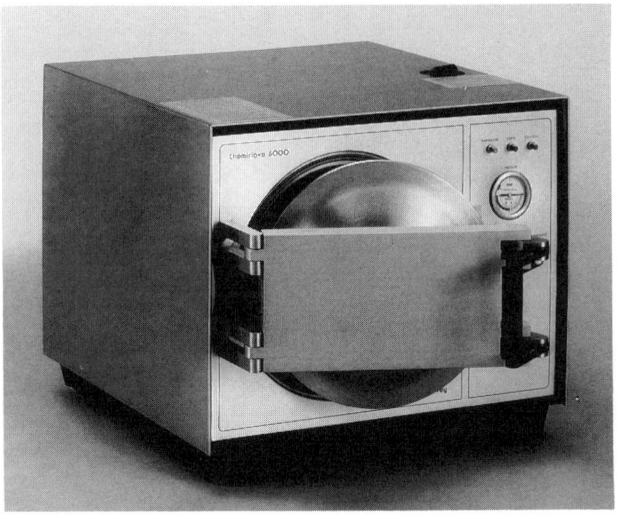

Figure 10-34. Harvey *Chemiclave* sterilizer. (*Courtesy MDT Corporation, Gardena, CA.*)

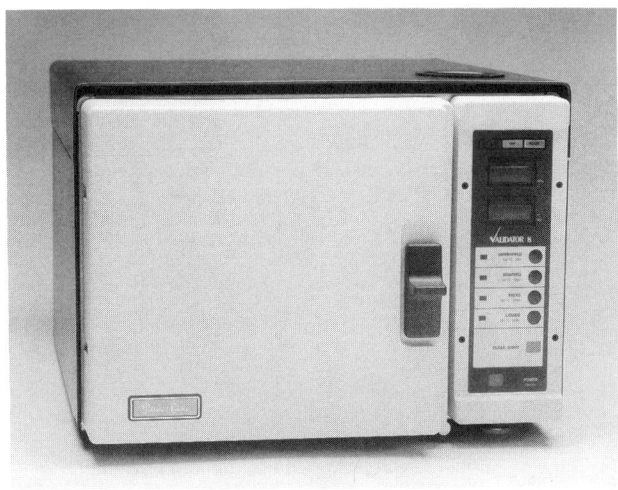

Figure 10-35. Autoclave sterilizer. (*Courtesy Pelton & Crane, Charlotte, NC.*)

a clean tray. Slots can be created within the cabinet to hold the trays or the cabinet can be designed to accommodate a prefabricated chrome rack to hold them (Figures 10-29 and 10-30).

Cassette Sterilization. This concept of sterilization, introduced a number of years ago, appears to be gaining in popularity for the 1990s. Its major advantage is the time saved by staff not having to handle instruments several times during the sterilization process.

Cassette sterilization requires that the majority of hand instruments be kept in a central sterilizing location, rather than being stored in cabinetry at each individual dental chair. Proponents of this concept feel that the simplest method of instrument transfer and sterilization involves the use of sterilization cassette systems (manufactured by Hu-Friedy Corporation). The sterilized cassettes contain all the instruments that would normally be in a tray setup. The sterilized cassette is brought into the operatory and opened, and instruments are used directly from the cassette. At the end of the procedure, dirty instruments are placed back into the individual compartments in the cassette for cleaning. The entire cassette (having drainage holes in all sides) is then placed into a powerful ultrasonic cleaning machine, after which the cassette is removed, drained, and placed into the steam or chemical sterilizer.

The advantages to the cassette system are that dental personnel have less risk of exposure to microorganisms, and time is saved in unpacking, cleaning, sterilizing, packing, and loading trays. In theory, one never has to open the cassette until it is needed in the operatory for a procedure.

Methods of Sterilization. There are various methods of sterilization, each with advantages and disadvantages, but most dentists will use an ultrasonic cleaner and a Harvey Chemiclave (unsaturated chemical vapor) or a steam autoclave.

Steam Autoclaving. This is a common form of sterilization that uses live steam under pressure. Because steam is water saturated, it has the disadvantage of rusting and corroding certain metals and dulling the cutting edge of many instruments.

Unsaturated Chemical Vapor. This method uses heat, a small amount of water, and chemicals under pressure. Because the resulting vapor is unsaturated with water, it does not harm cutting surfaces and does not rust or dull instruments. The disadvantage is that it cannot be used with liquids, certain plastics, agars, or items that cannot withstand a temperature of 131° Centigrade. The *Harvey Chemiclave* is a popular product of this type.

Dry Heat Sterilization. This procedure normally eliminates rusting and corroding caused by saturated steam, but it has limited usage because of the extremely high temperatures (350°F) and long exposure times required for each cycle (generally an hour).

A few construction issues should be noted here. With respect to electrical service, many sterilizers require a separate circuit. Regarding ventilation, steam and condensation from the sterilizer should be exhausted into the plenum or directly outdoors, if practical.

Occasionally a dentist will combine sterilization with a laboratory, provided sterilization is close to the operatories. This is not a good idea because sterilization is a cleaning process, and dental labs are dirty.

Dental Laboratory

The size of the laboratory will vary depending upon whether the dentist sends out most of the lab work or employs in-office lab technicians. If two workbenches are arranged so that they face each other, a dental engine, lathe (Figure 10-36), model trimmer (Figure 10-37), porcelain oven (Figure 10-38), casting machine, and other tools can be shared. If the workload demands it, two separate workstations could be set up so that one person does not interfere with the other. Upper cabinets should be positioned so that they are accessible to seated technicians without too much stretching. The sink should be positioned in a central location. If space is not available elsewhere, the air compressor and vacuum may be located in the lab to supply the lab and the operatories, unless it is located in a mechanical equipment room.

The type of vacuum used in the lab is a benchtop dust collector. Having no connection to the central suction used in the operatories, this small portable vacuum is used for collecting dry grinding and polishing dusts produced by the lathe or the handpieces.

The lab requires gas, compressed air, water, waste (acid-resistant drainage lines and sink with plaster trap), a plaster bin, and many electrical outlets (continuous plug strips should be mounted above the countertops). It is important to design the electrical service to accommodate the high usage requirements of various pieces of equipment. The lab may be located near the operatories to meet demands of immediate impression pouring, but if many noisy procedures are performed, it is wise to keep the lab a distance from the operatories. Since labs tend to be messy, it is desirable to have a door on the room so that patients cannot see into it.

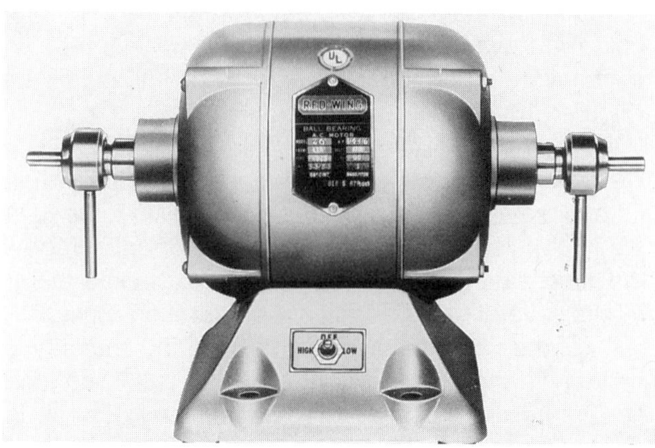

Figure 10-36. Dental lathe. (*Courtesy Handler Manufacturing Co., Inc., Westfield, NJ.*)

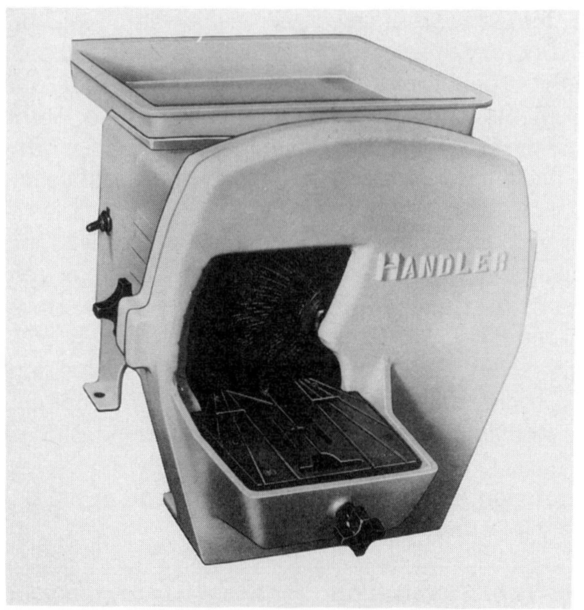

Figure 10-37. Model trimmer. (*Courtesy Handler Manufacturing Co., Inc., Westfield, NJ.*)

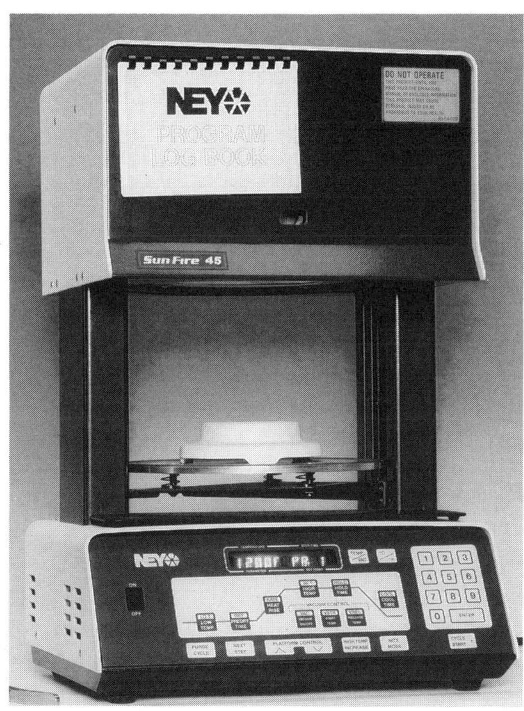

Figure 10-38. Porcelain oven. (*Courtesy J.M. Ney Co., Bloomfield, NJ.*)

Vanity Area

A mirror and shelf or vanity cabinet may be located in the corridor near the reception area if space permits. Thus a patient can comb hair or repair makeup while the receptionist is scheduling a future appointment (see Figures 10-6 and 10-27).

Patient Education

Many dentists have small patient education rooms that consist of a built-in countertop at a 29-inch height, stools or chairs, and several electrical outlets for audio-visual equipment — usually a TV monitor and VCR with videotapes. Patients may view presentations on how to floss teeth or reduce dental caries, or learn how a complicated dental procedure is performed. This saves the dentist and staff from continually having to repeat this information.

Sometimes this room is designed with freestanding furniture, which might be a table and chairs or a type of lounge seating. Oral surgeons often explain their surgical procedures in this room. Thus, the room might have a table with the surface housing a flush built-in light box for looking at X-rays and a cabinet with VCR and TV monitor (see Figure 10-76 and Color Plate 23, Figure 10-40).

Plaque Control

A plaque control room is a combination patient education/hygiene room and may be set up in different ways. One way is to equip it with two or three sinks (built into the countertop) and a wall-to-wall mirror so that a dental assistant can explain and demonstrate dental flossing and proper brushing techniques. Other offices use a standard dental chair in an operatory for this purpose.

Hygiene Operatory

The hygienist performs many duties. He or she takes X-rays, processes and mounts the film, performs dental prophylaxis, instructs patients on proper brushing and flossing techniques, discusses nutrition in regard to prevention of dental caries, and maintains the patient recall system (check-ups).

Many dentists dedicate one or more operatories to hygiene, while others schedule a hygienist perhaps two or three afternoons a week and use one of their standard operatories. In all cases, it is generally advisable to equip the hygiene operatories the same as the others. The use of antique dental chairs to reinforce a design theme should be avoided because it puts the hygienist at a functional handicap. A modern dental hygienist should have modern equipment.

Since the goal is positive reinforcement of good dental hygiene, this room should be attractively decorated so that a good impression lingers after the patient departs.

Analgesia and Anesthesia

The use of *analgesia* (medications that decrease sensitivity to pain but that do not put the patient to sleep) is not uncommon in dental practice. Local anesthetics, injected into the gum, make dentistry painless and require no special accommodation in the operatory. However, analgesia, usually a mixture of nitrous oxide (N_2O) and oxygen (O_2), requires special handling. These gases may simply be portable tanks that are wheeled into the operatory as needed or, more commonly, are centrally located in a small storage room either inside or outside of the suite and piped to each operatory. *Building and fire codes are very strict regarding where and how medical gases are to be stored.* In addition, tanks should be stored in a place that is easily accessible for servicing. Locating them near the private entrance to the suite (see Figure 10-17) allows easy exchange of tanks without the service person walking through the rest of the suite.

Medical gases stored in this manner are piped through degreased, sealed copper tubing (using only silver solder) to a flow meter in each operatory or surgery. If the tanks are stored in a remote location outside the suite, a zone shutoff valve assembly and alarm system must be located within the suite to monitor the supply. The alarm panel monitors the gas pressure and provides both an audible and visual alarm if line pressure fluctuates more than 20 percent in either direction. Nitrous tanks and valve are always placed to the left of the oxygen tanks and valve, as one faces them. This convention permits a firefighter to enter a smoky room and locate the more combustible oxygen tanks quickly.

The nitrous oxide conscious sedation system in Figure 10-41 has a clean-air scavenging system mask. One tube of the mask brings the fresh gas supply to the patient, and the other tube allows the exhaled nitrous oxide to be removed from the operatory by the central vacuum system. This eliminates the concentration of nitrous oxide in the operatory. The sedation system can be mounted in the operatory by three methods: post-mounted, wall/cabinet-mounted, or flush-mounted to a panel in the wall, as shown in Figure 10-41.

The use of *general anesthesia* (medication that puts patients to sleep) is confined mainly to oral surgeons, although intravenous sedation is also used by periodontists when doing implant surgery.

Special Plumbing and Electrical Requirements

The many variables in laying out an operatory and in selecting equipment demand close attention to the proper location of plumbing and electrical service. The space planner should work closely with a qualified, reputable dental equipment dealer in order to coordinate the location of utilities. These dealers also offer space planning services, either free with an equipment purchase, or for a small fee. It is wise to work with dealers in laying out equipment in the room. These are the people who will service the equipment after it is installed; therefore, it should be laid out according to their specifications.

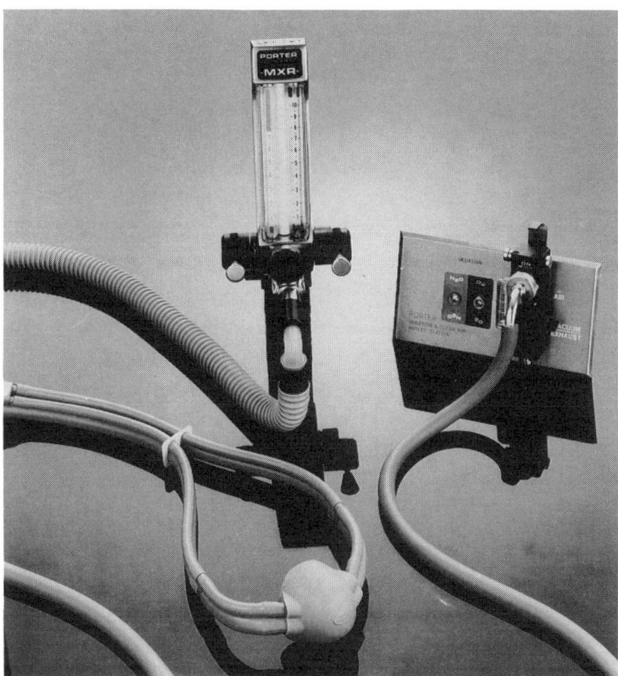

Figure 10-41. Nitrous oxide sedation system. (*Courtesy Porter Instrument Co., Hatfield, PA.*)

Most dental equipment has its own water supply and shutoff valve, but in addition, each operatory should have its own water and air shutoff valves so that repair work can be done in one operatory without closing down the entire office. The ideal location for these shutoff valves is in the cabinet under the sink in each room.

A *central water control* (solenoid valve) that will turn off all water throughout the suite should be located in the equipment room. It would be connected to a switch in the corridor near the staff entrance so that they may turn off all water at night and on weekends when they exit the suite.

Gas

Gas is used to heat certain impression materials. A dentist may want natural gas lines run into the operatories for a Bunsen burner. It is safer for the patient to locate the gas line in the rear wall behind the patient (rather than near the dental chair) to avoid hot materials dripping on the patient. Some dentists use a portable alcohol torch instead of gas, because running a gas line into a building is very expensive. Medical office buildings sometimes have a gas line in the building, and individual tenants must pay only for piping it to their suites.

Business Office

The business office of a dental suite is generally smaller than that of a similar-size medical office, since the procedures are often fewer and do not require the large amounts of paperwork associated with batteries of lab tests and X-ray films. Dental records are not as bulky as medical charts, and the X-ray films are considerably smaller.

The increasing popularity of dental insurance plans, including HMO prepaid dental plans for subscribers, may necessitate a larger business office to accommodate additional insurance and bookkeeping functions. Many dentists use computers for practice management as well as general ledger and billing. High-volume practices, such as pedodontics and orthodontics, process a lot of patients, and the business office must reflect this volume of transactions.

The file cabinet in Figure 10-42 works especially well in dental offices where it is desirable to make every foot of space count. This unit spins around in place to access filing on the two long parallel sides. The dental suite in Figure 10-78 uses this type of file cabinet.

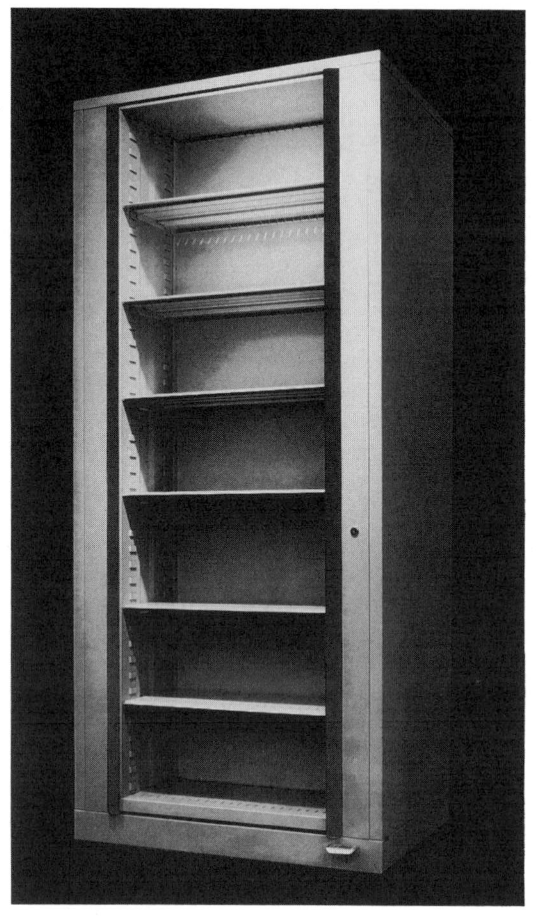

Figure 10-42. *Times-2 Speed Files. (Courtesy Richards-Wilcox/Gerard Metal Craftsmen, Gardena, CA.)*

The reader is referred to the Business Office section of Chapter 3 for a more complete discussion of this topic.

Staff Lounge

It is desirable to provide a staff lounge. This is a room, preferably with windows, where the staff can relax, have a cup of coffee, make a sandwich, and release some tension between patients' visits. This is especially important in hectic, high-volume practices and in surgical practices, where staff might be involved in long procedures. Patients can rarely assess the quality of the clinical care they receive, but they judge it, to some degree, by the attitude of the staff and the attention to detail in the interior environment. Thus, the staff must have their needs met in order to radiate good health and good cheer.

The staff lounge needs a built-in cabinet with sink and garbage disposal, under-counter refrigerator, microwave, and perhaps a cooktop. There should also be a table with chairs and perhaps some lounge seating. A closet for smocks or lab coats could be located here or in the corridor. The trend is for staff to wear uniforms only in the office; thus, dressing facilities may be a consideration.

Bathrooms

Many dentists prefer that the staff bathroom be located so that staff are not observed by patients when exiting the bathroom. The bathroom for patients might be located toward the front of the suite near the waiting room, or perhaps in the treatment area.

Waiting Room

The reader is referred to the Waiting Room section of Chapter 3 for a general discussion of waiting rooms. Dentists tend to have smaller waiting rooms than medical offices of the same square footage since the patient volume is lower. A family practice physician may see upwards of six patients per hour, while a general practice dentist may see only two or three, depending upon the complexity of the procedure and whether the appointment is primarily for examination and diagnosis or for restorative work. In cold-weather climates where people wear coats and galoshes and use umbrellas, a coat closet or coat rack should be located where it can be supervised by the business office staff. A patient should be able to enter the waiting room, proceed to the reception window to check in, then select a magazine and be seated without tripping on furniture or patients' feet.

It is important to make the patient feel like a welcome guest, rather than an intruder. To accomplish this, it is desirable to have the reception desk open without any glass and perhaps eliminate the door between the waiting room and the treatment area (see Figure 10-13). If a door is used, a French door with small panes of glass or a large panel of glass with sandblasted design would be appropriate. The reception desk should have a 42-inch-high stand-up-height shelf to provide privacy for the receptionist's work area. If it can be accomplished, the receptionist's primary work surface should be positioned so that he or she need not maintain eye contact with waiting patients, thereby being trapped into conversation.

Some dentists like patients to enter through one door, circulate through the treatment area and exit by another corridor, passing by a cashier/appointment desk on the way out. If this necessitates additional staff to separate the hello/good-bye functions, then it may not be advisable. The alternative is to provide a 42-inch-high stand-up-height shelf/desk in the exit corridor (Figures 10-6 and 10-43), allowing ample corridor width to accommodate this function. There should be a wall separating the reception area from the cashier/appointment area so that conversations about financial arrangements cannot be easily overheard by those in the waiting room.

The designer must carefully consider sound attenuation. It is advisable not to locate an operatory too close to the waiting room, so waiting patients can avoid overhearing the sound of a drill. The waiting room and corridors should have carpeting, and thought might be given to sound-absorbing wallcoverings or ceiling treatment.

Even though modern dentistry is relatively painless, many people carry with them remembrances of former times when this wasn't true. A visit to the dentist still inspires terror in many people, and the interior design of the suite should be directed toward creating a relaxing, soothing environment (Color Plate 23, Figure 10-39).

A patient wants to feel confident about being cared for by his or her dentist. If the office appears to be well organized, well cared for, with healthy live plants, and it lacks visual clutter, has current, high quality magazines, comfortable seating, and appropriate light for reading in the waiting room, chances are the patient will transfer that evidence of quality to the clinical setting.

As a rule of thumb, two seats in the waiting room should be provided for every operatory and hygiene

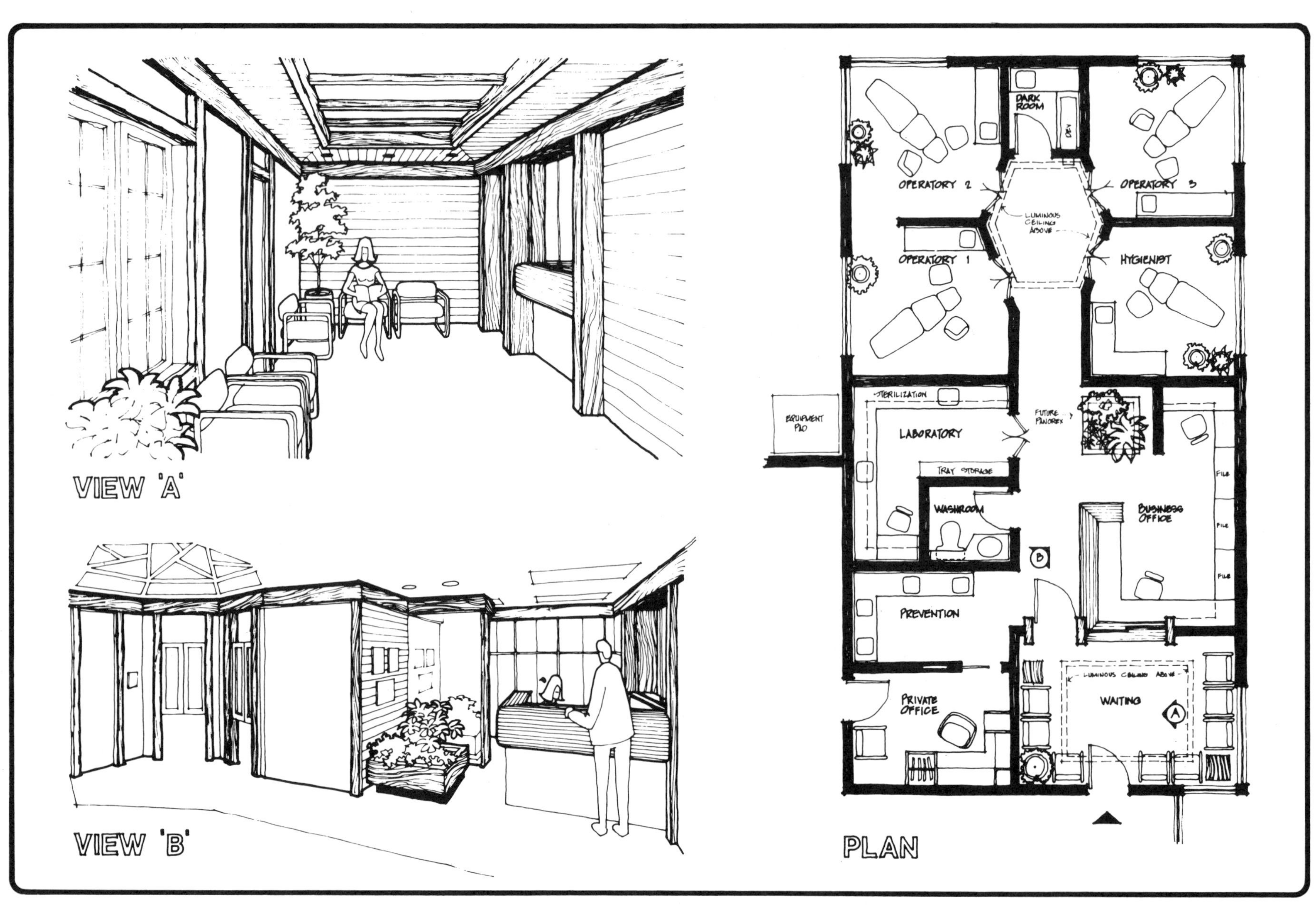

Figure 10-43. Suite plan for general dentistry. (*Courtesy T. Michael Hadley & Associates, AIA, Irvine, CA.*)

room. High-volume practices such as orthodontics and pedodontics, which are characterized by many short appointments, should have three to four seats per dental chair, if space permits.

Treatment Coordinator

Some offices have a treatment coordinator who handles patient relations and financial arrangements. In other offices, this person might be called the office manager or business manager. The duties vary, depending upon the needs of the individual practice, but generally this person manages the staff, handles any patient problems or complaints, acts as an executive assistant to the doctors, handles patient financial arrangements, and acts as office administrator. An ideal location for this office is near the reception or business office, so that when the office door is open, he or she can keep an eye on exiting patients. If a patient needs to discuss financial arrangements in privacy, the administrator's office is nearby.

This office need not be large, but must accommodate a desk, file cabinet, CRT (computer terminal), and two guest chairs. The feeling should be warm and nonthreatening.

Private Office

Dentists tend to have small private offices, sometimes as small as 8 × 10 feet. Patients rarely enter a dentist's private office, so it is used primarily to read mail, return phone calls, or relax between procedures. Sometimes, in order to save space, dentists will share a private office (see Figures 10-17 and 10-80).

X-ray

Some dentists equip all operatories for intraoral X-rays. Others confine X-rays to only one operatory or to a dedicated small room that is equipped with a panoramic X-ray, as well as an intraoral type. However, the panoramic X-ray unit is often placed in an alcove or niche in the corridor (see Figure 10-6). *Panoramic X-rays* provide a view of the complete mouth rather than just the limited area of the bitewing X-ray. This allows the dentist to assess abnormal bone configurations, cysts and tumors, impacted teeth, abscesses, TMJ problems, periodontal disease, and even sinus problems. The unit shown in Figure 10-44 requires an alcove 60 inches wide by 48 inches deep with a 90-inch minimum ceiling height. The unit can be adjusted to accommodate a patient standing or sitting. (The electrical requirements are as follows: single phase, 220 volts, 15 ampere service.)

Some dentists will have a *cephalometric* X-ray unit that provides images of the entire head and jaw different from the panoramic unit. Cephalometric X-ray units are used primarily by orthodontists. The panoramic/cephalometric X-ray unit shown in Figure 10-45 features two radiation sources, one for panoramic imaging and a separate tube-head for cephalometric radiography. It requires an alcove 80 inches wide, 48 inches deep, and a minimum ceiling height of 90 inches. X-ray facilities and the darkroom should be located near the hygienist's area.

The X-ray units shown in Figures 10-44 and 10-45 are DC (direct current), which account for less radiation scatter than AC (alternating current) units. Some manufacturers claim that there is no need to provide lead shielding in the walls, because the radiation scatter is

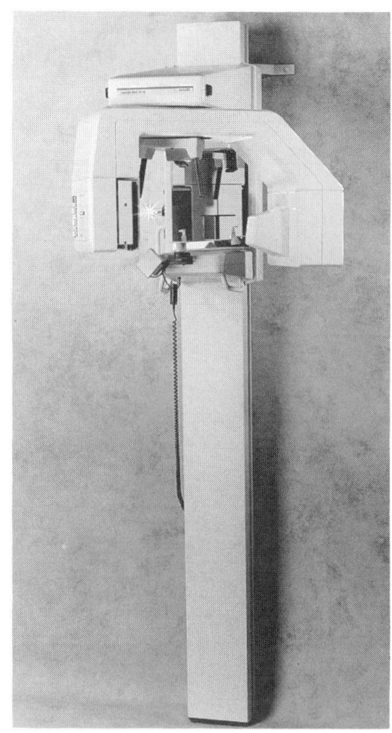

Figure 10-44. Panoramic X-ray unit. (*Courtesy Philips Dental Systems, Shelton, CT.*)

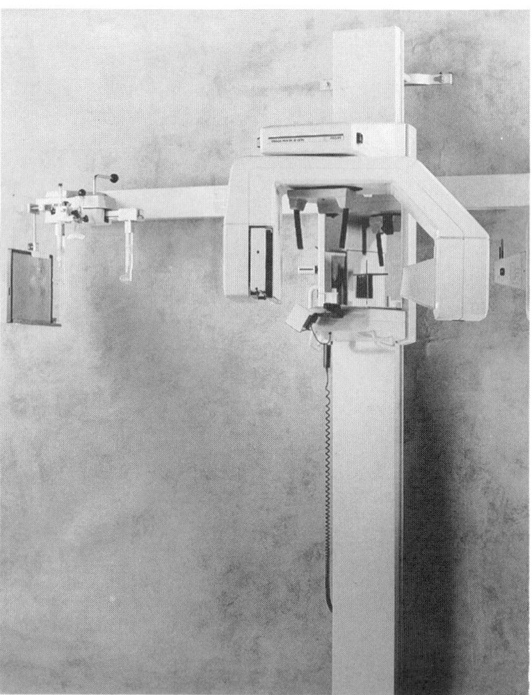

Figure 10-45. Panoramic/cephalometric X-ray unit. (*Courtesy Philips Dental Systems, Shelton, CT.*)

so minimal. They do recommend, however, two layers of gypsum board as "shielding" between rooms. These units are rated totally radiation safe at 2 meters (6 feet). In spite of this, many building codes and regulatory agencies insist on lead shielding.

If each operatory is equipped for intraoral X-rays, the X-ray head is located on the wall either to the side of the patient or, in an ambidextrous operatory, behind the patient. Sometimes an intraoral X-ray unit is shared by two operatories (Figure 10-46) by placing it in a cabinet that goes through the wall, between the operatories. The relationship of the X-ray mount to the position of the chair is critical since the arm will swing in several positions and will extend 5 or 6 feet. The wall that supports the X-ray mount must have additional reinforcement to support the weight, starting at 36 inches off the floor and terminating at a height of approximately 60 inches. The designer must check with the manufacturer or dental equipment installer to determine the proper amount of bracing for the unit.

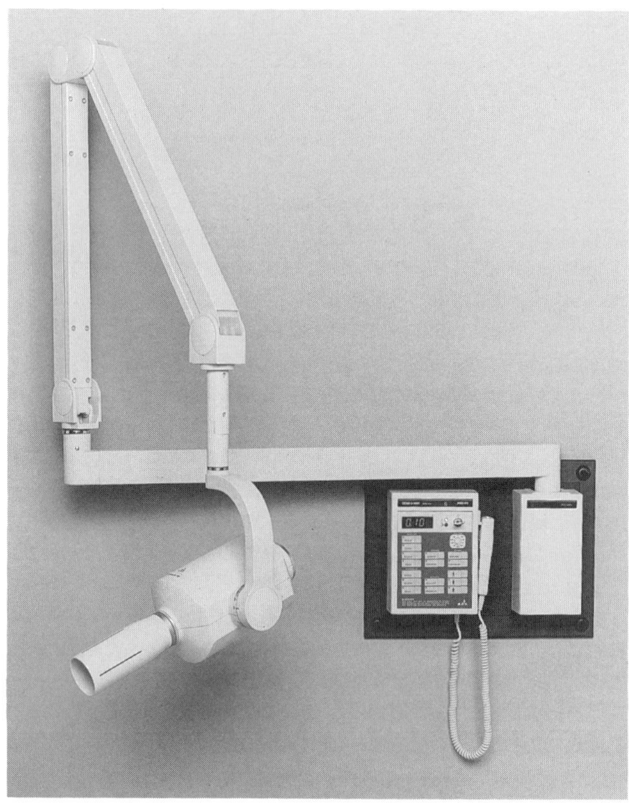

Figure 10-46. Intraoral X-ray unit. (*Courtesy Philips Dental Systems, Shelton, CT.*)

Each operatory must be equipped with an X-ray film illuminator (Figure 10-47), also called a view box. It

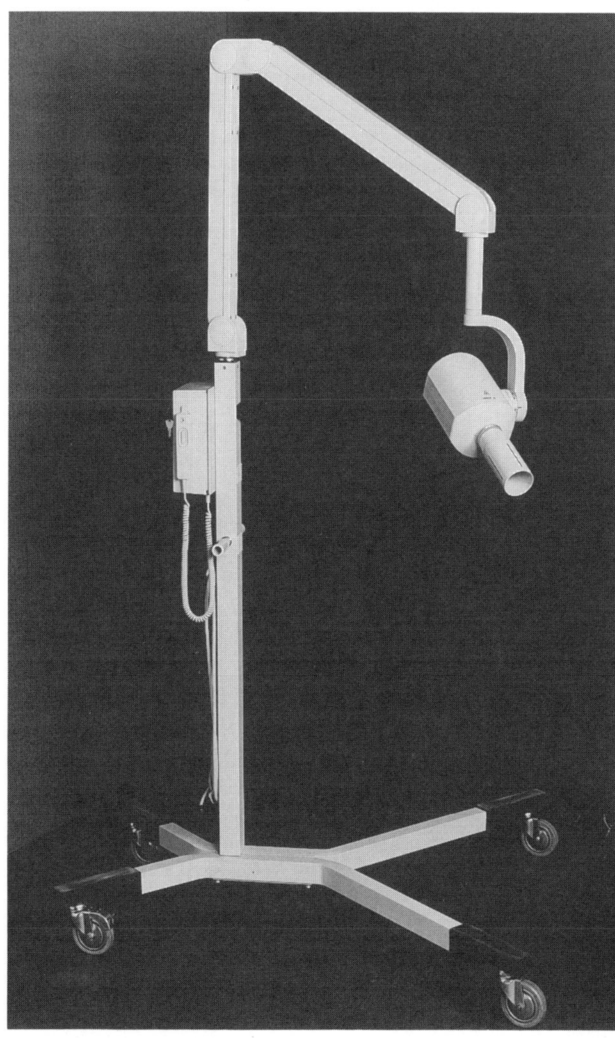

Figure 10-46a. Mobile X-ray unit. (*Courtesy Philips Dental Systems, Shelton, CT.*)

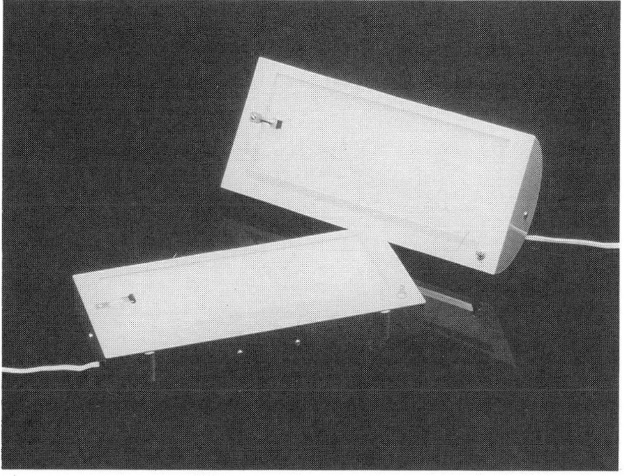

Figure 10-47. View box illuminator. (*Courtesy Clive Craig Co., Los Angeles, CA.*)

may be recessed in the wall over the fixed cabinet or it may be a portable tabletop model that sits on the counter. In custom dental cabinets, a view box may be built into the cabinet. These view boxes are small — approximately 6 × 12 inches.

Lead Shielding Requirements. Often, operatories in which intraoral X-rays are taken may not require lead shielding. However, it is always something that must be considered, and a radiation physicist must be consulted. If required, certain walls would have to be lined with lead to shield the operator and passersby from radiation scatter. The Bureau of Radiological Health or a local or state inspection agency must approve the plans and lead-shielding specifications. The physicist, in order to prepare a study, will require information on the location of the dental office within the medical building, the number of films made daily, and the type of equipment used, including the amount of radiation emitted. The radiation physicist's recommendations must then be strictly followed.

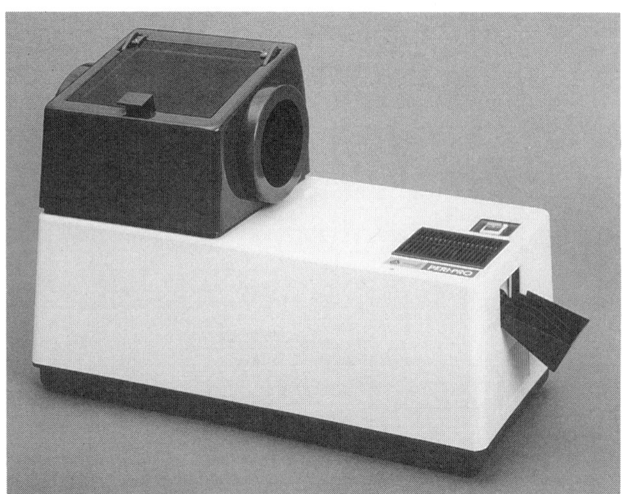

Figure 10-48. *Peri-Pro* automatic processor. (*Courtesy Air Techniques, Inc., Hicksville, NY.*)

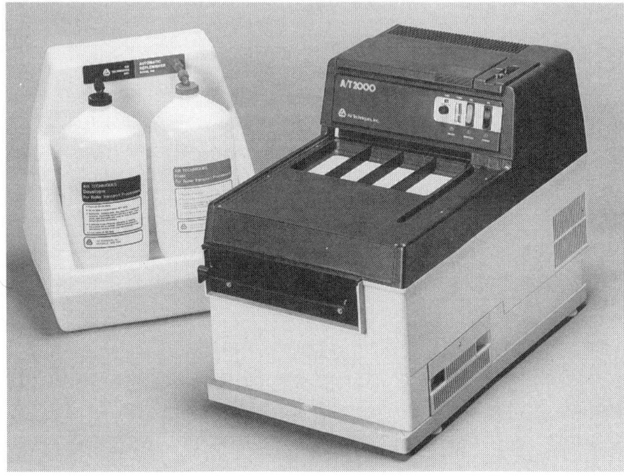

Figure 10-49. *AT/2000* automatic processor. (*Courtesy Air Techniques, Inc., Hicksville, NY.*)

Darkroom

A dental darkroom can be as small as 4 × 6 feet. Films may be developed manually or by an automatic processor. Most dentists use an automatic processor. The processor sits on a 30-inch-high counter. These are usually located in a darkroom, but most units are available with a daylight processing accessory, which allows film to be developed outside of a darkroom. In this case, the designer need provide merely a 4- × 5-foot alcove off the corridor for film processing.

The *Peri-Pro* (Figure 10-48) is a small unit 25 inches long × 10 inches deep × 8½ inches high, and it does only intraoral films. It does not require plumbing or a floor drain, because it is totally self-contained. It requires only a standard electrical outlet. The slightly larger unit, the *AT/2000* (Figure 10-49), processes intraoral, panoramic, and cephalometric films and is also available with a daylight film loader option. This unit is 15 inches wide × 25 inches deep × 18 inches high and has a small replenisher unit that sits on the countertop.

It should be noted that the daylight loader portion of the processor hangs off the edge of the countertop, requiring that the countertop be 25 inches deep. This unit does require cold water (¾-inch diameter male garden hose fitting) and an open vented drain. It does not require a floor drain, however, although local codes may require it whenever a processor has replenisher tanks. Codes vary widely with respect to waste drain requirements, and the designer must check local ordinances.

If the dentist starts out with a processor that does not require plumbing or a drain, it is advisable to plan for a future larger processor by installing a water line and drain during the general construction of the suite. It should be noted that the fixer and developer generally go down the waste drain, unless local codes prevent it. In some cities, the chemicals have to be collected in containers.

There should be a small area for storage in the darkroom or the processing alcove for bottles of developer and fixer. These plastic bottles are 1-quart size for the Peri-Pro and ½-gallon size for the AT-2000. There will also be a need to store packages of film. Unlike medical X-ray film, dental X-ray film is stored in lead-lined dispensing units, which are either wall-mounted in the operatory or stored in a drawer. Refrigerated storage for unexposed film should be provided if quantity purchasing of film is to be considered.

As with any processor, there needs to be a deep sink for occasionally washing the rollers (Figure 10-50). Perhaps it can be located under a hinged countertop, so that the sink is out of the way when not in use. The sink should be equipped with a sprayer. It is not necessary to provide backup manual tanks for duplicating X-rays. The daylight loader accessory is available with a film duplicator or dual-pack film can be exposed at the same time, providing a second copy at minimal expense.

Darkrooms often have a floor drain for overflow, but it really isn't needed with this type of automatic processor, although codes may require it for all processors. The darkroom or processing alcove should have an exhaust fan, and codes may require that the darkroom door have a lightproof louver ventilation panel. A darkroom door usually opens inward so that if someone tries to enter while developing is in process, the technician can put a foot against the door to prevent it. Darkrooms may have a red warning light over the door that is activated when the exhaust fan is started, and the safelight goes on inside the darkroom. A darkroom door need be only 24 inches wide functionally (however, codes for the handicapped stipulate a 36-inch width for all doors), and it must have a lightproof seal.

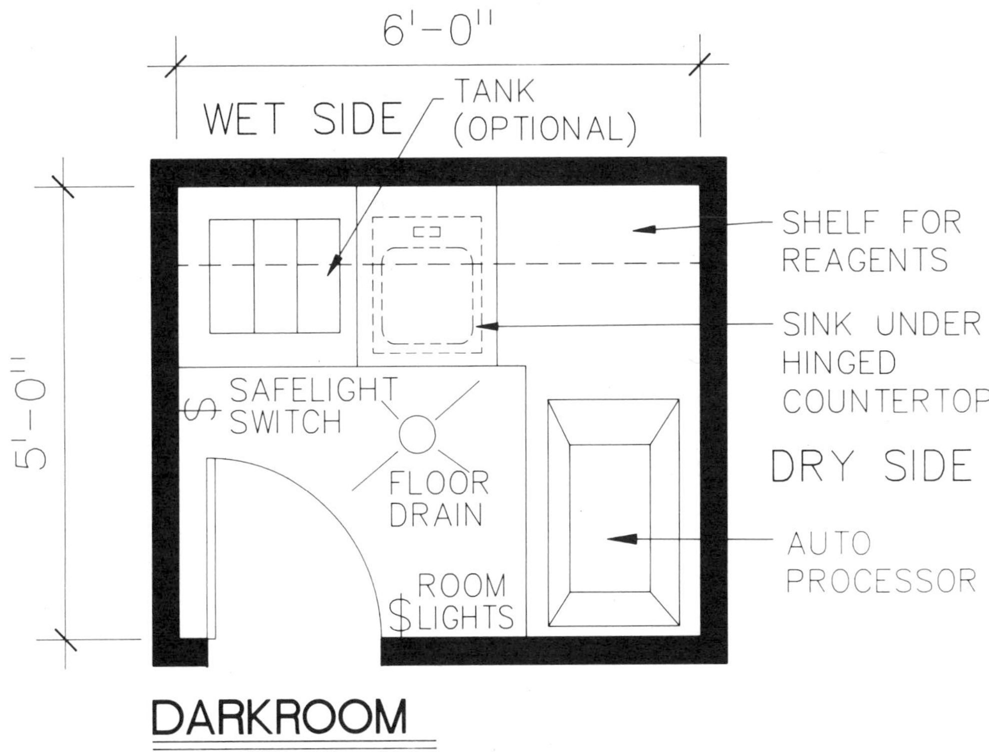

Figure 10-50. Layout of darkroom.

The darkroom must have two sources of light. A 100-watt incandescent light, either recessed or surface-mounted to the ceiling, for general work, and a safelight for working with exposed film. The safelight can be plugged into an outlet at 60 to 72 inches off the floor, and it can be activated by a pull chain or be wired into a wall switch. If the latter, the switch should be located away from the incandescent light switch so that the technician does not accidentally flip the wrong one while film is exposed. *Any recessed light fixtures, as well as the exhaust fan, must have light-sealed housings.*

A small viewing and sorting area should be provided outside the darkroom. This may consist of only a shelf with a view box illuminator for the technician to check the films.

Manual Processing. The requirements for manual processing are hot and cold water with a temperature control valve, a waste drain in the floor near the tanks, and a sink. The room should be set up with a wet and dry side (Figure 10-50) and should have two 4- to 5-foot-long counters either parallel to each other or at right angles. The wet side contains the sink and developing tank, while the dry side is used for loading and unloading film. Films may be hung in a rack over the wet side to air-dry or placed in an electric film dryer. The film dryer may be a countertop model or under-counter model. Either type requires an electrical outlet. A darkroom needs a timer, either electric or spring-loaded (wound manually). One outlet should be provided over the counter on both the wet and dry sides.

Normally countertops in a darkroom are 36 to 42 inches high, depending on personal preference. *Thirty inches is the maximum height if using an automatic processor.* A 6- to 10-inch-deep shelf mounted 14 inches above the countertop is convenient for bottles of X-ray chemicals. There is no need for closed storage in a darkroom. All shelves should be open.

A note of caution: Local codes normally require a vacuum breaker on piping to all darkroom tanks to prevent chemical waste from backing up into the water supply. (Temperature control valves sometimes have a built-in vacuum breaker.) Also, acid-resistant pipe is recommended since chemical waste is very corrosive.

Endodontists have a special need for manual processing of *working* X-rays. These are films made during the procedure to guide the dentist during treatment. Automatic processing takes too long to develop each of these single films, so the chairside assistant often slips into the darkroom, dips the film into small jars of chemicals and, in 30 seconds, has a processed film.

Lighting

Good lighting is mandatory in a dental operatory. It is critical to use full spectrum fluorescent lamps with a color rendering index (CRI) of 90 or more. The illumination should be free of shadows, and a *brightness ratio* of 10:1 should be maintained with the operating light. The operating light may slide in a track mounted in the ceiling (Figure 10-51), or it may be post-mounted to the dental chair (Figure 10-52). The quartz halogen operating light delivers a concentrated 1200 to 2500 footcandles of illumination at the oral cavity.

Thus the work counters and visual background of the room must receive 200 to 250 maintained footcandles to achieve a 10:1 brightness ratio with the 2500-footcandle operating light. Three four-lamp, surface-mounted fluorescent luminaires arranged in a U-shape around the chair (Figure 10-53) will meet this requirement. The reflectance of the floor, walls, and ceiling have an impact on the amount of perceived illumination, as will the ceiling height, the size and shape of the room, and the location of upper cabinets, if any.

Indirect fluorescent lighting around the perimeter of the room is aesthetically pleasing and keeps glare out

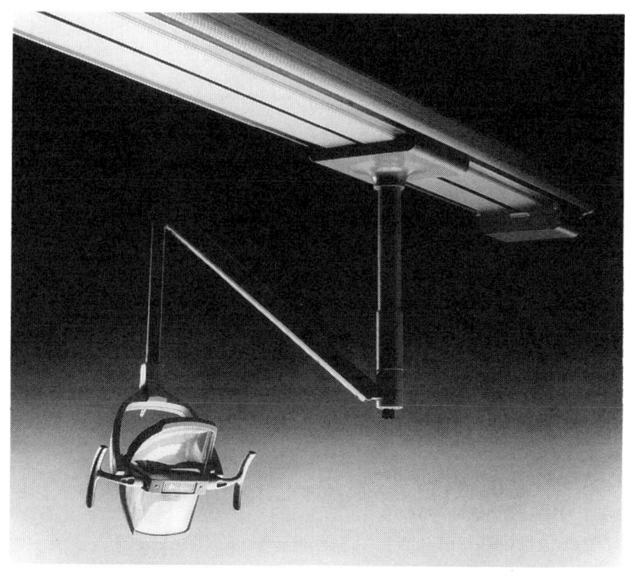

Figure 10-51. Track-mounted dental light. (*Courtesy Pelton & Crane, Charlotte, NC.*)

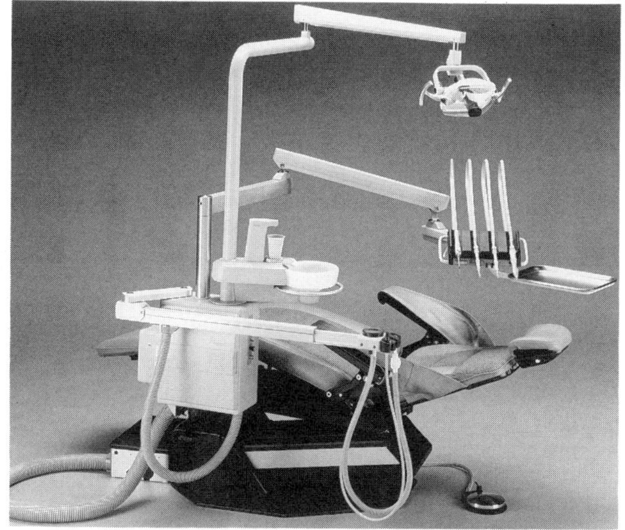

Figure 10-52. Dental light, post-mounted. (*Courtesy A-dec, Inc., Newberg, OR.*)

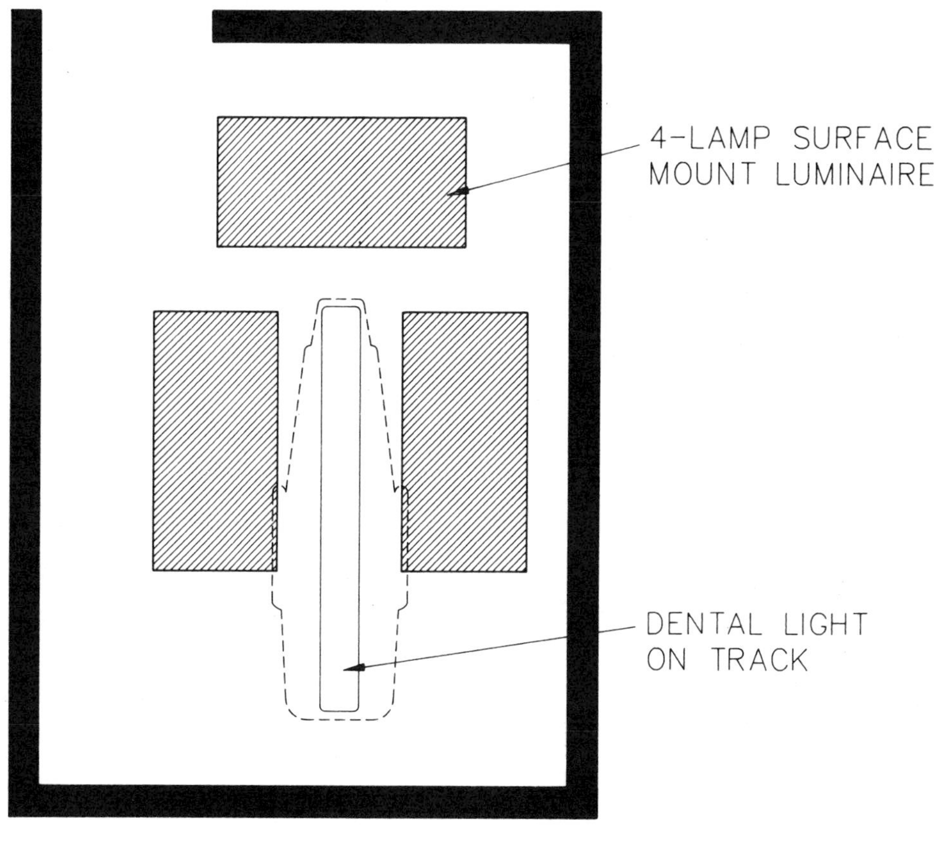

Figure 10-53. Operatory reflected ceiling plan.

of the patient's eyes. However, the number of lamps must still yield the 10:1 brightness ratio. This type of lighting lends itself to a self-contained individual room not broken by many openings and doors.

Dentists who use fiber-optic lights on their drills require bright rooms to prevent "optical bounce," a term that refers to the extreme opening and shutting of the iris of the eye due to extreme lighting differences. Optical bounce causes headaches and eye strain as the dentist shifts focus from a bright mouth to an overly dark room.

Operatories should not have busy wallcoverings with intense colors because the rooms are small, and reflection of the colors will make it difficult to match shades of teeth. Soft colors and patterns with little contrast reduce eye fatigue and make the room seem less confining. Many dentists prefer a northern exposure for shade matching in natural light.

Communication Systems

Many small offices do not have a communication system other than the telephone. In the interests of efficiency, however, a special system can save steps and reduce foot traffic. There are various types of communication systems available. Dealers who sell and install them can tailor a system to the needs of the individual office.

Telephone Intercom. The most basic system is the intercom button on the telephone. Each room would have to have a telephone to have the intercom facility. While this enables the receptionist to speak privately to the dentist in an operatory, it really does not fulfill the primary requirements for communication within a dental office.

Loudspeaker. This has the advantage that the dentist does not physically have to touch a telephone to receive a message, but it is unsatisfactory because it is noisy, and patients can hear messages. Also, it does not tell the dentist in which room the next patient is waiting.

Colored Signal Lights. A small panel of signal lights is mounted over operatory doors, in the lab, and in the sterilizing area, with a control panel in the business office and in the operatories. This system can tell the dentist which room to go to next or whether a phone call or emergency is awaiting his or her attention. It also provides a light to signal that the dentist needs assistance. The limitation of this system is that the lights may go unnoticed.

Buzzers and Chimes. A simple system of communication consists of a soft buzzer to indicate that the dentist needs assistance (and, if there are not more than three operatories, the room number might be indicated by the number of buzzes), and a chime to signal that the next patient is ready. In a small office, the staff knows which operatory the dentist is in, and the dentist usually knows in which operatory the next patient can be found without relying upon an auditory signal. However, this system is noisy and limited by the number of distinguishable sounds.

Combination System. The most effective communication system for a large office is a combination of all the above. A chime can be used for the phone. Signal lights, combined with a soft buzzer to call attention to the lights, can be used to indicate which dentist is in which operatory, tell the dentist which patient is next, to inform the staff of emergencies, direct staff without knowing where they are, inform staff of phone calls, allow staff to reply silently, and signal the number of patients awaiting each doctor. These systems may have quite sophisticated electronic design. Those that are microprocessor-controlled may be programmed for the communication needs of an individual practice. Figure 10-54 shows various models of these units.

Equipment Room

The space planner needs to think about locating the hot water heater, telephone terminal panel, medical gases, air compressor, vacuum pump, and provision for natural gas.

If the dental suite is located in a medical office building, occasionally there is a central mechanical equipment room on each floor to serve the tenants. This may allow the air compressor and vacuum pump to be housed in a remote location and piped to the dental suite, eliminating machinery noise and saving the tenant rent on square footage for a utility room within the suite. The building may also have a provision for natural gas, saving the tenant the cost of running a gas line into the building.

If the dental suite is located in a professional office building not specifically planned to accommodate dentists, the tenant usually has to bear the expense of piping gas into the building and allotting a room within the suite for the installation of equipment.

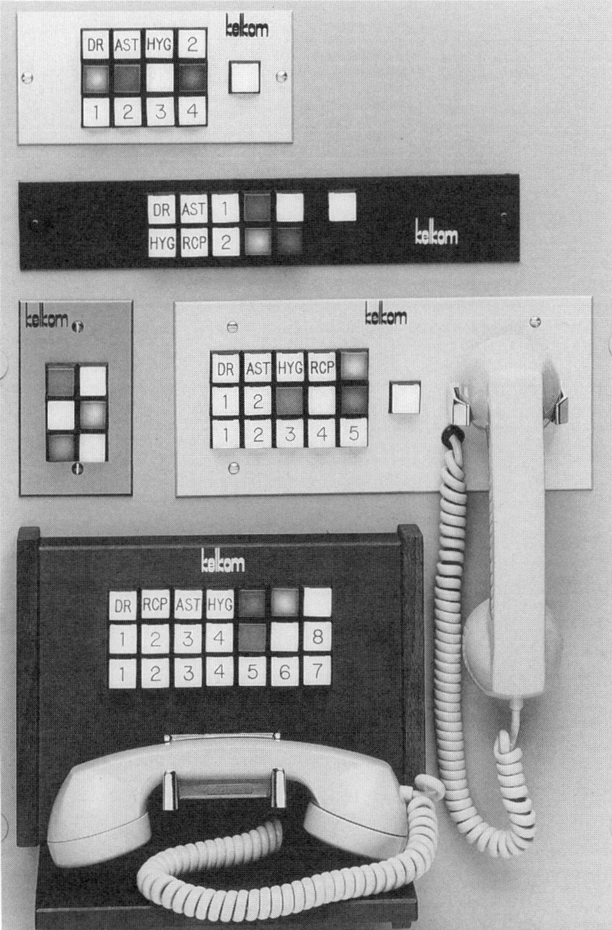

Figure 10-54. Communication systems. (*Courtesy Kelkom Systems, Redwood City, CA.*)

Table 10-2. Analysis of Program. Orthodontics

No. of Orthodontists:	1				2			
Waiting Room	14	× 20	=	280	16	× 22	=	352
Business Office/Recept.	12	× 16	=	192	12	× 16	=	192
Bookkeeping/Business Manager	10	× 12	=	120	10	× 12	=	120
Operatory Bay (4 chairs)	12	× 24	=	288	(9 chairs) 12	× 51	=	612
Quiet Room/X-ray	9-1/2	× 11-1/2	=	109	9-1/2	× 11-1/2	=	109
Audiovisual/Patient Education	6	× 12	=	72	6	× 12	=	72
Lab	8	× 12	=	96	8	× 12	=	96
Sterilizing Alcove	6	× 8	=	48	8	× 8	=	64
Darkroom	4	× 6	=	24	4	× 6	=	24
Staff Lounge	8	× 12	=	96	10	× 12	=	120
Toilet Rooms	2 @ 6	× 7	=	84	2 @ 6	× 7	=	84
Panoramic/Ceph X-ray	5	× 8	=	40	5	× 8	=	40
Private Office	10	× 12	=	120	2 @ 10	× 12	=	240
Storage	6	× 8	=	48	6	× 8	=	48
Mechanical Equipment Room	6	× 8	=	48	6	× 8	=	48
Subtotal				1665 ft²				2221 ft²
15% Circulation				250				333
Total				1915 ft²				2554 ft²

ORTHODONTICS

Orthodontics is the branch of dentistry that deals with straightening teeth and correcting bad bites (malocclusions). The majority of patients are children aged 12 to 18, although a sizable number of adults now avail themselves of these services. The orthodontic process is slow, often necessitating monthly visits for years.

Circulation

On the initial visit, the child is examined, and the orthodontist discusses the course of treatment with the parents in the private office. Some orthodontists have an elaborate office for making case presentations that includes a sliding panel which conceals a projection screen, operated by a remote control near the desk. The remote can control room lights and projector, as well. The room should also contain an illuminator for X-ray viewing, and perhaps a countertop for a VCR unit for patient education. The private office or consultation room should be comfortably furnished and have a pleasant ambience.

On subsequent visits the patient proceeds to a tooth brushing vanity and then to the operatory. After the first few visits, during which the major work is done, monthly follow-up visits are short. Orthodontics is a high-volume practice that benefits from a waiting room able to accommodate a large number of patients. Three or four seats should be provided for each dental chair, if space permits.

Operatory Bay

Orthodontists do most of their treatment in a large, communal operatory called a "bay," in which three to eight chairs are arranged with no separating walls between them. If space permits, the chairs may be arranged like spokes of a wheel with a sterilization station in the hub (Figures 10-55, 10-56, and Color Plate 24, Figure 10-57). But often chairs are arranged in a row parallel to each other (Figures 10-58, 10-59, and Color Plate 26, Figure 10-67). Chairs should be 3 feet from a wall, with 4 feet separating them from one another.

The location of fixed and mobile cabinets is critical so the orthodontist and assistant are able to move quickly from one patient to the next with instruments always within reach. The dental units, cabinetry, patient chairs, and dentist's and assistant's stools in Figure 10-59 are functional and have an uncluttered appearance. Even though the room has a great deal of cabinetry, the neutral color and clean lines keep it from dominating the room.

Orthodontists do not use as many dynamic instruments as general dentists, and it is not uncommon to see custom designed cabinets to the side or rear of the patient chair with instrumentation built-in. (Orthodontists do not use a high-speed handpiece.) The style of delivery is often over-the-patient, but could be rear delivery. Neither nitrous oxide nor oxygen would be needed, only suction and air.

In addition to the operatory bay, the orthodontist usually has a standard individual operatory, often referred to as a "quiet room," in which he or she may take X-rays, do the initial diagnostic examination, work on a noisy or obstreperous child, or treat an adult patient. This operatory may have special equipment lacking in the orthodontic units in the bay (Figure 10-60).

Laboratory

The laboratory should be large, with a storage bin for plaster and storage for the considerable number of plaster models accumulated. Sometimes as many as 4000 models, stored in cardboard boxes 3 × 3 × 3 inches, must be accommodated in the lab, or elsewhere in the suite, on shallow shelves. The reader is referred to the General Dentistry section of this chapter for further discussion of a dental laboratory.

Other Rooms

An orthodontist's office would have panoramic and cephalometric X-ray units, a darkroom, two toilet rooms, a fairly large business office, an audiovisual room and, perhaps, a private office for a bookkeeper or office manager. The reader is referred to the General Dentistry section of this chapter for layout information on X-ray units.

Waiting Room

The waiting room of an orthodontic office may be treated with great imagination since the patients are, for the most part, teenagers who often appreciate an office designed around a theme.

Figure 10-61 shows a waiting room designed several years ago with carpet-covered plywood platforms instead of individual chairs to increase seating capacity in an undersized room and, at the same time, appeal to the teenagers' preference for lounging about, rather than sitting upright in a chair. The walls are Levi blue denim and carry photo blowups of children in various stages of orthodontia — before (with crooked teeth), during (with the rubber bands and braces), and after (with straight teeth and beautiful smiles). The room, although unconventional, was a huge success and contributed to the orthodontist's popularity and the rapid growth of his practice. To further add architectural interest to the room, an artificial skylight fixture was centered over the platforms.

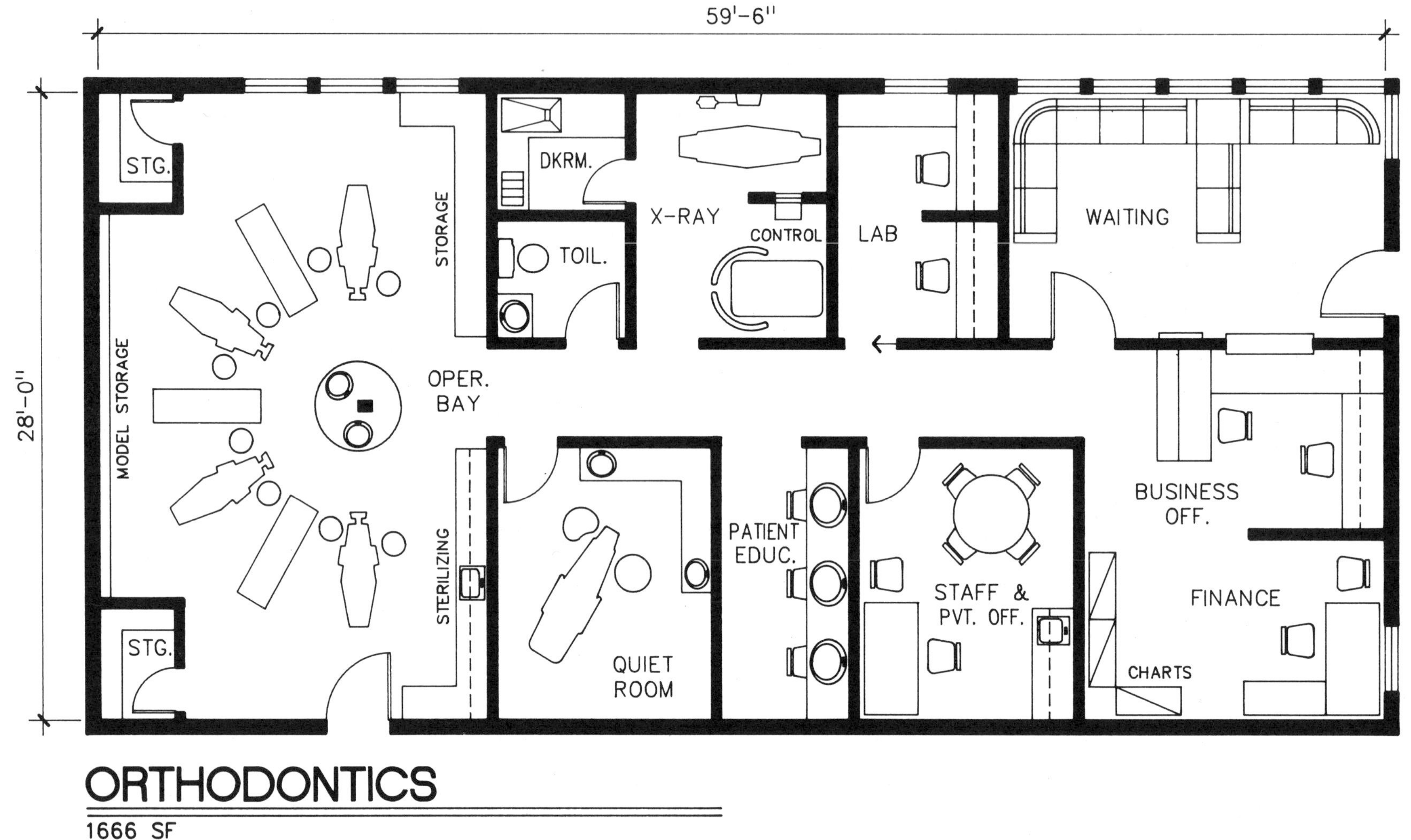

Figure 10-55. Suite plane for orthodontics, 1666 square feet.

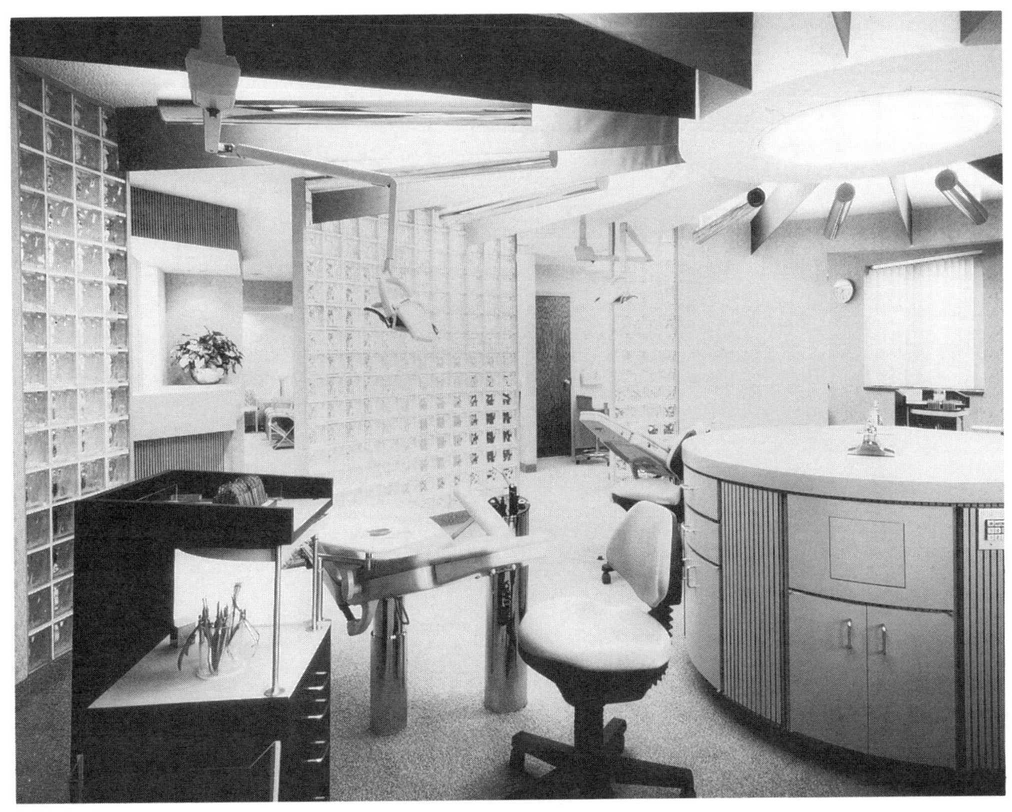

Figure 10-56. Orthodontic treatment bay. (*Courtesy Sue Walling, SW Design, Inc., Minneapolis, MN; Photographer: P.R. Siegrist.*)

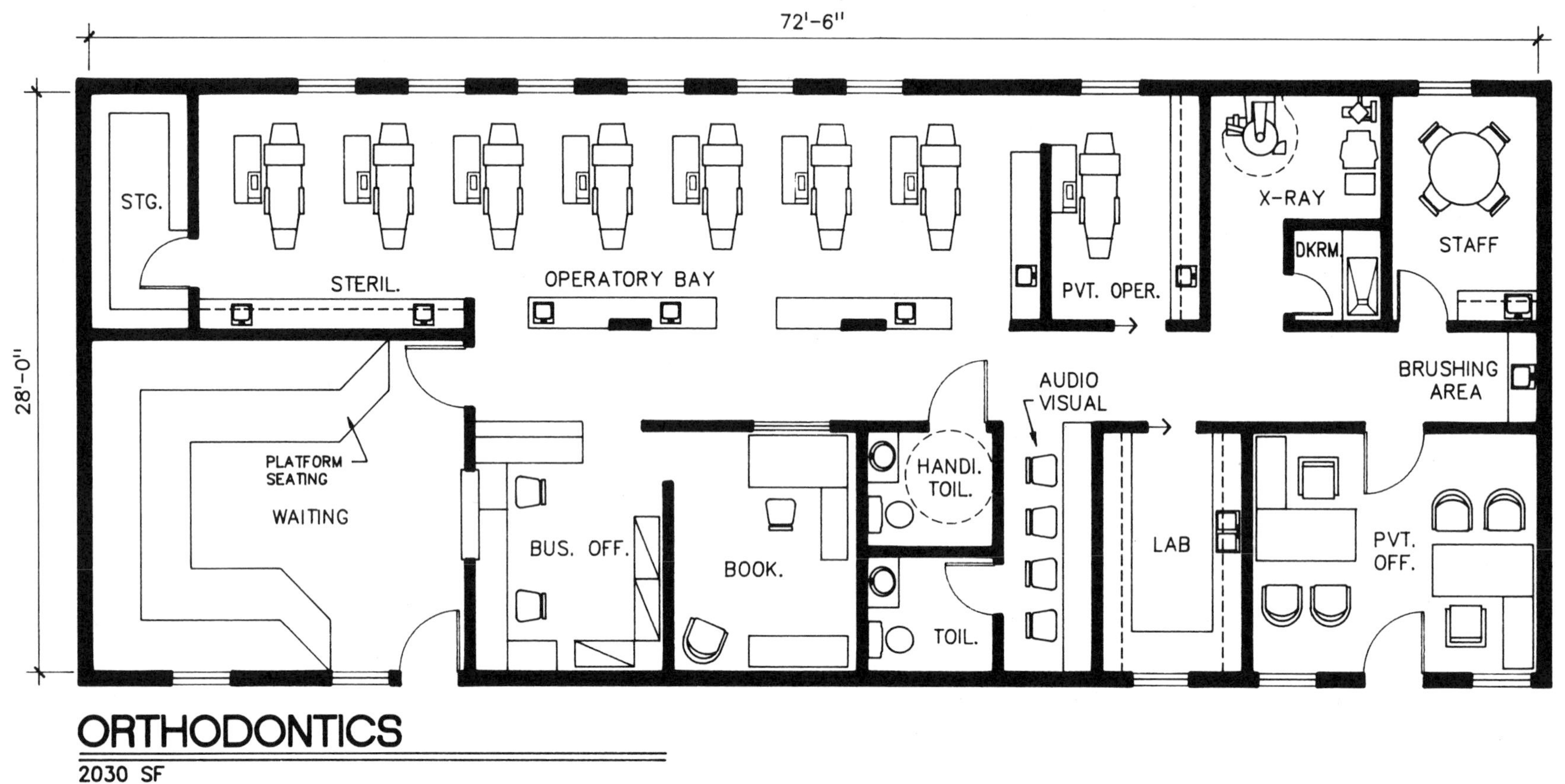

Figure 10-58. Suite plan for orthodontics, 2030 square feet.

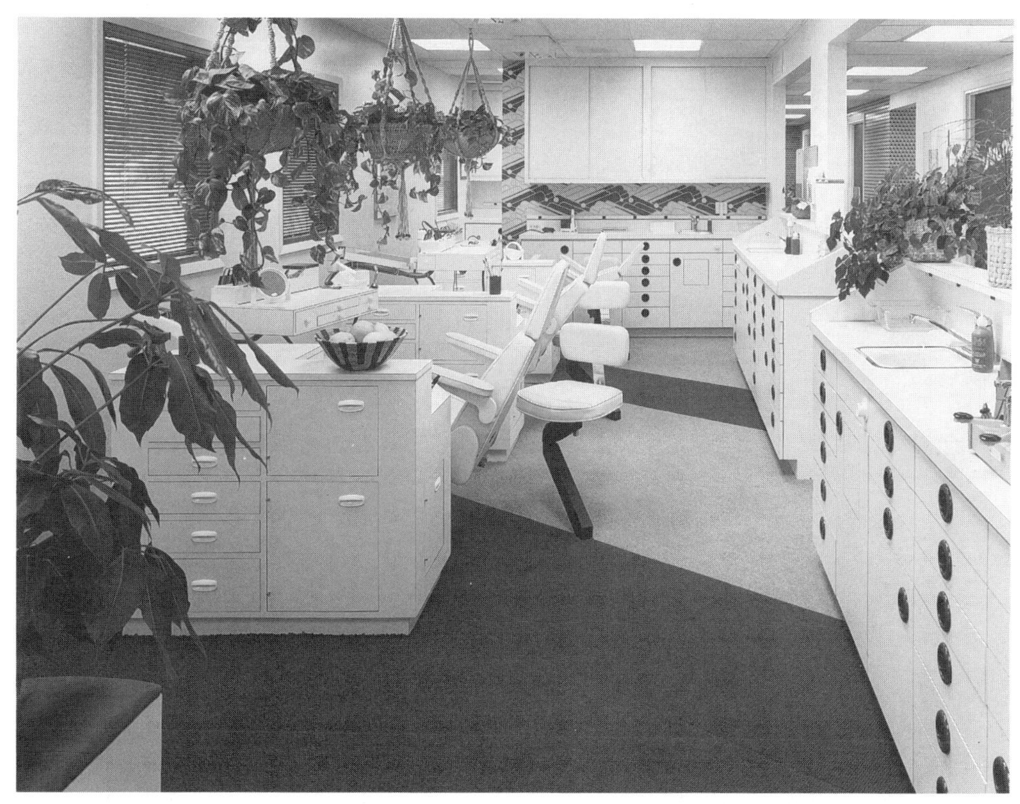

Figure 10-59. Orthodontic bay. (*Design: Jain Malkin Inc.; Photographer: Michael Denny.*)

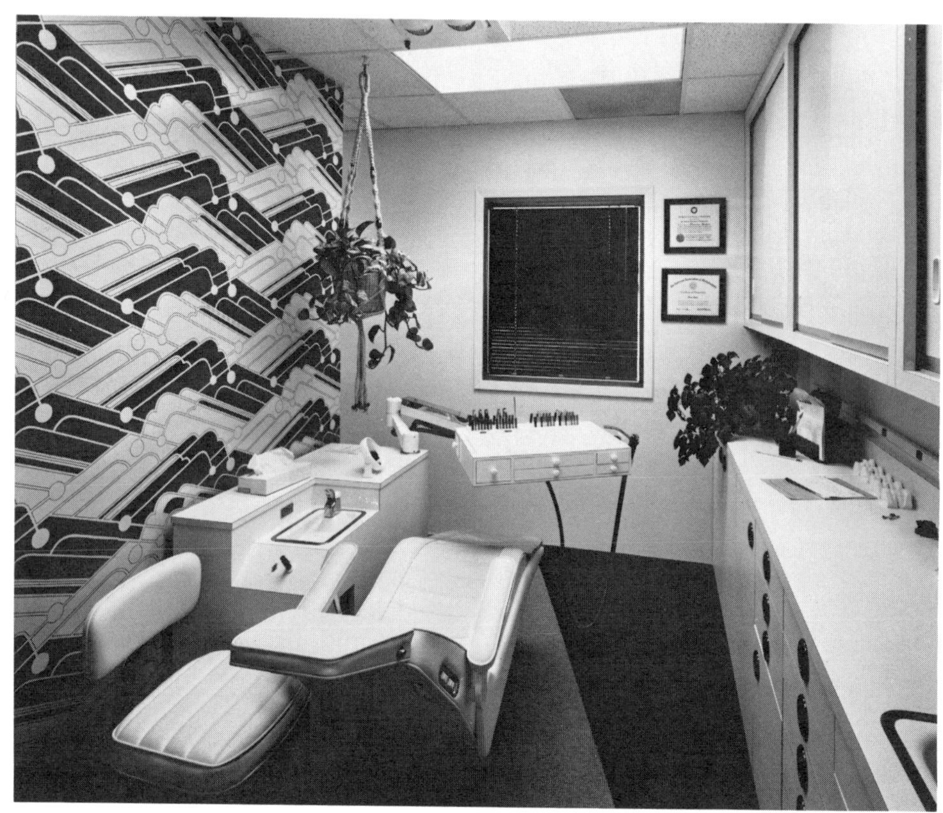

Figure 10-60. Quiet room. (*Courtesy Jain Malkin Inc.*)

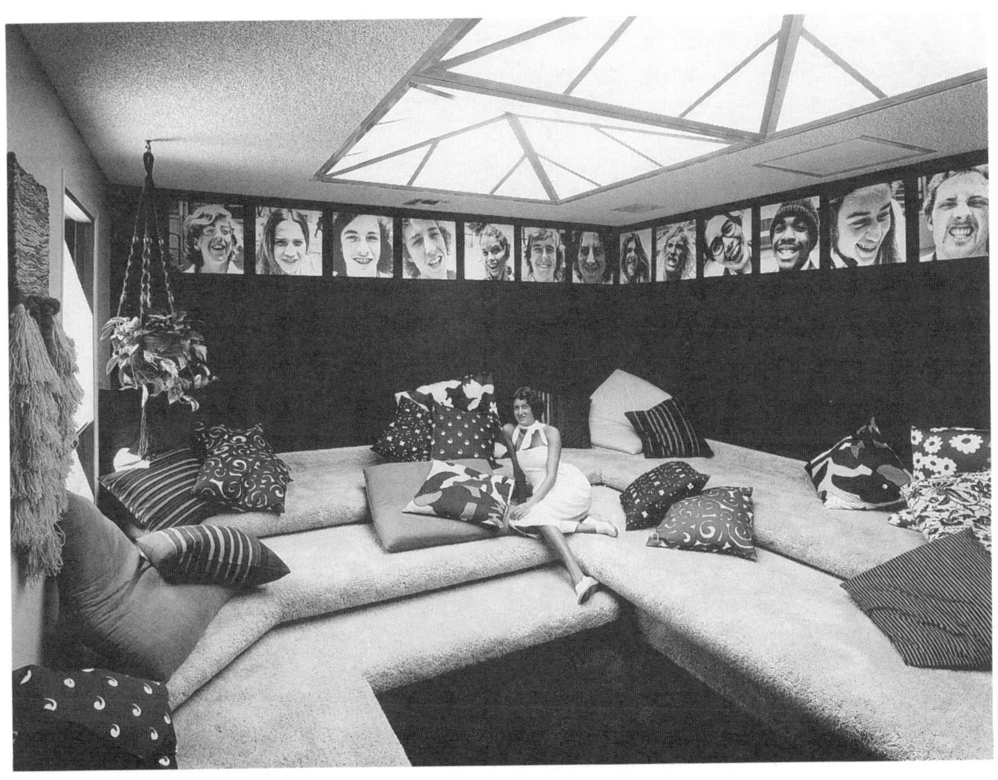

Figure 10-61. Waiting room, orthodontics. (*Design: Jain Malkin Inc.; Photographer: Michael Denny.*)

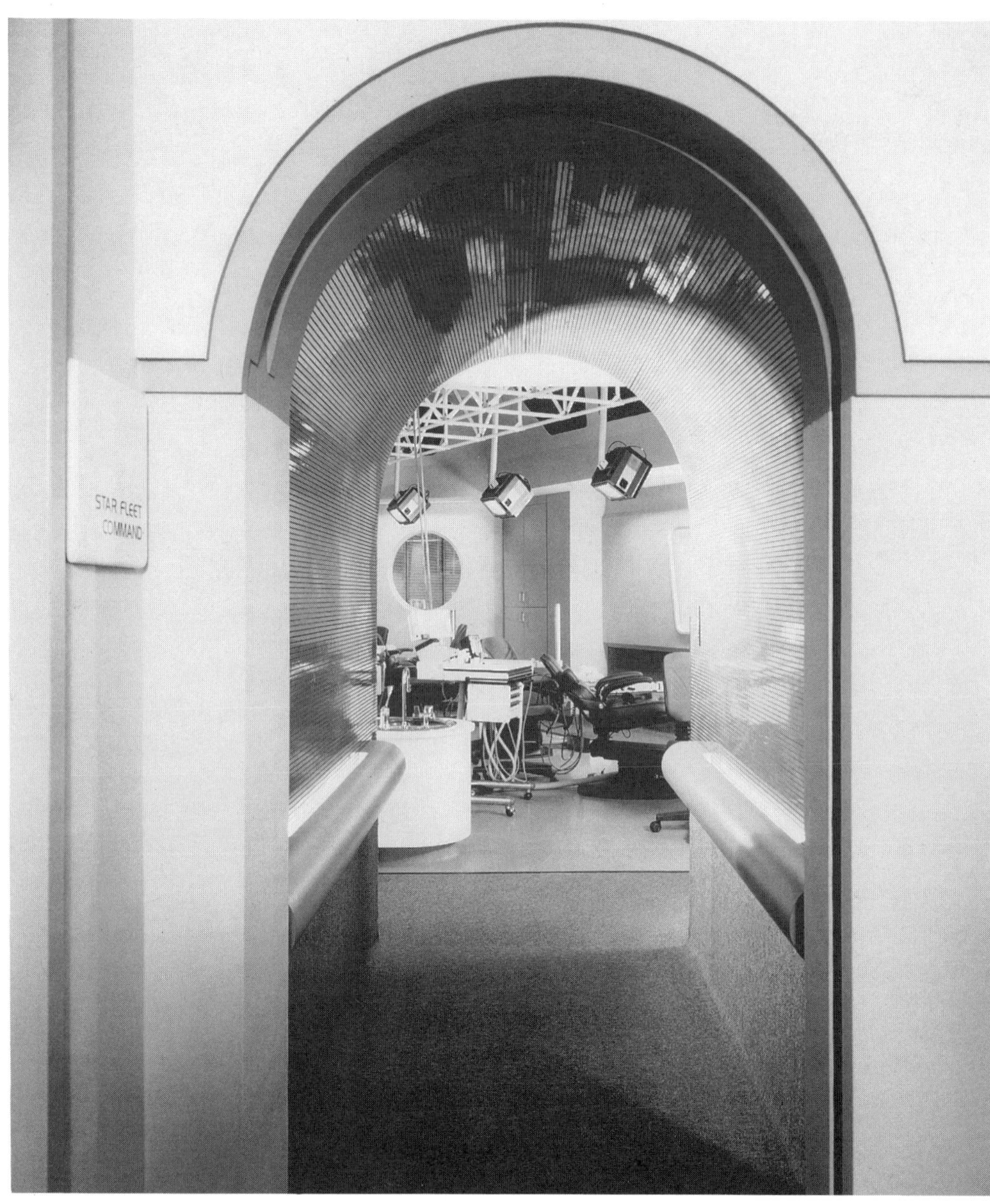

A truly imaginative office designed for children's dentistry is pictured in Color Plates 24 and 25, Figures 10-62, 10-63, and 10-64. Designed by Santa Monica, California, architect, Margo Hebald-Heymann AIA, this innovative office is a child's fantasy. The theme of outer space travel was expressed architecturally, not just cosmetically, as evidenced by the use of materials, the detailing, and lighting.

Patients register for their space adventure at the *pre-flight check-in* counter (Color Plate 25, Figure 10-63) and then entertain themselves in the "twenty-first century" outer lobby. There is a spaceship control panel, complete with space-age hardware, free video games, or films on a giant screen TV. At the time of treatment, an automatic door springs open to admit the child to a shiny, metallic *time warp tunnel* (Figure 10-65) through which he or she must pass to reach the main treatment area (Color Plate 25, Figure 10-64). The patient is ushered into a "flight chair" complete with overhead TV monitor, stereo headphones, and personal, individual remote controls.

A totally different theme treatment of an orthodontic office is shown in Color Plates 26 and 27, Figures 10-67 and 10-68. A tropical theme is expressed with bamboo detailing on the reception desk (Figure 10-69), blade fans, and stuffed tropical birds and iguanas perched in the soffit cut-outs and above the corridor "trellis" ceiling. Accent colors are those found in tropical flowers: magenta, melon, citron, and several shades of jungle greens.

Figure 10-65. Time warp tunnel. (*Architecture/Interiors: Margo Hebald-Heymann, AIA and Associates, Santa Monica, CA; Photographer: Marvin Rand, Marina del Rey, CA.*)

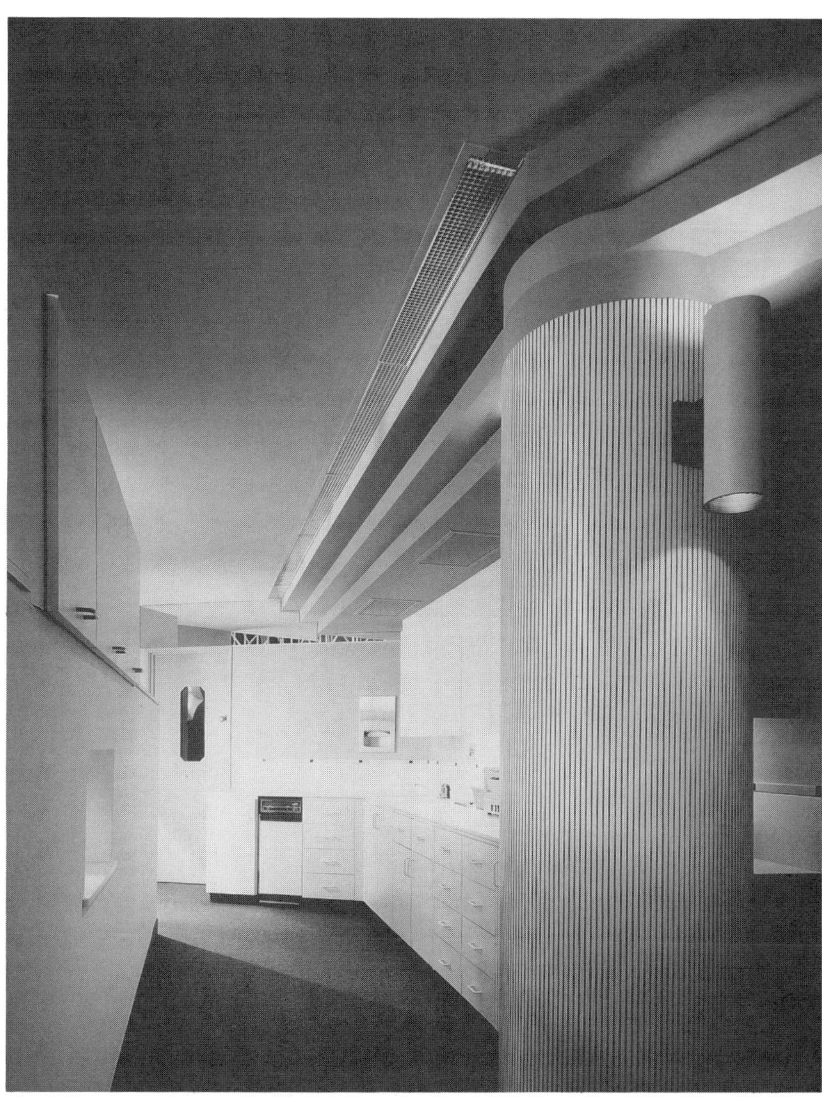

Figure 10-66. Sterilization area. (*Architecture/Interiors: Margo Hebald-Heymann, AIA and Associates, Santa Monica, CA; Photographer: Marvin Rand, Marina del Rey, CA.*)

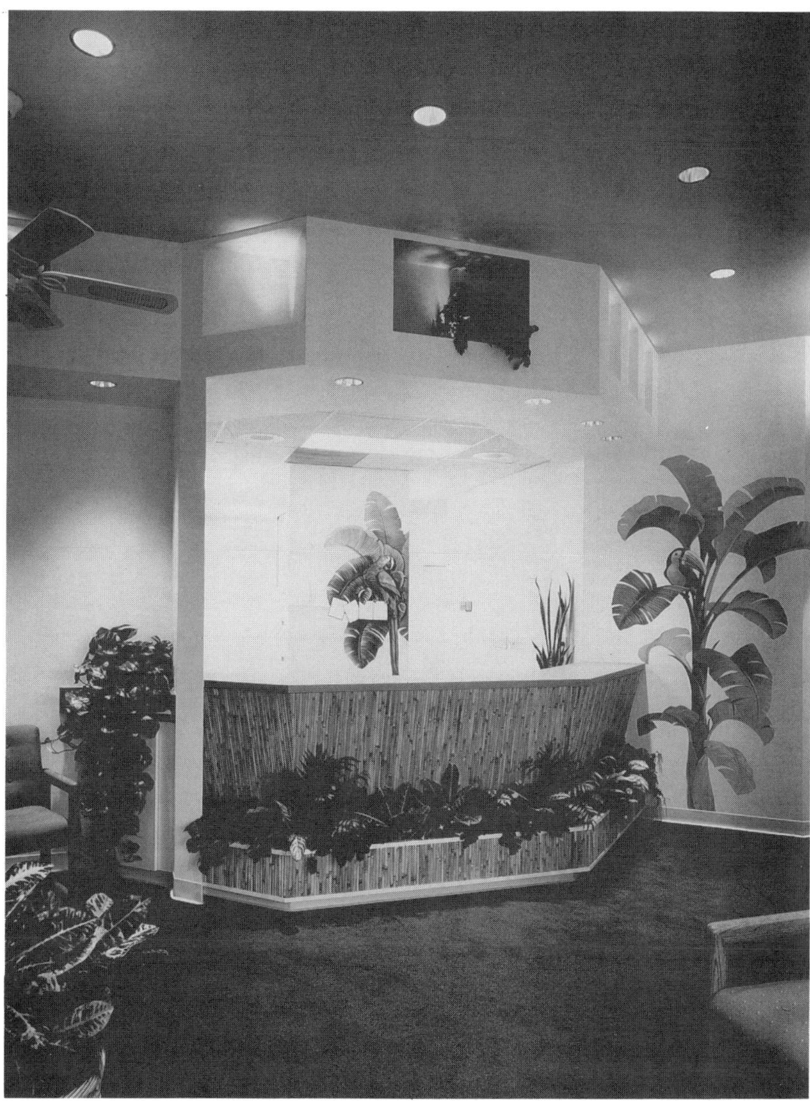

Figure 10-69. Reception desk, orthodontic office with tropical theme. (*Design: Jain Malkin Inc.; Photographer: John Christian.*)

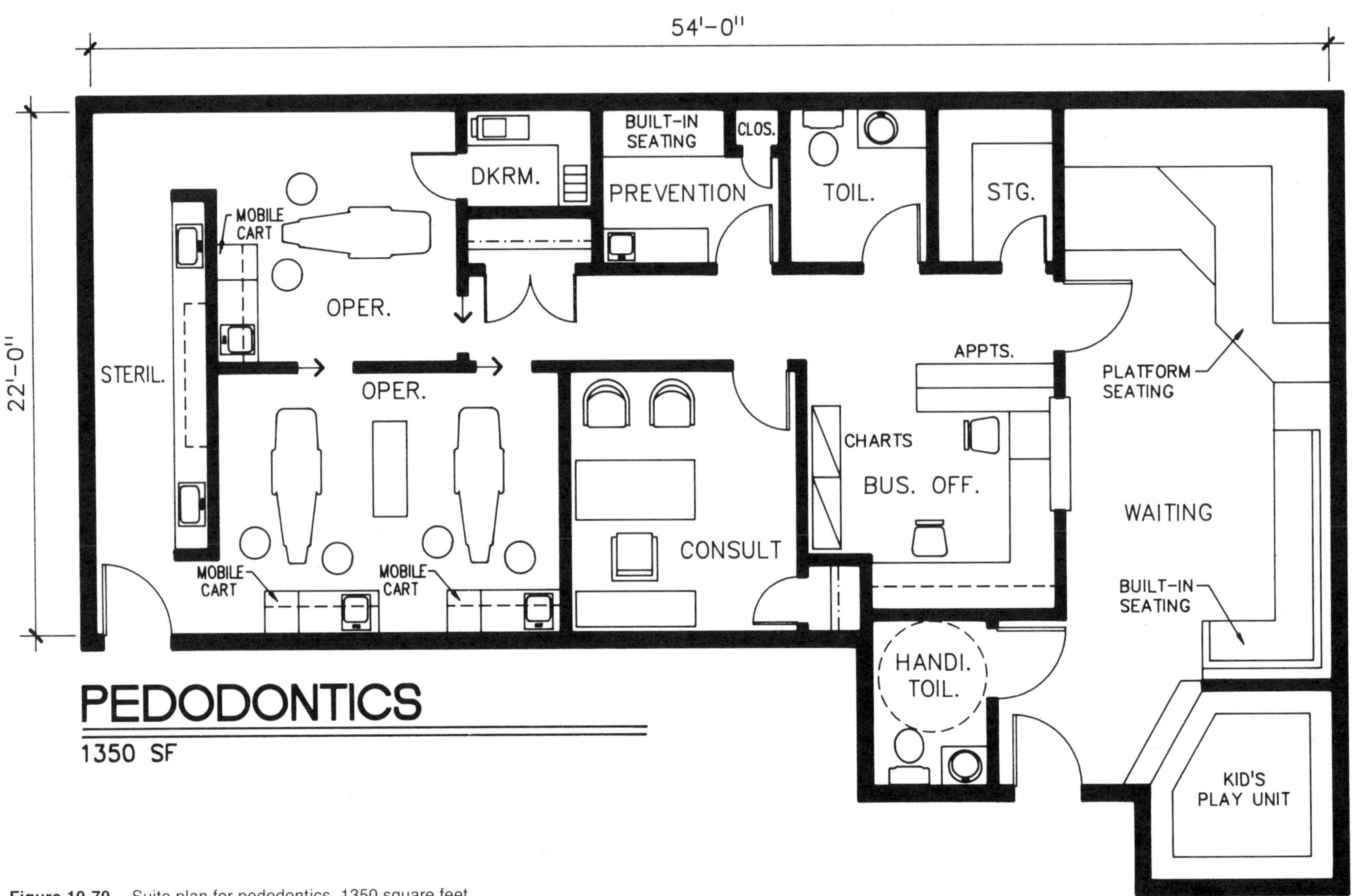

Figure 10-70. Suite plan for pedodontics, 1350 square feet.

PEDIATRIC DENTISTRY

Pediatric dentistry (also called *pedodontics*) is the branch of dentistry that specializes in children (Figure 10-70). It is based upon a philosophy of prevention. If the child's teeth are maintained properly from an early age, there will be fewer problems as the child grows older. Thus, children from the ages of 2 to 18 visit pediatric dentists. Since the children are so young, much of the instruction and care of the child's teeth is entrusted to the parent. The parent must learn how to floss and brush the toddler's teeth, until the child is old enough to do it.

Thus, a patient education room is required with a built-in bench so that the parent can be seated with the child's head in his or her lap and the child's body stretched out on the bench. The bench simulates a couch or bed at home, where plaque control is done with a dry toothbrush, without paste or water. The dental assistant sits near the parent and guides him or her during the procedure. A plywood bench or banquette, padded and upholstered with carpet (Figure 10-71), works well. The room should also have a built-in cabinet with sink, a large mirror, and good illumination (Figure 10-72).

Traffic Flow

A child and parent, on the initial visit, are escorted to the operatory, where the child's teeth are X-rayed and examined. Then the parent might visit with the pedodontist in the private office to discuss the course and cost of treatment.

Since the visits are typically short, this tends to be a high-volume practice. Thus, the circulation of patients should be direct and well planned, and things that little children should not touch should be behind closed doors. The waiting room must be large since each child

Table 10-3. Analysis of Program. Pedodontics

No. of Dentists:	1	
Waiting Room	14 × 20 =	280
Business Office/Recept.	12 × 16 =	192
Operatory Bay (3 chairs)	12 × 18 =	216
Quiet Room/X-ray	9 × 11 =	99
Sterilization	8 × 8 =	64
Lab	6 × 8 =	48
Darkroom	4 × 6 =	24
Staff Lounge	8 × 12 =	96
Toilet Rooms	2 @ 6 × 7 =	84
Prevention/Patient Education	10 × 12 =	120
Panoramic X-ray	5 × 8 =	40
Private Office	10 × 12 =	120
Storage	6 × 8 =	48
Mechanical Equipment Room	6 × 8 =	48
Subtotal		1479 ft^2
15% Circulation		218
Total		1697 ft^2

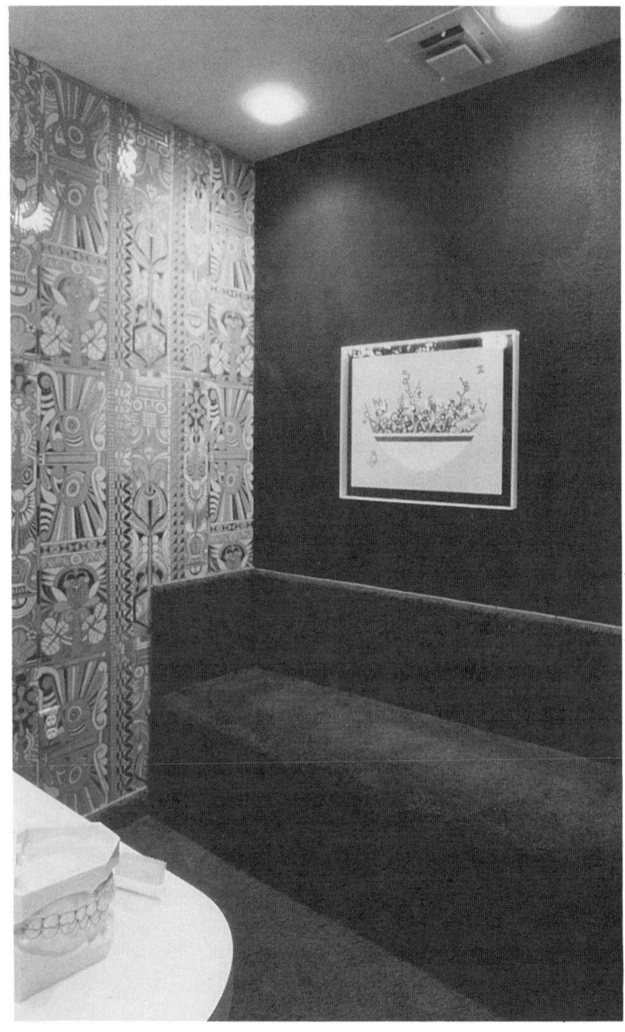

Figure 10-71. Pedodontic plaque control room. (*Design: Jain Malkin Inc.; Photographer: Michael Denny.*)

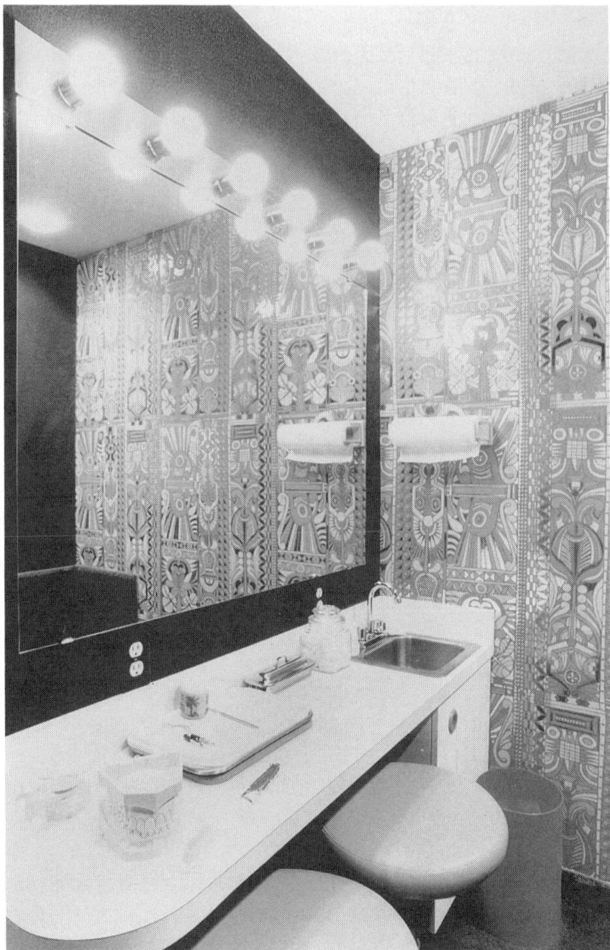

Figure 10-72. Pedodontic plaque control room (opposite side).

is accompanied by one or both parents and often, one or more siblings. A three-chair operatory bay may account for as many as 14 persons in the waiting room. The number of people in the waiting room is sometimes a function of the socioeconomic composition of the practice. Families with low incomes who cannot afford babysitters tend to bring all the children when one of them has to visit the dentist.

Waiting Room

This room can truly challenge the designer's imagination. It can be as fanciful as a fairy tale. Children get bored very quickly in a conventional waiting room. Therefore, they should be treated to something that captures their imagination and lets them climb around and expend their enormous energies. This has an added benefit: The children will associate a pleasant experience with a visit to the dentist, thus forging what may be a lifelong positive relationship with good dental care.

A built-in toy bin just under the cashier/checkout counter is welcomed by the children. While the parent is writing a check or arranging a future appointment, the child is kept amused by selecting a toy. If space permits, a toilet room may be provided in the waiting room area, in addition to the one in the treatment portion of the suite.

Operatory Bay

The pedo chair is a bit smaller than a standard dental chair (Figure 10-73). It is common in pedodontics, as in orthodontics, to have the chairs arranged in a communal bay. Peer group pressure seems to keep crying to a minimum. The room should have cabinetry similar to that of the orthodontist, and the room may be gaily decorated with artwork that appeals to children, located where they can see it.

Pediatric dentists usually use the same dynamic instruments as general dentists. The delivery of instrumentation may be over-the-patient, from the side, or from the rear. There is not a need for natural gas, except in the lab. Inhalation analgesia is fairly common in pedodontic practices. The gases would be centrally piped to each chair, generally in the cabinet directly behind the patient's head. A quick disconnect should be provided for connecting the analgesia equipment.

Other Rooms

The suite will require a business office and dental records area, darkroom, panoramic X-ray unit, storage room, sterilization area, small lab, quiet room, staff lounge, prevention/patient education room, private office, and at least three chairs, either in an open operatory bay or in individual operatories.

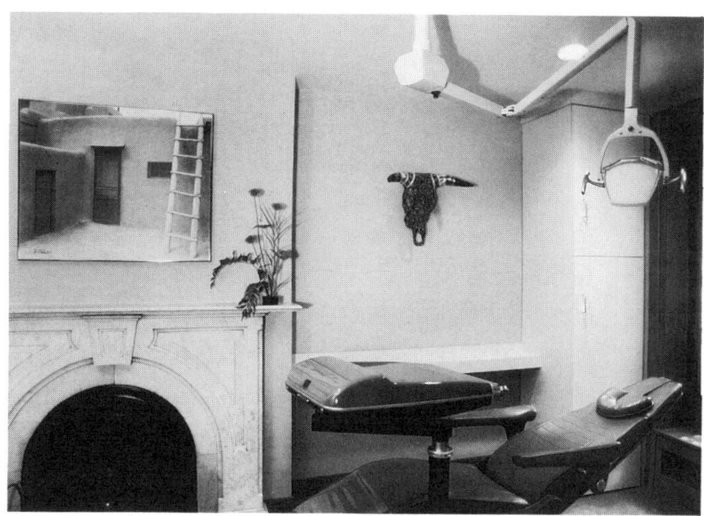

Figure 10-73. Pedodontic quiet room operatory. (*Courtesy Stuart Isler, D.M.D., New York, NY.*)

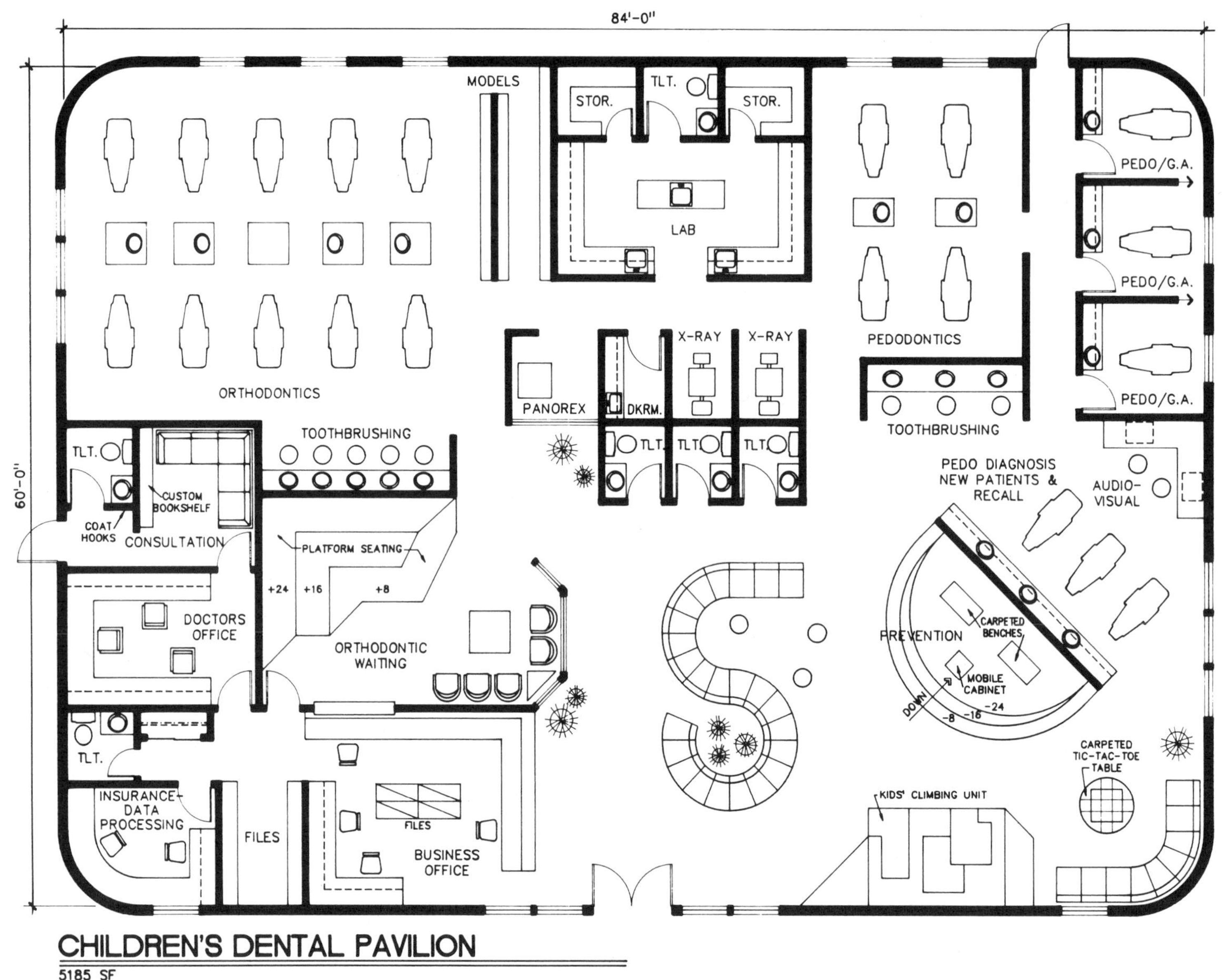

Figure 10-74. Suite plan for children's dental pavilion, 5185 square feet.

ORAL SURGERY

An oral surgeon's work consists primarily of *diagnosis* and *surgery.* On a patient's initial visit, a diagnosis will be made. Then the patient will be scheduled for surgery. A medical history must be taken for each patient. Some oral surgeons prefer to have the staff member take the patient history, perhaps in a private area in the business office, while others accomplish this in the consultation room. Most allow patients to complete their medical history while seated in the waiting room, using a clipboard. Similarly, some oral surgeons prefer to give post-operative instructions in the recovery room, while others like the patient and family members to sit near the front of the office to accomplish this prior to exiting (Figure 10-75).

Many oral surgeons use a consultation/patient education room located near the front of the suite to explain procedures to patients and to review X-rays (Figure 10-76). Depending upon individual needs, the room might have a table with a built-in light box, a TV monitor and VCR unit, and a cabinet with sink. This room can also double as a conference room for the staff.

For a solo practitioner, two small operatories will suffice for examination and diagnosis, and may be used for postoperative procedures and checkups, as well. One or both of these operatories will be equipped for taking intraoral X-rays. In addition, there is an alcove for a panoramic X-ray unit. A small darkroom and consultation room should be located near these operatories.

If all rooms, except treatment rooms, are located at the front of the suite near the waiting room, only surgical patients need enter the rear. Ideally, traffic would be separated so that the exam/diagnosis/X-ray functions are near the front of the suite, and the doctors' private offices, sterilization, recovery, and surgical operatories are at the rear of the suite, perhaps with an

Table 10-4. Analysis of Program. Oral Surgery

No. of Oral Surgeons:	1		2	
Waiting Room	12 × 14	= 168	14 × 16	= 224
Business Office/Recept.	12 × 14	= 168	14 × 16	= 224
Examination Operatories	2 @ 8 × 11-1/2	= 184	2 @ 8 × 11-1/2	= 184
Surgical Operatories	2 @ 12 × 12	= 288	4 @ 12 × 12	= 576
Prep/Cleanup[a]	6 × 8	= 48	6 × 8	= 48
Recovery Rooms	2 @ 5 × 8	= 80	4 @ 5 × 8	= 160
Panoramic X-ray	5 × 8	= 40	5 × 8	= 40
Sterilization/Lab[a]	8 × 8	= 64	10 × 10	= 100
Darkroom	4 × 6	= 24	4 × 6	= 24
Staff Lounge	8 × 12	= 96	10 × 12	= 120
Toilet Rooms	2 @ 6 × 7	= 84	3 @ 6 × 7	= 126
Private Office	10 × 10	= 100	2 @ 10 × 10	= 200
Storage	6 × 8	= 48	8 × 8	= 64
Mechanical Equipment Room	6 × 8	= 48	6 × 8	= 48
Subtotal		1440 ft^2		2138 ft^2
15% Circulation		216		321
Total		1656 ft^2		2459 ft^2

[a]These areas may be combined.

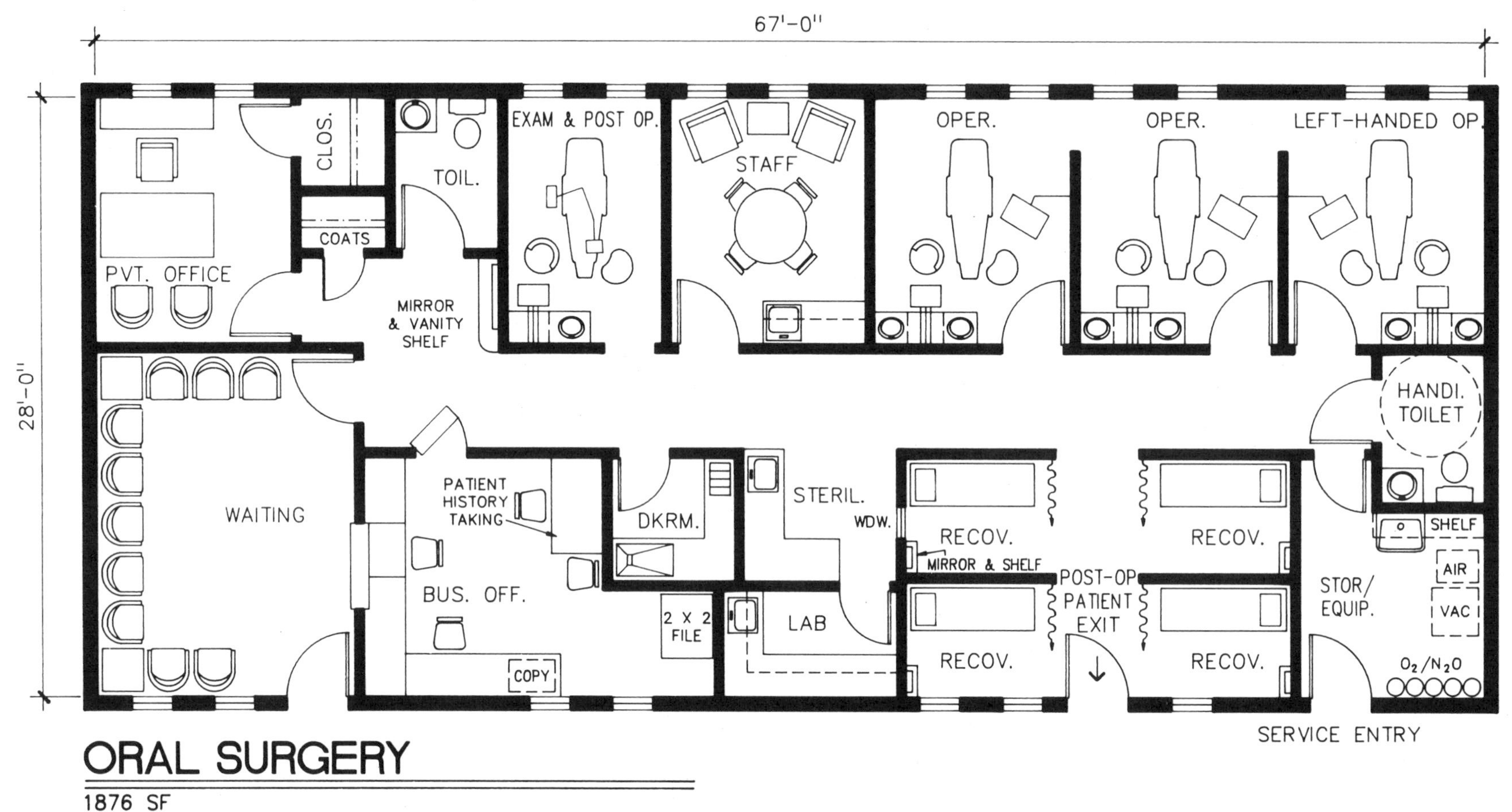

Figure 10-75. Suite plan for oral surgery, 1876 square feet.

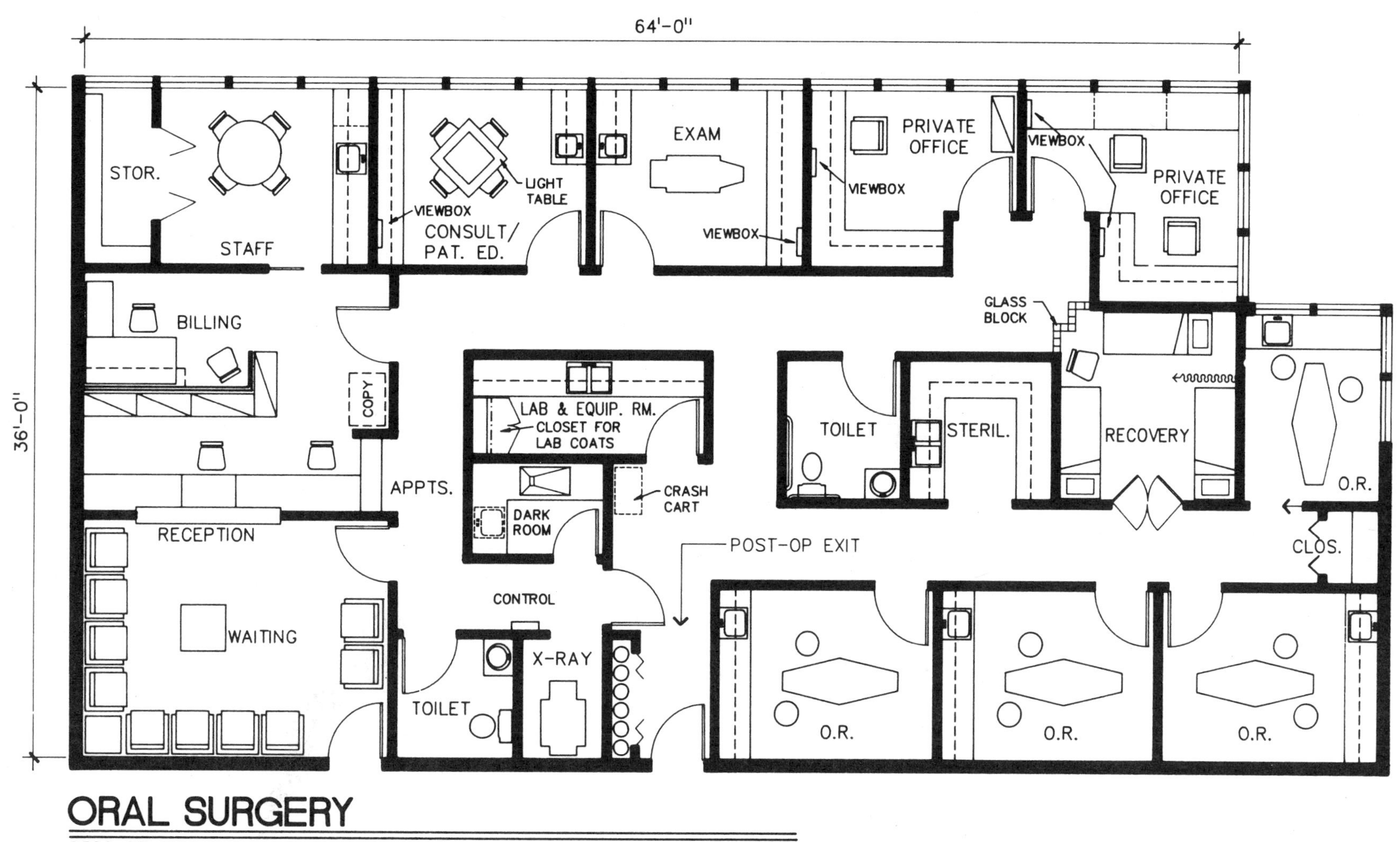

Figure 10-76. Suite plan for oral surgery, 2500 square feet.

exit for post-operative patients, so they don't have to walk through the waiting room (Figure 10-76).

A solo practitioner would generally have two surgical operatories in addition to the two exam/diagnosis operatories. A larger suite for three oral surgeons, where no more than two are practicing simultaneously, is shown in Figure 10-76. Typically, such a suite would have four surgical operatories, two exam operatories or perhaps, one exam and one consultation room, a small lab, two or three recovery beds, staff lounge, a good-sized reception office, and large sterilization area.

Some oral surgeons do not have any lab; others have a small one. If the suite lacks space for a dedicated equipment room, the air compressor and vacuum could be located in the lab.

X-ray

Some oral surgeons install X-ray machines only in the pre-op exam rooms; others place intraoral X-ray equipment in each operatory as well. In addition, an alcove for a panoramic X-ray is located near the front of the suite or examination area.

Surgical Operating Rooms

Oral surgeons usually work six-handed, using two assistants. One assistant handles the suction and retraction, and the other supports the patient's head and monitors the anesthesia. If a fiber-optic light is used, it would be handled by one of the assistants.

Surgical operatories are generally large, anywhere from 10 feet × 11 feet 6 inches to 11 × 12 feet. Many oral surgeons like the room designed with a full wall of base cabinets behind the patient's head. There is a sink, outlets for oxygen and nitrous oxide, an open area for storing the anesthesia cart (Figure 10-77), and perhaps an area for storing the assistant's mobile cart. There are a number of electrical outlets that must be properly located. The sink has foot-pedal controls or wrist-action faucets. Other equipment in the room includes a pulse oximeter, an automatic blood pressure machine, and possibly an EKG machine. The assistant, whether working off of a mobile cart from the rear, or using side delivery, would need suction and compressed air.

Oral surgeons use compressed nitrogen to drive high-speed surgical drills because it is a pure propellant, delivering very high, constant pressure. Compressed air is required for the other handpieces. The doctor may use a Mayo stand to hold the instrument tray or may work off of a mobile cart.

Medical gases must be piped into the room through degreased, sealed copper tubing (using only silver solder) to a flow meter in each surgery. Building and fire codes are very strict regarding where and how medical gases are stored. The reader is referred to the General Dentistry section of this chapter for further discussion of this topic.

Some oral surgeons use a special chair, while others use a standard dental chair with an armboard attachment for administering intravenous sedation. A resuscitation cart is nearby and close to electrical outlets to enable emergency equipment to be used immediately. Surgical operatories should have a nurse call buzzer.

Recovery

Before planning an oral surgery suite, the space planner must determine how the doctor transfers patients from the operatory to the recovery area. Many oral surgeons walk the patients with assistance, others use a wheelchair, and some may even use an operating room type gurney. The patient may remain on the gurney in the recovery room or may be transferred to a recovery bed. Sometimes oral surgeons do long, complicated procedures in a hospital or an ambulatory surgical center, rather than in the office. If a gurney is used in transferring patients, then surgical operatories, corridors, and recovery rooms have to be large enough to accommodate maneuvering. In addition, a place to store the gurney or wheelchair is required.

A solo practitioner with two operating rooms usually has two recovery beds. Generally, one recovery bed per operatory is sufficient. The bed may be an actual bed or a built-in platform with an upholstered foam rubber cushion. The area around each bed must be sufficient to allow staff good access to the patient's head in case resuscitation is required in an emergency.

There must also be a place for a companion to sit, a hook or locker for personal items, a vanity mirror and shelf, a tissue box, a wastebasket, and a blanket and pillow. There must be a suction and oxygen outlet near the head of each bed. A certain amount of privacy should be provided for each recovering patient, either by fixed partitions or a cubicle curtain. The recovery room should be near a toilet and also near a rear, private exit so that the patient does not have to pass through the waiting room after surgery. The recovery area must be located so that the staff can observe the patients while going about their clean-up and preparatory duties.

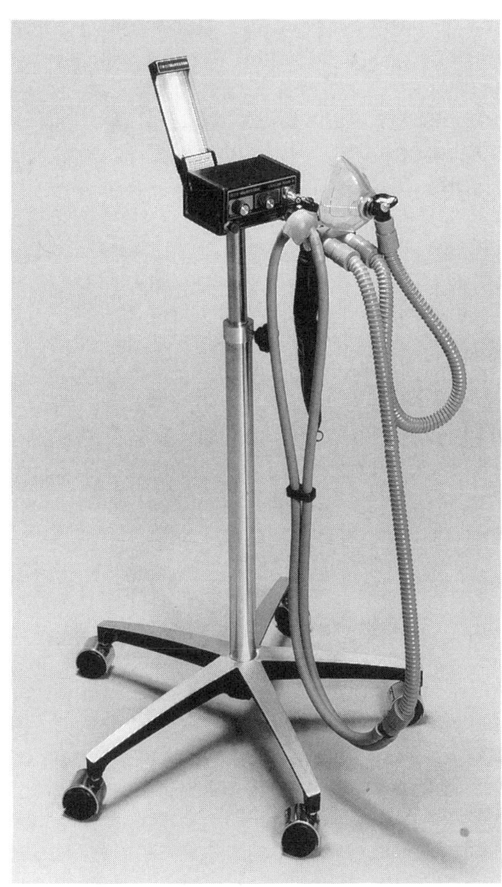

Figure 10-77. Anesthesia machine. (*Courtesy MDT Corporation, Gardena, CA.*)

Sterilization

This room should be fairly large, perhaps 8 × 10 or 10 × 10 feet, with 8 lineal feet of countertop on both the "dirty" and the "sterile" sides. A deep double sink with sprayer/scrubber attachment should be provided. A place for storing clean and dirty linen is required, plus storage for supplies, and a 3-foot wide sit-down desk space with telephone for doing paperwork and ordering supplies. The sink needs a plaster trap. There must be storage space for clean tray setups. The sterilization area must be centrally located between the surgical operatories and recovery area.

Other Rooms

A staff lounge is important due to the demanding nature of the work. The private office may be small, since patients usually do not enter. It is a place for the doctor to read mail, return phone calls, and take a break between procedures. The suite should contain at least two toilet rooms and a storage room. Due to the nature of the procedures, the volume of patients is low, so neither the business office nor the waiting room need be large. As with any surgical specialty, the office should be conservatively furnished using relaxing colors and avoiding flamboyance or frivolity. The surgeon's image should be that of a serious person, skilled and successful at his or her profession.

ENDODONTICS

This dental specialty is quite different from all others in that much of the work is emergent in nature. Endodontists deal with the root of the tooth, and therefore, all of their treatment is within the tooth and difficult to see. Much of the technique is done by tactile sense and numerous working X-rays are taken during treatment to help guide the dentist.

Some endodontists work six-handed as it allows them to increase their case load significantly. One assistant handles the air, suction, irrigation, and hands instruments to the doctor; the other changes burrs (drill bits) on the handpieces, reaches things, and does the charting. Assistants also clean the room after the procedure and seat the next patient.

The operatory in Figure 10-9, called the *optimal operatory,* works well for endodontic practice. The two openings to the room are essential since assistants occasionally leave the room during the procedure, either to develop X-rays or bring additional instruments. Sometimes a third assistant might be present during the procedure to handle a fiber-optic light, if used. A solo practitioner would have two treatment operatories with a third one for post-op visits or emergency care. Some may even have a fourth operatory for this purpose.

An endodontist would have an intraoral X-ray unit in every operatory, but there would be no need for a panoramic or cephalometric X-ray within the suite. An automatic processor would be used for developing some X-rays, but it takes too long to process the working X-rays done during treatment. For those, some assistants use baby food jars for the developer and fixer, enabling them to develop a single film in 30 seconds.

There should be one darkroom for every dentist, a need which is unique to this specialty. Therefore, if two dentists were working at one time, each would have a dedicated darkroom to enable the assistants to quickly develop working films during treatment. Some endodontists use a sonic device to measure the length of the root canal, thereby reducing or even eliminating the need for working X-rays during treatment. The reader is referred to the General Dentistry section of this chapter for additional discussion of X-ray and darkroom.

There is no need for a lab in an endodontic suite. The sterilization area should be designed as discussed under General Dentistry. An island design with two entrances is ideal, as shown in Figure 10-78. The other rooms of the suite would be similar to those required in general dentistry, including the business office, private office, staff lounge, waiting room, and so forth. There would be no special requirements in terms of interior design other than those discussed under General Dentistry. As with any dental operatory today, great care should be taken to control infection and follow OSHA guidelines.

PERIODONTICS

Periodontists treat gum disease and also do tooth implants, which involve bone grafts. Plaque control and hygiene are essential components of this practice. An ideal layout would be one that allows hygiene patients to be treated without walking through the surgery area. The suite plan in Figure 10-78 is an example. The hygiene and plaque control rooms are close to the waiting room. These patients, upon exiting, pass the cashier desk and exit through the waiting room. Surgical patients, on the other hand, have a separate circulation path. When exiting, they pass by a cashier/appointments desk and may exit either through the waiting room or the private exit.

Periodontic patients on the initial visit, after being examined, might meet with the office manager or treatment coordinator in the consultation room to discuss the course of treatment and make financial arrangements.

The suite shown in Figure 10-79 is for a solo practitioner, and that in Figure 10-80 is for two periodontists. Many periodontists believe that all operatories should be equipped in the same manner, enabling them to do surgical implants in any one of them. Others create a large surgical operatory for performing implant surgery, based upon design criteria recommended by Ingvar Branemark, a Swedish physician who pioneered the technique.

This involves a room designed to meet hospital standards for sterility. Special consideration is given to smooth, cleanable surfaces (walls, floors, and ceilings), no ledges on cabinets to collect dust, and an HVAC system that supplies the proper number of air changes per hour. A scrub area, sterilization/clean utility room, recovery area, and soiled linen/clean-up room are provided to support the surgery room. If the dentists use surgical gowns, a dressing area may be required.

Table 10-5. Analysis of Program. Periodontics

No. of Periodontists:	1	2
Waiting Room	12 × 14 = 168	14 × 16 = 224
Business Office/Recept.	12 × 14 = 168	14 × 16 = 224
Financial Arrangements	10 × 12 = 120	10 × 12 = 120
Office Manager	10 × 12 = 120	10 × 12 = 120
Plaque Control	8-1/2 × 11 = 93	2 @ 8-1/2 × 11 = 186
Hygiene Operatories	2 @ 8-1/2 × 11 = 186	4 @ 8-1/2 × 11 = 372
Surgical Operatories	2 @ 9-1/2 × 11-1/2 = 218	5 @ 9-1/2 × 11-1/2 = 546
Implant Operatory	12 × 12 = 144	12 × 12 = 144
Sterilization	10 × 10 = 100	10 × 12 = 120
Scrub/Workroom for Implants	8 × 10 = 80	8 × 10 = 80
Toilets	2 @ 6 × 7 = 84	3 @ 6 × 7 = 126
Recovery	8 × 10 = 80	10 × 10 = 100
Darkroom	4 × 6 = 24	4 × 6 = 24
Staff Lounge	10 × 12 = 120	12 × 12 = 144
Panoramic X-ray	5 × 8 = 40	5 × 8 = 40
Private Office	10 × 10 = 100	2 @ 10 × 10 = 200
Storage	6 × 8 = 48	8 × 8 = 64
Mechanical Equipment Room	6 × 8 = 48	6 × 8 = 48
Subtotal	1941 ft^2	2882 ft^2
15% Circulation	291	432
Total	2232 ft^2	3314 ft^2

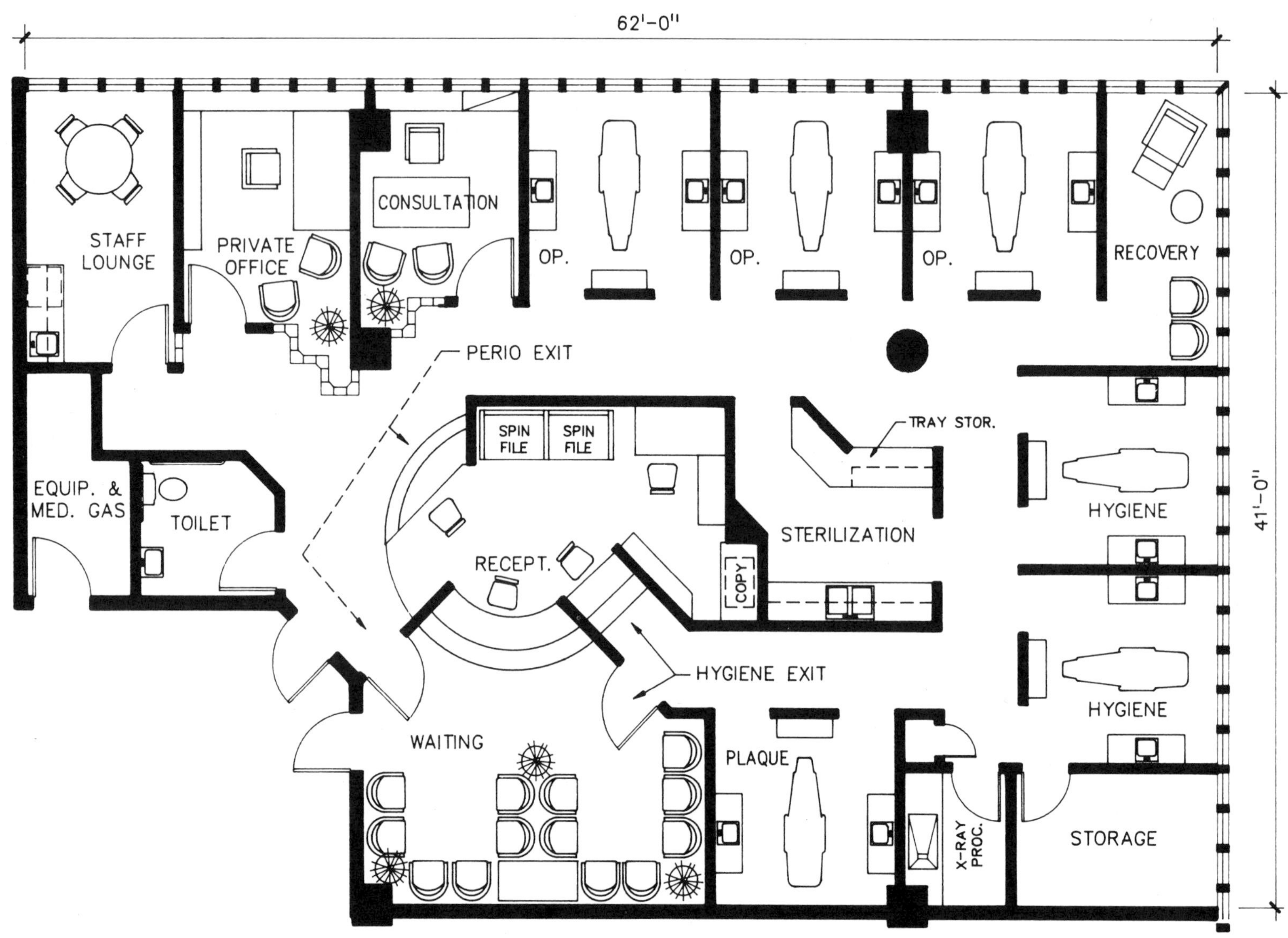

Figure 10-78. Suite plan for periodontics, 2270 square feet.

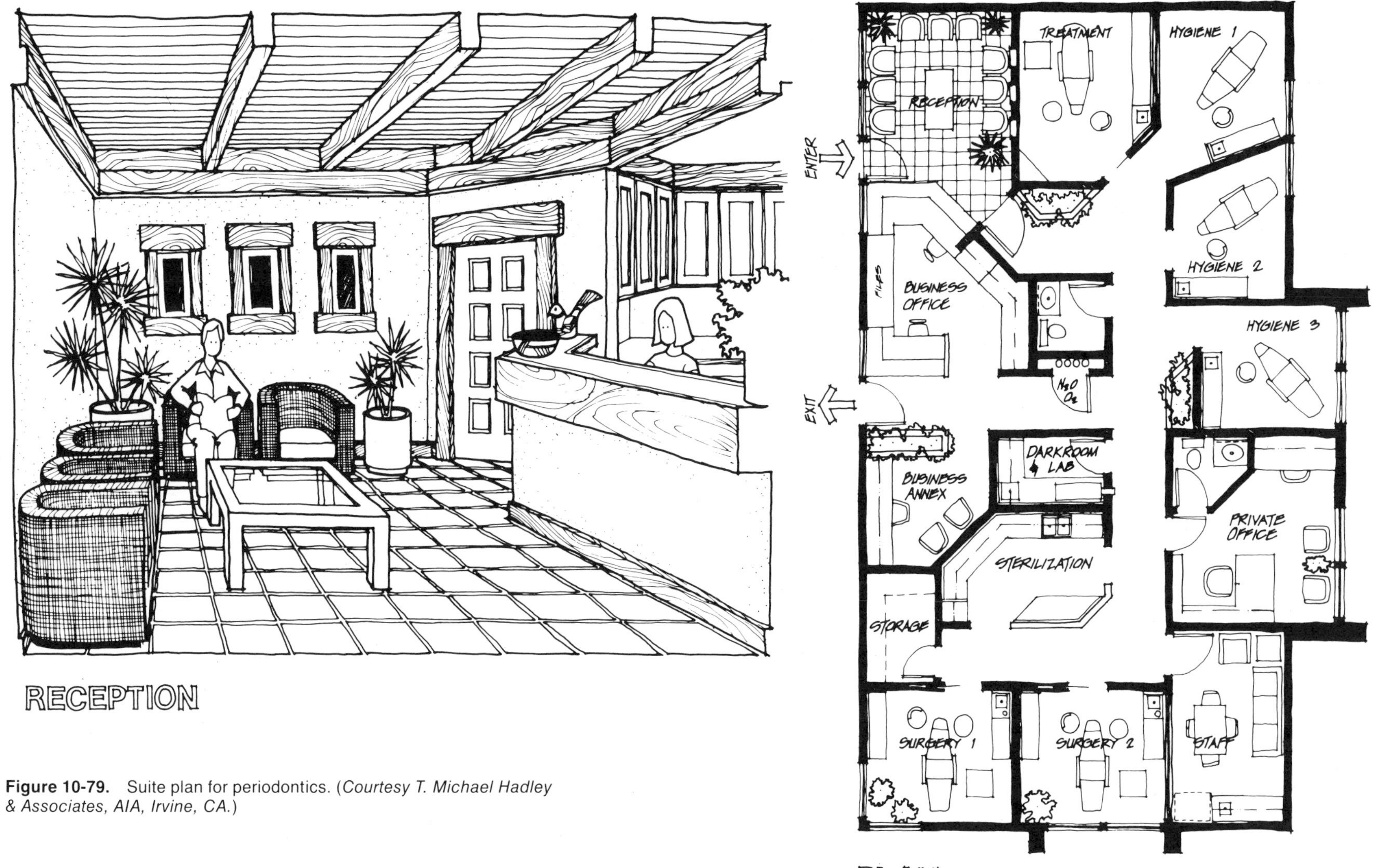

Figure 10-79. Suite plan for periodontics. (*Courtesy T. Michael Hadley & Associates, AIA, Irvine, CA.*)

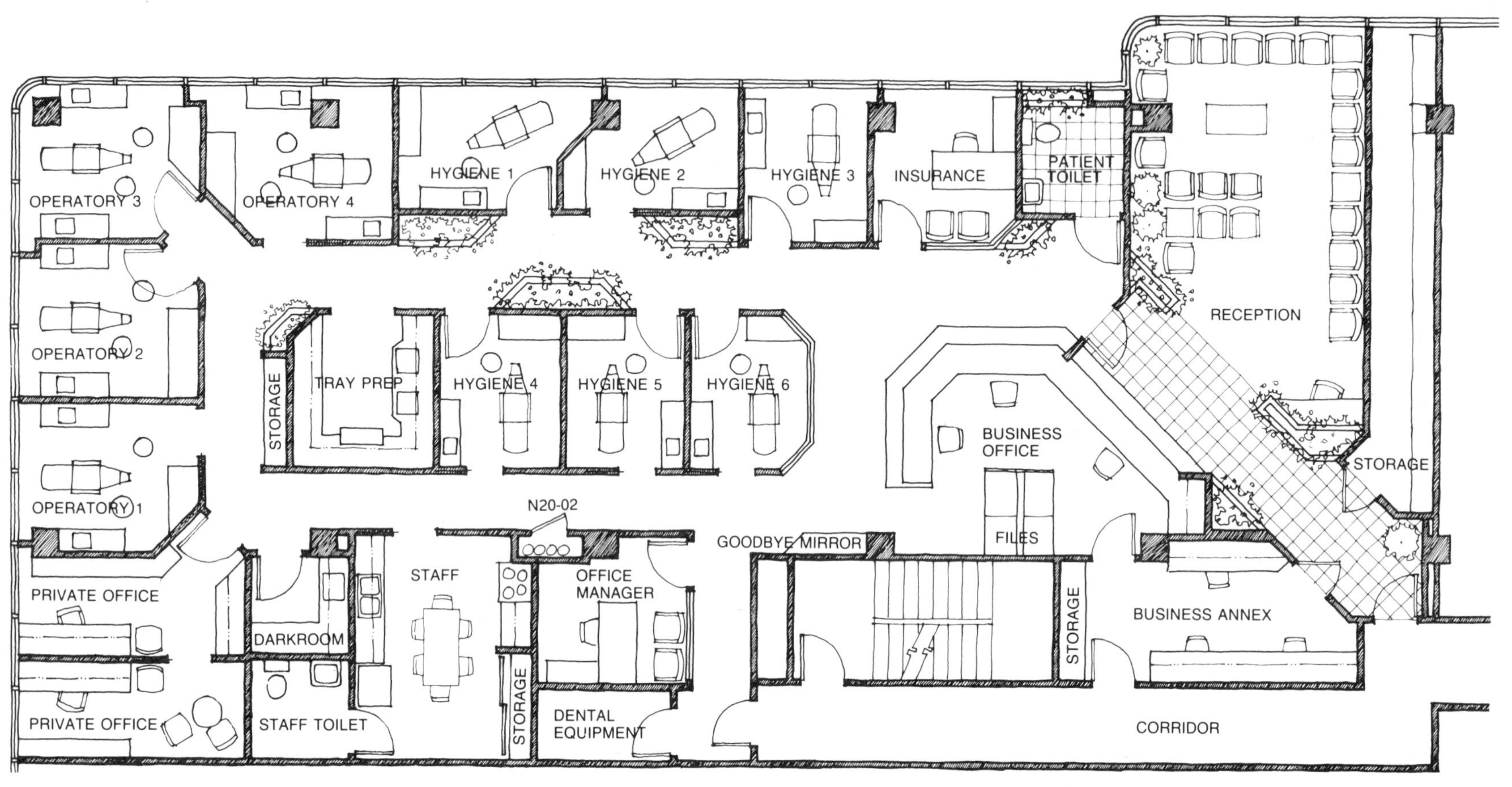

Figure 10-80. Suite plan for periodontics, 3782 square feet. (*Courtesy T. Michael Hadley & Associates, AIA, Irvine, CA.*)

Periodontists often work six-handed, especially when doing implant surgery. When intravenous sedation is used, blood pressure, pulse, and respiration must be constantly monitored.

A special handpiece is used when doing implants. It is portable and has to sit on something either behind or to the side of the patient. It has a stainless steel hook that holds a saline bag. The unit must be connected to compressed air or electric to drive it. These units are cooled with water. In addition, standard handpieces are also used.

The operatory in Figure 10-9 works well for periodontic offices. The operatories are equipped with nitrous oxide, oxygen, compressed air, and suction. The dentist might select over-the-patient, rear, or side delivery of instrumentation. Ideally, the dentist would use rear delivery, and the assistant, working to the left of the patient, would either work off of her own mobile cart or use a dual cart, shared with the doctor. A small recovery area with one or two recliner chairs is desirable.

All operatories may be equipped with intraoral X-ray units, most likely located on the rear wall. All other rooms in the suite would be similar to those required for general dentistry, including the business office, staff lounge, private office, and so forth. There are no special considerations with respect to interior design except if the doctor does a lot of implant surgery. Implant patients are generally elderly and would probably be more comfortable in an office that is calm and relaxing.

Color Plates 28 and 29, Figures 10-81 and 10-82, show a sophisticated periodontics office located in Beverly Hills, California.

SUMMARY

Much has changed in the practice of dentistry in the last ten years, causing many dentists to want to renovate their offices. Video display terminals located in dental treatment areas allow dentists to enter information on the patient's chart immediately and to schedule future appointments. Concern about infection control has mandated new design criteria for dental operatories. Consumers are more educated about health care and, in turn, are more selective about the professionals in whom they place their trust. Dentists, increasingly concerned about marketing, are engaging designers with special expertise in dental planning to help them create a functional office with an image that will appeal to their patients.

CHAPTER 11

The Impact of Color on the Medical Environment

INTRODUCTION TO COLOR THEORY

In early civilizations, man made color holy. He saw intimations of life's mysteries in the spectrum, and assigned it power — so that each color became emblematic of divine forces in a world that so integrated art, ritual, and myths with everyday life that each was suffused with the other. Color was a language in itself; hieroglyphic paintings of vibrant blues, reds, greens, and purples could be interpreted as clearly as words are today. Recent comparative cultural studies have shown similar symbolic uses of color among peoples who could not possibly have had contact with one another. Birren,* a noted color historian, has reported that the points of the compass in China, for example, were represented by black for north, white for west, red for south, and green for east, and that the people of ancient Ireland and also the Indians of North America used identical designations.

Now the old myths have been dismissed as superstition; color has been stripped of its early and specific symbolism; we can no longer precisely "read" a color painting. It is the task of psychologists and mythologists to plumb the depths of the human consciousness from which came those primal myths, and from which our dreams still come, so that we may arrive at a greater knowledge of our common inner life. It is also important to learn how color has always held humankind in its sway — so much so that we hallucinate color if deprived of it too long — and most important, to gauge scientifically its specific influences upon our behavior. The color gold no longer carries the power of the Egyptian sun-god, but research indicates that its perception does have an effect upon the entire human organism, not only the optic nerve. And the implications of this — the differentiated influences of colors, real and measurable — are manifold in regard to environmental design and just beginning to be recognized.

The history of color theory and research is long and variegated, with most of the early work done by philosophers and artists. Aristotle was the first to pose a systematic theory of color, one that is no longer considered relevant. In the early part of the eighteenth century the German poet Goethe expressed his views on color harmony and the symbolic values of color in his book, *Farbenlehre.* The most obvious weakness of Goethe's work was that of most color studies before the twentieth century; he dealt with hues, failing to con-

*Faber Birren, *Light, Color and Environment,* New York, Van Nostrand Reinhold, 1969.

sider saturation and brightness. Nevertheless, he did make an observation that — scores of studies and tests later — has been accepted as valid: that red, yellow, and orange — longer wavelength colors at the warm end of the spectrum — are exciting and "advancing" colors; they seem to come towards one and draw one out, while blue, green, and purple — shorter wavelength colors at the cool end of the spectrum — are "retreating" colors and induce a more quieting, inward-drawing response.

Artists have had their own theories of color and its effect, and they have often been penetrating and insightful, but always based on one person's trial and error, or impression, rather than vigorous scientific investigation. Nineteenth-century artist Odilon Redon made dazzling explorations into color. Other artists famous for their research in color theory include Paul Klee, Wasily Kandinsky, and Josef Albers. Dozens of others — among the more well known are Munsell, Ostwald, Chevreul, Bezold, and Wundt — toward the close of the nineteenth century and the beginning of the twentieth, postulated color theories and laws of harmony along less subjective lines than the often empirical studies of the artists. In the first quarter of the twentieth century, investigators even began testing color preferences for many different groups of people.

COLOR PREFERENCE TESTS

The obstacles confronting all of these color preference enthusiasts, however, were considerable: Color samples were not yet standardized, nor were their backgrounds, nor the light of their viewing conditions similarly controlled. Furthermore, there is difficulty inherent in any test of color and "affect," or feeling — since an individual does not respond to a hue as pure color, but as something that evokes myriad and unique associations with objects and with experiences, which are psychological processes that resist measurement. It is hardly surprising, then, that in 1925 one well-known researcher reviewed the mass of contradictory preference findings in his own and others' studies and declared that all hope of finding consistent reactions to color would have to be abandoned.

It was not. In the 55 years since that pessimistic dictum, a great variety of studies on color responses has been conducted. The number of color preference studies — on normal people, mentally disabled people, psychotics, males, females, the old, the young, in all parts of the world — is probably equal to the total of all other studies on "color and affect" combined. While the findings are often contradictory, certain agreement has been reached among numerous investigators. The difficulty in testing for color preference lies in not being able to control the many variables. Too many articles have been published on the results of market research, and these findings represent current fads rather than scientific investigation. Many of the "conclusions" extracted from these spurious studies are either obvious or dubious.

Color preferences develop as a reaction to culture, education, experience, and genetics. People see the world in different ways and process the environment according to their own needs and drives. Thus it has been postulated that there is a relationship between a person's color responses and his or her emotional state. But it is difficult to test reactions to color because so much depends on the subject's verbal assessment of what he or she sees, and colors are so symbolic, carrying highly personal connotations. If, as a child, a person had always been punished in a blue room, that person may dislike blue as an adult. Therefore any studies of color preference on "normal" subjects must be based on large samples so that individual biases due to highly personal experiences do not bias the results of the study, which may have been designed to test cultural color preferences, age color preferences, or some variable other than pathologically based color preferences or aversions. There is also the physiological problem that people often do not see a color alike. One person may see a dark green as having more yellow; one may see it as having more blue.

Because the color preferences of adults are so much a result of learning, many researchers have preferred to work with children to minimize the effects of learning and experience. Various studies have corroborated that young children prefer the warm, exciting colors of red and yellow, but when they get older they prefer cool colors — blues and greens — as they become less impulsive and more reflective and intellectual.

The researcher Ellis, however, noted in primitive societies a continuing preference for the brilliant hues of red and yellow from childhood into adulthood — and hypothesized that "the apparent trend away from yellow as a revered color among early Greeks and Romans was largely due to the taboo placed upon it by the Christian church, as the symbol of sin and gaiety." Another researcher in the preference field, T. R. Garth, conducted tests among children of six different groups — white, Negro, American Indian, Filipino, Japanese, and Mexican — and found that the preference differences were minimal among them; he concluded that the differences that do appear in adulthood are due to factors related to nurturing.

Eysenck, in a critical review of numerous other color preference studies conducted all over the world, and also of his own experiments, concluded that there is a high degree of agreement among investigators, and that a general order of preference is as follows: blue, red, green, violet, orange, and yellow. He furthermore concluded that there are no sex differences, apart from a slight preference among women for yellow over orange, and among men for orange over yellow.

How can such uniformity of color preference be explained? Researchers Guilford and Smith have attributed it to innate biological factors, while others have emphasized the role of culture, learning, and experience. The truth probably lies in a balance between the two, a combination of innate and cultural factors. In other words, it is not yet known exactly what determines color preferences, only that a marked similarity does exist among all peoples.

COLOR-FORM PREFERENCE

In child-development evaluation, various color-form preference categorization tests are among the most often used measures of the abstraction phenomenon — that ability to single out specific elements from a pattern on the basis of similar factors. The classic color-form preference of measure has been used mainly with young children, and it has demonstrated that most children reach the peak of color dominance around four and a half, that the median age of transition from color to form dominance is five, and that form dominance is usually established by the age of nine.

The Rorschach inkblot method has also been used, with its results consistently showing that pure color responses dominate among young children; color-form dominates in the older child; and from late childhood through adolescence and adulthood, form-color responses dominate. Explanations for the color-form dominance phenomenon include maturation, increased personality differentiation from the affective to the intellectual, increased meaningfulness of the environment in terms of utility, less concern for primitive characteristics, increased verbal skills, and introduction to reading and writing.

Furthermore, since 90 percent of the adult population is form-dominant, color-dominant persons have been considered deviates. One of the most commonly held theories is that since color is a primitive response, the adult color-dominant personality is impulsive, immature, egocentric, and less intelligent than his or her form-dominant and therefore mature, socially adjusted peers. Children who retain their color dominance after classmates have switched over, therefore, are considered regressive and are subjected to academic and cultural programs to change their orientation.

What is interesting, however, is that some recent studies of creativity have indicated that the color-oriented child is more likely to emerge as an artistic, creative adult, far more innovative than his or her form-dominant peers, who will tend to deal well with analytical work in the traditional mold. One of the ingredients of that creative ability is to be free of that mold, to see with fresh eyes and envision new relationships, untried combinations. If further studies support this theory, then it will be clear that a disservice has been done to those who have not fit the conventional mold, and who should be encouraged in their different way rather than pressed into a constricting and uniform shape.

One of the most interesting tests concerned with the connection between specific colors and emotion in children was performed by Alschuler and Hattwick at the University of Chicago. Noting that preschool children express themselves generally at the abstract, nonrepresentational level and reveal more of their affective lives than older children, they studied the expressive outlets of two-, three-, and four-year-old children in easel painting, crayons, clay, blocks, and dramatic play over an extended period of time. They concluded that color gave the clearest insights into the child's emotional life. Color preferences and color patterns gave clues to the child's emotional orientation. *Red,* found to be the most emotionally toned color, carried associations of both affection and love as well as aggression and hate. *Blue* was associated with drives toward control.

COLOR AND MENTAL DISORDERS

A variety of color tests — among them the Rorschach and the color pyramid test, devised by Swiss psychologist Max Pfister in 1950 — are used as diagnostic tools in determining normality/abnormality. Because so many tests involving color preference, response, and placement have been made on the mentally and emotionally ill, with such a plethora of conflicting results, it is clear that the data must be interpreted cautiously and in conjunction with those from other tests. The most abused area here is probably preference, as some have not hesitated to link preference for specific colors to specific disorders, in irresponsible and unproven attribution. Eric P. Mosse, as quoted in Birren, reveals:

> We generally found in hysterical patients, especially in psychoneuroses with anxiety states, a predilection for green as symbolizing the mentioned escape mechanism. . . . Red is the color of choice of the hypomaniac patient giving the tumult of his emotions their 'burning' and 'bloody' expression. And we don't wonder that melancholia and depression reveal themselves through a complete 'blackout.' Finally, we see yellow as the color of schizophrenia. . . . This yellow is the proper and intrinsic color of the morbid mind. Whenever we observe its accumulative appearance, we may be sure we are dealing with a deep-lying psychotic disturbance.

Birren, a noted color historian, disagrees. "Yellow may be looked upon as an intellectual color associated both with great intelligence and mental deficiency." He claims that schizophrenics prefer blue. The contradictions are legion. A study done by Warner, in which 300 patients were tested including diagnosed anxiety neurotics, catatonic schizophrenics, manics, and depressives, found in most cases no significant correlation of preference with psychiatric disorders.

How does the Rorschach contribute to clinical diagnosis? Rorschach's hypothesis was that color responses are measures of the affective, or emotional, state, and he noted that neurotics are subject to "color shock," (rejection) as manifested in a delayed reaction time when presented with a color blot. He also stated that red evoked the shock response in neurotics more often than did other colors. Schizophrenics also suffer color shock when presented with the chromatic or color cards (following the black and white cards) of the Rorschach. Birren postulates that color may represent an unwanted intrusion into their inner life.

In the realm of color research, however, nothing goes uncontested, and the Rorschach is no exception. Two major criticisms of it are the lack of work with normal subjects as a criterion against which pathological groups could be compared, and also the basic postulate that the way in which a person responds to color in inkblots reflects his or her typical mode of dealing with, or integrating, affect. In fact, researchers Cerbus and Nichols, in trying to replicate Rorschach's findings, found no correlation between color responsiveness and impulsivity, and no significant difference in use of color by neurotics, schizophrenics, and normals. Nevertheless, the weight of evidence still favors the Rorschach color-affect theory.

Color and Depression

Almost unanimous agreement exists regarding the depressive's total lack of interest in color. However, some studies indicate that depressed people prefer dark colors of low saturation, and others claim they prefer bright, deeply saturated colors. Probably both conclusions are accurate, since color can be either a stimulant or compensation for lack of excitement and dreariness as well as a reflection of one's inner state. Seen in another manner, the depressive's attraction for bright colors may be an expression of homeostasis — the organism's subconscious striving for balance or equilibrium.

Compton Fabric Preference Test

Another test done with the mentally ill that deserves mention is the Compton fabric preference test. Sharpe* reports that Compton tested the fabric and design preferences of a group of hospitalized psychotic women, in terms of the relationship between concepts of body, image boundary, penetration of boundary, and clothing preference. It was anticipated that persons with mental and emotional problems would be likely to suffer some aberrated form of body image, and it was found that persons with weak body boundaries tended to reinforce them with fabrics of strong figure-ground contrasts and brighter, more highly saturated colors — thus allowing them to feel less vulnerable to penetration, in a sense armored by the "strength" of the color and pattern.

BIOLOGICAL EFFECTS OF COLOR

At the dawn of civilization, color was a biological necessity for locating food and observing predators. It is nature's survival kit for plants and animals — it attracts, camouflages, and protects them. Today color permeates our entire existence. Every aspect of our life involves color: Traffic is directed by color; instrument panels are regulated by color; electrical wires are color coded; advertising is printed in color; medicines and capsules are in color; office file folders have colored

*Deborah T. Sharpe, *The Psychology of Color and Design,* Nelson Hall Co., Chicago, 1974, p. 71.

tabs; clothing has color; uniforms have color; the list is infinite. Biological or physiological reactions to color are the most susceptible to testing and the most valuable from a pragmatic point of view, particularly in relation to design. Kurt Goldstein, a highly regarded researcher, attributes the ambiguity of so much research on color to the fact that the tests were not performed from a "biological point of view"; for color, he has stated, affects the behavior of the entire organism.

Goldstein is criticized primarily for having worked with a small sample of brain-damaged people, but he presumes — and later studies appear to support his position — that these sensations occur in "normals" also, but are brought to the fore in extremely sensitive persons, such as artists, or in psychotics or neurotics. One of his most famous examples of color and effect is that of a woman who had cerebellar disease and resultant disturbance of equilibrium; when she wore a red dress, her symptoms increased to the point of her falling down.

Other effects of *red* that Goldstein noted in other patients were myopic refraction, abnormal deviation of the arms when held out from the body, errors in cutaneous localization, and again, increased loss of equilibrium. In all of these cases, *green* had the opposite effect, that of reducing the already present abnormal conditions. Goldstein states, "The stronger deviation of the arms in red stimulation corresponds to the experience of being disrupted, thrown out, abnormally attracted to the outer world." Green stimulation resulted in withdrawal from the outer world and meditation.

Goldstein also noted a large variety of differential motor reactions displayed by his patients under the effects of red and green. Movements executed with the same intention were performed much more exactly in green than in red light; handwriting, for example, was nearer to normal with green ink than with red. And estimates of length, as well as weight and time, were better under green light than red.

Other investigators have noted that blood pressure and respiration increased during exposure to red light, but decreased in blue illumination. Red light has been said to reduce the pain of rheumatism and arthritis. It dilates the blood vessels and produces heat in the tissues. Birren postulates that the red color of mercurochrome may be effective in the healing of wounds due to its absorption of blue light. Blue light aids headaches and lowers blood pressure, and its tranquilizing effect may even aid insomniacs. Blue light is currently used with high success in the treatment of jaundice — bilirubinemia — in newborns. Yellow has been said to stimulate the appetite and to raise low blood pressure associated with anemia.

Finally, supporting the work of Goldstein and others, tests done with GSR (galvanic skin response, commonly called the lie-detector test) produced significant relationships between GSR and the colors that have been rated high in excitatory value, mainly reds and yellows.

COLOR AND PERSONALITY

Another major area of color research has focused on the interaction between color and personality. Many of these "tests" take the form of informal questionnaires in popular magazines — both irresponsible and exploitative. More serious tests include the Rorschach inkblot, and the color-form tests discussed previously. Although color has been associated with personal characteristics since antiquity, it was not until the publication of the Rorschach, in Switzerland in 1921, that a systematic exploration of the relationship between color responses and personality, or emotional pattern, was begun.

In Germany in the mid-1930s, Jaensch developed a personality-type theory correlating "systems of emotion" with "systems of color vision." Jaensch began by observing that in daylight vision there is increased sensitivity for red and yellow, and in twilight vision there is increased sensitivity for green and blue. He went on to classify individuals according to their predominance of warm or cold vision systems.

Persons of the "warm color type" supposedly meet the external world with warm feelings; those of the "cold color type" are closed off from their surroundings and inwardly integrated. Before puberty, Jaensch asserted, most individuals are of the "outward integration" type, but in maturity the distinction between Nordic and Mediterranean types appears: Nordic being of the cold system, Mediterranean of the warm. As spurious as Jaensch's theories seem, they have not been universally repudiated by those concerned with color research. Birren, noted author of dozens of books and articles on color, corroborates Jaensch's findings but substitutes "blond complexion type" for Nordic and "brunet" for Mediterranean, perhaps to make the "theory" seem more universal. Whatever the label, such notions seem far too generalized to be taken seriously.

Others have recognized the potential for opportunism and exploitation in color, since it strikes the public imagination, and its maze of contradictory research offers "scientific findings" to support practically any theory or commercial gimmick. In 1969, a book appeared by Max Luscher called the *Luscher Color Test,* which subsequently reached the ranks of the best-seller list, and which relates the various personality characteristics to a person's ranking of several series of colors. The reader is led to believe that through these projective devices he or she can determine his or her personality structure, his or her strengths or weaknesses, within just a few minutes.

Some believe that this kind of instrument, used in conjunction with many others, can be useful; others question any validity. What is inarguable, however, is that the *Luscher Color Test,* issued as a popular test, is grossly misleading, although Luscher's test seems to be highly regarded by many professionals in the field. His book, *The 4-Color Person,* tantalizes readers of the September 1979 *House & Garden* with an "intriguing color quiz"[*sic*], which promises to reveal the key to the reader's "four dominant feelings of self — self-confidence, self-respect, self-satisfaction, and self-development." Various categories (furniture, modern art, music, architecture, etc.) of preference are listed. Upon scoring the quiz, the reader becomes aware that the four preference choices of each category have been related to red, yellow, blue, or green, depending upon the assumed "affect" qualities of each color. Thus a preference for a "mobile by Calder" registers a point for yellow (self-development, imagination, independence); a preference for "Chopin," a point for blue (romance, trust, love, and peace); a taste for "cymbidium orchids" rates a point for green (self-respect, responsibility, persistence); and a preference for "riding a bike" over "joining a car pool" rates a red (passion, vitality, self-confidence).

Such personality quizzes are too simplistic and do not take into account those who have broad interests and catholic tastes. A gardener, for example, might prefer cymbidium orchids over daisies, because he or she has a greenhouse and has had good luck with that plant. Sometimes the questions on these tests are ridiculous: Would you rather read a book to a sick friend, eat in an Italian restaurant, or go dancing? Do you prefer filet mignon, duck flambé, imported cheeses, or homemade soup? Do you prefer florals, geometrics, or batik fabrics? A sophisticated person may like all of the choices equally depending upon the proper context. Such examples of popularized color theory are analogous to newspaper astrology. Home-decorating magazines frequently carry articles that offer such illuminating clues to one's inner life as, "If you like red, you

are a strong personality with a craving for action, and are compatible not only with other reds but 'sun yellow' and 'wild iris.'"

Researchers have even hypothesized that people express their personalities through the clothes they wear. Sharpe reports, "An overview of the research suggests that the more *secure* individual tends to favor colors that range from neutral to cool (green, blue, beige and gray), of medium value tending toward dull, whereas the more *insecure* individual tends to select warm, bright colors (red, yellow) that range from the extremes of light and dark."*

Such generalizations are narrow since they overlook many obvious reasons people dress as they do (education, upbringing, climate, budget, artistic expression, professional impact) and do not take into account the many people for whom clothing is completely unimportant, or those who economically cannot afford to express themselves sartorially, or that large group of people who wear anything that is "fashionable" at the moment regardless of whether it suits them. Perhaps those to whom clothing is unimportant are secure, since their self-image is not dependent upon others' visual assessment of them. Those who cannot afford to buy the clothes they might like to buy may fall anywhere along the secure-insecure scale. Those who must continually buy and wear what is fashionable at the moment perhaps are the most insecure, since this expresses a strong desire to be accepted and to conform. Thus it seems that clothing is not a valid indicator of personality: There are too many variables.

COLOR AND HARMONY

In the last two decades many of the old color taboos have been lifted, and the archaic "laws" have become obsolete — especially that of *complementary* colors (mainly, those diametrically opposite one another on the spectrally ordered color wheel) — as the only basis for color harmony. According to traditional colorists, complementary colors equaled harmony equaled balance; the modern school of colors added: non-complementary colors equaled asymmetry equaled tension.

But adherence to such rigid formulas began to give way in the sixties, when the color revolution, paralleling others, exploded in bursts of psychedelic light, furthering a lasting acceptance of a vastly wider range of color combinations, as well as more vivid, brilliant color. The psychedelic movement helped to create among designers a more eclectic approach, one that accepts the dictates of neither school but rather relies on creating the color environment most appropriate to the specific situation, taking into account the size of the space, its architectural form, the proposed use of the space, age of the occupants, natural light, and the tasks to be performed there.

Color harmony is not just a function of the relationship of hues but depends largely upon the quantity of color, the intensity, balance, and weight. Certain color combinations create tension or movement. The goal of color is not always harmony; sometimes it is used to excite, stimulate, manipulate, create tension, or expand or contract a space.

THE COLOR WHEEL

The old color wheel (Color Plate 30, Figure 11-1), based on arbitrary paint-mixing color qualities, has been replaced by a new color wheel (Color Plate 30, Figure 11-2) in which colors are based on the true color perception qualities of vision. The new color wheel has additional advantages in that it is accurate in explain-

*Sharpe, ibid., p. 69.

ing subtractive, additive, and partitive color mixing. Thus in the new color wheel, the complement of yellow is blue, not violet. The complement of green is magenta, not red. Although it has been widely accepted (based on the old color wheel) that red is the complement of green and vice versa, this is usually incorrect. The afterimage of green is magenta and the afterimage of red is cyan (blue).

The three color mixing systems are defined as follows.

Subtractive. Transparent colors placed on top of each other or in front of each other form a third color. Yellow and blue mixed make green. The mixed color is always darker than any of the component colors.

Additive. The cumulative effect of colored lights mixed together. The mixed color is always lighter than the lightest component color. Yellow and blue light equal white.

Partitive. The averaging of several colors as in pointillism style paintings. Adjacent spots in three-color printing and color TV are "mixed" by the eye and read as solid colors. The total effect of a fabric woven of different-color threads is a color different from any of the component threads individually. The mixed color has the average brightness of all the colors mixed.

It is not within the scope of this chapter to discuss in detail the highly technical aspects of color theory or the rationale that supports the development of the new color wheel. The reader is referred to an extraordinarily fine and highly readable book on the subject, *The Theory and Practice of Color,* by Frans Gerritsen (New York, Van Nostrand Reinhold, 1974).

LAWS OF PERCEPTION*

Sensitivity to Light and Color

The human eye can distinguish up to 9 million colors with normal vision and mutual combinations of the three eye primaries, blue, green, and red (short, medium, and long wavelengths, respectively) and the three eye secondaries, yellow, magenta, and cyan. Color is light energy after it hits the eye. *Rods and cones,* the light *receptors,* are located in the retina. There are many more rods than cones. The rods are clustered on the periphery of the retina and the cones in the center, generally speaking. Since the cones are concentrated in the center of the retina, color sensitivity *decreases* toward the periphery of the retina until it reaches the edge where only light and dark can be discriminated. *Translating this into a more practical application, the greatest values (brightnesses) and the warm, active colors (yellows, red, and oranges) should be placed in the center of attention. Lower brightnesses and cool, unsaturated colors (dark green, dark blue, dark brown) should appear on the periphery of the visual field.* This knowledge is particularly important for the design of graphic signage, posters, large paintings, exhibitions, displays, and interior design. One may lead people from one room to another by the skillful arrangement of successive values and colors.

*A good deal of the material presented under *Laws of Perception* has been adapted from *The Theory and Practice of Color,* by Frans Gerritsen, New York, Van Nostrand Reinhold, 1974.

Simultaneous Contrast

Simultaneous contrast is the change in appearance of a color due to the influence of a surrounding contrasting color: Larger color masses influence smaller ones. If two spots of a neutral gray are surrounded by a larger area of white and black, respectively, the gray surrounded by white will *appear* to have less brightness than the gray surrounded by black. This happens because the local adaptation of the eye is less sensitive to high brightness in a bright surrounding, thus more sensitive to low brightness or value. Against the bright white background, then, the gray will be evaluated as having less brightness than it actually has. However, against a black background, the eye will be less sensitive to low brightness and will evaluate the gray spot as being very bright. This is true not just of white and black but of most colors in which a strong contrast exists (Color Plate 31, Figure 11-3).

Successive Contrast and Afterimage

When the eye adapts to the value and color of an environment, this will influence the brightness and color of what is seen directly thereafter. For example, if the eye adapts to a blue background of a stage set, and a performer wearing a yellow costume suddenly appears, the costume will appear much brighter yellow than if the eye had not first adapted to yellow's complementary color, blue. If one concentrates on a green surface and then looks away at a white one, an afterimage of magenta will appear. One is, in effect, seeing the white surface *minus* the green to which the eye has already adapted. Looking at a certain color produces an *afterimage* of its complement (Color Plate 31, Figure 11-4). A practical application of this principle is the surgical operating room, where walls and garments are always blue-green because the eye is concentrated on a red spot (blood), and when surgeons look up from their work, they see afterimages of blue-green. If walls and garments were white, they would see green spots before their eyes every time they looked away from their work. Thus blue-green walls and gowns act as a background to neutralize these afterimages.

Another example of afterimage can be experienced if one walks through a corridor that has yellow walls, a warm-toned floor, and incandescent (warm) light — essentially a yellow-hued environment. When leaving the corridor, perhaps entering a lobby, one will see afterimages of blue, the complement of yellow. *This is very important for interior design.* An understanding of this concept can prevent a designer from creating undesirable color relationships.

Metameric Color Pairs

Metameric color pairs are those that are alike only under certain conditions. For example, if two color chips of turquoise blue paint fabricated by two different paint manufacturers seem identical under incandescent light, they may appear vastly different from each other under a different source of light, due to the absorption curves of the color surfaces. The vast number of chemical formulas and varying compositions of pigment and binder will produce colors that, although they may appear to match another color in a certain light, actually have different short and long wavelength areas. Thus the colors would look quite different under a different source of light, due to the differences in absorption.

A practical application of this principle occurs daily in the offices of architects and interior designers. Frequently the carefully selected paint colors specified by an architect or designer will be met by the contractor's request for a substitution of manufacturer. While seemingly harmless, provided the substituted manufacturer has a high-quality comparable product, the possibility of "mixing to match" the designer's original palette of colors is almost impossible.

It is highly unlikely that the two manufacturers would use the same chemical formula and exactly the same type of pigment. The colors will probably be "mixed to match" under cool white fluorescent light in the paint store. While they may appear to match perfectly there, they will not match in the incandescent light or warm white fluorescent of the job site. *The pigment molecules of one formulation will be sensitive to and absorb different wavelengths than the other formulation.* Colors that have identical chemical formulations will look identical in all sources of light, even if the samples were mixed at different times. It is critical that colors always be evaluated under the lighting conditions where they will be used.

Reflectance

Colors of a room are influenced by the reflection of natural light entering the room as well as by artificial sources of light. An example of the first condition is a room with a large expanse of window facing a garden. The green grass will absorb most of the long wavelengths of the daylight (the reds and oranges) and permit the short wavelengths (greens and blues) to be reflected through the window onto the walls of the room. If the walls are white, they will have a green tint. The green tint can be neutralized by painting the reflection wall a *complementary* color in the magenta or red family.

An example of the second condition (artificial light) is a corridor with red carpet, white walls, and white ceiling, with recessed incandescent light fixtures. The carpet absorbs most of the wavelengths of the artificial light except for the long waves of the red-orange spectrum. Thus the floor reflects an intense red light on the ceiling, making it appear red. A way to avoid this condition is by lighting the ceiling from below.

Purkinje Effect

The Purkinje effect was named after its discoverer, a Czechoslovakian physician, who observed that at twilight, color impressions are shifted to favor the short wavelength area of the spectrum. Thus reds, oranges, and yellows become colorless, and darker, greens and blues become clearer.

Color Constancy

This phenomenon refers to the relationship between the eye and the brain to translate visual information in a constant manner. For example, if one looks at a piece of white paper while standing in front of a red wall under daylight, the paper will still appear white, but a colored photograph would show the paper to be pink. In other words, intellectually the brain knows the paper is white and so translates it as white in spite of perceptual information to the contrary.

Advancing and Receding Colors

Goethe's observation, mentioned earlier, that warm colors seem to advance while cool colors recede, can be explained by optic laws. Red — being only slightly refracted by the lens of the eye — focuses at a point behind the retina, and the lens, in order to see it clearly, grows more convex, thus pulling the color forward. Blue, on the other hand, is more sharply refracted and causes the lens to flatten out, thus decreasing its size by pushing its image back.

Figure-Ground Reversal

This phenomenon is a principle of Gestalt psychology and refers to the optical illusion apparent particularly in geometric patterns in which the figure seems to be in front of the background. Obviously, both figure and ground are printed on the same surface. Warm colors (red, orange, yellow) tend to be seen as figure since they advance, and cool colors (green, blue, purple) as ground since they recede. But whether a color is seen as figure or ground also depends on the value (light advances, dark recedes) and the saturation (high advances, low recedes).

COLOR SYMBOLISM

Emotional evaluations of color are a function of time, place, culture, nationality, age, fashion, and even gender. Colors conjure up highly personal images and meanings, making it difficult to predict and understand preferences. Furthermore, emotional evaluations of colors are made in relation to an object. While "apricot" may be a fashionable color this year for residential interiors, it is unlikely to be considered tasteful in an automobile or a toaster. People usually like colors associated with pleasurable experiences. Those who like modern art usually like the brilliant colors found in such paintings. Those who prefer the old masters often favor a more subdued palette.

The symbolic nature of color is expressed in color names, which are often made up of the basic color plus an adjective: *black magic, snow white, spice beige, chocolate brown, shocking pink, red hot, true blue (loyal).* Paint manufacturers often express sheer whimsy in naming colors such as "persimmon" for an olive green or "touch of love," which tells one nothing about the color.

Colors, through the ages, have come to be associated with certain emotions or personality traits. Some of the more common follow.

Blue: Tranquility, cool, solitude, intelligence, soothingness, truth, divinity, quiet, melancholy, calm, sincerity, generosity, serenity, hope, conformity, control, suppression of feelings, constancy, accomplishment, devotion, introspection.

Yellow: Joy, gaiety, harvest, brilliance, morbidity, cowardice, disease, fruition, regality, hope, jaundice.

Orange: Warmth, glow, sociality, friendliness, good cheer, good nature, gregariousness.

Red: Heart, blood, tragedy, cruelty, war, heat, hatred, power, bravery, love of life, courage, fire, fury, purgatory, passion, beauty, truth, shame, destruction, anger, danger, stop, love, excitement.

Green: Peace, youth, hope, victory, jealousy, life, nature, immortality, safety, conventionality, good adjustment, balance.

Orange-Brown: Deceit, distrust, inconstancy, treachery.

Red-Brown: Strength, solidity, vigor, sadness, maturity, simplicity, sturdiness, reliability, rationality.

White: Truth, innocence, purity, virginity, chastity, modesty, humility, light, love, temperance, friendship.

Black: Evil, gloom, death, terror, horror, darkness, crime, melancholy, secrecy, mystery, wickedness, witchcraft, mourning, solemnity, potency, social status.

Gray: Penance, humility, sadness, age, sobriety, death, fear, dreariness, bleakness, sterility, maturity, emotionlessness, isolation.

PRACTICAL APPLICATIONS OF COLOR PSYCHOLOGY

Where does all this investigation — preference and personality, color shock and loss of equilibrium — bring us in terms of design? Clearly, much of the research that has been reviewed here is as yet inconclusive. Many conclusions propagated about the effect of color and its link to emotional patterns have not been scientifically proven; so the real investigation of the effect of color upon human behavior has only just begun. The early state of the science notwithstanding, however, certain practical applications in design do suggest themselves.

1. *Reds and yellows,* for example, should be used in settings where creative activity is desired; *greens and blues* in areas that require more quiet and extended concentration — and the appropriate combinations of these colors in classrooms, hospitals, and offices.
2. Cool colors should be used in the surroundings of the hysterical, hypertensive, and anxious, red, in the depressive's environment. Highly saturated colors should be avoided with autistic schizophrenics, as should red with those afflicted — like Goldstein's classic case — with organic brain disease.
3. Rousing, bright colors should be used with the aged rather than pastels, which are barely visible to those with failing eyesight.
4. Strongly contrasting figure-ground patterns and extremely bright colors should be avoided in the rooms of psychotic patients since these — when not worn by the patients but impinging upon them from their environment — might be thought to have an overwhelming, even intimidating, and threatening effect.
5. The knowledge of color preference and usage can be employed in cultural liaisons and trade with foreign countries. Knowing which colors are taboo and which carry religious or symbolic associations in each country is mandatory for expanded marketing and trade relations.
6. Under *warm* colors, time is overestimated; weights seem heavier; objects seem larger; rooms appear smaller. Under *cool* colors, time is underestimated; weights seem lighter; objects seem smaller; rooms appear larger. Thus, cool colors should be used where monotonous tasks are performed to make the time seem to pass more quickly, and red, for example, should be used in an employees' restroom to reduce the amount of time spent there.
7. Under *warm* colors with high illumination, there is increased alertness and outward orientation — good where muscular effort or action are required such as a physical therapy gym. Under *cool* colors and low illumination, there is less distraction and more opportunity to concentrate on difficult tasks, an inward orientation is fostered. Noise induces increased sensitivity for cool colors, probably because the tranquility of these colors compensates for the increased aural stimulation. One becomes less sensitive to warm colors under noise, since they offer additional stimulation rather than less.

COLOR AND ITS EFFECT ON OUR PERCEPTION OF SPACE

The various laws of perception discussed previously can be translated into the following guidelines for interior design and architecture.

1. To prepare people for the color of a room they are about to enter, the entry should be painted a *complementary* color.
2. Color modifies architectural form — it can expand, shorten, widen, lengthen, and give the illusion of lowering or raising a ceiling. Color can change the appearance of the environment to lift the individual out of reality.

3. Bright colors seem lighter in weight. Ordered from "heavy" to "light" they are: red, blue, purple, orange, green, yellow.

4. Bright objects are overestimated in size. Yellow appears the largest, with white, red, green, blue, and black in descending order.

5. A light object appears larger against a dark background. A dark object will appear smaller against a light background.

6. The wall opposite a window should generally be kept light, or it will absorb much of the daylight.

7. A window wall and frame should be light so as not to contrast too much with daylight sky — high contrast can result in headaches and eye strain.

8. If a red wall is placed next to a yellow wall, the yellow wall will appear greener than it actually is due to the afterimage of red: cyan. The blue afterimage of the yellow will cause the red to appear more purple.

9. Warm colors advance; cool colors recede.

10. Light colors and small patterns visually enlarge a space. Dark colors and large patterns make it appear smaller.

11. The absence of variety in the visual environment causes sensory deprivation. Those who are confined to nursing homes, hospitals, and institutions desperately need changes in lighting, accent walls, and artwork in order for their nervous systems to function properly. Monotonous white walls devoid of interesting graphics or artwork deprive the brain of the constantly changing stimulation it requires to remain healthy.

12. In low levels of light (under 30 footcandles), object and surface colors will appear normal when the light surface is slightly tinted with pink, orange, or yellow. As higher light levels are reached, a normal appearance for object colors will be found with cooler light; it is best to stay warm at low levels and go cooler at high levels* (Kruithof's principle).

Light, Color and Environment, by Faber Birren, New York, Van Nostrand Reinhold, 1969, p. 25.

Since lighting and color influence each other greatly, the reader is referred to Chapter 13 for additional information.

SUMMARY

Old strictures are loosening, and more attention is being focused on the environment's vital influence and the powers inherent in design. In the past, different disciplines were rigidly separate; social scientists concentrated on the influence of the social environment; psychologists were absorbed with rat behavior and isolated stimuli in the sterile confines of their laboratories; and designers and architects strove, in the main, for aesthetically pleasing functionality. What is now emerging, however, is a more interdisciplinary, holistic approach, for we have begun to perceive people in their total environment, to realize that behavior is influenced by space, structure, color, lighting, activity, and other participants, as well as by our own inner being — in sum, that everything has its effect in an environmental process that works as a kind of circular feedback. With this understanding, design becomes in a sense akin to social action: We can either stimulate learning or dull the requisite desire and concentration; enhance recuperation or impede it; encourage vital social interaction or hinder it; improve mental and emotional well-being or further listless torpor. While an awareness of these influences through emerging research in the field is important for *any* design, be it private home or public facility, it is *crucial* in the planning of societal structures — schools, hospitals, mental and penal institutions, factories, office buildings — that contain large masses of people over sustained periods of time, thus giving shape to the moments and course of their lives.

CHAPTER 12

Interior Finishes and Furniture

The interior design of a medical or dental office is critically important to the patients' assessment of the physician or dentist and the level of anxiety patients experience. Patients can rarely assess the quality of the clinical care provided. Nevertheless, a judgment is made based upon interactions with staff and an evaluation of the interior environment. Visible attention to detail in office design generates feelings of confidence about the health care professionals who work there and the services that are provided.

This chapter will discuss specifications of interior finish materials and furniture items that are particularly well suited to medical and dental offices. Photographs of individual rooms displaying a great attention to detail are scattered throughout the chapters of this book and in the color plates.

All too often, medical and dental interiors are designed to residential standards, with materials not intended to withstand the stress of a high-volume office. A door that, in a residence, may be opened and closed 3000 times a year, may be opened and closed 100,000 times a year in a medical office. Similarly, shag or cut pile carpet designed for residential use does not hold up well. It is difficult to clean and may show wear sooner than a commercial carpet.

If budget permits, all walls should receive a commercial vinyl wallcovering (see Chapter 15 for classification characteristics). Gypsum board walls make a good substrate for application of vinyl wallcoverings provided they have not been textured. A light texture is desirable, however, if the walls will be painted, since texture helps to conceal drywall taping and nail heads. A heavy stucco or sand finish texture is to be avoided, since it collects dirt and is difficult to clean. Special wall treatments such as wood paneling, grasscloth, or woven fabrics should not be used in examination or treatment areas, but may be used in limited areas such as consultation rooms and waiting rooms.

Certain high-profile suites such as plastic surgery may demand unusual interior finishes to achieve their marketing goals; however, sanitation and flammability considerations must not be overlooked. There are two issues here. First, if a product specified does not meet the minimum flammability standard for a particular usage, the physician may be denied Medicare reimbursement or the facility may be denied state licensing. For example, putting a hardwood floor in the operating room of an office-based surgery suite will prevent that physician from getting reimbursed for the use of the facility. (In order to gain Medicare certification and reimbursement from many of the third-party payers, the surgery suite must meet NFPA 101 Life Safety Code, which stipulates fire ratings, among other things, for all areas of an office-based surgery suite.)

The second issue is potential liability in case of fire faced by the designer who specifies interior finish materials. If, after a fire, it is determined that any of the materials within the office did not meet the minimum flammability requirements, the designer is certain to be included in the lawsuit. These are the two main reasons that designers should be extremely cautious and diligent in determining which, if any, local or state codes apply to the selection of interior finishes for their specific medical or dental project.

The Uniform Building Code, in use in various cities, classifies medical office buildings as a Group B occupancy. As of this writing, interior finishes having a flame-spread index of 75 or less would be suitable for all areas within the suite (with the exception of surgery suites, where patients may be unconscious). Some areas of the suite may have finishes with a flame-spread rating in excess of 75, provided the area is not an enclosed vertical exitway (stairwell) or an exit corridor.

A suspended acoustic tile ceiling is more suitable than a gypsum board ceiling because it gives access to the electrical and mechanical equipment above it and is easier to clean. Where sanitation is of extreme importance, a plastic-coated acoustic tile or an enameled gypsum board ceiling should be used.

Flooring may be carpet, vinyl composition tile (VCT), sheet vinyl, ceramic tile, or a combination of all four. The least expensive flooring is VCT, which is very durable, but it does need to be waxed and buffed. Sheet vinyl is recommended for wet areas such as bathrooms if the budget does not allow for ceramic tile. Sheet vinyl is also recommended in minor surgeries or anywhere sanitation is a concern because it has fewer seams than VCT and may be installed with a self-coved base. Tarkett, a Swedish manufacturer, markets several high-quality sheet vinyl floorings suitable for operating room suites and other treatment areas where cleanliness is important. It also offers a cushioned sheet vinyl that does not compress under the weight of heavy equipment. The Tarkett products are extremely flexible and malleable, allowing them to be coved up around inside and outside corners, pipes, floor sinks, or other obstructions, creating a seamless floor. Seams may be either chemically welded or heat welded.

There is an attractive wood flooring product called *GenuWood,* manufactured by Perma-Grain Products (Media, Pennsylvania) that meets a Class A flame-spread rating. It has a 20 mil layer of clear vinyl over the wood veneer, making it easy to clean, although it is not a seamless installation.

Also new is a class of woven wallcoverings made of polyolefin that carries a Class A flame-spread rating, is mildew resistant, remarkably durable, and has the luxurious appearance of fine linen fabric. These wallcoverings may even be used in patient areas of hospitals. Even though these fabrics appear to be delicate, they are extremely tough and may even be cleaned with a bleach solution. Maharam *Tek-Wall,* Design Tex *Stone Wall,* and Armorweave *Polaris Plus* are products of this type.

CARPET

It is not uncommon to find entire medical or dental offices carpeted. Apart from any considerations previously discussed regarding infection control, carpet, if selected properly, is easy to maintain and adds warmth to the office appearance. It provides a much-needed acoustic function as well, and it prevents serious accidents caused by people slipping.

When discussing carpet fibers, it is important to keep in mind that the fiber composition of a carpet style is only one of several performance factors to consider in the specification process. *Yarn weight, pile height, twist count, camouflage texture,* and *color* can have a much greater combined impact on the suitability and performance of carpet than fiber selection alone. Therefore, a careful evaluation and comparison of all specifications should be made prior to selecting a particular carpet.

Although polypropylene (Olefin) fibers have shown some recent strength in the lower-end market, and wool fiber has gained some ground in the very high end, nylon has continued to grow as the fiber of choice for most health care facilities. Superior performance characteristics such as resiliency, abrasion resistance, cleanability, stain resistance, and texture retention have virtually eliminated other fibers such as polyester and acrylic.

Type 6.6 nylon (Du Pont, Monsanto) is approximately 17 percent harder than Type 6 (BASF, Allied Chemical). All other things being equal, this could affect performance characteristics accordingly; however, pattern, camouflage, color, and other factors can largely overcome this differential.

In areas where the use of caustics and bleaching agents is common, solution-dyed nylons may be the best option. These yarn systems do not necessarily have better general stain resistance, but are substantially more colorfast than conventionally dyed nylons and permit the use of a bleach cleaning agent. Because the yarn is pigmented before tufting or weaving, the color consistency from roll to roll is excellent.

Antimicrobial treatment (Sylgard), designed to inhibit the growth and reproduction of microorganisms, has been established as a significant enhancement to carpet manufacturing. Molds, mildew, fungi, and other microorganisms cannot multiply, cause odors, or discolor the carpet. Potential infection and allergic reaction to these organisms is eliminated, although the control of odor and mustiness is perhaps the most visible advantage of these treatments.

Fluorochemical treatments (Teflon) for enhanced stain resistance are an important aspect of any specification for carpet in a medical environment. These treatments, which may be effectively applied at several points in the manufacturing process, greatly reduce the surface tension of the fiber, and thus its propensity to attract soil and absorb stains. (Teflon may even be applied in the field, immediately after installation, with the same degree of efficacy.) This enhancement may be the most important in the medical environment, since much more carpet is replaced each year because of food and protein stains than for most other reasons combined. Remember, nylon fibers do not wear out. Maintaining the appearance of the carpet through using fluorochemical treatments and good maintenance can make a significant difference in the useful life of the carpet.

For maximum performance, consider these specifications:

	CUT PILE		LOOP PILE
	BCF	**Spun Nylon**	**BCF**
Yarn weight*	38 oz.	42 oz.	32 oz.
Pile height*	.375	.375	.250
Twist count*	5.5 × 5.5	5.5 × 5.5	—

*Minimum requirements

BCF = bulk continuous filament

Static control in carpet fibers is now all but taken for granted. Any "branded" nylons such as *Antron, Ultron, Zeftron,* and *Anso* will contain a small percentage of conductive filaments capable of reducing static discharge to below the level of human sensitivity (3.5 KV). Some mills offer additional static control (1.5 KV) by using a conductive backing and latex as well. This can be important for use with sensitive computer equipment.

Carpets with a synthetic backing (instead of jute) are desirable particularly where there is a possibility of water leakage. The synthetic backing will not rot or leach out its color, as does jute. When jute gets wet, the dye in it sometimes leaches to the carpet surface, which is very difficult to remove. Dental suites are often prone to plumbing accidents, so it would be especially important to use a carpet with a synthetic backing there.

A *level loop* pile is the most serviceable for high-traffic areas, although a combination loop and cut pile will work well in most medical or dental facilities. A number of high-traffic commercial cut piles are available that perform quite well, although solid colors may not camouflage soil.

Contrary to what was said previously about appropriate pile heights, pediatric waiting rooms often do well with a fairly thick cut pile or even a *saxony* texture yarn. This is because parents may be embarrassed to report accidents, and it may be days before urine or drops of milk or grape juice are discovered — dried and caked. A high pile tends to hide these discolorations well and, if all else fails, the carpet tufts can be be snipped to remove the stain.

Carpet in a medical or dental office is best installed glued directly to the slab with no pad. This provides a firm footing, making it less likely that people will trip. Direct glue-down is the recommended installation method in hospitals and many other commercial facilities as well. In offices, it sometimes eliminates the need for acrylic chair mats since it is firm enough to allow chairs and carts to roll freely. Where a pad is desired, as in a consultation room, a rubber slab pad is preferable to a foam waffle pad, which tends to "bottom out." *Omalon* is a high quality brand of pad that works well where pad is desired in a commercial facility.

Although for years direct glue-down has been the preferred method of installation in commercial facilities, there is considerable evidence to indicate that a *double glue* method may become equally popular in coming years. This new installation technique extends the appearance life of carpet by keeping the pile from packing down and losing texture. With this method, a special ⅛-inch-thick carpet cushion (pad) is glued to the floor, and, in turn, the carpet is glued to the pad. It is made possible with advancements in adhesives combined with a specially engineered high-density pad. One such cushion is called *Tread-Mor,* manufactured by Sponge-Cushion, Inc., for its *Dubl-Stik* installation method.

FURNITURE

Offices located in cities with inclement weather must provide an area near the entrance to the waiting room for removing boots, rubbers, and winter apparel. An umbrella caddy and coat hooks (some low enough for children) are also necessary. For the comfort of those waiting, it is desirable that the coat area be visible from the waiting room. Offices in southern California and other areas with a temperate climate usually do not have entry vestibules or coat closets.

To eliminate the clutter of magazines strewn about the room, waiting rooms ought to have a magazine rack. Wall-hung units are most functional. While these may be custom designed, those shown in Figures 12-1, 12-2, and 12-3 are available in a number of options with respect to size and finish.

Most offices need to display and dispense many health care education pamphlets and brochures. The brochure rack shown in Figure 12-4 comes in various sizes and may be placed near the nurse station or in the waiting room.

The doors of medical exam rooms require a chart rack. Those in Figures 12-5, 12-6, and 12-7 function well and are available in a number of accent colors. Some are sized for a standard medical chart, others for radiology films, and yet others are a combination size, with a pocket for each. It is a nice amenity to provide an individual magazine rack in each exam room such as that shown in Figure 12-10. Exam rooms also require coat hooks and hangers. Those shown in Figure 12-9 come in attractive colors and are soft to the touch.

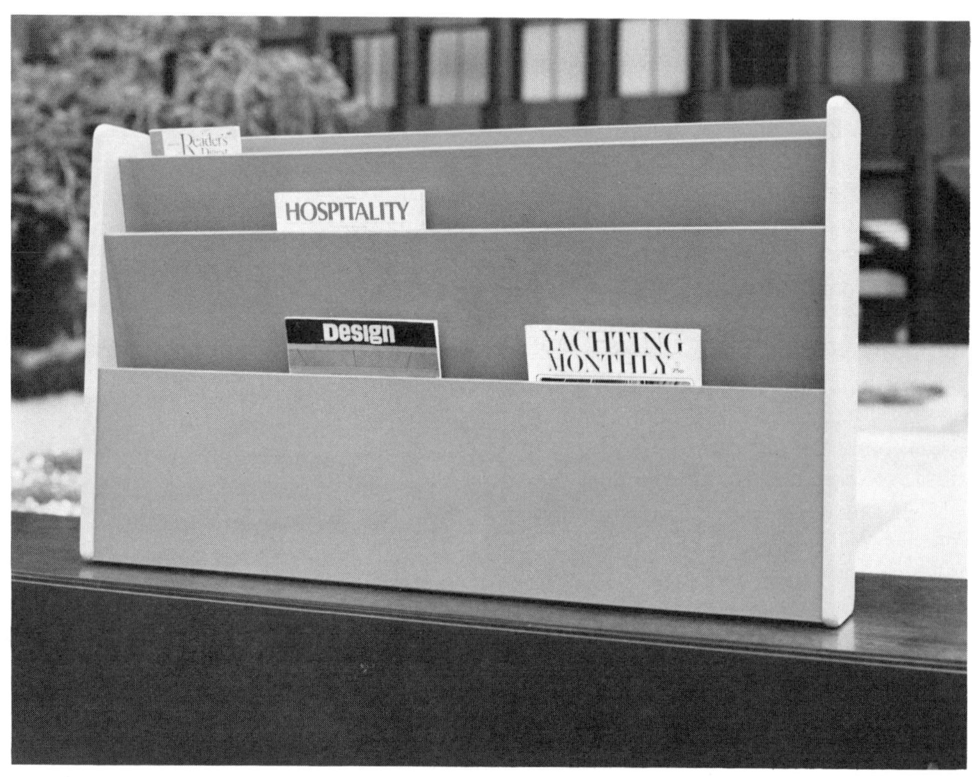

Figure 12-1. Magazine rack. (*Courtesy Peter Pepper Products Co., Compton, CA.*)

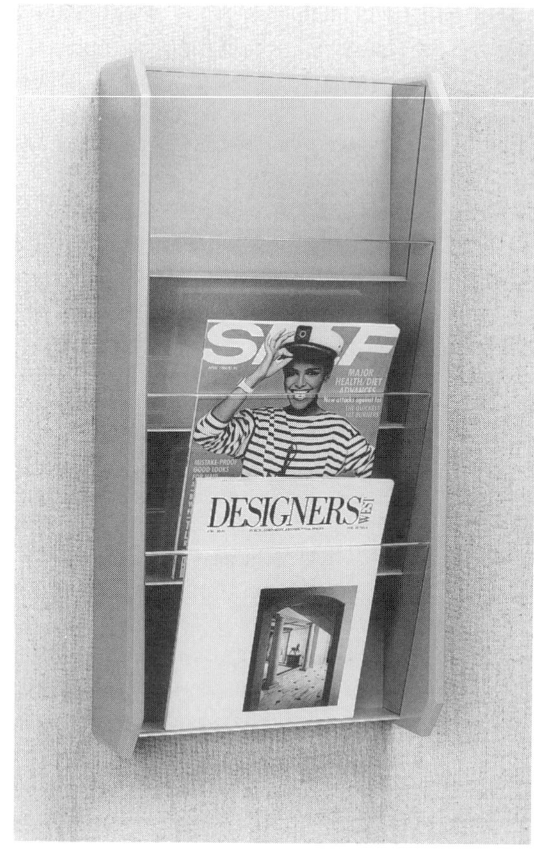

Figure 12-2. Magazine rack. (*Courtesy Peter Pepper Products Co., Compton, CA.*)

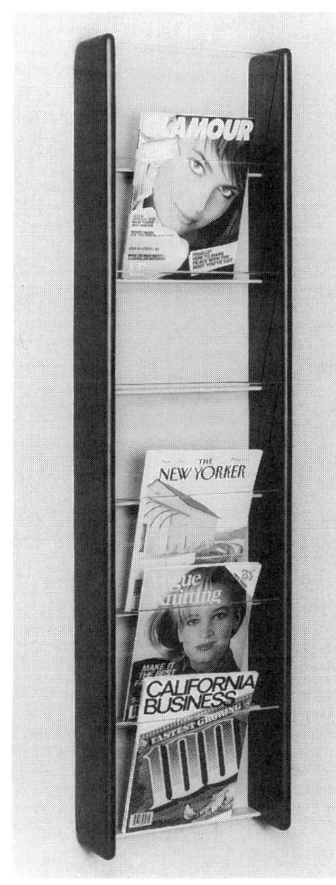

Figure 12-3. Magazine rack. (*Courtesy Peter Pepper Products Co., Compton, CA.*)

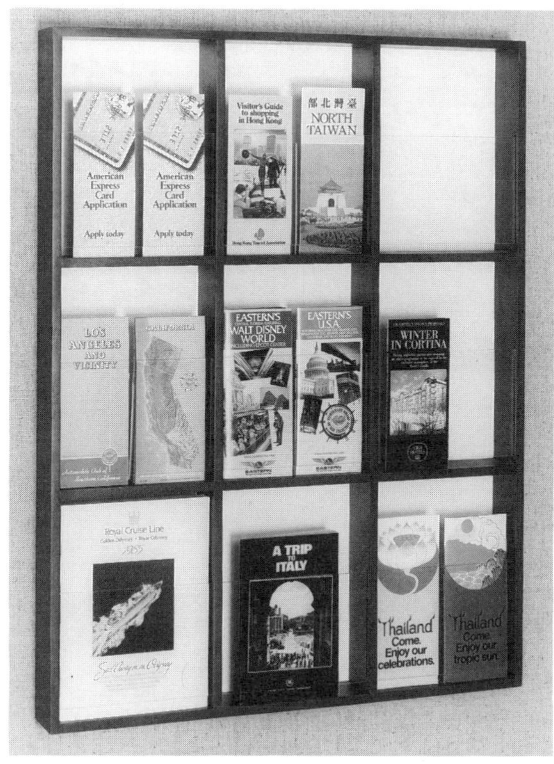

Figure 12-4. Brochure rack. (*Courtesy Peter Pepper Products Co., Compton, CA.*)

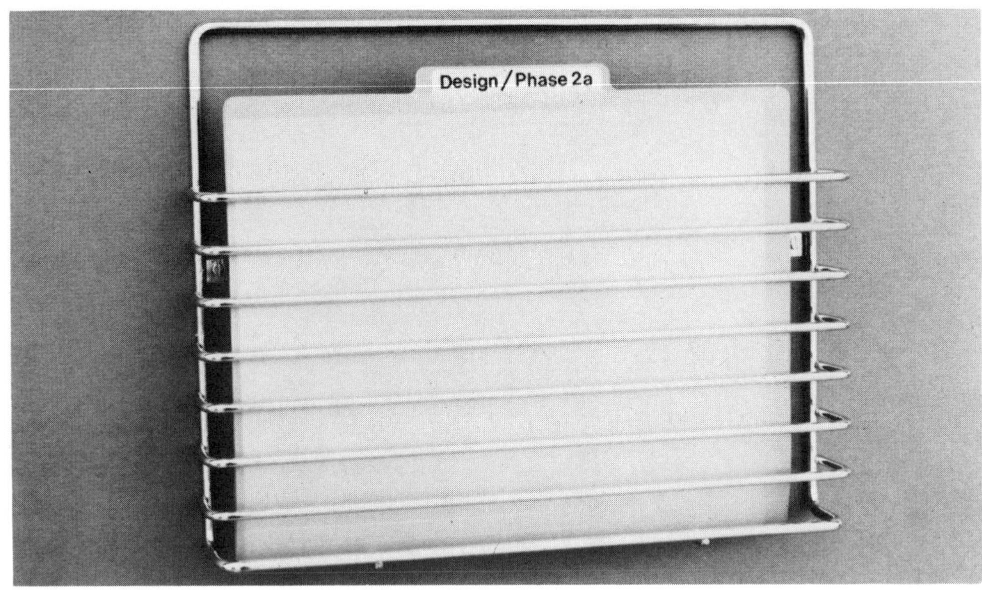

Figure 12-5. Chart rack. (*Courtesy Peter Pepper Products Co., Compton, CA.*)

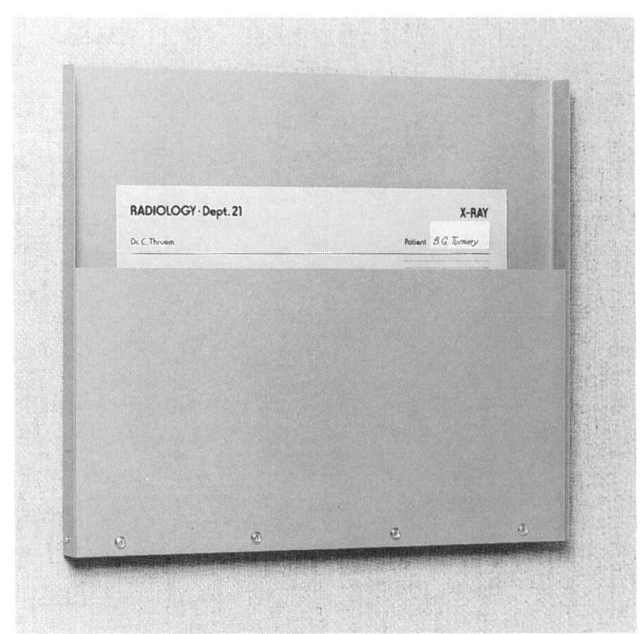

Figure 12-7. Chart rack for radiology films. (*Courtesy Peter Pepper Products Co., Compton, CA.*)

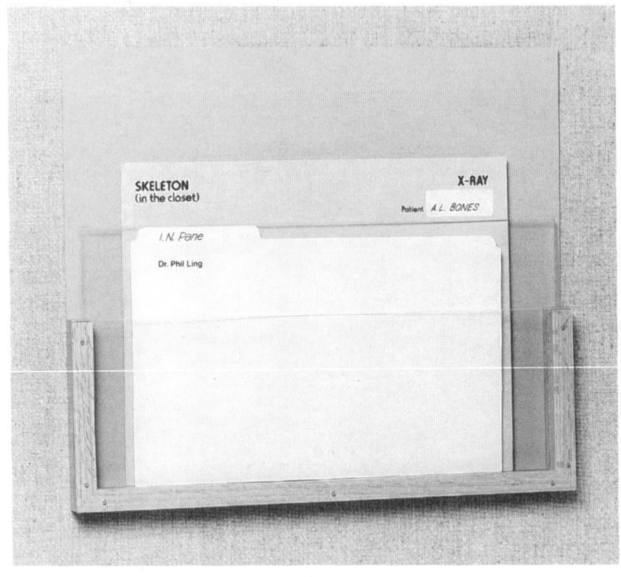

Figure 12-6. Combination medical chart/X-ray rack. (*Courtesy Peter Pepper Products Co., Compton, CA.*)

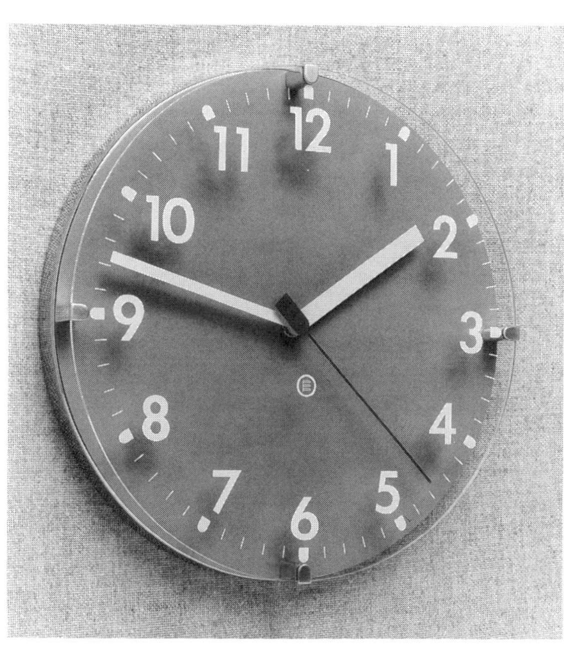

Figure 12-8. Clock. (*Courtesy Peter Pepper Products Co., Compton, CA.*)

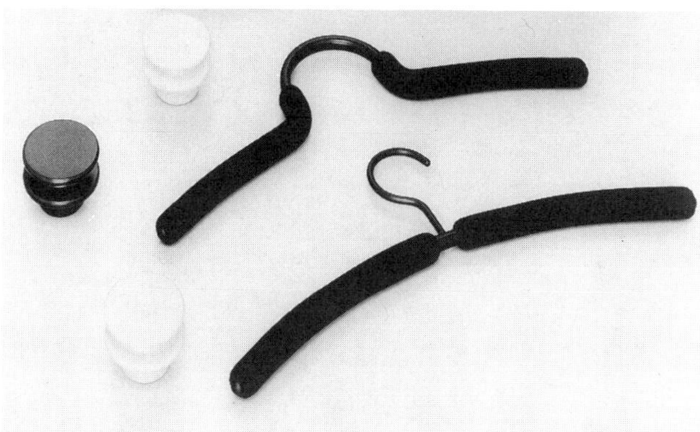

Figure 12-9. Clothes hooks and hangers. (*Courtesy Peter Pepper Products Co., Compton, CA.*)

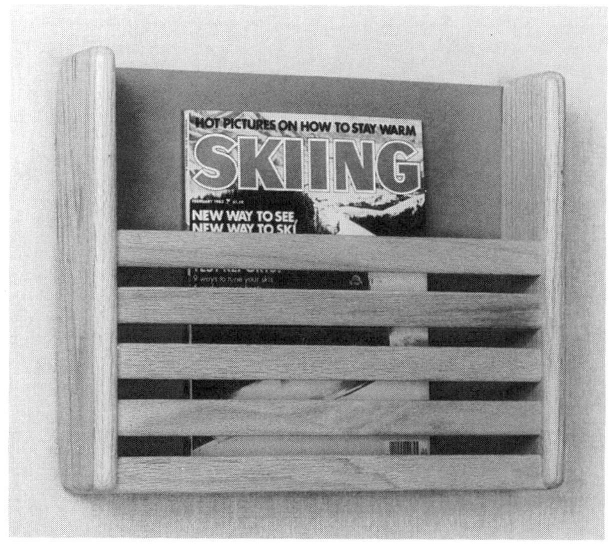

Figure 12-10. Magazine rack for exam room. (*Courtesy Peter Pepper Products Co., Compton, CA.*)

Decorative accessories that are also functional add color to a business office or nurse station. The perpetual calendar in Figure 12-11 and the clock in Figure 12-8 are examples.

There is great latitude in selecting waiting room seating. The main criteria are that a suitable number of individual chairs with arms be provided and that the chairs not be too low or hard to get out of. The seating in Figures 12-12, 12-13, and 12-14 includes examples of chairs that are well suited to medical and dental waiting rooms. Each of these is well balanced, so that it will not tip when someone pushes against one arm only. The modular seating in Figures 12-12 and 12-13 is also available in individual chairs, plus a number of other configurations. The modular seating in Figure 12-15 has a soft, residential appearance, but features excellent lumbar support, a variety of armrest styles, and field-changeable upholstery covers.

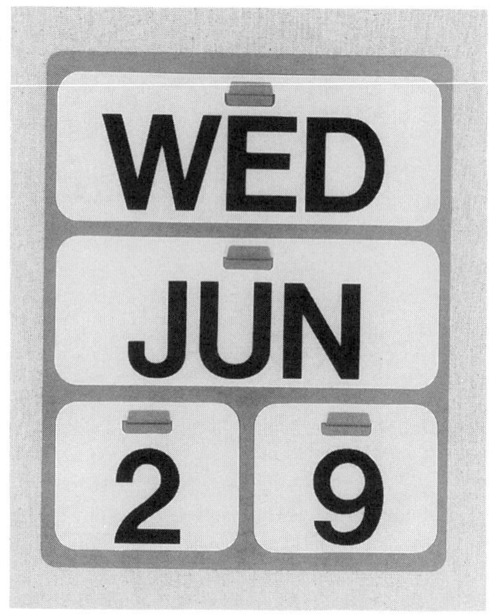

Figure 12-11. Perpetual calendar. (*Courtesy Peter Pepper Products Co., Compton, CA.*)

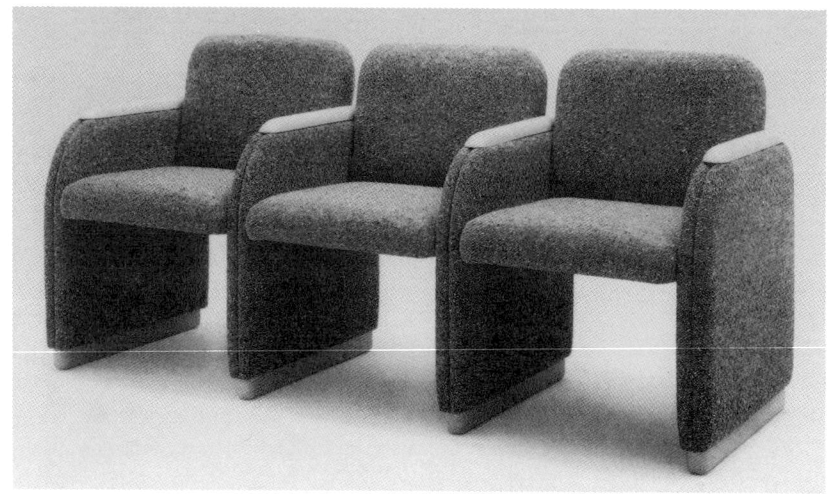

Figure 12-12. Waiting room seating. (*Courtesy Condi, Compton, CA.*)

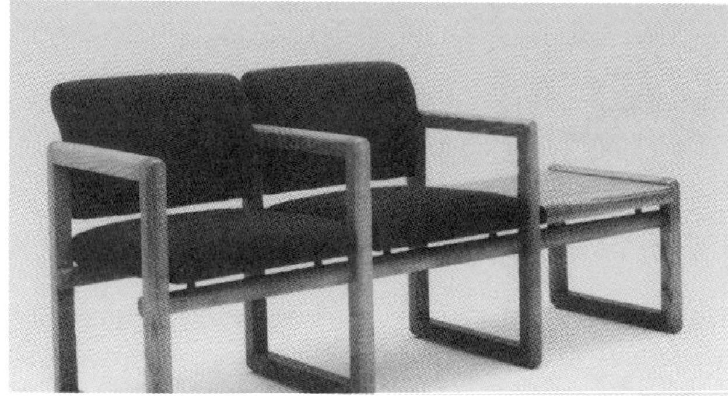

Figure 12-13. Modular seating. (*Courtesy Condi, Compton, CA.*)

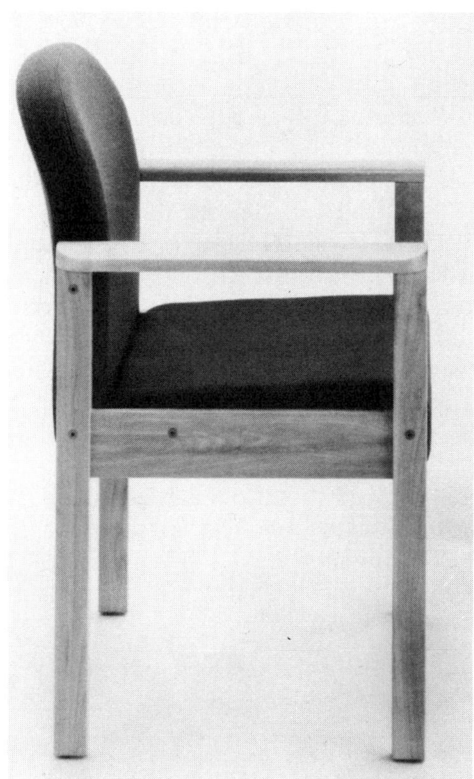

Figure 12-14. Waiting room chairs. (*Courtesy Thonet Industries, York, PA.*)

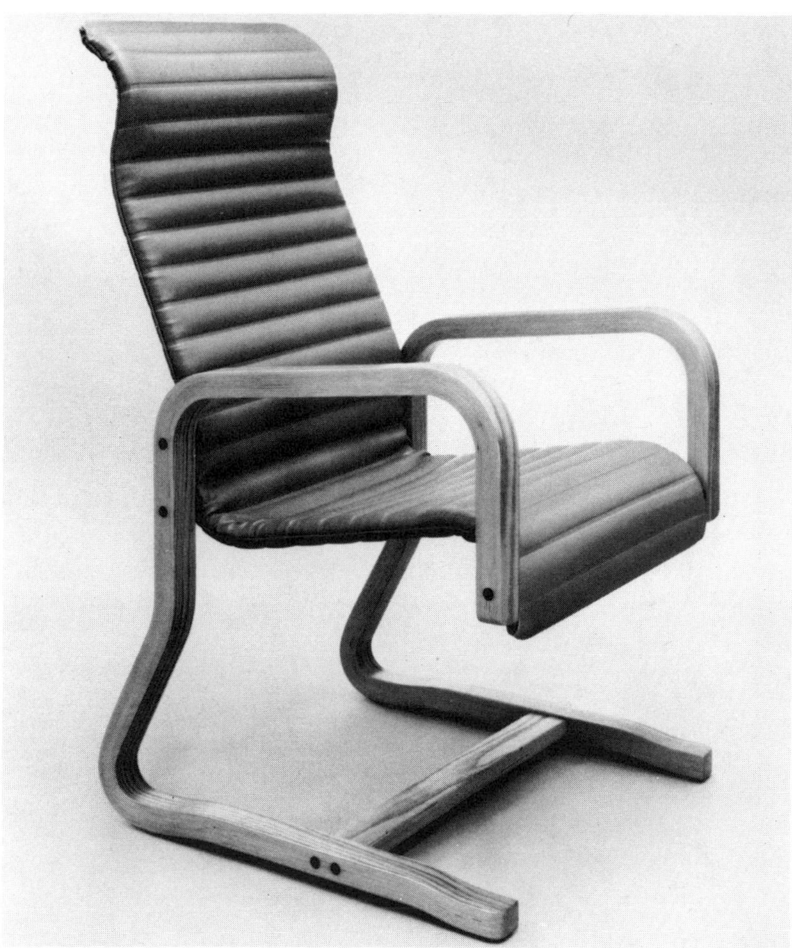

Figure 12-16. High-backed chair for geriatric patients or those with orthopedic problems. (*Courtesy Thonet Industries.*)

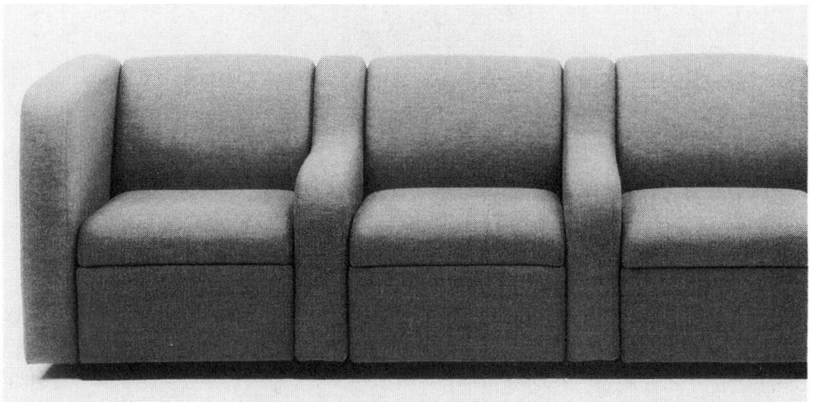

Figure 12-15. Modular seating. (*Courtesy Roger Leib, Add Interior Systems, Inc., Los Angeles, CA.*)

Practices with a number of geriatric patients or patients with arthritic or orthopedic problems may wish to provide some high-backed seating such as that shown in Figures 12-16, 12-17, 12-18, and 12-19. The chair shown in Figure 12-18 has a rocking motion or flex that is quite soothing.

It is important for the parents' and staff's sanity to keep children well occupied — patients and siblings alike. A small table or work counter will provide space for coloring or for playing games. Proper storage for toys will encourage the children to replace toys after use.

Educational exhibits or artwork can be put to good use in a medical waiting room. The subject matter may provide useful information about the facility or its physicians or history, or explain birth defects, sports injuries, or other medical conditions.

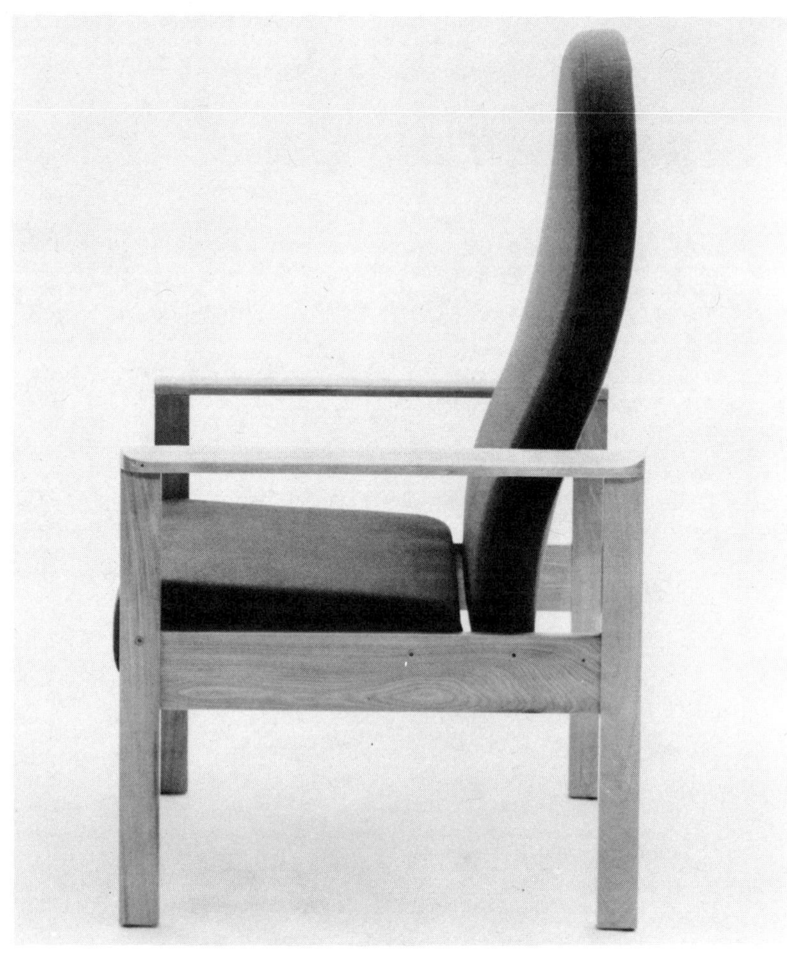

Figure 12-17. High-backed chair. (*Courtesy Thonet Industries.*)

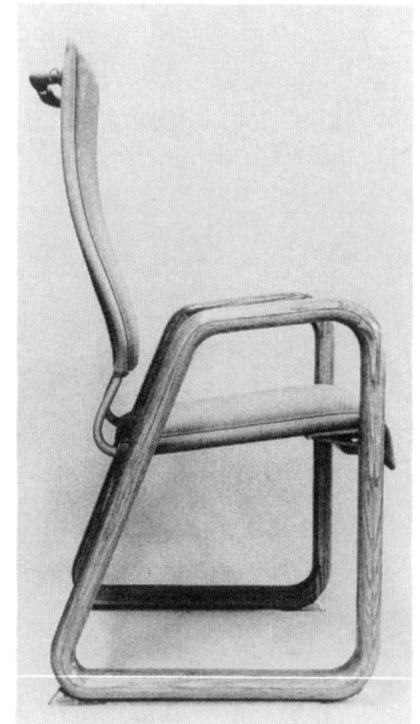

Figure 12-18. High-backed chair. (*Courtesy Roger Leib, Add Interior Systems, Inc., Los Angeles, CA.*)

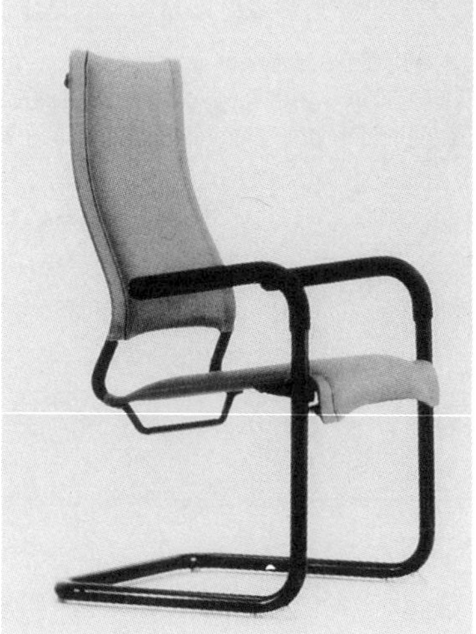

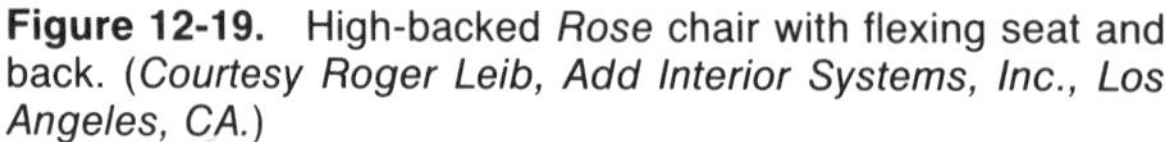

Figure 12-19. High-backed *Rose* chair with flexing seat and back. (*Courtesy Roger Leib, Add Interior Systems, Inc., Los Angeles, CA.*)

CHAPTER 13
Lighting

BIOLOGICAL EFFECTS OF LIGHT

Traditionally, lighting engineers and those in the design professions have been concerned with lighting in terms of vision or aesthetics. Until recently, the biological significance of light has been overlooked. Incandescent and fluorescent lamps are fabricated according to the assumption that people will be exposed to sunlight as a normal part of each day and not be confined to a habitation of artificial illumination. These lamps emit a narrow spectrum of light that does not include ultraviolet.

Fluorescent light is light without heat, whereby ultraviolet radiation is converted into radiation of a longer wavelength. (Since the human eye is not sensitive to UV radiation, these wavelengths are lengthened by phosphors to which the eye is sensitive.) Different phosphors create different tints of fluorescent light. Thus fluorescent lamps, in simplistic terms, are nothing more than glass tubes, the inner surface of which has been coated with phosphor powders, which, when excited by ultraviolet energy created within the arc stream, give off visible light. Most fluorescent lamp tints cost the same to manufacture, although due to marketing demand, cool white always costs less than more appealing colors.

If people are to be confined for long periods away from sunlight, a balanced light that emits a fairly full spectrum of wavelengths is desirable. The illumination of our environment acts both to induce and time glandular and metabolic functions affecting, among other things, milk produced, the quality and quantity of eggs laid, and stimulation or inhibition of sexual activity. Light dilates blood vessels, thereby increasing circulation. Sudden exposure to bright light stimulates the adrenal gland. Our biological time clocks — our circadian rhythms — are manipulated by light. Studies have shown that subjects who are forced to live in darkness for prolonged periods suffer sensory deprivation. The loss of environmental cues that tell the body what to do throws body systems out of kilter.

As populations increase and pollution keeps pace, those in urban centers will increasingly be forced to live in indoor environments. People confined to nursing homes or institutions who are not able to get outdoors similarly depend on their indoor environment to supply well-balanced light that includes some ultraviolet. Those who design such environments will have to be aware of not only the biological effects of light, but also the psychological effects as well as the visual quality of the light.

Perhaps the optimal solution for lighting offices, homes, restaurants, hospitals, and hotels would be a system of changing light levels and tints. Since natural light changes throughout the day (warm and rosy at dawn and dusk, bright with a bluish cast at midday), should we not try to imitate these day-night cycles in our indoor environments?

TECHNICAL DATA

The sensations that we call color and light are our psychological interpretations of certain portions of the electromagnetic spectrum. How well we see colors depends on how closely the ingredients of artificial light sources match the ingredients of sunlight. Artificial sources of light have varying degrees of each color — some have more warm wavelengths and some more cool. An incandescent bulb, for example, is high in orange and red and low in blue and violet; thus, it imparts a warm glow, but it is far from the color of daylight. The most efficient lamp is probably the sodium vapor lamp, but its color rendition is so distorted that it cannot be used in interior environments.

Fluorescent lamps are far more energy efficient than incandescent. Typically, fluorescents produce about 72 lumens (the amount of light generated at the light source) per watt, compared with 17.5 lumens per watt produced by a 100-watt general service incandescent lamp. The fluorescent has an average life of 15,000 hours versus 750 hours for the average incandescent. Furthermore, it takes 60 gallons of oil to burn one 100-watt bulb continuously for one year. With energy shortages having become a fact of life, it seems irresponsible to use more than a smattering of incandescent just for special effects when fluorescent will not suffice.

Fluorescent lamps have been improved in recent years, and more than 20 different colors are available. However, careful selection must be made after consulting manufacturers' lamp specification catalogs, because bulbs of the same wattage do not necessarily have equal lumen counts. There are often other quantitative differences about a particular lamp from one manufacturer to another.

Fluorescent lamps are selected on the basis of lumen output, color temperature, and color rendition. The color temperature is expressed in degrees Kelvin. The higher the color temperature, the bluer the appearance and the closer to daylight; the lower the color temperature, the redder the appearance. The color rendering index (CRI) describes the ability of a lamp to render objects as they would be seen in outdoor sunlight, which has a CRI of 100. Thus a lamp with a CRI of 80 renders the object 80 percent as accurately as outdoor sunlight. Below is a list of the most commonly used fluorescent lamps plus a few unique ones.

Cool White lamps are approximately 4100°K with a CRI of 68. They intensify white, gray, blue, and green and do not blend well with incandescent.

Cool White Deluxe lamps are 4100°K with a CRI of 89. Their color rendition is a big improvement over Cool White lamps, but the lumens per watt are reduced considerably, so more of them are needed to achieve the same level of illumination as with Cool White. They produce a very light pinkish-white color.

Warm White lamps are approximately 3000°K with a CRI of 56. They slightly distort all colors and have a pink glow, but mix well with incandescent.

Warm White Deluxe lamps are 3000°K with a CRI of 71. They greatly intensify warm colors, are not as pink as standard Warm White, and blend well with incandescent.

Daylight lamps are 6500°K and usually have a CRI of 75, but Duro-Test Corp. makes one with a CRI of 92. This lamp produces a cold blue-white light, not enhancing to warm colors and incandescent light, but useful in a room where a large quantity of natural light is present.

Standard White lamps are 3500°K with a CRI of 64. These lamps fall between Cool White and Warm White, so they are a good middle-of-the-road choice where budget does not permit a higher-quality lamp. The one with the highest CRI number is best. These lamps blend adequately with incandescent light.

Vita-Lite lamp is 5500°K with a CRI of 91. This is a

high-quality lamp made only by Duro-Test Corp. It is a bright white lamp that simulates the full color and ultraviolet spectrum of sunlight.

Ultralume 3000 lamp is 3000°K with a CRI of 85. Made by Phillips, this lamp enhances warm colors and has better color rendition than Warm White Deluxe.

Optima 32 lamp is 3200°K with a CRI of 82. Manufactured by Duro-Test Corp., this is a general purpose lamp with the warmth of incandescent, but better color rendition.

Optima 50 lamp is 5000°K with a CRI of 91. Made by Duro-Test Corp., its usage is recommended where visual acuity is required and where color matching is performed.

SP35 lamp is 3500°K with a CRI of 73. Made by General Electric Co., this lamp renders skin tones very well, making it ideal for medical offices. It has the good color rendering properties of Cool White Deluxe and Warm White Deluxe, but has considerably more light output. Cool White Deluxe has 56 lumens per watt, while SP35 offers 83 lumens per watt. The SP35 complements both cool and warm color palettes, producing a crisp light midpoint between Cool White and Warm White.

SPX35 is 3500°K with a CRI of 82. Manufactured by General Electric Co., it is an enhanced version of the SP35, which is more expensive, but makes colors appear more vivid.

Compact fluorescent lamps are 2700°K with a CRI of 81. Manufactured by many lamp companies, this new type of fluorescent is a small twin tube in a U-shape, available in 7-watt, 9-watt, and 13-watt lamps. The color rendition is very similar to incandescent, but tends to be a bit more pink, rather than yellow. The 7-watt lamp is equivalent to a 40-watt incandescent; the 9-watt lamp, to a 60-watt incandescent; and the 13-watt, to a 75-watt incandescent. These lamps are very popular because they combine the high efficiency and long life of fluorescent lamps with good color rendition. Their size allows them to be used in downlights, wall sconces, and other types of fixtures that previously required incandescent bulbs.

Low-voltage lamps are of many types, the most common of which is the MR-16. These are 12-volt quartz halogen lamps that average 3000°K and render colors vividly. The beam can be precisely focused to enhance textures or an art object, or to add drama to a room. Low-voltage lamps accomplish a desired level of illumination with fewer watts than required by incandescent lamps, making them energy efficient. Additionally, the miniature size of the lamp allows it to be used in fixtures much smaller than those which accommodate incandescent bulbs. MR-16s give a clean, white light that enhances all colors.

For comparison, an incandescent lamp is 2800°K, and daylight (although it does vary with the time of day, the time of the year, and whether the sky is sunny or cloudy) is arbitrarily established at 6500°K. The reader is encouraged to write to the Duro-Test Corp. in North Bergen, New Jersey, and to Westinghouse in Bloomfield, New Jersey. Both manufacturers have excellent technical literature on their lamps. The General Electric Co. in Nela Park, Ohio, also publishes a number of interesting booklets.

ENERGY CONSERVATION

Worse than not enough light is too much light. More is not better. The designer, if not qualified to do the lighting calculations, may wish to retain a lighting consultant or an electrical engineer. A high level of general illumination tends to wash out textures and colors. Much more interesting, not to mention energy efficient, is an interplay of high and low levels of illumination. In offices, we now light the task, not the entire room.

Lighting, skillfully handled, can set up a rhythm of patterns, light, and shadow which can transform an otherwise commonplace interior into something quite spectacular.

Another practical way to prune watts is to install fixtures with dimmer controls. (Fluorescents must be ordered specifically with dimming ballasts.) An attempt to save electricity by removing two of the four lamps in a four-lamp fixture without changing the ballast saves nothing. One should specify only acrylic lenses, never polystyrene, which is less expensive but yellows with age.

The maintenance of light fixtures is extremely important to their performance. Technical equations permit one to calculate the *light loss factor,* which takes into account temperature and voltage variations, dirt on the lens, lamp depreciation, maintenance procedures, and atmospheric conditions. The ceiling height and the reflectance of walls and floor also affect the footcandle level (the measurement of light that reaches a given surface). Thus when one speaks of a requirement of 100 *maintained* footcandles at a given task, one must start with a number of lamps somewhat in excess of that measurement to take into account the light loss factor and the interior finishes of the room.

MEDICAL OFFICE ELECTRICAL AND LIGHTING REQUIREMENTS

The electrical and lighting requirements for medical and dental offices differ greatly with the specialty and are discussed somewhat under each chapter. Chapter 10 discusses thoroughly the requirements of dental operatories, so that information will not be repeated here. Figure 13-1 shows the recommended electrical outlets for the pediatric suite first introduced in Figure 3-78. Figure 13-2 shows a typical reflected ceiling plan and switching diagram for the same pediatric suite.

Exam rooms need a maintained light level of 100 footcandles. This can be achieved by two four-lamp (2- × 4-foot) luminaires, either recessed (lay-in) or surface mounted. Physicians who require a high-intensity light for examinations will have a portable lamp or other light source for that purpose.

Nurse stations also require a maintained illumination of 100 footcandles. A lower light level is appropriate for waiting rooms (30 to 50 footcandles), and the concentration of illumination should be where people are reading. The lighting may be indirect downlights or fluorescent luminaires, or perhaps an artificial skylight. Figure 13-3 shows an entry foyer of an orthopedic surgery suite, using incandescent lights tucked away in the exposed truss joists to create a sculptural interplay of light on the walls. A nurse station, the internal core of this orthopedic surgery suite (Figure 13-4), has a wood ceiling to add warmth and recessed fluorescent downlights that, instead of giving uniform illumination, create pools of light and interesting drama.

The reader is referred to Color Plate 5, Figure 4-13, for an example of low-voltage lighting in the waiting room of a women's clinic. The lighting is crisp and white, and precisely focused, adding drama to the room rather than a wash of overall illumination.

Figure 13-5 shows the very narrow waiting room and reception desk of a dental clinic in a remodeled brownstone in Manhattan. To open up the room and add interest, different levels of gypsum board create a multilevel ceiling. Fluorescent lamps with theatrical gels add washes of color to the walls and ceiling.

Corridors need only about 20 footcandles of illumination, and the light certainly need not be confined to the ceiling. In fact, lighting mounted on the walls of a corridor often gives better color rendition to interior fin-

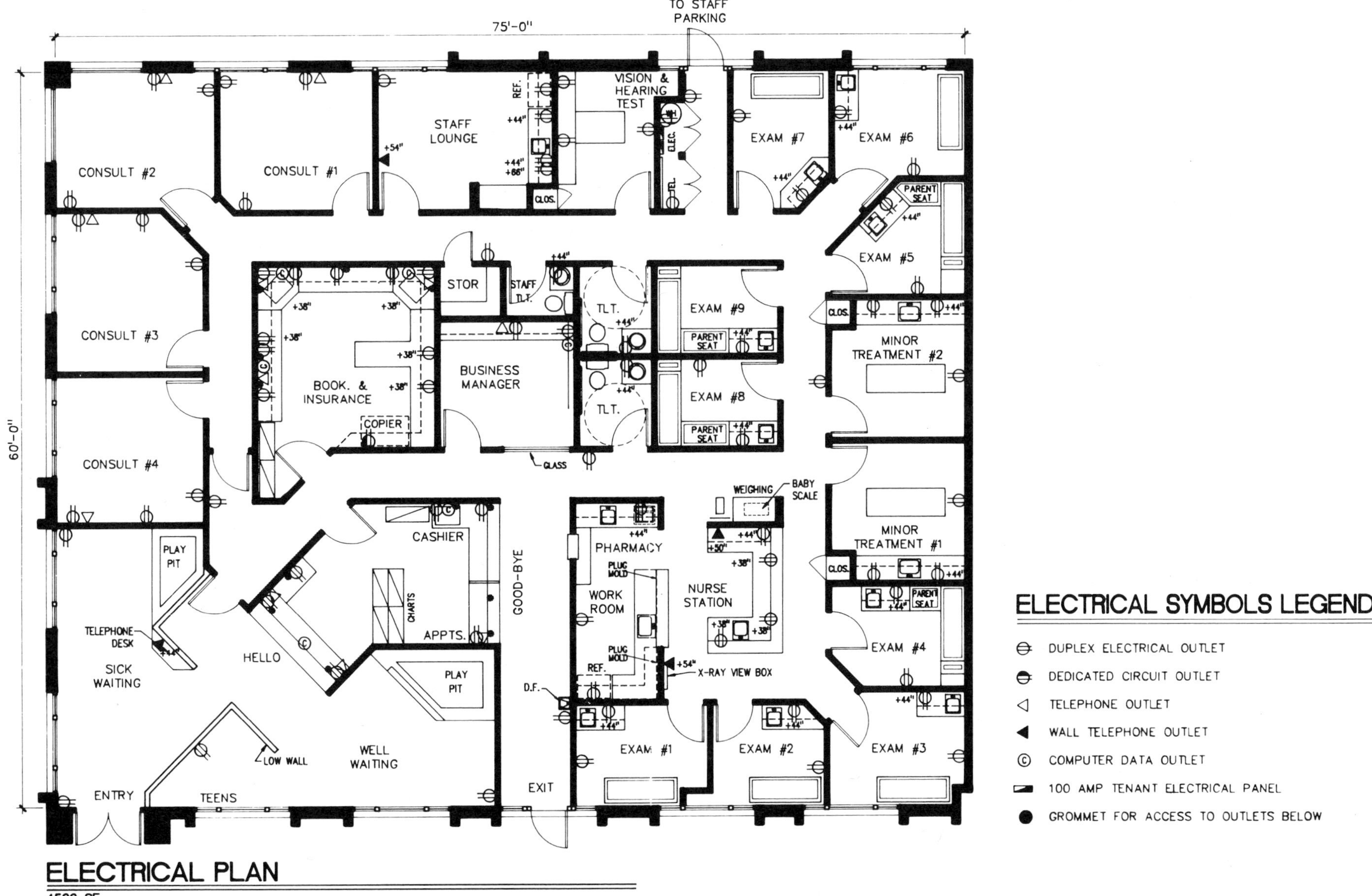

Figure 13-1. Electrical plan for pediatric suite Figure 3-78.

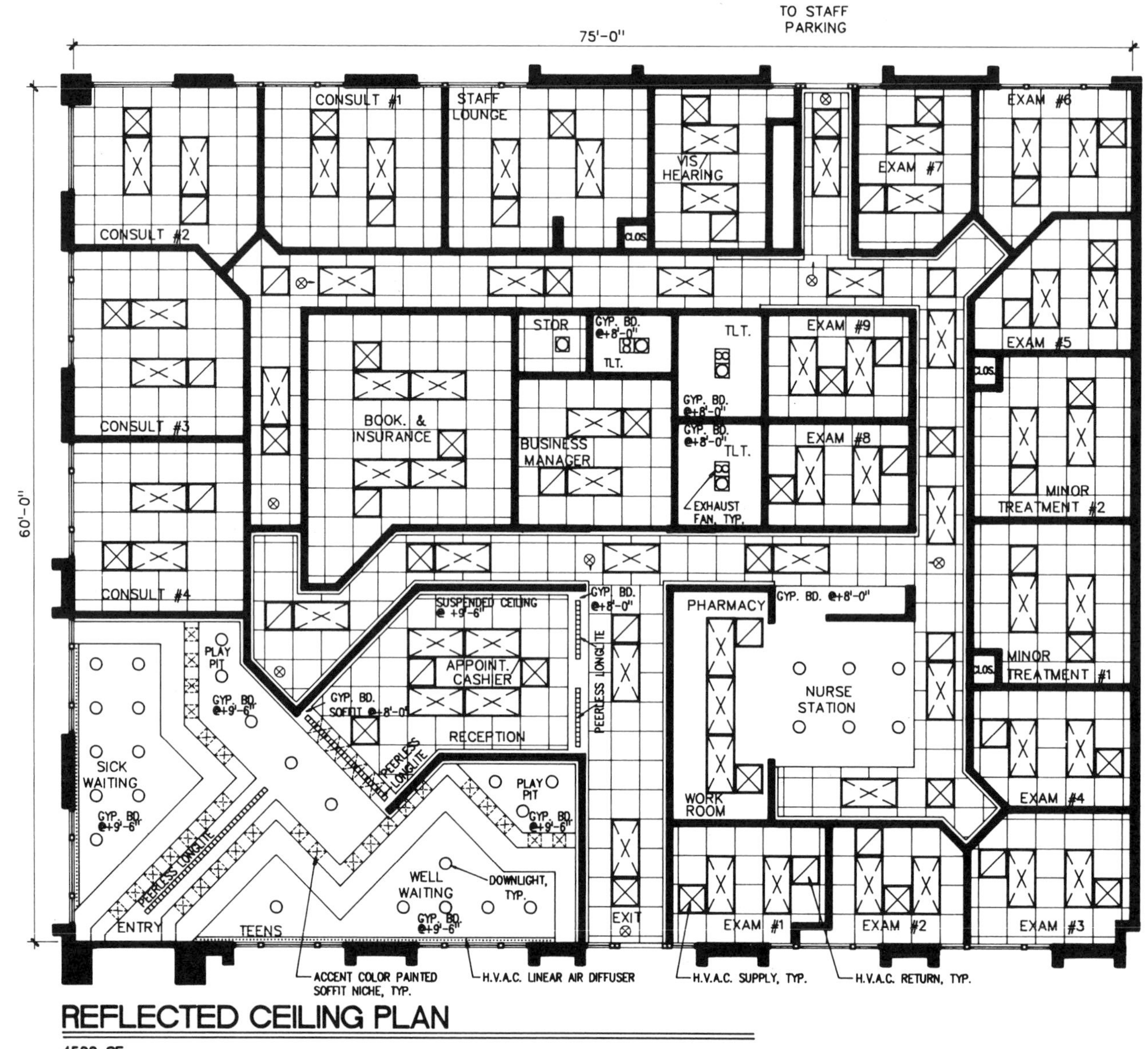

Figure 13-2. Reflected ceiling plan for pediatric suite Figure 3-78.

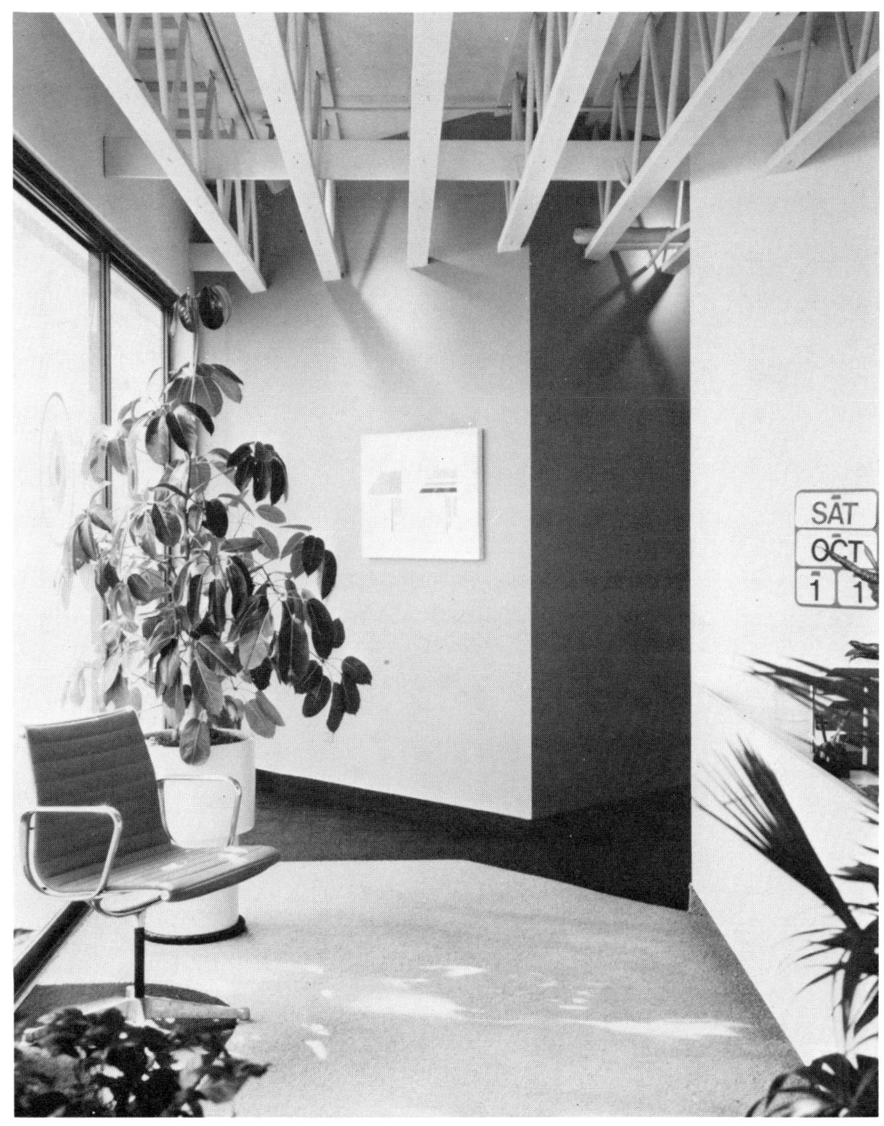

Figure 13-3. Entry foyer, orthopedic surgery suite. (*Courtesy Jain Malkin Inc.*)

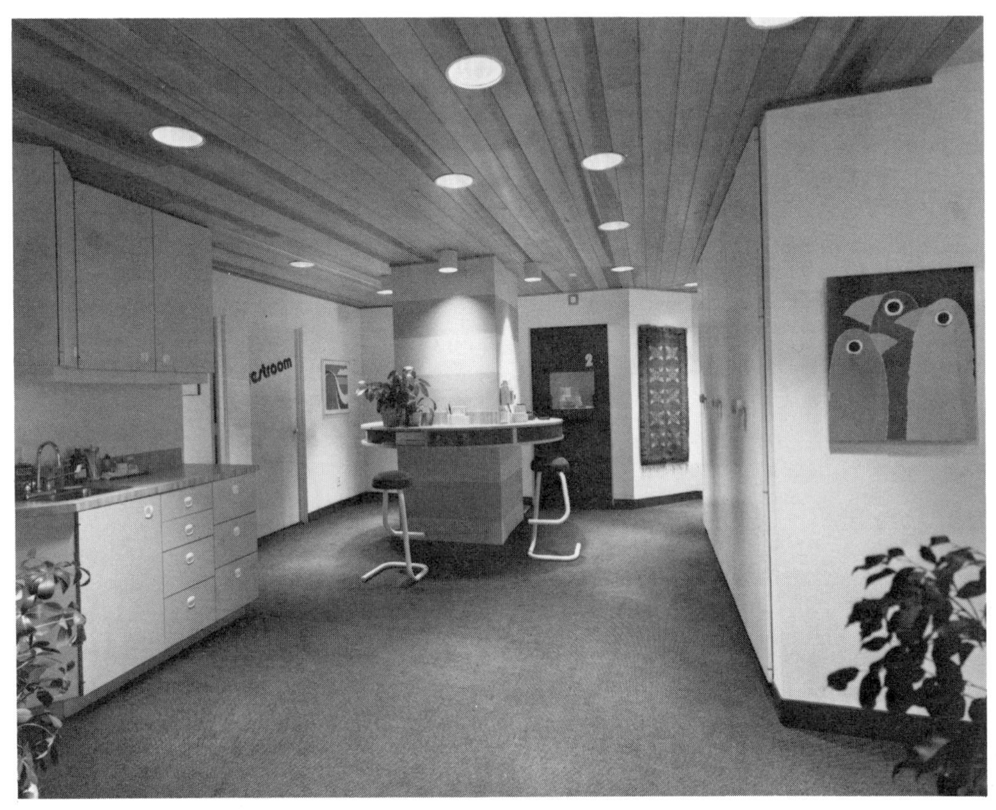

Figure 13-4. Nurse station, orthopedic surgery. (*Courtesy Jain Malkin Inc.*)

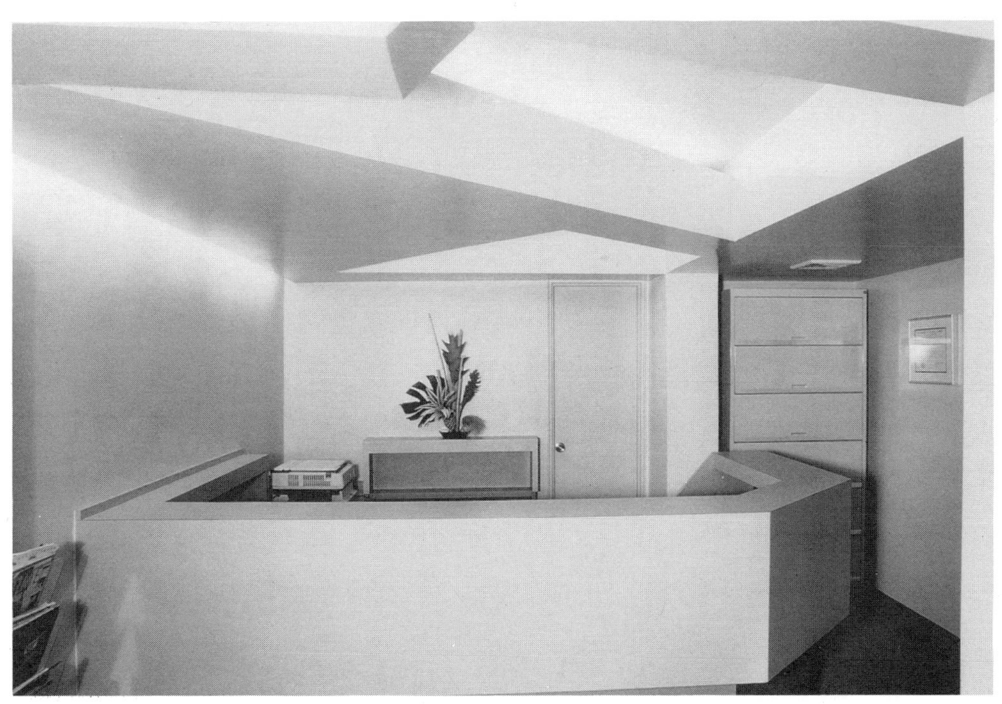

Figure 13-5. Ceiling/lighting, dental office reception room. (*Design: Jain Malkin Inc.; Photographer: Stuart Isler, D.M.D., New York, NY.*)

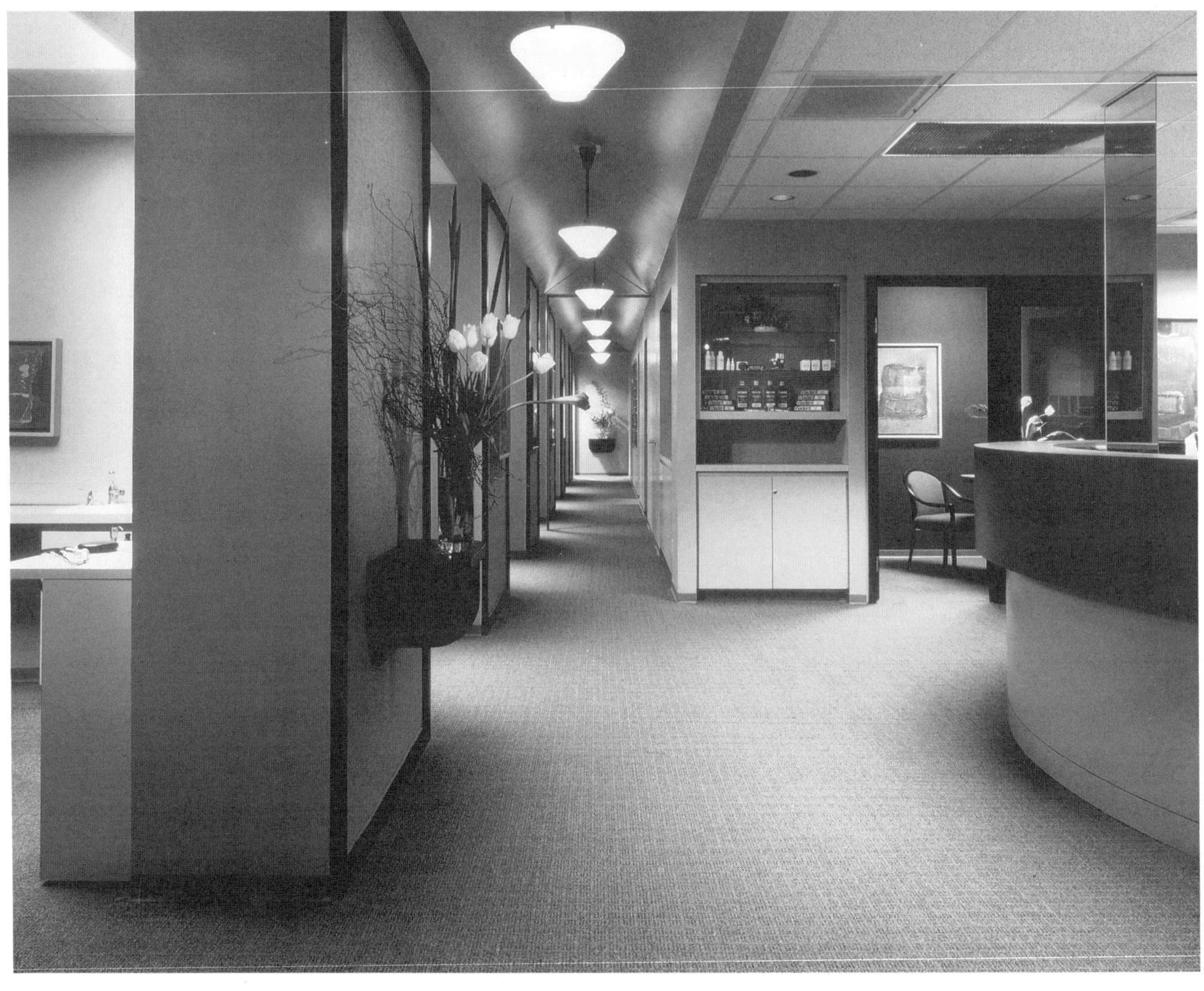

Figure 13-6. Corridor, general dentistry office. (*Courtesy Carmel Repp Ltd., Interior Design Associates, San Diego, CA; Photographer: Kim Brun.*)

ishes than would those same lights mounted on the ceiling. Also, there is more glare when lights are mounted on the ceiling. Figure 13-6 shows the corridor of a dental suite. The vaulted ceiling and Italian pendant light fixtures create a residential ambience with a European flavor. The corridor in Color Plate 32, Figure 13-9, provides indirect lighting without glare.

The reader is referred to Color Plate 15, Figures 6-14 and 6-15, for lighting treatment of a 30,000-square-foot group practice clinic. The corridor is especially interesting, with recessed light niches punctuating it and overall illumination provided by a fluorescent light cove near the ceiling. Wall sconces (with compact fluorescent lamps) further enhance the nonclinical appearance of the corridor. The waiting room features a variety of light sources: overhead fluorescents with low-glare parabolic lenses, ceiling-mounted focusable accent lights, and cove lighting within the tiered gypsum board soffits.

Figure 13-7 shows a lighting treatment for exposed truss joists where there is no place to hide electrical wiring or bury the housing for a recessed fixture. A light track fastened to the chord of the joist lends itself well to the informality of the exposed truss architectural style.

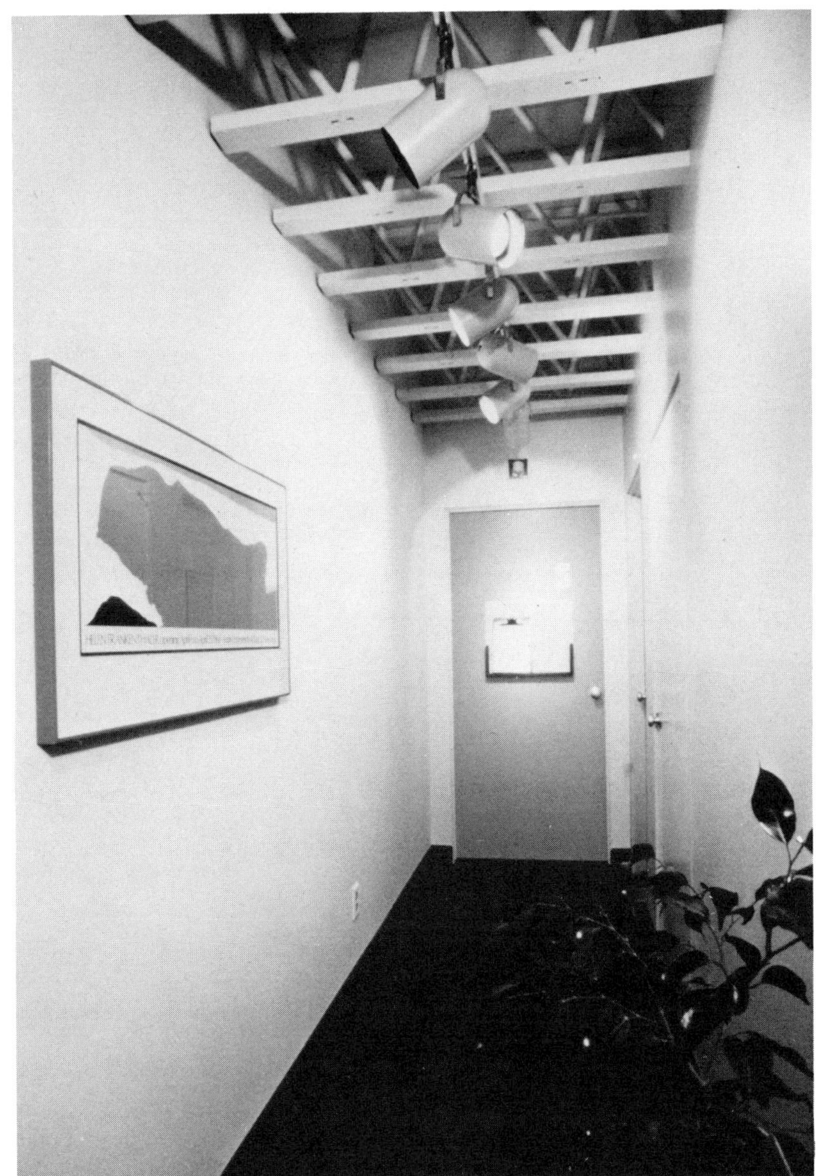

Figure 13-7. Corridor lighting. (*Courtesy Jain Malkin Inc.*)

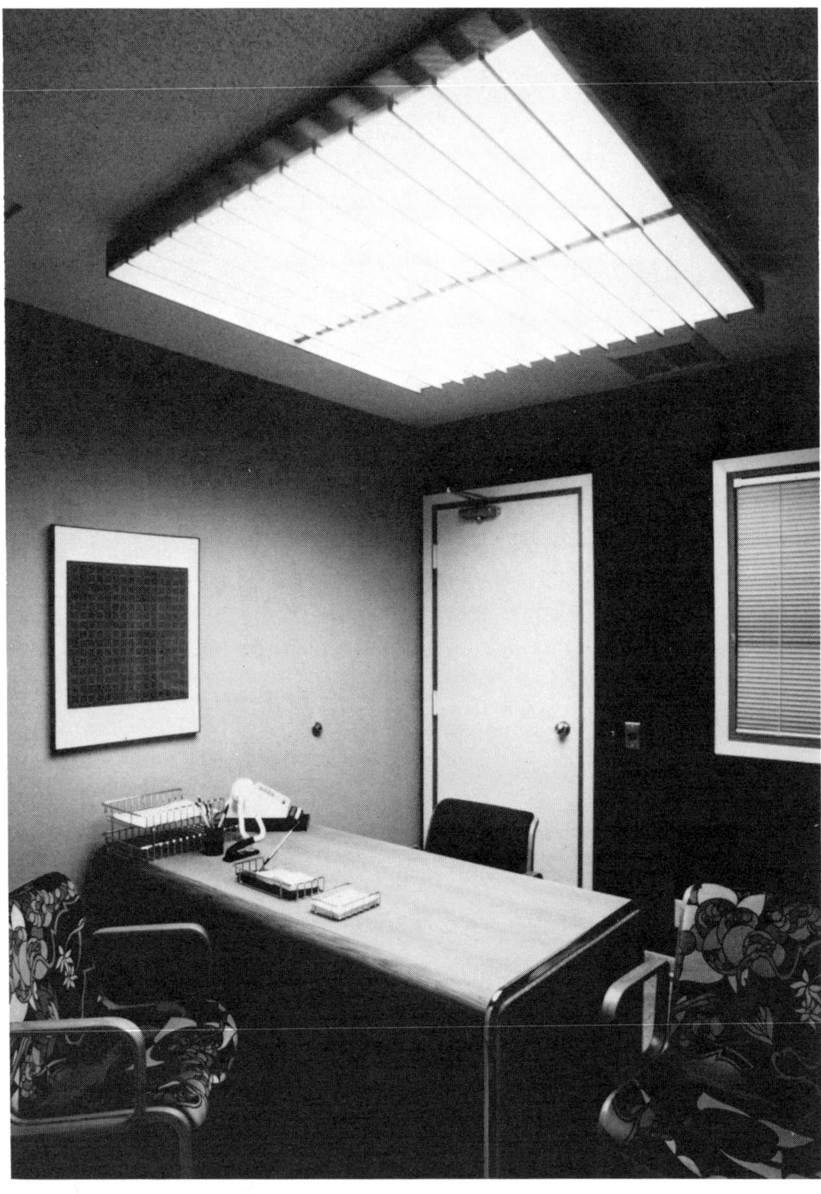

Figure 13-8. Consultation room lighting.

The consultation room requires approximately 50 footcandles of light concentrated over the desk. Figure 13-8 shows two oak-framed surface-mounted fluorescents butted together to form a larger and more imposing fixture unit. Additional lighting in a consultation room may be used to accent diplomas or artwork if the room is large enough to handle additional lighting.

Minor surgery rooms require from 100 to 150 maintained footcandles, depending on the detail of the procedures performed. Most minor surgery rooms will have a ceiling-mounted high-intensity surgical light in addition to two four-lamp fluorescents.

The lighting requirements of specialized rooms such as ophthalmology refracting rooms or radiology rooms are discussed under these specialities, as are any special considerations concerning the type or level of illumination for the individual suite as a whole.

CHAPTER 14

Construction Methods and Building Systems

HEATING, VENTILATING, AND AIR CONDITIONING (HVAC)

The mechanical requirements of medical and dental offices are quite specialized in that the physical comfort of staff and patients is very important, and there are a great many variables in terms of room function, often within a small area. An *examination room,* for example, is typically 8 × 12 feet in size, and the patient (who spends more time in the room than the doctor) is usually undressed. The *waiting room,* by contrast, is designed to accommodate many people, and often they have sweaters or coats on their laps, which add to their body warmth. Not only does this room have a higher density (one person per 16 to 20 square feet compared with one person per 96 square feet in an exam room), but the occupants themselves generate heat.

A *nurse station* or *business office,* where fully clothed persons are busily moving about, has yet a different requirement. The *dental operatory,* typically 100 square feet, usually has three occupants and a high level of illumination. These rooms each have different comfort requirements in terms of temperature and varying load characteristics. The lighting load for a waiting room will be approximately 2 watts per square foot; for an examination room, 3.3 watts per square foot; for a dental laboratory, 10 watts per square foot; for a nurse station or business office, 2.5 watts; and for corridors, 1 to 1.5 watts per square foot.

The factors that must be considered in designing a functional HVAC system are:

1. Lighting load
2. Room occupancy
3. Equipment load
4. Comfort level based on room function

The capacity of the mechanical system should take into account requirements of such special tenants as a sports medicine facility, ambulatory surgical center, or clinical lab.

The type of HVAC system (equipment and method of distribution) may vary, but often it is a ducted air system that supplies heated, cooled, and fresh air. The system should be designed with maximum concern for sound control. Thus each room may have its own supply and air return; undercutting doors and the use of transfer grilles for return air are to be avoided. Sound carried through the ducts of a ventilation system can be reduced in a number of ways.

A certain amount of sound will naturally be absorbed in the duct wall lining, and some will pass through the duct walls into the plenum. Additional insulation, duct linings, or package attenuation units can produce an even greater degree of sound control. However, a certain amount of white noise produced by the mechanical system is desirable for masking conversation from room to room.

Performance Spec

It is advisable to write a performance spec for the HVAC system to define goals about room zoning and after-hours operation (physicians often work late and on weekends), and to analyze equipment costs, projected energy use, and operating costs.

The need for after-hours HVAC operation must not be underestimated. Surgeons who live far from the hospital may sleep in their offices if called to the hospital late at night for an emergency. Others may open their offices on weekends to treat a sick patient. Extended evening and Saturday hours are fairly common for many dental and medical practices, to accommodate people who work.

CONTROL OF ODORS

To prevent spreading odors from radiography/fluoroscopy rooms, darkroom, toilets, cast room, laboratory, or other areas, the ventilation system should be designed so that negative air pressure, relative to adjoining corridors, is maintained. This can be accomplished by exhausting more air from these rooms than is supplied to them, and by reversing this procedure in the corridors. *Air from fluoroscopic radiography rooms should not be recirculated when these rooms are in use, unless adequate odor removal equipment is incorporated in the ventilation system.*

PLUMBING

Plumbing in a medical or dental facility is not essentially different from that in other types of commercial buildings, but by their very nature, medical office buildings have a high density of plumbing fixtures, and provisions must be made to locate them anywhere except along the perimeter of the building. No area should be too far from drainage to accommodate ¼ inch per foot slope within the given plenum depth. Plaster traps should be supplied in sinks for cast rooms, clinical laboratories, barium prep areas, dental laboratories, and sometimes in minor surgery rooms. Darkrooms and clinical laboratories should have acid-resistant waste piping.

MEDICAL GASES

Certain suites — dentists, oral surgeons, plastic surgeons — require medical gases. Building and fire codes are very strict regarding where and how medical gases are stored. Gases may be in mobile tanks that are wheeled from room to room as needed, or gases (nitrous oxide and oxygen) may be stored in tanks in a nearby room designed for that purpose and piped through degreased, sealed copper tubing (using only silver solder) to a flow meter in each room where gases are needed. If gases are located outside of the suite, a pressure gauge must be located within the suite to monitor the supply. The reader is referred to the General Dentistry section of Chapter 10 for a complete discussion of this topic.

Certain suites require compressed air and central

suction. Usually each tenant will have a vacuum pump and air compressor located in a small mechanical equipment room within the suite, but some medical buildings provide these utilities and pipe them to the suites. Vacuum piping is PVC Schedule 40. Suites requiring these utilities include dentists, oral surgeons, clinical laboratories, and dental laboratories.

SOUND CONTROL

Sound control is of utmost importance in a medical office, especially in examination rooms and consultation rooms. Unfortunately, all too many medical buildings are constructed with profit rather than function as the prime motivation, and partitions terminate at the finished ceiling and have no sound-attenuating properties. There are, however, several ways to reduce sound transmission without spending great sums of money:

1. All partitions should terminate 6 to 8 inches above the suspended ceiling. Thus each room has its own ceiling, rather than dropping the suspended acoustic ceiling over the entire suite, with only the demising walls continuing above it.
2. Sound can be absorbed near its source through the use of carpet, wallcoverings, draperies, and acoustic ceiling tile.
3. Solid-core doors should be used.
4. Fiberglas batting should be added inside partitions between studs.
5. To control passage of sound through walls, floors, and ceilings, acoustical holes should be avoided, such as those created by use of pocket doors or when electrical outlets on opposite sides of a partition are positioned too close to each other, when doors are poorly fitted, when plumbing pipes or heating ducts are improperly fitted, or when partitions do not make proper contact with the ceiling.
6. A certain amount of white noise from the ventilation system will mask soft conversation from room to room.
7. A piped-in music system will also mask normal conversation. An AM-FM tuner or cassette deck located in the business office with speakers in the waiting room and corridors is preferable to the well-known brand of prerecorded background music.
8. Certain rooms, such as psychiatrists' consultation rooms and audio rooms for hearing tests, need a high level of sound control. There are a number of ways to create a sound-attenuating partition. Creased Thermafiber insulation, application of sound board, and isolation through the use of resilient channels are three methods commonly used.

MEDICAL OFFICE COMMUNICATION SYSTEMS

The reader is referred to Chapter 10 for a discussion of communication systems for the dental office.

Many offices of more than 1500 square feet have some sort of interoffice communication system other than the telephone intercom. There are three conditions for which some sort of signal is required:

1. To tell the doctor which room has the next patient
2. To call the doctor to the telephone
3. To call a nurse or aide when the doctor is in the examining room

A small panel of signal lights mounted above exam room doors can indicate to the doctor when a patient has been prepared for examination. When the patient is ready, the nurse turns on the light code for a particular doctor. When the doctor enters the room, he or she turns off the light. This system requires additional modification for large busy practices, since several patients may be prepared and waiting for an individual doctor who will need some way of knowing the sequence.

The receptionist who handles the phone must know in which room each doctor can be found. A toggle switch for each doctor must be located in each exam, treatment, or consultation room the doctor uses. When the doctor enters the room, he or she trips the switch, which lights a panel located at the reception desk.

Some offices do not use signal lights. A variety of "homemade" systems may be devised, one of which follows. Assume, for our example, a group of three orthopedists: Each physician is assigned a color and a set of Plexiglas chips 4 × 5 inches in size. Each chip has a large number, 1 to 3 (since each has the use of three exam rooms). The chips are stored in a wall-mounted rack at the centrally located nurse station. When a nurse readies a patient, she puts that doctor's color chip in a slot on the door; thus each doctor knows, by the color of the chip, if the patient in that room is his or hers and, by the number, the order in which to examine the patients.

In order to call a nurse or aide when the doctor is in the exam room, a signal light can be used, but it may not be noticed — a distinct disadvantage. A preferred system is an annunciator panel, although it is limited by the number of sounds a person can reasonably discriminate. Each doctor would have a distinctive buzz or chime. When the nurse hears the signal, she consults a panel to determine what room the doctor is in, and proceeds to that room.

There are a variety of other interoffice communication systems available. Dealers who sell these products also install them. They can design a system to suit the needs of the individual office and can furnish the designer with the electrical specifications.

FIRE PROTECTION

Special consideration must be given to the type of fire extinguishing system used in such suites as radiology or clinical labs, which contain a great deal of expensive computer-based equipment. Sprinklers would do considerable damage. Halon gas is preferable.

CHECKLIST

The following is a checklist of odds and ends to jog the designer's memory. It is not intended as a complete inventory of requirements.

Code Review

- Occupancy load
- Number of required exits, separation of exits
- Illuminated exit signs
- Radiation shielding
- Fire separations
- Handicapped bathrooms and other accessibility requirements

Partitions

- Sound control
- Continuation above suspended ceiling
- Fiberglas batting
- Verify construction of partitions with contractor when planning offices in a building not designed by the space planner. (One may find that the contractor, in order to come in with a low bid, based his bid on a 2½-inch studs, giving a finished wall that has to be "thickened" wherever plumbing occurs.)
- Verify or specify texture of finished wall

- Spec eggshell finish for walls for durability and cleanability
- Spec special ceiling heights, if required
- No texture for walls that will receive wallcovering

Doors

- Hollow versus solid core
- Pocket doors
- Gate or Dutch doors
- Door closers
- Hardware, keying of locks
- Door finish: painted or stained, plastic laminate
- Door stops
- Type of door frame
- Spec width and height of doors
- Spec carpet height (plus pad, if any) for cutting doors

Plumbing

- Plaster traps
- Wrist- or foot-pedal control faucets
- Acid-resistant waste pipes
- Spec sizes of sinks; china or stainless steel
- Vacuum breakers (darkrooms)
- Separate shutoffs for each fixture
- Floor drains in cystoscopy, darkrooms, hot-water heater room
- Temperature regulators in darkrooms

Communication Systems

- Telephones
- Intercom
- Signal lights
- Annunciator panel
- Music system: provide speakers
- Locate telephone terminal panel (requires electrical outlet)

Mechanical Systems

- Locate air compressor and vacuum
- Locate medical gases, natural gas
- Locate hot-water heater (if electric, requires outlet) and floor drain
- Exhaust fans (bathrooms, darkrooms, labs, cast rooms)

Casework

- Spec style of construction, types of drawer glides, hardware, hinges
- Detail typing wells in business office
- Trash slots in exam cabinets, as required
- Spec wood blocking in walls (or ceiling) to support X-ray view boxes, cassette pass boxes, dental operatory lights and X-ray heads, special light fixtures, casework, and certain pieces of medical equipment

Lighting

- Do switching diagram
- Spec dimmers as required (fluorescent fixtures require dimming ballasts)
- Spec color fluorescent lamps
- Spec lamp wattages
- Spec lenses of fixtures
- Spec color of grid (spline) suspended acoustic ceiling
- Spec acoustic tile

Electrical

- Note special outlets, 220-volt lines, floor receptacles
- Spec height of outlets
- Outlets over countertops should run horizontally
- Locate circuit breaker panel
- Locate intercom and phone, note wall phones

Miscellaneous

- Locate scale spaces, as required, noting any that are to be recessed in the slab
- Illuminated exit signs
- Fire extinguishing equipment

CHAPTER 15

Researching Codes and Reference Materials

Codes are designed to ensure life safety. As health care services have become more complex and sophisticated, the design and construction of these facilities have become more specialized. Paralleling the increasing sophistication in health care is the development of numerous codes and standards designed to limit risk and make buildings relatively safe.

The problem is that codes occasionally contradict one another, and the language is frequently subject to interpretation. Often, the level of protection is a value judgment. The minimum standards per code may be inadequate for a facility serving the elderly, for example. Or the corollary may be true: The minimum standards may occasionally be excessive for a particular project. The cost of implementing them may make the project unfeasible. Thus codes must be evaluated in terms of: (1) *What is an acceptable level of risk in terms of life safety?* (2) *Is the cost of that level of protection warranted or within the budget for the facility?* and (3) *Are the codes or standards applicable to that facility redundant?*

Further complicating these issues is the fact that codes are written by one body and enforced by another. The local agent, who is responsible for interpretation and compliance, does not always understand the intent of the codes, and agents within the same office may disagree on interpretations. Nevertheless, codes are an important part of medical work, and designers need to be familiar with them. If anything, the next ten years will bring more codes and regulations, not fewer.

Codes cover the general areas outlined in the following sections:

FIRE PROTECTION

1. *Flammability of Materials:* especially carpet, wallcoverings, draperies, upholstery fillings and fabrics, carpet and wallcovering adhesives.
2. *Exiting Requirements:* number of exits, travel distances between doors of exit, corridor separations, sizes of doors and stairwells, construction of doors and walls, illumination of fire exits.
3. *Storage:* how and where medical gases are to be used and stored; storage of combustible solid supplies.
4. *Fire-Fighting Equipment:* locations of wet and dry standpipes; chemical fire extinguishers; and in high-rise buildings, smoke evacuation shafts and central control station for fire department use.
5. *Electrical Systems:* standards for wiring, equipment, emergency power systems.
6. *Fire Detection Devices:* locations of sprinklers, smoke detectors, and alarms.

HANDICAPPED

(Both federal and state codes provide for the handicapped.)

1. Location of ramps, curb cuts, parking stalls; placement of exits and design configurations.
2. Dimensions of elevators and restrooms, door widths, and placement of restroom fixtures and accessories.

SANITATION

1. Cleanability of wallcovering, flooring, and other interior finishes.
2. Asepsis (ability to support bacteria) of interior finish materials.

MINIMUM CONSTRUCTION REQUIREMENTS

1. Minimum sizes of rooms and minimum sizes of various departments (within a hospital, for example), location and number of windows, minimum ceiling heights, relationship of various rooms to one another.
2. Planning and programming decisions with regard to function.
3. Accommodation of equipment: spaces for gurneys, drinking fountains, public telephones. Minimum requirements for laundries, kitchens, laboratories, operating rooms, etc.

ENERGY CONSERVATION/ ENVIRONMENTAL IMPACT

State and local codes govern energy conservation and the ecological impact of a proposed building on its environment.

The above code classifications may fall under the jurisdiction of city, county, state, or federal codes, in addition to the following nationally recognized standards:

Life Safety Code (published by the National Fire Protection Assn.)
National Electrical Code (published by the National Fire Protection Assn.)
The Rehabilitation Act of 1973 (concerns the handicapped)
Building Officials and Code Administrators (BOCA)
Joint Commission on Accreditation of Hospitals
Guidelines for Construction and Equipment of Hospitals and Medical Facilities (published by the U.S. Department of Health and Human Services)
National Bureau of Standards (U.S. Department of Commerce)
American Society for Testing and Materials (ASTM)
Underwriters' Laboratories

Recognized state building codes include:

Uniform Building Code (used by many western states)
Southern Standard Building Code
National Building Code

Some states have their own building code; others use a regional code that serves several neighboring states.

CERTIFICATE OF NEED

Prior to building a state-licensed health care facility or remodeling or expanding an existing one, the local health systems agency (HSA) must endorse the project and, in some states, a Certificate of Need (CON) must be obtained from the state. The CON is designed to prevent duplication of highly specialized facilities and equipment and to keep a lid on rising health care costs. States receiving federal funds under the National Health Planning and Resource Development Act of 1974 were required to introduce CON programs. As of this writing, however, a number of states have abandoned their CON programs.

CODES RELATING TO MEDICAL OFFICE BUILDINGS

Code requirements for medical and dental offices are minimal compared to those for hospitals. The local building code will determine the type of construction for a particular medical building and site, the zoning requirements, and the fire zone.

Although state building codes vary, the following items are generally pertinent to planning individual medical and dental offices within a medical office building.

- Minimum width of corridors
- Number of exits
- Handicapped bathrooms
- Separation of exits
- Maximum length of dead-end corridors
- Minimum ceiling heights
- Construction of partitions
- Fire separations
- Radiation shielding
- Fire detection devices or sprinklers

Some of these items apply only to suites in excess of a specified square footage. Suites having an occupant load of 30 or more (generally 3000 square feet or larger), for example, in the *Uniform Building Code,* 1985 edition, must have at least two exits "separated by a distance equal to not less than one-half the length of the maximum overall diagonal dimension of the area to be served measured in a straight line between exits," and no more than a 20-foot dead-end corridor.

With an occupancy load of 100 or more, the suite would have to have corridors of one-hour fire-resistive construction. Codes applying to medical office buildings deal mainly with fire prevention and exiting in case of fire, as well as handicapped accessibility. The following principles are easy to understand in terms of space planning and construction.

Isolation of Risk

If a facility is divided into section by corridor separations, fire-resistive stairwell enclosures, and sealed vertical openings, the fire may be contained and prevented from spreading.

Required Exits

The number of exits is based on the proposed occupancy load or the number of people using the space. Approved exits must lead directly out or to other means of egress, and doors may have to open in the direction of egress (depending on the occupant load). Exits may not be through kitchens, storage rooms, or spaces used for similar purpose. Thus people will not be trapped in a building, and all exits will be clearly marked and accessible in case of fire.

Separation of Exits

When more than one exit is required, each must be separated by a specified distance proportional to the size of the space to provide alternate access if one is blocked by fire.

Stairs and Doors

Stairwells with fire-resistive enclosures and self-closing fire doors are intended to be smoke-free evacuation towers in case of fire. The stairs must be sufficiently wide to enable people on stretchers to be evacuated if necessary.

Fire Warning or Extinguishing Devices

Sprinkler systems are required in many facilities, particularly in laboratories, boiler rooms, large storage areas, or hazardous areas that are often unoccupied. Smoke or heat detectors and alarms are good warning devices where sprinklers are not feasible.

FLAMMABILITY TESTING

Building codes, regulations, and local ordinances are designed to restrict the use of flammable materials on walls, floors, and ceilings of buildings. The flammability characteristics of various interior finish materials influence the behavior of a fire. Although it is impossible to make a building and its furnishings absolutely "fireproof," it is desirable to limit the risk to a reasonable standard by ensuring that the major interior finishes will not support flame or generate smoke. The NFPA 101 Life Safety Code specifies the flame-spread, smoke density, and fuel-contributed standards for floors and walls of hospitals.

Carpet

The flame retardance of a carpet is a significant factor in its selection for a health care facility. Carpet fibers have different melting points: Acrylics melt at 420°F to 490°F; nylons, 415°F to 480°F; modacrylics, 275°F to 300°F. Polypropylene fuses at 285°F to 330°F; wool, which does not melt, scorches at approximately 400°F. Four factors affect the flammability of a carpet:

1. Type of face yarn
2. Type of construction and texture
3. Pile density
4. Underlayment or pad

There are three tests of carpet flammability:

The Pill Test (Dept. of Commerce #DOCFF-1-70). A methenamine pill (a timed burning tablet) placed on the carpet is used to determine if a carpet will burn when ignited by a small incendiary source. Since April 1971 all carpet sold in the United States must pass the pill test.

The Steiner Tunnel Test (E-84). This has been the standard test of carpet and wallcovering flame-spread, although its validity for testing the flammability of carpet in a realistic situation has been widely disputed. This test is required by the U.S. Department of Health and Human Services for all carpets installed in hospitals receiving Hill-Burton Act funds. The carpet sample is mounted on the ceiling of a tunnel and exposed to a front flame. The results are published as a flame-spread rating.

Flooring Radiant Panel Test. This is the newest and most accurate test for carpet flammability. Local fire marshals in some cities are still unfamiliar with this test and insist upon a tunnel test rating. However, many new commercial carpets now have only radiant panel test ratings; thus, in a couple of years, this test will probably replace the Steiner tunnel test. The radiant panel test evolved from extensive corridor fire test programs. The test measures the *critical radiant flux* (the minimum radiant energy necessary for a fire to continue to burn and spread) in watts per square centimeter (watts/cm^2). The lower the number, the greater the capacity for flame propagation.

0.45 watts/cm^2 is the minimum critical radiant flux recommended within corridors and exitways of hospitals and nursing homes.*

0.22 watts/cm^2 is the minimum critical radiant flux recommended within corridors and exitways of other occupancies except one-family and two-family dwellings.*

These values provide a level of safety for a carpeted hospital corridor equal to or in excess of that now provided in the NFPA 101 Life Safety Code. Smoke density is as important as flame-spread, since many people are killed by the smoke generated by a fire.

**Flammability Testing for Carpet,* by I. A. Benjamin and S. Davis, Washington, D.C., The National Bureau of Standards, U.S. Dept. of Commerce, April 1978.

Wallcoverings

Interior finish materials (including wallcoverings) are grouped into three classes, according to their flame-spread and smoke development characteristics. Codes qualify rooms by occupancy and specify which class of finish is applicable.

Class A Interior Finish. Flame-Spread 0-25, Smoke Developed 0-450.
Class B Interior Finish. Flame-Spread 26-75, Smoke Developed 0-450.
Class C Interior Finish. Flame-Spread 76-200, Smoke Developed 0-450.

Where Class C is specified, Classes A and B are permitted; where Class B is specified, Class A is permitted.

Wallcoverings are also classified according to weight and texture. Smooth surfaces — less apt to support bacterial growth or collect dirt — are required for operating rooms, recovery rooms, and sterilization areas. Textured wallcoverings may be used in waiting rooms, corridors, offices, and examination areas.

It is the designer's responsibility to verify the codes pertinent to a particular project. If local codes stipulate minimum flammability standards for finishes in a room, an exit corridor, or an area of a medical suite, then swatches of all interior finish materials must be attached to a copy of the laboratory test data (supporting the flame-spread classification claimed) and submitted to the state fire marshal for approval.

Wallcovering Specifications. Fabric-backed vinyl wallcoverings are classified into three general categories:

Type I. In accordance with federal specification CCC-

W-408a, Type I must weigh a minimum of 7 ounces per square yard and may weigh up to 13 ounces per square yard. It usually has a lightweight scrim backing. Type I materials are acceptable for light commercial use such as offices and corridors with moderate traffic.

Type II. In accordance with federal specification CCC-W-408a, Type II must weigh a minimum of 13 ounces per square yard and may weigh up to 22 ounces per square yard. It usually has an Osnaburg or drill tear-resistant fabric backing. Type II materials are suitable for general commercial use in public corridors of hospitals, lobbies, waiting rooms, dining rooms, cafeterias, and other areas of high traffic and above-average abuse.

Type III. In accordance with federal specification CCC-W-408a, Type III must weigh in excess of 22 ounces per square yard. It usually has a broken twill fabric backing for maximum strength and tear resistance. Type III materials are suitable for areas receiving exceptionally hard wear and abrasion such as elevators, stores and shops, hospital corridors, and stairwells.

Codes affecting medical and dental office occupancies generally do not stipulate weight of wallcoverings; however, codes for hospitals do.

Wallcoverings in high-traffic areas can be ordered with a *Tedlar coating* to give walls even greater protection. Tedlar is a registered trade name for a tough preformed film of polyvinyl fluoride, which is laminated to the face of the vinyl wallcovering to make it resist stains such as lipstick, ballpoint pens, silver nitrate, and other indelible substances. Even harsh solvents and cleaning solutions will not mar the Tedlar coating, making it ideal for use in psychiatric hospitals, pediatric wards, and other institutional facilities where walls are subject to graffiti and high abuse.

Appendixes

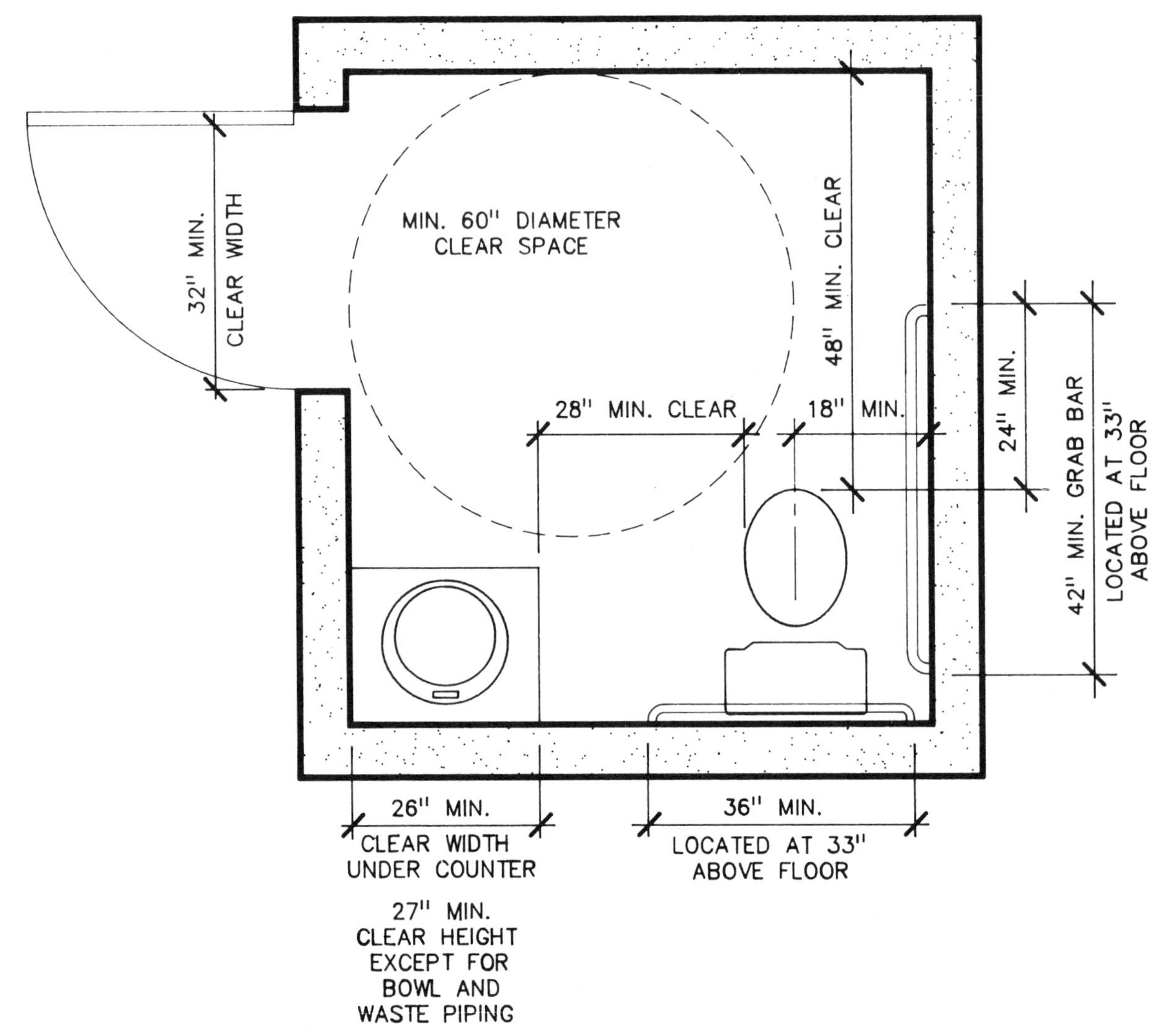

HANDICAPPED TOILET

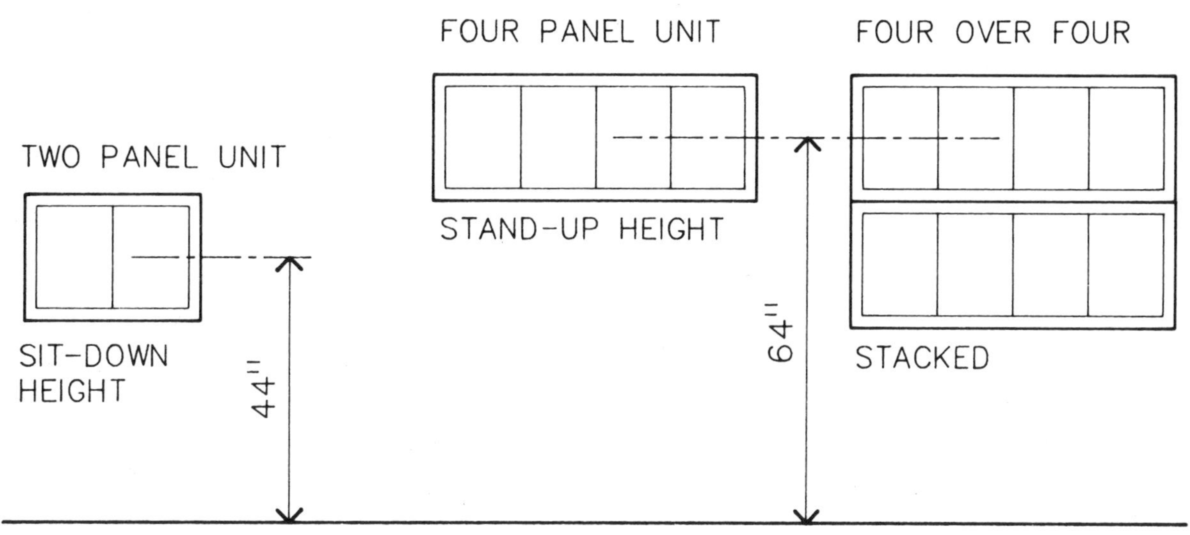

SUGGESTED MOUNTING HEIGHTS FOR VIEW BOX ILLUMINATORS

APPENDIX 2

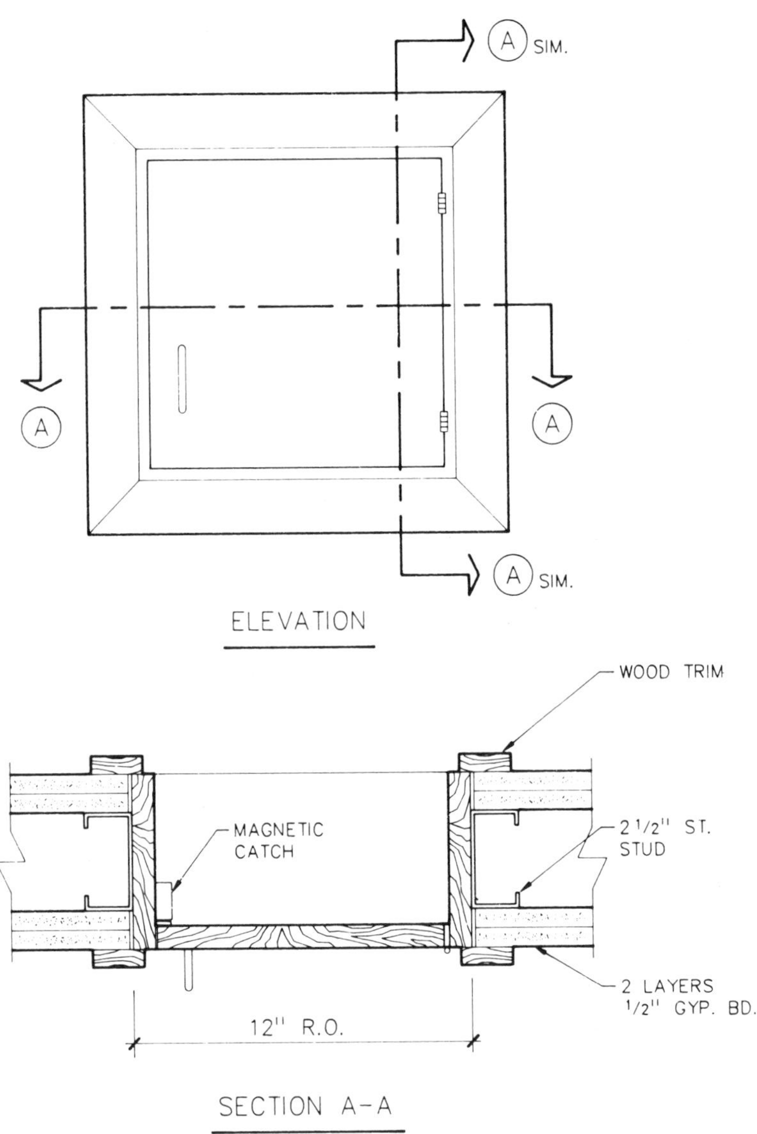

APPENDIX 3

SPECIMEN PASS-THROUGH

APPENDIX 4: MEDICAL SPACE PLANNING QUESTIONNAIRE

Date: ____________

Physician group name: ____________

Telephone no.: ____________

Questionnaire filled out by: ____________

Medical specialty: ____________

Size of present office: ____________ SF ____________

Anticipated size of new office: ____________ SF ____________

Suite location requirements within building: ____________

PROPOSED STAFF

Administration:

Reception ____________

Insurance ____________

Bookkeeping ____________

Office manager ____________

Other ____________

____

____

Medical:

Physicians ____________

Aides ____________

R.N.s ____________

1

L.V.N.s ____________

Nurse Pract. ____________

Other ____________

____

____

PROPOSED BUSINESS OFFICE

Medical records:

No. chart file cabinets required ____________

Size chart file cabinets required ____________

If you do not use freestanding chart file cabinets, please describe what you do use (e.g. custom built), and tell us how many lineal feet you require for this type of chart filing

____

____

____

We shall assume that the figures you give us include the projected growth you want to include in laying out the new office.

Computer Systems:

Describe which of your staff members will require a CRT at their workstations. Which of these will also require a typewriter?

____

____

____

____

2

Describe the size and brand of computer(s) and printer(s) you intend to use. Do you have a CPU (central processing unit) that requires a separate room with air conditioning? Does it require a raised floor for cable runs?

____

____

____

____

Bookkeeping:

If everything in your office is not done on computer, then describe the bookkeeping system you use (e.g., pegboard, ledger cards, Burroughs posting machine, etc.).

____

____

____

____

____

Specialized Equipment:

Type of photocopy machine ____________________

Floor stand __________ or countertop model __________

FAX machine ________________________.

Other equipment (please describe) ________________

____

3

____

____

PATIENT PROFILE

Average number patients/day ____________________

Office hours: From __________ to ________________

Composition of patients (describe age, sex, ethnic background):

____

____

____

____

PROPOSED SUITE REQUIREMENTS

It would be very helpful if you could give us approximate sizes and number of rooms needed. To guide you, we have listed in parentheses typical sizes of each room that suit most medical specialties.

Exam rooms (8 × 12) ____________________

Minor surgery/treatment (12 × 12) ________________

Consultation rms./Drs.' offices (12 × 12) ____________

Lab (8 × 10) ________________________

Nurse stations (6 × 8) ____________________

Combined with lab? __________

Separate? __________

Storage ____________________________

4

Conference with library (12 × 16) ____________

Staff lounge (10 × 12) ____________

Patient education room (8 × 10) ____________

Toilets ____________

Waiting room (estimate 20 SF per person) ____________

____

Children's play area ____________

Business Office:

Reception: No. of people ____________

Cashier/Appts.: No. of people ____________

Bookkeeping: No. of people ____________

Insurance: No. of people ____________

Office manager ____________

Describe the overall size of the business office, and stipulate whether the bookkeeper, insurance clerk, and office manager are included in one room, or will they have separate offices?

____

____

____

____

____

5

SPECIALIZED ROOMS

EKG ____________

Pulmonary function ____________

Procto/Sigmoid ____________

Endoscopy suite ____________

Cast room(s) ____________

Audio room ____________

Allergy test rooms ____________

X-ray ____________

Types of films ____________

Viewing area ____________

Darkroom ____________

Barium prep ____________

Film filing ____________ lineal feet

Automatic processor ____________

Physical therapy ____________

Office-based surgery suite (give details) ____________

____

____

Ophthalmology:

Field room ____________

Mydriatic room ____________

6

No. refraction rooms ______________________

Data collection room ______________________

Office-based surgery ______________________

Optical dispensing ______________________

Miscellaneous rooms ______________________

____

____

MISCELLANEOUS

Do you need medical gases (nitrous oxide, oxygen) or vacuum?

____

____

Thank you.

7

APPENDIX 5: DENTAL SPACE PLANNING QUESTIONNAIRE

Date: ____________

Dental group name: ____________

Telephone no. ____________

Questionnaire filled out by: ____________

Dental specialty: ____________

Dental equipment dealer: ____________

Salesperson to contact: ____________

Size of present office: ____________ SF ______

Anticipated size of new office: ____________ SF ______

Suite location requirements within building: ____________

PRACTICE METHODS

Is doctor right-handed? ________ or left-handed? ________

Type of present delivery system: ____________

____

Type of new delivery system:

Over the patient

Specify chair-mounted ________ or post-mounted ________ for dentist.

Specify chair-mounted/post-mounted ____________ or mobile cart ____________ for auxiliary.

Ambidextrous delivery (over the toe of chair) ____________

1

Side

Specify split cart _____ wall-mounted _____ or cabinet ________.

If wall-mounted or cabinet for dentist, will auxiliary be same or use mobile cart? ____________

Rear

Specify dual-purpose cart ______ fixed cabinet ______.

Do you practice two- ________ four- ________ or six-handed ________ dentistry?

PROPOSED STAFF

Administration:

Reception ____________

Casher/appts. ____________

Insurance ____________

Bookkeeping ____________

Office manager ____________

Other ____________

____

____

Describe the overall size of the business office, and stipulate whether the bookkeeper, insurance clerk, and office manager are included in one room, or will they have separate offices?

____

____

2

Clinical:

Dentists ______

Auxiliaries ______

Hygienist ______

Lab techs ______

PROPOSED BUSINESS OFFICE

Dental Records:

No. chart file cabinets required ______

Size chart file cabinets required ______

If you do not use freestanding chart file cabinets, please describe what you do use (e.g., custom built), and tell us how many lineal feet you require for this type of chart filing.

We shall assume that the figures you give us include the projected growth you want to include in laying out the new office.

Computer Systems:

Describe which of your staff members will require a CRT at their workstations. Which of these will also require a typewriter?

3

Describe the size and brand of computer(s) and printer(s) you intend to use. Do you have a CPU (central processing unit) that requires a separate room with air conditioning? Does it require a raised floor for cable runs?

Bookkeeping:

If everything in your office is not done on computer, then describe the system you use (e.g., pegboard, ledger cards, Burroughs posting machine, etc.).

Specialized Equipment:

Type of photocopy machine ______

Floor stand ______ or countertop model ______

FAX machine ______

4

Other equipment (please describe) ____________________

____

____

____

PATIENT PROFILE

Average number patients/day ____________________

Office hours: From __________ to __________

Composition of patients (describe age, sex, ethnic background):

____

____

____

____

PROPOSED SUITE REQUIREMENTS

It would be very helpful if you could give us approximate sizes of rooms.

Waiting room (estimate 20 SF per person) ____________________

____

Children's play area ____________________

No. and size of operatories ____________________

If Pedo or Ortho, do you want an operatory bay? __________ If so, how many chairs? __________ How many private operatories or "quiet rooms" do you want? __________

5

Hygiene room(s) ____________________.

Do you use a fully equipped standard operatory for hygiene?

____

Is it dedicated to hygiene or also used for dental treatment?

____

____

X-ray:

Equip each operatory with head mounted on side wall ______ or rear (for ambidextrous operatory)? ____________________

Panoramic ____________________

Cephalometric ____________________

Darkroom __________ Type of processor __________

Lab:

Specify types of lab work done in-house: ____________________

____

and what types you send out: ____________________

____

Size of lab: ____________________

Sterilization ____________________

Patient education room __________ with sink __________

Staff lounge ____________________

Toilets ____________________

6

Brushing cabinet ______________________ (for Pedo or Ortho)

Vanity alcove (to repair makeup upon exiting suite) ______________

Storage ______________________________________

Dr.'s private office __________ Shared ______________

with toilet __________ with shower ______________

Equipment room:

Inside suite ______ Outside suite ______ On roof __________

For Oral Surgeons Only:

No. recovery beds ______________________________

No. examination operatories ______________________

No. surgical operatories __________________________

Clean-up/dirty workroom __________________________

Clean linens/prep ______________________________

Private exit for post-surgical patients ______________

MISCELLANEOUS

Nitrous Oxide and Oxygen

Portable tanks ____________ Piped through wall ____________

Tray/Tub Storage

In sterilization area ______________________________

In sterilization area with pass-through to operatory ____________

In operatory cabinet ______________________________

In corridor cabinet close to operatory ______________

7

Operating light

On dental unit ______________ Ceiling track ______________

Post-mounted ______________________________________

Vacuum

Cuspidor ______ Wall outlet ______ In mobile cabinet __________

On dental unit ______________________________________

Sterilization

Autoclave ________ Ultrasonic ________ Dry heat ____________

Harvey Chemiclave ____________ Cassette system ____________

Asst.'s Cart

Electric ________ Gas ________ Air ________ Suction ______

Dentist's Cart

Electric ________ Gas ________ Air ________ Suction ______

Sinks in operatories

Wall-mounted ____________ Built into cabinet ______________

One ______ or two ______ Rear wall ______ or side ________

Utility requirements

Water ________ Compressed air ________ Gas ____________

Do you use nitrogen? ______________________________

Thank you.

8

Index

INDEX NOTE: An *f.* after a page number refers to a figure; a *t.* refers to a table.

AAAAPSF (American Association for Accreditation of Ambulatory Plastic Surgery Facilities), 142, 144
AAAHC (Accreditation Association for Ambulatory Health Care), 267, 270
Accreditation Association for Ambulatory Health Care (AAAHC), 267, 270
ADA (American Dental Association), 333
Albers, Josef, 409
Allergy, 148–154
  consultation room, 153
  examination room, 148–149, 153
  injection protocol, 148
  interior design, 148, 153, 154*f.*
  laboratory, 153
  nurse station, 148, 153
  patient history interview, 148–149
  patient volume, 148
  pediatric, 148, 152–154*f.*
  program analysis, 149*t.*
  reaction room, 148
  schematic diagram, 149*f.*
  skin test room, 149
  suite plan:
    2172 square feet, 150*f.*
    2470 square feet, 152*f.*
    3600 square feet, 151*f.*
  treatment room, 153
  waiting room, 148, 153*f.*, 154*f.*
Altieri, Peter, 306
Ambulatory surgical center, 265–293
  access, 271–272
    disabled, 271
    entrance, 272
    service, 272
    staff, 272
    vehicle, 271
Ambulatory surgical center (*Cont.*):
  accreditation, 267, 269
  administration, 293
  advantages of, 265–266
  air compressor, 288
  business office, 273–274
  codes, 269–270
    electric shock, 269
    explosion, 269
    fire, 269, 277
    infection control, 269–270, 277, 282, 285
    power failure, 269, 277
  CON program, 267, 453
  discharge area, 270–271, 273, 291
  dressing room, 271, 288, 295*f.*
  emergency care facility, 271, 281*f.*
  endoscopy room, 277–278
  Health Systems Agency review, 267, 453
  hospital transfer agreement, 269
  insurance, 267–268, 271
  interior design, 268, 273–275, 288
  licensure, 266–269
  lighting, 273, 275, 286, 288
  location of, 268–269
  marketing of, 268
  mechanical requirements, 445
  medical gases, 282, 285, 288
  medical records, 273–274
  Medicare certification, 267–268
  minor surgery room, 286
  nurse station, 274, 290–292
  operational protocols, 270
  patient flow, 270–271
  patient pick-up area, 271
  pediatric patients, 275
    recovery room, 292

Ambulatory surgical center (*Cont.*):
Phoenix Surgicenter, 265
post-anesthesia recovery, 270–271, 274–275, 290–291
lighting, 291
room size, 290
pre-op holding, 270–271, 274–275
reception, 272–273
recovery lounge, 271, 273, 291–292
interior decorating, 292
lighting, 292
space planning, 270
staff area, 288–290
staff flow, 270
staff lounge, 272
storage room, 277, 285, 287
suite plan:
7312 square feet, 281*f.*
12,744 square feet, 278–279*f.*
surgical core, 275–277, 280–293
central corridor, 275, 290
scrub area, 276
surgical procedures performed at, 268
waiting room, 272–274
capacity, 273
waste disposal, 269, 272, 290
workrooms, 286–288
clean, 287
janitor's closet, 288
lighting, 286
soiled, 286, 287*f.*
sterilization, 286
(*See also* Operating room)
American Association for Accreditation of Ambulatory Plastic Surgery Facilities (AAAAPSF), 142, 144
American Dental Association (ADA), 333
American National Standards Institute (ANSI):
document Z-136.1 (1986), 284
document Z-136.3 (1988), 285
American Registry of Radiologic Technologists, 197
ANSI (*see* American National Standards Institute)
Aristotle, 408
Association of Operating Room Nurses, 270, 288
Audio test room, 91, 105, 110–111
sound control, 447
Back office (*see* Consultation room; Examination room; Laboratory; Nurse station; Treatment room)
Birren, Faber, *Light, Color and Environment,* 408, 411–414, 421
Blood drawing, 50, 52, 67, 241, 245, 248
chair, 246*f.*
Bookkeeping, 28–33, 38
computer systems, 29–32, 258
dental, 369, 383
general surgery, 169
group practice, 258
health maintenance organization, 250–251
internal medicine, 67
radiology, 195
safe, 33
sports medicine, 299
traditional methods, 30, 32–33
ledger cards, 30–33
pegboard, 30, 32
Branemark, Ingvar, 403
Bucky (wall-mounted film holder), 212
Building systems (*see* Construction methods; Space planning)
Bureau of Radiological Health, 375
Business office, 25, 26, 28*f.*, 29, 39
ambulatory surgical center, 273–274
dental, 369–370, 383, 395, 397, 402
dermatology, 128
dictation, 34*f.*, 35
furniture, 430
gate door, 26, 29
general surgery, 166, 169
group practice, 264
insurance records, 32–33, 67, 169, 267–268, 271, 369
internal medicine, 67, 264
lighting, 445
mechanical requirements, 445
medical transcription, 34*f.*, 35, 67
office manager, 35–36, 67
orthopedic surgery, 175
otolaryngology, 105
pediatrics, 84
physical therapy, 329
psychiatry, 155

Business office (*Cont.*):
radiology, 195
sports medicine, 299–300
urology, 169
women's health center, 28*f.*
workstation, 33*f.*
(*See also* Bookkeeping; Medical records; Reception)

Cardiopulmonary laboratory, 65–66
Carpet, 423–425
in allergy suite, 153
in ambulatory surgical center, 268, 274, 288, 292
antimicrobial treatment, 424
backing of, 424
in darkroom, 206
in dental suite, 333, 361, 371, 393, 424
in dermatology suite, 133
fiber composition, 423
flammability testing, 454–455
Flooring Radiant Panel Test, 455
The Pill Test, 454
The Steiner Tunnel Test, 454–455
fluorochemical treatment, 424
in general surgery suite, 169
installation techniques, 425
in magnetic resonance imaging suite, 235
in mammography suite, 226
in neurology suite, 163
in obstetrics and gynecology suite, 102
in orthopedic surgery suite, 185
in pediatrics suite, 82, 91, 425
in physical therapy suite, 325
in plastic surgery suite, 147
in radiation oncology suite, 228
in radiology suite, 195
sound control and, 447
specifications, 424
in sports medicine suite, 299–300
static control, 424
in waiting room, 425
in women's health center, 104
Cassette pass box, 203*f.*, 205
CAT (computed axial tomography) scan (*see* Computed tomography)
CDC (Centers for Disease Control), 270, 333
Center for Sports Medicine, The (San Diego, California), 306–307
suite plan, 296*f.*
Center for Sports Medicine and Orthopedics (Phoenix, Arizona), 303–306
suite plan, 305*f.*
Centers for Disease Control (CDC), 270, 333
Certificate of need (CON) program, 267, 453
Circulation (*see* Patient flow; Staff flow)
Clinical laboratory, 240–248
administrative area, 244
air compressor, 447
air conditioning, 247
automated analyzers, 50*f.*, 243–244
blood drawing, 241, 245, 248
chair, 246*f.*
central communication center, 245
dressing room, 244
glass-washing area, 247
in group practice, 248–249
interior design, 248
lighting, 248
mechanical requirements, 445
plumbing requirements, 446
power requirements, 248
program development, 240
schematic diagram, 241*f.*
space expansion, 247
specimen accessioning, 246
sterilization area, 247
suite plan, 242*f.*
technical modules, 241, 243
chemistry, 241, 243–246
hematology, 241, 243, 245*f.*
histology, 243
serology-microbiology, 243
urinalysis, 243
toilet room, 244
utility requirements, 247
ventilation, 247
waiting room, 244, 248
waste disposal, 246–247
Codes, 423, 451–456
for ambulatory surgical center, 269–270
certificate of need, 267, 453

Codes (*Cont.*):
construction code review, 448
for darkroom, 378
disabled persons protection, 452
energy conservation, 452
environmental impact, 452
evaluation of, 451
fire protection, 451
flammability testing, 454–456
carpet, 454–455
wallcoverings, 455–456
for medical gases, 368, 446
medical office building, 453–454
doors, 454
exists, 453–454
fire warning system, 454
isolation of risk, 453
stairs, 454
minimum construction requirements, 452
NFPA 56F, 288
NFPA 70, 269, 277
NFPA 99, 269, 277
NFPA 101, 127, 141–142, 266–269, 422, 454–455
for office-based surgery, 422
sanitation, 452
Uniform Building Code, 423
Color, 408–421
additive, 416
advancing, 418–419
afterimage, 417
biological effects of, 412–413
color constancy, 418
color-form preference, 410–411, 413
color mixing systems, 416
color preference tests, 409–411
color pyramid test, 411
color theory, 408–409, 414
applications of, 420
color wheel, 415–416
complementary, 415, 418, 420
Compton fabric preference test, 412
depression and, 412
figure-ground reversal, 419
harmony and, 415
Kruithof's principle, 421
Color (*Cont.*):
laws of perception, 416–419
light sensitivity, 416
lighting and, 421, 434
mental disorders and, 411–412
metameric color pairs, 417–418
noncomplementary, 415
of operating room, 417
paint colors, 417–419
partitive, 416
personality and, 413–415
of physical therapy gym, 420
psychedelic movement and, 415
Purkinje effect, 418
receding, 418–419
reflectance, 418
research studies on, 408–414, 418, 420
simultaneous contrast, 417
space perception and, 420–421
subtractive, 416
successive contrast, 417
symbolism, 419
of toilet room, 420
Communication system, 447–449
dental suite, 380–381
Compton fabric preference test, 412
Computed tomography (CT), 187–188, 190, 224–226
control room, 225–226
diagnostic viewing room, 226
equipment, 224*f.*, 225
film processing, 202
lighting, 225–226
medical records, 226
pass box, 226
procedure room, 225
view box illuminator, 224
Computer systems for business office, 29–32, 258, 424
CON (certificate of need) program, 267, 453
Construction methods, 445–450
air compressor, 446–447
checklist, 448–450
casework, 449
communication system, 449
construction code review, 448
doors, 449

Construction methods, checklist (*Cont.*):
electrical system, 450
lighting, 449
mechanical system, 449
partitions, 448–449
plumbing, 449
communication system, 447–449
fire protection, 448
HVAC system, 445–446
performance spec, 446
sound control, 446–447
medical gases, 446
minimum construction requirements, 452
odor control, 446
piped-in music system, 447
plumbing, 446, 449
sound control, 447
(*See also* Codes; Space planning)
Consultation room, 39, 43, 45, 48–49
allergy, 153
dental, 336, 382, 395
dermatology, 128
general surgery, 166
interior design, 422
internal medicine, 48, 55, 66
lighting, 444
neurology, 48, 163
obstetrics and gynecology, 102
ophthalmology, 127
oral surgery, 397, 400, 402
orthopedic surgery, 175, 181, 182*f.*
otolaryngology, 105
patient intimidation and, 3
pediatrics, 48, 91
personal memorabilia in, 4, 48, 141, 155
plastic surgery, 138, 141, 142*f.*
psychiatry, 155, 447
radiology, 200–201, 203*f.*
sound control, 447
sports medicine, 299
for surgeon, 48–49
urology, 169
women's health center, 104
Council on Dental Therapeutics, 333
CP29 Lighting for Health Care Facilities (Illuminating Engineers Society), 282
CT (*see* Computed tomography)

Darkroom, 53–55
codes for, 378
decentralized, 201, 204
dental, 336, 376–378, 383, 395, 397
developer tanks, 206
door, 206, 208
dry side, 204–205
electrical requirements, 204–205
equipment, 208*f.*, 209*f.*
exhaust vent, 205
film processor, 205–206, 208
interior design, 206
internal medicine, 67
lead shielding, 189, 197–198
lighting, 206
odor control, 214, 446
orthopedic surgery, 175, 182
otolaryngology, 105
pass box, 203*f.*, 205
plumbing requirements, 446
portable, 204
radiology, 197, 201–202, 204–210
sink, 205
storage, 206
waste disposal, 208, 210
water supply, 205, 208
wet side, 204, 206
(*See also* X-ray room)
Dentistry, 332–381, 407
ambidextrous operatory, 343
bookkeeping, 369
business office, 369–370
communication system, 380–381
buzzer, 380
chime, 380
colored signal lights, 380
combination system, 380–381
loudspeaker, 380
telephone intercom, 380
consultation room, 336

Dentistry (*Cont.*):
darkroom, 336, 376–378
layout, 377*f.*
manual processing, 378
dental assistant, 339
equipment, 334, 335*f.*, 348, 354*f.*, 355*f.*, 359*f.*, 379*f.*
storage room, 381
four-handed, 345
gas lines, 369
group practice, 338*f.*
hygiene operatory, 367–368
infection control, 333–334, 344–346, 356, 407
interior design, 333–334, 361, 368, 370–371, 424
laboratory, 336, 365–366, 447
equipment, 366, 367*f.*
plumbing requirements, 446
lighting, 378–380, 436, 441–443, 445
operatory reflected ceiling plan, 379*f.*
marketing plan, 332, 407
medical gases, 368, 369*f.*, 446
medical records, 369
operatory delivery systems, 346, 348
over-the-patient, 340*f.*, 344, 348, 353*f.*
rear, 340*f.*, 344, 346, 350*f.*
side, 340*f.*, 344, 346–348
split cart, 340*f.*, 346
12 o'clock column, 346, 351*f.*
operatory design, 343, 345
air compressor, 356–357, 447
casework, 344
central suction, 356
doors, 344, 357, 359
electrical requirements, 368
layout, 340*f.*, 342*f.*, 345–346, 348
mechanical requirements, 445
modular casework, 344, 347*f.*,
number of operatories, 345
plumbing requirements, 368–369
psychological considerations, 361
sink, 344, 357
size, 343–345
tray setup, 359, 360*f.*
tubs, 359, 360*f.*
work surface, 344

Dentistry (*Cont.*):
operatory instrumentation, 346
of assistant, 344
of dentist, 344
evacuation system, 346
handheld, 346
handpiece delivery system, 346
three-way syringe, 346
patient education, 367
patient flow, 336, 337*f.*
patient volume, 371
plaque control room, 367
private entrance, 339
program analysis, 339*t.*
reception, 336, 367, 371, 441*f.*
schematic diagram, 336*f.*
six-handed, 345
space planning, 332–333
staff flow, 336, 337*f.*, 339, 345
staff lounge, 370
sterilization area, 336, 361, 365
cassette sterilization, 365
dry heat sterilization, 365
equipment, 361, 364*f.*
steam autoclaving, 365
tray setup, 361, 365
unsaturated chemical vapor, 365
suite plan, 358*f.*, 363*f.*, 372*f.*,
1400 square feet, 349*f.*
1664 square feet, 362*f.*
2528 square feet, 338*f.*
3680 square feet, 352*f.*
4500 square feet, 338*f.*
toilet room, 336, 370
vanity area, 367
view box illuminator, 345, 374–375
waiting room, 336, 358*f.*, 371, 373, 441*f.*
x-ray room, 336, 347*f.*, 373–375
lead shielding, 374–375
(*See also* Endodontics; Oral surgery; Orthodontics; Pediatric dentistry; Periodontics)
Dermatology, 128–135
business office, 128
consultation room, 128

Dermatology (*Cont.*):
  equipment, 135*f.*
  examination room, 128
    windows, 43
  interior design, 133
  laboratory, 128
  laser surgery, 132
  minor surgery room, 128, 132–133
  Mohs' histographic surgery, 133
  program analysis, 128*t.*
  psoralen ultraviolent light, 133
  schematic diagram, 129*f.*
  storage room, 128, 133
  suite plan:
    1344 square feet, 130*f.*
    2048 square feet, 131*f.*
    4384 square feet, 134*f.*
    group practice, 255*f.*
  toilet room, 128
  waiting room, 128, 135*f.*
Diagnostic medicine (*see* Clinical laboratory; Computed tomography; Magnetic resonance imaging; Nuclear medicine; Radiography/fluoroscopy room; Radiography room; Radiology)
Dictation, 34*f.*, 35
Disabled persons, 22, 185, 271, 452
Dressing room, 40
  ambulatory surgical center, 271, 288, 295*f.*
  clinical laboratory, 244
  obstetrics and gynecology, 93
  orthopedic surgery, 40
  otolaryngology, 40, 110
  plastic surgery, 146
  radiation oncology suite, 228
  radiography/fluoroscopy room, 211
  radiology, 189, 193, 195, 211, 228
  sports medicine, 301
  urology, 169
  women's health center, 104

Ear, nose and throat (*see* Otolaryngology)
ECG (electrocardiography) room, 56–59, 66–67
Echocardiography, 57, 66
EKG (electrocardiograph) room, 56–59, 66–67
Endodontics, 332, 402
  darkroom, 378
  working x-rays, 378
  (*See also* Dentistry)
Endoscopy, 67, 69, 71*f.*, 72
  in ambulatory surgical center, 277–278
  layout, 70*f.*
  recovery room, 72
  workroom, 69, 72
ENT (*see* Otolaryngology)
Essential Electrical Systems (NFPA 99), 269, 277
Examination room, 38–45, 48
  for adolescent patients, 78
  allergy, 148–149, 153
  cabinets, 41–42, 95, 106
  corridors, 39, 91, 182
  dermatology, 43, 128
  door placement, 40–41, 93
  electrical requirements, 43–44, 95, 106, 119, 121
  furniture, 425, 429*f.*
  general surgery, 166
  instrument console, 119
  interior design, 422
  internal medicine, 55–56
  layout, 42*f.*
  lighting, 119, 121, 436, 445
  mechnical requirements, 445
  neurology, 159, 163
  obstetrics and gynecology, 43, 44, 93, 95, 97*f.*, 98*f.*
  ophthalmology, 112, 115, 119, 121–123, 127
  oral surgery, 397, 400
  orthopedic surgery, 40, 44–45, 175, 178*f.*, 179, 182
  otolaryngology, 40, 44, 105–106, 109
  patient flow, 38–39
  patient privacy, 4
  pediatrics, 44, 45, 77–79, 82, 86–88*f.*
    number of rooms, 77–78
  plastic surgery, 136, 137, 141*f.*
  psychiatry, 158*f.*
  sink, 41–42, 78, 93, 105, 119
  size, 39, 78–79, 445
  sound control, 447
  sports medicine, 299
  table, 40–41, 44–45, 79, 82, 95

Examination room (*Cont.*):
urology, 169
windows, 43, 95
women's health center, 104
writing desk, 43, 95
(*See also* Dressing room; Treatment room)

Facial plastic surgery, 105, 111
outpatient surgery room, 110
suite plan, 107*f.*
Family practice, 92
patient volume, 371
suite plan, 51*f.*
(*See also* General practice)
Farbenlehre (Goethe), 408–409, 418
FASA (Federated Ambulatory Surgical Association), 267, 269
FASC (*see* Ambulatory surgical center)
Federated Ambulatory Surgical Association (FASA), 267, 269
Figure-ground reversal, 419
Fire extinguisher, 33
Flooring, 422–423
in operating room, 422–423
sheet vinyl, 423
vinyl composition tile (VCT), 423
(*See also* Carpet)
Fluorescent light (*see under* Lighting)
Fluoroscopy room, 186, 200, 211
(*See also* Radiography/fluoroscopy room)
Ford, John, 265
4-Color Person, The (Luscher), 414
Freestanding ambulatory surgical center (*see* Ambulatory surgical center)
Front office (*see* Business office)
Furniture, 425–432
in ambulatory surgical center, 288
brochure rack, 425, 427*f.*
for business office, 430
chairs, 431*f.*, 432*f.*
chart rack, 425, 428*f.*
for children, 432
choosing, 4–5
clock, 429*f.*
in examination room, 425, 429*f.*

Furniture (*Cont.*):
magazine rack, 425–427, 429*f.*
modular seating, 430, 431*f.*
for nurse station, 430
for orthopedic surgery suite, 431*f.*, 432
for patient education, 425, 432
perpetual calendar, 430*f.*
in waiting room, 425, 430, 432

Galvanic skin response (GSR), 413
Garth, T. R., 410
General dentistry (*see* Dentistry)
General practice (G.P.), 19–54
group practice, 250, 264
program analysis, 261*t.*
suite plan, 263*f.*
laboratory, 52
nurse station, 52
program analysis, 21*t.*
schematic diagram, 20*f.*
suite plan:
1536 square feet, 27*f.*
4140 square feet, 46*f.*
waiting room, 22
x-ray room, 52–53
General surgery, 164, 166–169
bookkeeping, 169
business office, 166, 169
consultation room, 166
examination room, 166
interior design, 169
minor surgery room, 166
nurse station, 166
physician schedule, 166
program analysis, 166*t.*
reception, 169
schematic diagram, 166*f.*
suite plan:
1152 square feet, 167*f.*
2747 square feet, 168*f.*
toilet room, 166
waiting room, 166
Gerritsen, Frans, *The Theory and Practice of Color,* 416
Goethe, Johann Wolfgang von, *Farbenlehre,* 408–409, 418

Goldstein, Kurt, 413, 420
G.P. (*see* General practice)
Group practice, 249–264
  advantages of, 249
  clinic sinage system, 251, 254*f.*
  clinical laboratory, 248
  dentistry, 338*f.*
  general practice, 250, 264
    program analysis, 261*t.*
    suite plan, 263*f.*
  health maintenance organization, 250–251
  internal medicine, 161, 164, 250
    business office, 264
    laboratory, 264
    suite plan, 263*f.*
    waiting room, 264
  lighting, 443
  multispecialty, 250, 256–260
    bookkeeping, 258
    decentralized plan, 260
    medical records, 256
    patient flow, 260
    program analysis, 262*t.*
    reception, 257–258, 260
    satellite plan, 256*f.*, 257
    suite plan, 257–259*f.*
    waiting room, 257
  pharmacy, 330
  radiography room, 256
  radiology, 249, 256
  schematic diagrams, 251*f.*, 252*f.*, 256*f.*, 257*f.*
  single-specialty, 250–255
    centralized plan, 251, 253*f.*
    decentralized plan, 251, 252*f.*, 255*f.*
    dermatology suite plan, 254*f.*
    island plan, 251
    obstetrics and gynecology suite plan, 253*f.*
    program analysis, 261*t.*, 262*t.*
Group practice HMO model, 251, 258
GSR (galvanic skin response), 413

Hall, Edward T., 3
Hand surgeon, 179
Health club (*see* Sports medicine)
Health maintenance organization (HMO), 250–251
  bookkeeping, 250–251
  dentistry plan, 369
  group practice model, 251, 258
  Independent Practice Association, 251
Health Planning and Resources Development Act (1974), 267
Health systems agency (HSA), 267, 453
Hearing test room (*see* Audio test room)
HMO (*see* Health maintenance organization)
Holter monitoring, 57–58, 60*f.*, 66
Hot lab, 218, 220, 222
  bench-top shields, 222
  electrical requirements, 222
  equipment, 220–223*f.*
  vial shields, 220, 222
HSA (health systems agency), 267, 453
Huxtable, Ada Louise, 3

Illuminating Engineers Society, 286
  CP29 Lighting for Health Care Facilities, 282
Independent Practice Association (IPA), 251
Infectious waste disposal (*see* Waste disposal)
Inhalation therapy, 66–67
Insurance records, 32–33, 67, 141, 169, 267–268, 271, 369
Interior design:
  for allergy suite, 148, 153, 154*f.*
  for ambulatory surgical center, 268, 273–275, 288, 292
  ceilings, 423
  for clinical laboratory, 248
  for darkroom, 206
  for dental suite, 333–334, 361, 368, 370–371, 383, 390, 395, 402
  for dermatology suite, 133
  flammability standards, 422–423
  flooring, 422–423
    sheet vinyl, 423
    vinyl composition tile (VCT), 423
  for general surgery suite, 169
  for internal medicine suite, 72
  for magnetic resonance imaging suite, 232, 235
  for mammography suite, 226
  for neurology suite, 163
  for obstetrics and gynecology suite, 102
  for operating room, 285–286, 422–423

Interior design (*Cont.*):
for ophthalmology suite, 127
for orthopedic surgery suite, 185
for otolaryngology suite, 111
for pediatrics suite, 77, 82–86, 91
for physical therapy suite, 314, 317, 322
for plastic surgery suite, 147–148, 422
for psychiatry suite, 155
for radiation oncology suite, 228
for radiology suite, 195
sensory deprivation, 421
for sports medicine suite, 299–302
for urology suite, 169
for waiting room, 23
for women's health center, 103–104
(*See also* Carpet; Color; Furniture; Lighting; Psychology; Wallcoverings)
Internal medicine, 54–72, 92
business office, 67
cardiopulmonary laboratory, 65–66
consultation room, 48, 55, 66
darkroom, 67
echocardiography, 57, 66
electrocardiograph (EKG) room, 56–59, 66–67
endoscopy, 67, 69–72
examination room, 55–56
group practice, 250, 261, 264
business office, 264
laboratory, 264
suite plan, 263*f.*
waiting room, 264
Holter monitoring, 57–58, 60*f.*, 66
inhalation therapy, 66–67
interior design, 72
laboratory, 55, 67
physician schedule, 55
proctology room, 67
program analysis, 56*t.*
pulmonary function laboratory, 62–63, 65–66
reception, 67
schematic diagram, 55*f.*
storage room, 56
suite plan:
2384 square feet, 64*f.*
5984 square feet, 68*f.*

Internal medicine (*Cont.*):
tech work area, 66
vascular laboratory, 60, 61*f.*
waiting room, 22, 67
x-ray room, 52–53, 56, 67
Intravenous pyelogram (IVP), 212
IPA (Independent Practice Association), 251
IVP (intravenous pyelogram), 212

Joint Commission on Accreditation of Hospitals (JCAH), 267

Kandinsky, Wasily, 409
Klee, Paul, 409
Kruithof's principle, 421

Laboratory, 50, 52
allergy, 153
blood drawing, 50, 52, 67, 241, 245, 248
cardiopulmonary, 65–66
dental, 336, 365–367, 383, 395, 400, 446–447
dermatology, 128
general practice, 52
group practice, 248, 264
internal medicine, 67, 264
obstetrics and gynecology, 50, 99, 102
odor control, 446
otolaryngology, 50, 105
pulmonary function, 62–63, 65–66
specimen pass-through, 50, 99, 104
STAT, 248
toilet room, 50
urology, 169
vascular, 60, 61*f.*
(*See also* Clinical laboratory; Hot lab)
Laser surgery:
controls, 284–285
dangers of, 282–283, 285
in dermatology suite, 132
equipment storage, 285
in operating room, 282–285
in ophthalmology suite, 124–126
room wallcoverings, 286
water supply, 285

Lead shielding:
in darkroom, 189, 197–198
in dental suite, 374–375
in mammography suite, 226
in nuclear medicine suite, 214, 218, 220, 222
in radiation oncology suite, 228
in radiology suite, 213
in ultrasound suite, 214
in x-ray room, 53, 374–375
Lie-detector test, 413
Life Safety Code (NFPA 101), 127, 141–142, 266–269, 422, 454–455
Light, Color and Environment (Birren), 408, 411–414, 421
Lighting, 433–444
ambulatory surgical center, 273, 275, 286, 288, 290–292
biological effects of, 433
business office, 445
clinical laboratory, 248
color and, 416, 421, 434
computed tomography suite, 225–226
construction checklist, 449
consultation room, 444
corridor, 436, 442*f.*, 443, 445
darkroom, 206
dental suite, 371, 378–380, 436, 441–443, 445
dimmer switch, 436
electrical plan, 436, 437*f.*
energy conservation, 435–436
light loss factor, 436
examination room, 119, 121, 436, 445
fluorescent light, 433–436
compact fluorescent, 435
cool white, 434
cool white deluxe, 434
daylight, 434
low-voltage, 435
optima, 32, 50, 435
SP35, 435
SPX, 35, 435
standard white, 434
ultralume, 435
vita-lite, 434–435
warm white, 434
warm white deluxe, 434
group practice suite, 443
Lighting (*Cont.*):
incandescent light, 433–435
light fixture maintenance, 436
magnetic resonance imaging suite, 232, 234
mammography suite, 226
minor surgery room, 444
neurology suite, 163
nurse station, 436, 440*f.*, 445
operating room, 277, 282, 285, 290*f.*
ophthalmology suite, 119, 121, 127
orthopedic surgery suite, 436, 439*f.*, 440*f.*
pediatric suite, 436–438
physical therapy suite, 322
plastic surgery suite, 147
psychological effects of, 433
radiography/fluoroscopy room, 214
radiology suite, 200
reception, 436, 441*f.*
reflected ceiling plan, 436, 438*f.*
sports medicine suite, 302
technical data, 434–435
ultraviolet radiation, 433
waiting room, 4, 436, 443, 445
women's health center, 104, 436
Luscher, Max:
The 4-Color Person, 414
Luscher Color Test, 414

Magnetic resonance imaging (MRI), 187–188, 229–239
case study, 235, 237
cryogenic replenishment, 232, 234
dewars, 232, 234
environment's effect on magnet, 229, 232, 234
equipment, 229–231*f.*, 235*f.*, 236*f.*
film processing, 202
floor loading, 232, 234–235
fringe magnetic field, 232
Gauss field, 229, 232, 233*f.*
HVAC system, 232, 234
interior design, 232, 235
lighting, 232, 234
magnet transport access, 229, 234
magnetic field influence, 232, 234
magnet's effect on environment, 229, 232
planning considerations, 229, 232, 234–235

Magnetic resonance imaging (MRI) (*Cont.*):
power requirements, 232, 234
RFI shielding, 232, 234
shims, 232, 235
space planning, 229, 232, 234–235
suite plans, 236*f.*, 237*f.*, 239*f.*
Tesla field, 232, 234
Mammography, 187, 226–228
film processing, 202, 226
interior design, 226
lead shielding, 226
lighting, 226
Mayo Clinic, 45, 249
Medical gases, 446
codes for usage, 368, 446
in dentistry, 368, 369*f.*, 400, 401*f.*, 446
in operating room, 282, 285, 288
in plastic surgery, 446
Medical office building (MOB) codes, 453–454
Medical office building (MOB) design (*see* Construction methods; Space planning)
Medical records, 36–38
in ambulatory surgical center, 273–274
in clinical laboratory, 246
color-coding of, 36–38
for computed tomography, 226
in dentistry, 369, 395
in group practice, 256
in internal medicine, 67
in ophthalmology, 127
in orthopedic surgery, 175, 182
in physical therapy, 329
in radiology, 36, 195, 201, 202*f.*
in sports medicine, 295, 299
storage units, 36, 37, 39–41*f.*
pruning of, 37–38
Medical specialties, 92
subspecialties, 92
(*See also* Allergy; Dermatology; General surgery; Neurology; Neurosurgery; Obstetrics and gynecology; Ophthalmology; Orthopedic surgery; Otolaryngology; Pain treatment center; Plastic surgery; Psychiatry; Urology; Women's health centers)
Medical transcription, 34*f.*, 35, 67
Menninger Clinic, 249
Minor surgery room, 47
ambulatory surgical center, 286
dermatology, 128, 132–133
general surgery, 166
lighting, 444
obstetrics and gynecology, 97, 98*f.*, 102
ophthalmology, 112
orthopedic surgery, 181
otolaryngology, 105, 110
plumbing requirements, 446
sports medicine, 299
women's health center, 104
MOB (medical office building) codes, 453–454
MOB (medical office building) design (*see* Construction methods; Space planning)
Mohs' histographic surgery, 133
Mosse, Eric P., 411
MRI (*see* Magnetic resonance imaging)

Nader, Ralph, 2
National Electrical Code (NEC; NFPA 70), 269, 277
National Health Planning and Resource Development Act (1974), 453
NEC (National Electrical Code; NFPA 70), 269, 277
Neurology, 159–163
consultation room, 48, 163
diagnostic procedures, 159, 161–163
electroencephalogram (EEG), 159, 161–162
electromyography (EMG), 161*f.*, 163
evoked potential, 161*f.*, 162
spinal tap, 162
examination room, 159, 163
interior design, 163
lighting, 163
program analysis, 162*t.*
schematic diagram, 159*f.*
suite plan, 160*f.*
Neurosurgery, 164
suite plan, 165*f.*
NFPA 56F, 288
NFPA 70 (National Electric Code), 269, 277

NFPA 99, 269, 277, 288
NFPA 101 (*Life Safety Code*), 127, 141–142, 266–269, 422, 454–455
Nuclear medicine, 187, 190, 214–223
  equipment, 216*f.*, 218–233*f.*
    structural support, 223
  film processing, 202
  hot lab, 218, 220, 222
    bench-top shields, 222
    electrical requirements, 222
    equipment, 220–223*f.*
    vial shields, 220, 222
  lead shielding, 214, 218, 220, 222
  nuclear stress test, 218
  room layout, 216*f.*, 217*f.*
  scans, 215–216
  SPECT, 216
  storage, 220
  ventilation studies, 218
Nurse practitioner, 49, 92–93
Nurse station, 38, 49–50, 52
  allergy, 148, 153
  ambulatory surgical center, 274, 290–292
  furniture, 430
  general practice, 52
  general surgery, 166
  lighting, 436, 440*f.*, 445
  mechanical requirements, 445
  obstetrics and gynecology, 49–50
  orthopedic surgery, 52, 175, 436, 440*f.*
  otolaryngology, 105
  pediatrics, 82, 84
  plastic surgery, 136
  sports medicine, 299
  women's health center, 104

Obstetrics and gynecology (OB-GYN), 92–102
  consultation room, 102
  dressing room, 93
  examination room, 93, 95, 97*f.*, 98*f.*
    cabinets, 43, 95
    door placement, 93
    electrical requirments, 44, 95
    sink, 93
    table, 95
Obstetrics and gynecology (OB-GYN), examination room (*Cont.*):
    windows, 95
    writing desk, 95
  group practice:
    program analysis, 262*t.*
    suite plan, 253*f.*
  interior design, 102
  laboratory, 50, 99, 102
  minor surgery room, 97, 98*f.*, 102
  nurse practitioner, 49, 92–93
  nurse station, 49–50
  patient education, 95, 97
  patient flow, 93
  program analysis, 95*t.*
  schematic diagram, 93*f.*
  suite plan:
    1373 square feet, 100*f.*
    1536 square feet, 101*f.*
    3136 square feet, 96*f.*
    3750 square feet, 94*f.*
  toilet room, 99, 102
  waiting room, 22, 93, 102
  waste disposal, 97, 99
  (*See also* Women's health center)
Occupational Safety and Health Administration (OSHA), 333
Office-based surgery (*see* Outpatient surgery room)
Office manager, 35–36, 67
Operating room, 274, 276–277, 280–286
  accessory items, 285
  cabinets, 277
  color of, 417
  electrical systems, 277, 285
  endoscopy procedures, 277
  equipment storage, 285
  HVAC system, 277, 280–282, 285
    Steriflo, 281–282
  interior design, 285–286, 422–423
  laser surgery, 282–285
    controls, 284–285
    dangers of, 282–283, 285
    water supply, 285
  lighting, 277, 282, 285, 290*f.*
  mechanical system, 277, 280–282
  medical gases, 282, 285, 288

Operating room (*Cont.*):
oral surgery, 397, 400, 401*f.*
planning issues, 277
procedure room, 277
size, 276–277
sterilization room, 277, 286
Ophthalmology, 111–128
automated refraction, 122–123
consultation room, 127
contact lens, 112, 115
data collection room, 122–123
dispensing physician, 113–115
equipment, 117–120*f.*, 124*f.*
examination room, 112, 115, 119, 121–123, 127
fluorescein angiography, 126
insurance records, 127
interior design, 127–128
laser surgery, 124–126
lighting, 119, 121, 127
medical records, 127
minor surgery room, 112
mydriatic area, 122
optical dispensing, 112, 115
outpatient surgery room, 126–127, 141
patient volume, 111–112
program analysis, 112*t.*
refraction room, 112, 115, 119, 121–122, 127
chair, 119
electrical requirements, 119, 121
instrument console, 119
sink, 119
schematic diagram, 111*f.*
suite plan:
1872 square feet, 113*f.*
2780 square feet, 116*f.*
4610 square feet, 114*f.*
tangent screen, 123–124
visual fields, 123–124
Optician, 112, 115
Oral surgery, 332, 397–402
air compressor, 447
business office, 397, 402
consultation room, 397, 400, 402
darkroom, 397
Oral surgery (*Cont.*):
examination room, 397, 400
interior design, 402
laboratory, 400
patient education, 367, 397
patient flow, 397
program analysis, 397*t.*
reception, 400
recovery room, 397, 400–401
staff lounge, 402
sterilization area, 397, 400–402
storage room, 400, 402
suite plan:
1876 square feet, 398*f.*
2500 square feet, 399*f.*
surgical operating room, 397, 400
equipment, 400, 401*f.*
medical gases, 368, 400, 446
toilet room, 402
waiting room, 397, 402
x-ray room, 397, 400
(*See also* Dentistry)
Orthodontics, 382–391
audiovisual room, 383
bookkeeping, 383
business office, 369, 383
consultation room, 382
darkroom, 383
interior design, 383, 390
laboratory, 383
operatory bay, 382–383, 385*f.*, 387*f.*, 395
patient flow, 382
program analysis, 382*t.*
quiet room, 383, 388*f.*
reception, 390, 391*f.*
sterilization area, 391*f.*
suite plan:
1666 square feet, 384*f.*
2030 square feet, 386*f.*
toilet room, 383
waiting room, 373, 382, 383, 389*f.*, 390
x-ray room, 383
(*See also* Dentistry)
Orthopedic surgery, 173–185
business office, 175

Orthopedic surgery (*Cont.*):
cast room, 175, 179–182
cabinet, 181*f.*
odor control, 446
plumbing requirements, 446
consultation room, 175, 181, 182*f.*
corridors, 182
darkroom, 175, 182
dressing room, 40
equipment, 173*f.*
examination room, 175, 178*f.*, 179
electrical requirements, 44
table, 44–45
furniture, 431*f.*, 432
hand surgeon, 179
interior design, 185
lighting, 436, 439*f.*, 440*f.*
medical records, 175, 182
minor surgery room, 181
nurse station, 52, 175, 436, 440*f.*
patient education, 182, 184*f.*, 185
physical therapy room, 175
physician schedule, 173
program analysis, 175*t.*
group practice, 262*t.*
room adjacency, 182
schematic diagram, 173*f.*
staff lounge, 175
storage room, 175
suite plan:
1728 square feet, 177*f.*
2368 square feet, 176*f.*
4464 square feet, 183*f.*
7040 square feet, 174*f.*
tech work area, 184*f.*
toilet room, 175, 185
waiting room, 22, 175, 185
waste disposal, 181
x-ray room, 175, 182
(*See also* Sports medicine)
OSHA (Occupational Safety and Health Administration), 333
Otolaryngology (ENT), 104–111
audio test room, 105, 110–111
business office, 105
Otolaryngology (ENT) (*Cont.*):
consultation room, 105
darkroom, 105
dressing room, 40, 110
equipment, 109*f.*
examination room, 105–106, 109
cabinet, 106
electrical requirements, 44, 109
sink, 105
facial plastic surgery, 105, 107*f.*, 110–111
interior design, 111
laboratory, 50, 105
minor surgery room, 105, 110
nurse station, 105
outpatient surgery room, 105, 110
program analysis, 106*t.*
recovery room, 105, 110
schematic diagram, 106*f.*
suite plan:
1940 square feet, 107*f.*
2025 square feet, 108*f.*
waiting room, 105
x-ray room, 105
Outpatient surgery room:
codes for, 422
design, 144–145
flooring, 422
ophthalmology, 126–127, 141
otolaryngology, 105, 110
plastic surgery, 136, 141–142, 144, 146*f.*
(*See also* Ambulatory surgical center; Oral surgery)

Pain treatment center, 164
Paramedical suite:
pharmacy, 330–331
(*See also* Physical therapy)
Patient education, 25–26
dentistry, 367, 393–395, 397
furniture for, 425, 432
obstetrics and gynecology, 95, 97
orthopedic surgery, 182, 184*f.*, 185
plastic surgery, 137, 141
women's health center, 99*f.*, 103

Patient flow, 38–39
ambulatory surgical center, 270–271
dentistry, 336, 337*f.*, 382, 393, 397
group practice, 260
obstetrics and gynecology, 93
plastic surgery, 136
radiology, 189–190
urology, 169
Pediatric dentistry, 393–396
business office, 369, 395
consultation room, 395
darkroom, 395
interior design, 395
laboratory, 395
medical records, 395
operatory bay, 395
patient education, 393–395
patient flow, 393
program analysis, 393*t.*
quiet room, 395
staff lounge, 395
sterilization area, 395
storage room, 395
suite plan:
1350 square feet, 392*f.*
5185 square feet, 396*f.*
toilet room, 395
waiting room, 373, 390, 393, 395
x-ray room, 395
(*See also* Dentistry)
Pediatrics, 72–92
audio test room, 91
business office, 84
consultation room, 48, 91
corridor, 91
examination room, 77–79, 82, 87*f.*, 88*f.*
for adolescent patients, 78
electrical requirements, 44
number of rooms, 77–78
sinks, 78
size, 78–79
table, 45, 79, 82, 86*f.*
interior design, 77, 82–86, 91, 425
lighting, 436–438
nurse station, 82, 84
Pediatrics (*Cont.*):
program analysis, 76
reception, 76*f.*, 83*f.*, 84, 86*f.*, 90*f.*
schematic diagram, 73*f.*
storage room, 91
suite plan:
1440 square feet, 75*f.*
1680 square feet, 81*f.*
2183 square feet, 74*f.*
2915 square feet, 82*f.*
4500 square feet, 89*f.*
waiting room, 22, 23, 73, 76–80, 85*f.*
Pedodontics (*see* Pediatric dentistry)
Periodontics, 332, 403–407
program analysis, 403*t.*
reception, 405*f.*
suite plan, 405*f.*
2270 square feet, 404*f.*
3782 square feet, 406*f.*
use of medical gases, 368
(*See also* Dentistry)
Pfister, Max, 411
Pharmacy, 330–331
display space, 330
in group practice, 330
prescription volume, 330–331
suite plan, 331*f.*
toilet room, 331
workstation, 331
Phlebotomy (*see* Blood drawing)
Phoenix Surgicenter, 265
Physical therapy, 314–329
adjustments, 327*f.*, 329
business office, 329
continuous passive motion (CPM), 317, 327–329
electrical requirements, 329
electrical stimulation, 323*f.*, 327
equipment room, 317
exercise gym, 324–326, 328*f.*, 329*f.*
color of, 420
hot or cold, 317–320
hydrotherapy, 314–317
interior design, 314, 317, 322
iontophoresis, 327
lighting, 322

Physical therapy (*Cont.*):
linen storage, 317
locker room, 329
massage, 322
medical records, 329
mobilization, 327*f.*, 329
in orthopedic surgery suite, 175
program analysis, 315*t.*
staff lounge, 329
storage room, 329
suite plan, 321*f.*
therapist, 329
toilet room, 329
traction, 327
transcutaneous electrical nerve stimulation (T.E.N.S.), 317, 327, 328*f.*
ultrasound, 317, 322, 323*f.*, 327
waiting room, 329
(*See also* Sports medicine)
Plastic surgery, 136–148
American Association for Accreditation of Ambulatory Plastic Surgery Facilities, 142, 144
beauty salon, 146
consultation room, 138, 141, 142*f.*
dressing room, 146
examination room, 136, 137, 141*f.*
facial, 105, 107*f.*, 110–111
freestanding surgical center, 141
interior design, 147–148, 422
lighting, 147
nurse station, 136
outpatient surgery room, 136, 141–142, 144, 146*f.*
patient education, 137, 141
patient flow, 136
physician schedule, 136–137
private entrance, 137
program analysis, 138*f.*
reception, 136
recovery room, 136, 137, 146, 147*f.*
schematic diagram, 137*f.*
suite plan:
2520 square feet, 140*f.*
2720 square feet, 143*f.*
2765 square feet, 139*f.*
2772 square feet, 144*f.*
Plastic surgery (*Cont.*):
use of medical gases, 446
waiting room, 136, 146
Preventive medicine, 250
Primary care, 19
(*See also* General practice; Internal medicine; Pediatrics)
Private entrance, 38, 48
for dental suite, 339
for plastic surgery suite, 137
Private office (*see* Consultation room)
Proctology room, 67
Psoralen ultraviolet light (PUVA), 133
Psychiatry, 155–158
business office, 155
child, 155
consultation room, 155
noise control, 447
examination room, 158*f.*
group therapy room, 155
interior design, 155
program analysis, 156*t.*
schematic diagram, 156*f.*
storage, 158*f.*
suite plan, 157*f.*
waiting room, 22, 155
Psychology, 1–5, 39
body language, 4
of color, 408–415, 420
consumerism and, 2, 102
cultural differences, 3
in dental practice, 361
first impressions, 2, 21–22
lighting and, 433
patient intimidation, 3–4
patient satisfaction, 1–2
perceived status difference, 3–4
privacy, 1, 4
territorial boundaries, 1, 3
waiting, 2–3
Psychology of Color and Design, The (Sharpe), 412, 415
Pulmonary function laboratory, 62–63, 65–66
room layout, 65–66
Purkinje effect, 418
PUVA (psoralen ultraviolet light), 133

Radiation oncology, 186–187, 226, 228
dressing room, 228
interior design, 228
lead shielding, 228
tech work area, 228
waiting room, 228
Radiography/fluoroscopy (R/F) room, 189, 190, 197, 210, 212*f.*, 213*f.*
barium prep area, 211
plumbing requirements, 446
dressing room in, 211
lighting, 214
odor control, 214, 446
table, 197, 213
toilet room in, 210–211
Radiography room, 189–190, 197–198, 210–212
door, 213
electrical requirements, 210
equipment, 210–212
film processing, 202
group practice, 256
size, 210
storage, 212–213
toilet room in, 212
wall-mounted film holder (bucky), 212
(*See also* Darkroom)
Radiology, 52, 186–210
bookkeeping, 195
business office, 195
cassette pass box, 203*f.*, 205
consultation room, 200–201, 203*f.*
diagnostic imaging modalities, 186–188
dressing room, 189, 193, 195
emergency precautions, 214
film filing, 197, 201, 202*f.*
film processing, 201–210
daylight system, 201, 202, 204–207, 209–210, 226
integrated film processor, 201–202, 204, 207*f.*
single-film cassette, 202
transportable film magazine, 202
film reading room, 200
fluoroscopy room, 186, 200, 211
intravenous pyelogram, 212
lead shielding, 213
lighting, 200
Radiology (*Cont.*):
mammography, 187, 202, 226–228
medical records, 36, 195, 201, 202*f.*
patient privacy, 4
planning considerations, 188–190, 193, 210, 213
equipment, 188–189
functional relationships, 189*f.*, 193
patient flow, 189–190
staff floor, 190
radiation oncology, 187, 226, 228
reception, 190
referring physician viewing, 200
schematic diagram, 193*f.*
space planning, 188–190, 193, 210, 213, 224–225
suite components, 193, 195, 197–210
suite plan:
2420 square feet, 194*f.*
2990 square feet, 196*f.*
6660 square feet, 191*f.*
6900 square feet, 192*f.*
tech work area, 189, 195, 197–198
control area, 197–199
ultrasound, 186–187, 190, 202, 214, 215*f.*
view box illuminator, 197, 200–201
waiting room, 190, 195
(*See also* Computed tomography; Darkroom; Magnetic resonance imaging; Nuclear medicine; Radiography room; Radiography/fluoroscopy room; X-ray room)
Reception, 4, 23–26
ambulatory surgical center, 272–273
dental, 336, 367, 371, 390, 391*f.*, 400, 405*f.*, 441*f.*
family practice, 260*f.*
general surgery, 169
group practice, 257–258, 260
internal medicine, 67
lighting, 436, 441*f.*
pediatrics, 76*f.*, 83*f.*, 84, 86*f.*, 90*f.*
plastic surgery, 136
radiology, 190
sports medicine, 299–300, 302
women's health center, 25*f.*, 103–104
Recovery room:
ambulatory surgical center, 270–271, 273–275, 290–292
endoscopy, 72
oral surgery, 397, 400–401

Recovery room (*Cont.*):
  otolaryngology, 105, 109–110
  plastic surgery, 136, 137, 146, 147*f.*
  urology, 169
Redon, Odilon, 409
Reed, Wallace, 265
R/F room (*see* Radiography/fluoroscopy room)
Root canal (*see* Endodontics)
Rorschach inkblot method, 410–413

San Diego Sports Medicine Center (San Diego, California), 302–303
Scharbauer, Pamela, 308
Scheduling (*see* Patient flow; Staff flow)
Sensory deprivation, 421
Sharpe, Deborah T., *The Psychology of Color and Design,* 412, 415
Single photon emission computed tomography (SPECT), 216
Space planning, 6–18
  amenities, 15
  building feasibility study, 14
  building leasing, 14, 16–17
  building shell design, 6–11
    configurations, 15
    core services, 6
    floor area efficiency, 6–7
    intermediate columns, 11
    moment-resistant steel, 7
    perimeter columns, 11
    stairwells, 6–7
    structural support, 7, 11
  building standards, 15
  hospital-based MOB, 17–18
  medical suite functions, 20–21
  planning module, 11–14
    ceilings, 14
    suite bay depths, 12, 14
    windows, 14
  politics of, 16–17, 23
  private entrance, 38, 48
  rentable space, 6
    11,256 square feet, 13*f.*
    11,484 square feet, 7*f.*
    12,360 square feet, 10*f.*

Space planning, rentable space (*Cont.*):
    13,500 square feet, 9*f.*
    19,200 square feet, 8*f.*
  tenant improvement allowances, 15–16
  windows, 43
  work letter, 16
  (*See also* Construction methods)
Specialized medicine (*see* Medical specialties)
Specimen pass-through, 50, 99, 104, 244
SPECT (single photon emission computed tomography), 216
Sports medicine, 294–313
  access, 295
  aerobics area, 295, 299, 300, 302, 307*f.*
  bookkeeping, 299
  business office, 299–300
  case studies, 302–313
  The Center for Sports Medicine, 306–307
    suite plan, 296*f.*
  Center for Sports Medicine and Orthopedics, 303–306
    suite plan, 305*f.*
  consultation room, 299
  dressing room, 301
  examination room, 299
  fitness gym, 295, 297*f.*, 299–300, 302
  goals, 294
  hydrotherapy room, 295, 300–302, 310*f.*
  indoor track, 309*f.*
  interior design, 299–302
  internal layout, 295, 299–300
  lighting, 302
  linen storage, 301
  locker room, 298–301
  marketing plan, 294–295, 300
  mechanical requirements, 445
  medical records, 295, 299
  minor surgery room, 299
  nurse station, 299
  physical therapy, 295, 300–302
  pool, 299–300
  reception, 299–300, 302
  San Diego Sports Medicine Center, 302–303
  shower room, 299–301
  sound control, 300

Sports medicine (*Cont.*):
spa, 299, 301
steam room, 300–301
toilet room, 301
treatment room, 299, 302
user mix, 295
ventilation, 300–301
waiting room, 300
Western Montana Sports Medicine & Fitness Center, 308–313
sections, 313*f.*
suite plan, 311*f.*, 312*f.*
wet areas, 300–301
Staff flow, 190, 270, 336, 337*f.*, 339
Staff lounge, 54
ambulatory surgical center, 272, 288–290
dental suite, 370, 395, 402
orthopedic surgery suite, 175
physical therapy suite, 329
STAT laboratory, 248
Steriflo system, 281–282
Storage room, 54
ambulatory surgical center, 277, 285, 287
dental, 381, 395, 400, 402
dermatology, 128, 133
internal medicine, 56
nuclear medicine, 220
orthopedic surgery, 175
pediatrics, 91
physical therapy, 317, 329
psychiatry, 158*f.*
radiography room, 212–213
sports medicine, 301
Summer, Robert, 3
Surgeon, schedule of, 55
Surgery:
consultation room, 48–49
freestanding surgical center, 141
Mohs' histographic, 133
waiting room, 22
(*See also* Ambulatory surgical center; General surgery; Laser surgery; Minor surgery room; Neurosurgery; Oral surgery; Orthopedic surgery; Outpatient surgery room; Plastic surgery)

Tech work area:
internal medicine, 66
orthopedic surgery, 184*f.*
radiation oncology, 228
radiology, 189, 195, 197–199
Technician, 195, 197
Technologist, 195, 197
Theory and Practice of Color, The (Gerritsen), 416
Toilet room:
clinical laboratory, 244
color of, 420
dental, 336, 370, 383, 395, 402
dermatology, 128
flooring, 423
general surgery, 166
laboratory, 50
obstetrics and gynecology, 99, 102
odor control, 446
orthopedic surgery, 175, 185
pharmacy, 331
physical therapy, 329
plastic surgery, 147
in radiography/fluoroscopy (R/F) room, 210–211
in radiography room, 212
specimen pass-through, 244
sports medicine, 301
urology, 169
in waiting room, 24, 73
Traffic flow (*see* Patient flow; Staff flow)
Treatment room, 47
allergy, 153
interior design, 422
sports medicine, 299, 302
(*See also* Examination room; Minor surgery room)

Ultrasound, 60*f.*, 186–187, 190, 202, 214, 215*f.*
film processing, 202
lead shielding, 214
in physical therapy, 317, 322, 323*f.*, 327
Uniform Building Code, 423
Urology, 169–172
business office, 169
consultation room, 169
cystoscopy room, 169

Urology (*Cont.*):
dressing room, 169
examination room, 169
interior design, 169
laboratory, 169
patient flow, 169
program analysis, 170*t.*
recovery room, 169
schematic diagram, 170*f.*
suite plan:
1504 square feet, 171*f.*
1984 square feet, 172*f.*
toilet room, 169
waiting room, 169
waste disposal, 169
x-ray room, 169
USDHHS Guidelines for Construction and Equipment of Hospitals and Medical Facilities, 277, 282
Use of Electricity in Patient Care (NFPA 99), 277

Vascular laboratory, 60
layout, 61*f.*
Venipuncture (*see* Blood drawing)
View box illuminator, 180*f.,* 197, 200–201, 224, 345, 374–375

Waiting room, 21–24
allergy, 148, 153*f.,* 154*f.*
ambulatory surgical center, 272–274
chair arrangement, 77
children's area, 23, 76, 78–80*f.,* 85*f.*
clinical laboratory, 244, 248
dental, 336, 358*f.,* 371, 373, 382, 383, 389*f.,* 390, 393, 395, 397, 402
dermatology, 128, 135*f.*
first impression of, 2, 21–22
functions of, 22
furniture, 425, 430–432
general practice, 22
general surgery, 166
group practice, 257, 264
interior design, 23, 422, 425
internal medicine, 22, 67, 264
lighting, 4, 436, 443, 445
mechanical requirements, 445

Waiting room (*Cont.*):
number of seats, 22–23, 77, 264
obstetrics and gynecology, 22, 93, 102
orthopedic surgery, 22, 175, 185
otolaryngology, 105
pediatrics, 22, 23, 73, 76–80, 85*f.*
physical therapy, 329
plants in, 4
plastic surgery, 136, 146
psychiatry, 22, 155
radiation oncology, 228
radiology, 190, 195
seating arrangements, 3
sick baby, 73
size, 22–23
sports medicine, 300
surgery, 22
toilet room in, 24, 73
urology, 169
well baby, 73
(*See also* Reception)
Wallcoverings, 422
in ambulatory surgical center, 268, 274, 288, 292
in consultation room, 422
in dental suite, 333–334, 371, 380
in examination room, 422
flammability testing, 423, 455–456
im mammography suite, 226
in obstetrics and gynecology suite, 102
in operating room, 286
in ophthalmology suite, 127–128
in orthopedic surgery suite, 185
in pediatrics suite, 77, 82
in physical therapy suite, 314
in plastic surgery suite, 147
sound control and, 447
specifications, 455–456
in sports medicine suite, 302
in treatment room, 422
in waiting room, 422
Waste disposal:
in ambulatory surgical center, 269, 272, 290
in clinical laboratory, 246–247
in darkroom, 208
in obstetrics and gynecology suite, 97, 99

Waste disposal (*Cont.*):
in orthopedic surgery suite, 181
in urology suite, 169
Western Montana Sports Medicine & Fitness Center (Missoula, Montana), 308–313
sections, 313*f.*
suite plan, 311*f.*, 312*f.*
Women's health center, 102–104
business office, 28*f.*
consultation room, 104
dressing room, 104
examination room, 104
interior design, 103–104
lighting, 104, 436
minor surgery room, 104
nurse station, 104

Women's health center (*Cont.*):
patient education, 99*f.*, 103
reception, 25*f.*, 103–104
suite plan, 105*f.*
(*See also* Obstetrics and gynecology)

X-ray room, 52–53
dental, 336, 347*f.*, 373–375, 383, 395, 397, 400
general practice, 52–53
internal medicine, 52–53, 56, 67
lead shielding, 53, 189, 374–375
orthopedic surgery, 175, 182
otolaryngology, 105
urology, 169
(*See also* Darkroom; Radiology)
Xerography, 226